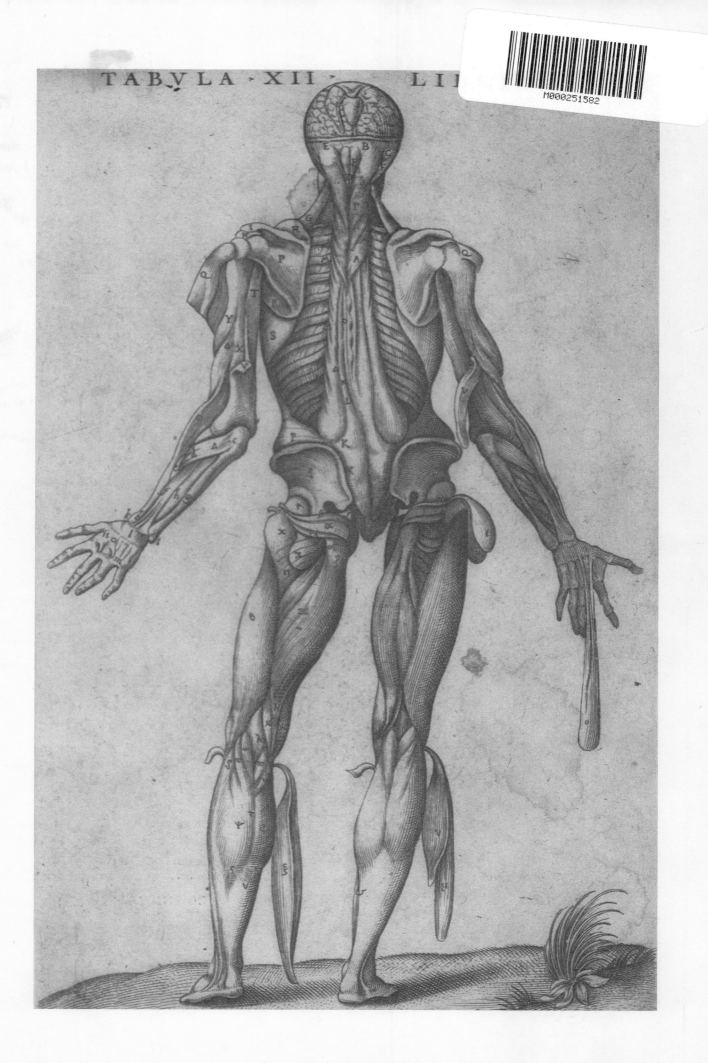

Best wishes, John McCain
& [signature]

McCRAW and ARNOLD's ATLAS
of Muscle and Musculocutaneous Flaps

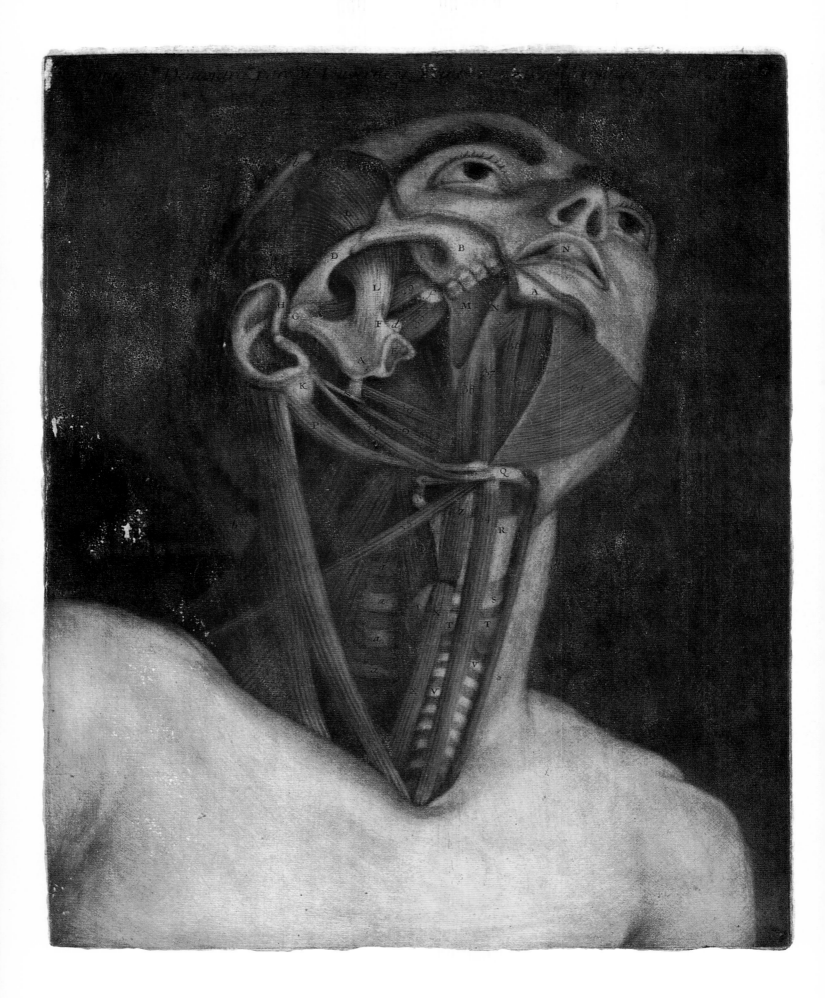

McCRAW AND ARNOLD's ATLAS
of Muscle and Musculocutaneous Flaps

John B. McCraw, M.D., F.A.C.S.
Professor of Plastic and
   Reconstructive Surgery
Eastern Virginia Medical School
Norfolk, Virginia

Phillip G. Arnold, M.D., F.A.C.S.
Consultant in Plastic and
   Reconstructive Surgery
Mayo Clinic
Rochester, Minnesota

Contributing Authors

David G. Dibbell, M.D.
G. Patrick Maxwell, M.D.
J. Brien Murphy, M.D.

Peter Pairolero, M.D.
Christoph Papp, M.D.

Case Contributors

Thomas Arganese, M.D.
George Irons, M.D.

William Magee, M.D.
Harvey Rosen, M.D.

Hampton Press Publishing Company, Inc.
Norfolk, Virginia

The reader should recognize that the procedures described in this Atlas may be fallible for reasons not described herein. This work represents the experience and the considered opinions of the authors.

The choice of an Atlas format and the chosen task of providing broad coverage of the many procedures necessitates an abbreviated textual content. The authors acknowledge the following limitations:

Based on cadaver dissections, appropriate descriptions were prepared for each procedure. These may not be completely correct anatomically, and are subject to reader interpretation.

The methods described have worked in the hands of the authors, but this may not be the experience of the reader.

No attempt has been made to list every possible source of technical error, risk, or complication.

The work is incomplete in regard to expected developments and risks, present and future.

The text is abbreviated and does not constitute a comprehensive course in these procedures. It may be advisable for the reader to undertake formal instruction in the technical aspects of these procedures prior to their application.

When product names, trade names, trademarks, etc., appear in the text of this publication not identified as such it is not to be taken as a sign that such names, as understood by the Trade Marks and Merchandise Marks Act, are in the public domain and may be used freely by anyone.

Illustrations for the frontispiece and endpapers provided by and used with the permission of the Foundanzione G. Sanvenero-Roselli, Milan, Italy.

Produced by Ann McMellin

Designed by Germaine Clair
Typeset by Teagle and Little, Inc.
Printed by Teagle and Little, Inc.
        Norfolk, Virginia

International Standard Book Number: 0-939789-00-0
Library of Congress Catalog Card Number: 86-82307

To Paul W. Black, M.D. and Leonard T. Furlow, Jr., M.D.
Mentors, Colleagues, and Dear Friends

CONTENTS

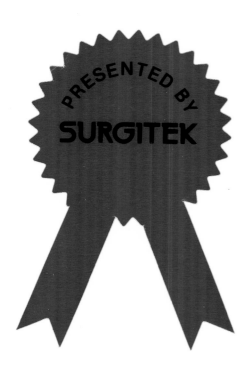

PRESENTED BY SURGITEK

FOREWORD

About two years ago, I asked John McCraw to mark out a few of his favorite musculocutaneous flaps on a cadaver for a book I was writing, to illustrate the importance of laboratory research in clinical surgery. Months, and then years went by, but nothing came from Norfolk. I have always been adequately intrigued by "Quick-Draw" McCraw to keep at least one eye on him and to suspect that during any long period of silence, he must be cooking something up. He was! In fact, he reversed my earlier request, with the same cavalier ease that he flips a cadaver flap, into a request for a Foreword to this book of flaps. As it turned out, McCraw, Arnold, Dibbell, and Murphy had already been five years into the making of this book, culling through well over 100,000 photographs, to obtain the final color pictures. Surprisingly, a less comprehensive version of this book was finished in 1980. Yet the authors postponed a possibly premature publication until a consensus opinion could be evolved in regard to the context of each flap, amongst the many choices of flaps available.

My immediate response to McCraw's request (for a Foreword) was that I have always been wary of "cookbooks," not because they have no immediate value, which they often do, but because such books set up a routine and an inherent "gospel" which tends to promote mental stasis. After study of numerous completed chapters of this book, it became evident to me that the essence of this book is anatomy. And, as it takes hundreds of millions of years to alter anatomy, there seemed to be a good chance that the data presented here will serve as a guide of relatively permanent value.

The seed of this remarkable Atlas was sewn when McCraw first studied intra-cellular calcium transfer in "island" rectus femoris muscle flaps in frogs in 1968. At the time, he was an Orthopaedic resident and an amateur physiology fellow at Duke. As a basic scientist, he was an admitted failure because the measured intra-cellular calcium transfer was no different between "island" muscle flaps and in-situ muscle flaps. He had wrongly anticipated a difference because of the expected ischemic differential between the two flap treatments. At least he became conversant with the concept of the "island" muscle flap, even if it was in the humble frog. Little did he know that he would face even greater failures (and successes) in humans in the years to come.

He then finished general surgery in Gainesville and graduated to a plastic surgery residency under Josh Jurkiewicz, who had already unleashed the creative genius of Luis Vasconez into the clinical applications of muscle flaps in the leg. Luis was impressed by the early work of Ralph Ger, and Luis promptly involved McCraw because of his Orthopaedic background and interest in anatomy. Their comfort with muscle flaps led to the experimental study of musculocutaneous flaps in dogs, a study which could justifiably be transferred to human use. Residency came to an end, but the collaboration continued.

McCraw joined Dave Dibbell at the Wilford Hall USAF Hospital, and between 1973 and 1975 a dozen or more usable myocutaneous flaps were defined. This information was freely shared with a triangle of friends, which included the Atlanta group and P.G. Arnold at the Mayo Clinic, over the next several years. From there, each group went on to make independent and unique contributions. By 1978, McCraw and Dibbell offered their first experimental and clinical reports, which included a staggering 168 cases of myocutaneous flaps. Very soon, Arnold's ingenious new developments and applications at the Mayo Clinic made these numbers pale by comparison.

These authors and their talented colleagues continued to work together in nine consecutive Norfolk Flap Workshops, and each year the teachers learned as much from the other teachers as the students learned from the teachers, at a time when the field was changing monthly. This book was finally composed in an attempt to solidify the material presented at these many workshops. At first, the questions were as naive as: "can you use this flap for cancer? can it be used for infections? and, can it be used just to fill a hole?" The obvious answers were: "Yes, yes, and yes." Gradually, the questions became more and more sophisticated in regard to advantages, disadvantages, complications, and the rational choice of flaps, once the anatomy was known. Fortunately, the authors learned what the students wanted to know, in order to intelligently apply this new information — hence, this Atlas.

Now we are presented with a spectacular array of vivid fresh cadaveric dissections. The authors are to be commended for the uncommon feat of actually rendering cadavers colorful and exciting! The most commonly used muscle and musculocutaneous flaps are outlined, dissected in understandable stages, and transposed through their expected arcs of rotation. The clinical cases accurately portray the normal uses of these flaps, and the demonstrations of the inevitable complications are brutally honest. The text presents a concise account of pertinent anatomy, specific flap uses, regional flap comparisons, advantages, disadvantages, complications and pitfalls, as well as a short discussion about the donor site. This presentation has been so expertly executed that it will make it relatively easy for other surgeons to use these most helpful flaps.

In our conversations, McCraw did state: "These cases cannot be presently duplicated by any other local method of reconstruction, and I doubt that they will be in the near future. Nevertheless, I do hope that they will be superseded, if ever, when I am in heaven so that someone else can write about it." It does seem likely that these authors will have exchanged their scalpels for harps before these flaps are surpassed, unless, that is, the cross-grafting barrier is broken. Then, these local flaps will be discarded in favor of cadaveric microneurovascular "free" flaps to replace the exact missing unit at no physical expense to the patient. Even then, the anatomy depicted here will be pertinent.

This master guide book should be in the possession or within the reach of all reconstructive surgeons, both for their personal use and for the education of their patients, because it is the definitive work on the subject.

D. Ralph Millard, Jr.
Miami, Florida

PREFACE

What can we make of the current popularity of muscle and musculocutaneous flaps? Could this be just another passing fancy, or will this survive all of our surgical careers? We believe the latter, but seemingly fundamental advances can be ephemeral and can cloud our distant vision. This abbreviated presentation of our perceptions of the presently available muscle and skin-muscle flaps is offered, primarily, as an anatomical record which should not be outdated. Even if we develop totally reliable microvascular transfers which can be completed rapidly, these classic anatomical and rudimentary physiologic observations will still be pertinent.

We have tried to place each flap into the context of other similar flaps. In the process we may have discredited certain flaps and resurrected others, but we have tried to avoid any unwarranted flap ''flattery.'' Ian McGregor explored this issue in his discussion of Ian Taylor's ''extended deep inferior epigastric flap'' article in the *Journal of Plastic and Reconstructive Surgery* (Dec. 1983):

> One might be forgiven for believing that the recent flood of papers describing new myocutaneous flaps must surely be subsiding to a trickle. This paper by Taylor and co-workers, however, demonstrates that a persistent scrutiny of the vascular patterns of superficial muscles and the skin overlying them is still capable of revealing new potential flaps or extensions of existing flaps. The question, of course, might be asked whether more flaps are required, or whether a plethora does not exist already. To this the answer must be that when any flap is described, its ultimate value and its sphere of applicability cannot be gauged with any degree of accuracy. It is only with the passage of time and wide usage that possible value becomes actual and the method establishes its 'pecking order' in the flap hierarchy — in the front line or in the reserves. Clinical situations arise where, for one reason or another, a preferred technique cannot be used, and it is then that the availability of an armory of alternatives becomes more essential to provide a surgical 'defense in depth.'

This pre-eminent Professor of the British Commonwealth, and beyond, has offered this sage advice, which we have tried to follow. As Dr. Millard has mentioned in the Foreword, we have delayed publication of this Atlas for a period of years to validate Mr. McGregor's test of worth — the passage of time and wide usage.

P.G., Dave Dibbell, and I decided in 1979 to ''do'' this book. We chose to wait until our combined experience could allow us to offer good and lasting solutions to some difficult reconstruction problems. Until recently the appropriate flap choices were quite debatable. Some problems still evade our best judgment and remain unsolved. However, on the issues which we have addressed, we feel comfortable with our comparisons of the available flaps and in our descriptions of their ''personalities.'' New and better solutions will evolve, but this Atlas should be a good building block.

This book is called McCraw and Arnold's Atlas because only the two of us ended up writing the book. What was intended to be a simple recitation turned out to take seven years of nights and weekends. Yes, it was painful, but we both survived. Suffice it to say, our wives and families suffered more than we did. In the end P.G. wanted to call it McCraw and Arnold's Last Atlas so no publisher would ever ask us to produce another book.

Many people created the environment that allowed us to produce this book. The genesis of this book ultimately lies with our professors of surgery, Dr. Hugh Stephenson, Jr. and the late Dr. Nathan Womack, who initially encouraged us in the pursuit of surgery as a career and in basic research as a path to scientific expansion. We can never repay our debt to Dr. Leonard Furlow, Jr. and Dr. Paul W. Black for allowing us to emulate their surgical skills and personal caring. These two men not only conveyed concepts to us; they taught us how to think. Our surgical lives continue to be strongly influenced by them, but more importantly, our personal lives are brightened by their friendship — one of our special privileges. It was also our good fortune to be students of Dr. Maurice J. Jurkiewicz. Dr. ''J'' will undoubtedly be remembered in the surgical history of the Twentieth Century as a distinct pioneer in fostering surgical creativity in clinical experimentation which is balanced by human respect and compassion, in the context of the strictest ethical, moral, and scientific standards. The continuing financial support for many years of basic research was provided by the Taylor Foundation of Norfolk, Virginia, and by our friends Steve and Mary Lewis Campbell. The Campbells' encouragement and guidance ultimately facilitated the formation of the Hampton Press Publishing Co. and the completion of this Atlas. Our families, associates, and friends have seen us consumed by this project for many years. There is no way we can properly express our appreciation for the help and support they have given to us. Finally, our colleagues afforded us an unparalleled opportunity to pursue an earnest commitment to the new horizons of muscle flap surgery.

We are indebted to Dave Dibbell, Pat Maxwell, Brien Murphy, and Ann McMellin for the many hours they devoted to dissecting and photographing the fresh cadavers. Two years were spent completing the flap dissections using a green background, but the artistic vision of Pat Maxwell interceded. This complete set of ''green'' photographs was discarded and replaced with a better ''black velvet'' set over the next five years. The scarcity of time and fresh cadavers prolonged the agony because it was necessary to photograph each flap dissection several times. Hence, each cadaver photograph used in the book represents several hundred photographs that were not used. The final photographs were completed in August 1986.

The contributions of Peter Pairolero, to the serratus and the intrathoracic chapters of this Atlas and to the development of these procedures, is significant and should be recognized. P.G. is grateful for his collaboration and for his friendship.

We would like to offer a special thanks to the plastic surgery residents and fellows at the Eastern Virginia Graduate School of Medicine over the past six years. Memory precludes a complete listing of all those who tirelessly helped with the cadaver dissections, but we must recognize Chris Papp, Hallene Marragh, Tom Arganese, Al Fleury, Bruce Freeman, Brien Murphy, Mike Norris, David Teasley, Mike Vincent, and Ivor Kaplan. The hours spent by John Grossman and Jeff Posnick in helping to compile the bibliography are also appreciated. Above all else, this time in the laborotory was fun and has left us with fond memories of the camaraderie with our friends.

This Atlas would certainly never exist without the endless ebullience and creativity of Ann McMellin. She deserves our sincerest thanks for overseeing every aspect of the production, printing, and publication from start to finish. Germaine Clair, who designed the Atlas with consideration of the practical needs of the reader and while maintaining our commitment to artistry and excellence, has contributed to many aspects of this project. For the actual production of the Atlas, our thanks to Greg Jordan and the numerous people at Teagle and Little printers who adeptly implemented our vision, and especially to Elawna Sisley, who, somehow, knew where everything was during the entire project. Several secretaries gave special attention to compiling the text. They include Vicky Martin, Laurie Blaine, Judith Tessmer, Billi Jo Hardesty and many Kelly Girls. Their contributions were essential to the success of the project.

This *Atlas* should not be considered as the ultimate answer, nor even complete. It is a guide to work from and it should be supplemented by personal dissections, formal training and individual experience. Still, there may never be a ''final answer.'' Flap surgery is a little like playing a chess game designed by a sardonic Nature, who does not reveal all the rules of the game. What is flap *delay*? What is vascular *spasm*? Why should *cold* be harmful, when it is helpful in so many other conditions? What can we do to remedy a *dying flap*? How can we ever see ''inside'' the *physiology of the microcirculation*? At the present time, we are only moving through the early stages of anatomical description. We still have just a rudimentary knowledge of the physiologic reasons for our successes or failures. Maybe in the future this same sardonic Nature will reveal the rules of this ''chess game.'' Then, we will have an opportunity to understand both the physiology and anatomy of muscle flaps. We envy the surgeons who will be afforded this view.

John B. McCraw
Norfolk, Virginia

BASIC PRINCIPLES OF MUSCLE FLAP SURGERY

This "back to the basics" chapter may be of little help to the active practitioner of muscle flap surgery, but even the most experienced of us has faced the disappointed patient or the problem caused by our own faulty logic. Nine years of Flap Dissection Workshops has instructed the faculty as much as the participants. Each year, more time has progressively been devoted to discussions of basic principles and complications. The presentation by Luis Vasconez on Complications is the perennial favorite. Luis calls his talk "That's Not Plastic Surgery," and his first sentence is always: "I didn't borrow these cases." He follows with the *Four Laws of Vasconez* pertaining to flap survival:

1. Some do, some don't.
2. All of the flap survived, except for the part needed to cover the defect.
3. If plan A is a complete failure, do not make plan B exactly the same as plan A.
4. It always happens to me.

If an expert in muscle flap surgery can do this so self-effacingly, so must we all. Let's consider several important factors, beginning with the central figure — the patient.

PATIENT EDUCATION

The questions: "Did you have to use plastic surgery?" or "Did you have to use plastic?" occur all too often and reflect a lack of understanding of the fundamental role of the reconstructive surgeon. Once instructed that the basis for the specialty is tissue transfer, it is easier for the patient to understand our place in his care. First we must clarify our role as a consultant in wound healing, tissue transfer, form and function. It is still the perception of many patients that the reconstructive surgeon is simply one who is technically meticulous and who deals in surgery that relates as much to appearance as to function. It is also not unusual for the patient to be surprised to learn that his trusted internist or personal surgeon is not as thoroughly versed as the reconstruction surgeon in the complicated problems of wound healing and wound repair.

The intended goals of a reconstructive surgical procedure are better accepted if the patient understands the *reasons for considering various options,* e.g. a flap, a skin graft or secondary healing. For instance, a painful skin graft becomes more palatable once the patient recognizes that it will shorten the time of healing and provide a more durable surface than an epithelialized scar. When a flap is needed, the reasons for choosing from among muscle, musculocutaneous and cutaneous flaps should also be carefully delineated. The donor site deformity, the expected quality of the reconstruction, as well as the overall morbidity all need to be thoroughly understood by the patient. When the "built-in" risk of failure is high, e.g. the recurrence of a long-standing osteomyelitis or the potential loss of an extremity with the failed coverage of a vascular prosthesis, the patient must recognize and accept these risks in advance of any surgical efforts.

Patients should understand that *no restorative surgery can return them to complete normality* and that imperfections of contour or function may require later revisions. On the other hand, the patient must recognize that the current methods of reconstruction offer reasonable solutions to some difficult problems and that these methods escaped our comprehension and exceeded our surgical capabilities a mere ten years past. The present methods of breast reconstruction offer a good example of the vastly improved quality of our reconstructive capabilities. Even so, the surgeon should help the patient understand that these imperfect reconstructions must be contrasted with the mastectomy deformity or with older types of reconstructions, rather than with the normal breast. The distinct benefits of our current surgical methods can easily outweigh the inherent imperfections, the attendant morbidity, the expected risks; and the reconstructive burden can be diminished for both the patient and the surgeon. As a final note on communication with patients, we must all remember our personal dread of surgery upon ourselves. Imagining the "great surgeon" in their place is a real source of empathy for patients undergoing these major procedures. We must be sure that this empathy transcends that trite quip: "Of course every operation is a major operation, if you're having it." We can do better than that.

PATIENT SELECTION

The most significant factor in patient selection is an understanding by the surgeon of the *patient's perceptions of the anticipated surgery,* after the patient has been thoroughly informed and apprised of the various options. This transfer of information is difficult because it requires us to blend a technical education with a humanistic approach. What is legally called "informed consent" is practically impossible to obtain literally because patients remember very little of what they have been told and also because they optimistically place themselves in the uncomplicated, "good result" category of patients. It is very clear that the patient should not be considered as a candidate for any surgery, regardless of the legal niceties, unless he is able to "intelligently concur" with the known risks, benefits, and alternatives. He must also accept the expected length of hospital stay, the need for prolonged follow-up, and the reasonable possibility of unusual complications and secondary revisions.

Medicine has now evolved from a system of condescending physician "paternalism" to one of active patient "consumerism" in an effort to restore some personal control for the patient. In today's litigious environment surgeons are reluctant to persuade and even more loathe to coerce the decision of any patient. We presume that the patient, after receiving a monochromatic factual litany of the various options, is fully capable of making an intelligent choice between profoundly different procedures without the benefit of any prior knowledge or surgical experience. This is patently unfair to the patient because it deprives him of any basis for a reasonable judgment. We also presume that, once the choice is made by the patient, we are absolved of any responsibility as to the appropriateness of the choice. Hence, when things go awry, it has to be the patient's fault. Nothing could be more reminiscent of the Cultural Revolution in China. We don't need peasants acting as surgeons, no matter what the legal or governmental stresses might dictate. We need actively to direct patients away from any and all bad choices which are influenced by the rush of the moment, expediency, or by their inexperience in making complex reconstructive surgical decisions. Likewise, patients may refuse what is considered to be the appropriate treatment for any number of psychological reasons. For example, the paraplegic's refusal of a total thigh flap, when that is the only possible option, is a way of reasserting control over his condition of dependency. Such open recalcitrance can also be a manifestation of secondary depression which arises from a feeling of helplessness and hopelessness. Similarly, the patient who insists on an immediate breast reconstruction, so that she'll have "two normal breasts" when she awakes from the anesthetic, is overtly denying the existence of either the breast cancer or the mastectomy. This patient will have no way of knowing that her goal is unrealistic unless her choices are carefully guided. The surgeon who participates in this denial "play acting" and allows himself to be manipulated away from the reality of the situation only reinforces these feelings.

The surgeon thereby sets himself up to produce an impossible goal in trying to fulfill the patient's inflated expectations. When he does not achieve the anticipated goal, he is perceived as either deceitful or incompetent, to the eventual detriment of the patient-doctor relationship.

Patients frequently become angry about their disease, because of bitterness about their fate, guilt that they somehow caused the disease or fear for the well-being of loved ones in the case of their absence. This anger is easily "displaced" toward the physician, who may be blamed for the entire chain of events. The doctor must recognize and resolve this anger prior to any reconstruction intervention or it will evolve into patient dissatisfaction and even more anger — the common denominator of malpractice claims. Two recent lawsuits can be cited to illustrate the full spectrum of this "displaced" anger toward the reconstructive surgeon.

Case #1

A thirty-two-year-old nurse consulted her general surgeon for a very large neglected adenocarcinoma of the breast. The tumor was intentionally neglected by the patient because she was afraid that a biopsy would be malignant and would result in the loss of her breast. The general surgeon recommended a massive resection of breast skin in order to obtain an adequate extirpation as well as a soft tissue reconstruction with a latissimus dorsi myocutaneous flap rather than a skin graft. The operation was a technical success, but the patient failed psychologically. She sued both surgeons because of her anger about the disease, the deforming operation, and the general surgeon's fee. Even though she remained friendly with the plastic surgeon, *he was sued because his ability to correct a massive defect with a flap caused the general surgeon to perform a larger and more deforming mastectomy* than he would have performed in the absence of a plastic surgeon. Faulty logic, yes, but reasonable enough to the plaintiff lawyer who was in search of "deep pockets." The uninsured general surgeon precipitated the legal action because of his abrasive, uncaring personality and his relentless pursuit of his surgical fee. Since the general surgeon was "bare" and had no tangible assets, he was released from the suit. After days of tiring courtroom proceedings and seemingly unfair press coverage, the suit was decided in favor of the defendant plastic surgeon. Was this suit avoidable? Definitely. The young plastic surgeon was pleased with the fine surgical result, and his patient appeared to be happy and appreciative. What went wrong? The plastic surgeon thought of himself as only a consultant in the case, presuming that the patient was well prepared for both the extirpative and reconstructive operations, and that the judgment of the general surgeon was correct. During the trial, evidence was introduced to the effect that the extensive mastectomy was not indicated, that a large flap was no better than a skin graft and that the additive reconstructive procedure unnecessarily scarred the back. Naturally, these opinions were refuted by the defense. The general surgeon was portrayed as incompetent, negligent, abrasive, greedy and slothful. The naive young plastic surgeon was painted with the same brush of vicarious liability. Instead of recognizing the patient's preexisting anger and ill-preparation, the plastic surgeon participated in the case as a "flap technician" rather than as a physician. In his eyes, she was the general surgeon's patient, and he was just "helping out." He paid for this judgmental error dearly even though the case was "won." In fact, both sides lost.

Case #2

A sixty-eight-year-old florist was healthy and working until the day he was admitted to the hospital for a femoral artery thrombectomy. Four months later he was still in the hospital, having undergone numerous unsuccessful vascular reconstructive procedures by highly competent vascular surgeons. The foot was adequately revascularized by a femoral-popliteal and a popliteal-posterior tibial Gortex® graft. The Gortex® graft became exposed in the mid-calf, and the skin on the dorsum of the foot was lost because of an occluded anterior tibial artery. The exposed Gortex® graft in the calf was successfully covered with a soleus muscle flap. Multiple attempts to skin graft the dorsum of the foot were unsuccessful, and since no local or distant flaps were reasonable considerations, it became necessary to amputate the foot. *The plastic surgeon was sued for the loss of the foot.* The patient was embittered by the prolonged hospitalization and the loss of his foot, but he couldn't bring himself to be angry with his good friend, the vascular surgeon. He then directed his anger toward the plastic surgeon. His deteriorating psychological condition was compounded by the fact that he had lost his floral business and that the hospital expenses had drained him of his life savings. The plastic surgeon ignored the psychodynamics of the existing situation and didn't emphasize the gravity and complexity of his proposed reconstructive salvage attempts. It was shown in court, to the satisfaction of the jury, that the reconstructive surgeon was responsible for saving the leg, not for losing the foot. How much easier it would have been to have settled these matters prior to the successful muscle flap operation in the calf. The plaintiff left the courtroom still feeling angry and injured, and further in debt. The plastic surgeon left feeling innocent and falsely accused — a victim of the "unfair" legal system. The plastic surgeon also was left with a permanent legal blemish on a previously untarnished record — a fact which could subsequently hurt his ability to maintain his hospital credentials.

Declining or deferring participation in the care of a patient is something which is difficult for any surgeon because we view ourselves as simply trying to "help" the patient. The surgeon should strongly consider not undertaking any surgical reconstruction when the negative factors of psychological instability, unrealistic goals, disagreement with treatment modalities, or expected future non-compliance with instructions are suspected. In this situation, it is fair to explain to the patient that you are not capable of achieving a result which is acceptable to yourself and expected by him. Once this important caveat is established, the discussion should be rationally and amicably ended. Another simple and helpful method of pre-operative evaluation is an analysis of the rapport which is established at three minutes and maintained at thirty minutes after initiation of the patient interview. If one is comfortable with the patient quickly, and if this mutual understanding remains established at thirty minutes, one can rely on this as an extremely valuable prognosticator of future understanding and cooperation. If any of these non-surgical details is left unresolved before surgery, it will be hard for the patient to accept the traumatic experience involved with some of these difficult reconstruction endeavors.

WOUND PREPARATION

Although muscle flaps are known to facilitate the decontamination of minimally infected wounds, their capabilities are certainly limited and must be assisted by appropriate *wound preparation*. Quantitative wound cultures are frequently used to monitor problem wounds because they are both accurate and quantitative. A reasonable effort should be made to obtain a pre-operative quantitative bacteriological count of less than 10^5 bacteria per gram of tissue, but the test can be over-used and should not replace clinical judgment. Burn wounds may provide the exception to this rule, but as experience provides improved clinical judgment, quantitative cultures tend to be employed in an inverse proportion to the worth of this clinical judgment. One experienced surgeon has said: "The main time that I get quantitative cultures is when I forget to tell the resident not to get them." Quantitative cultures have little or no place in frank osteomyelitis or in infected ulcers because a satisfactory culture cannot be obtained without a vigorous operative debridement. Furthermore, the test results can be spurious as a result of a poorly selected biopsy site.

The *type of topical care* is less important than the interest of the doctors and nurses in preparing the wound.

Professor Robert Chase once said: "The best way to get a wound to granulate is to get a third year medical student interested in it" — succinct, but sage advice. Wet-to-dry dressings are the most commonly used form of dressing, but they are difficult to properly perform. The modern nurse is no longer well versed in this type of wound care unless he or she has had a special experience or a particular interest in wound care. The wet-to-dry dressing frequently fails because it is allowed to completely dry out. When this happens, the dressing serves little more purpose than a simple dry dressing. Iodoform gauze packing is an even more pernicious form of dressing. The chemical agent effectively "pickles" or "fixes" the margins of the wound so that capillary ingrowth and secondary healing are thwarted. Only its medicinal smell belies its usefulness.

Enzymes have been used for many years, but they are not necessarily any more effective than diligent saline dressings. Most of the enzyme preparations have been singularly disappointing, with the exception of Travase.® Travase® can be helpful in removing the final adherent slough if it is less than one mm in thickness. The ointment must be applied in a very thick coat and covered with a moist dressing which is neither totally wet nor allowed to dry. In every case it is imperative to change the dressing frequently. If this agent has not had a significant effect in three to four days, it probably will not contribute much more with time. Debrisan® is another agent which can be helpful in reducing the bacterial count in weeping wounds, but it is not helpful in the usual dry venous or arterial ulcer. It is simple to use, but it can trap surface bacteria if it is not completely removed at each dressing change. The *Waterpik*® is the best method to remove this material, and it usually does not cause any significant discomfort. One wonders whether the debridement accomplished by the Waterpik® itself is not the more significant agent in allowing the humoral defenses to gain the upper hand over the existing surface bacteria. *Systemic antibiotics* have not been particularly helpful unless the wounds are frankly infected. Even then, antibiotics may not achieve a sufficient tissue concentration at the wound surface. Osteomyelitis is more appropriately treated by operative debridement since it is never cured by antibiotics alone. Short term administration of systemic antibiotics is probably completely superfluous in the surgical process of eradicating osteomyelitis, but long term I.V. antibiotics have been helpful in conjunction with surgical debridement and closure.

Deep wounds are more difficult to deal with because they are not amenable to the usual topical agents. Whenever they can be used, in-and-out irrigation systems have offered some impressive results. Diluted Betadine® is commonly used in lieu of saline, but it is difficult to tell whether or not it is any more effective than saline. Even diluted Betadine® instillation may cause harm by "drying out" the wound. Saline flushing of the wound surface certainly seems to be just as effective in diluting the bacterial population. In either case, the volume of the fluid is the critical factor in the process.

Whirlpool treatments are relatively ineffective and slow in debriding deep wounds unless the Waterpik® is used simultaneously. The major advantage of the whirlpool is related to the diligent dressing changes offered by the physical therapist. It also provides a convenient bath. The major disadvantage is that the surgeon is allowed to remove himself from these seemingly mundane chores, and when the patient is "out of sight and out of mind," everything moves more slowly. A progress notation of "still going to whirlpool," when translated, equates with "still spending somebody's money." One of the most effective methods of cleaning a dirty wound, whether it is a sternotomy wound or an osteomyelitic cavity, is the bathroom shower. A Waterpik® can also be used at the same time as the shower. The high pressure pulsations probably speed along the process, but the large volumes of fluid in the irrigation seem to make the critical difference. It doesn't matter whether tap water or saline is the agent or whether the irrigation is performed by the patient himself or by a highly trained professional. The point is to get the patient actively involved.

TIMING

The *timing of the muscle flap coverage* is preferably deferred until the wound is clean. If the dressings are green and the wound is slick, shiny and stinks, you don't need quantitative cultures to guide you. Xenograft and allograft "take" can be used as predictive factors in burn wounds, but they are seldom used in muscle flap closures. Multiple debridements may be necessary, prior to definitive wound closure, but it is not always essential to remove a foreign body such as a metallic implant to prepare the wound adequately. Some deep ulcers and osteomyelitic defects can only be prepared by repeated vigorous operating room debridements. The decision as to whether or not a muscle flap should be immediately elevated and inset is a matter of practiced surgical judgment. There are no "rules," and there should be no recriminations involved with the expense of one or more operative debridements to successfully prepare a difficult wound.

In the case of complex, open tibial fractures, the recent trend is to provide early and complete muscle coverage in the *"golden period"* of the first five days. After this brief interlude, the incidence of chronic osteomyelitis increases dramatically. The fear of closing these wounds and creating a "closed space" infection is based on the faulty surgical logic of the 1930's. Empirical observation finally has dispelled this myth even though it prevails at times in current practice. A reasonable extension of the concept of early local muscle coverage of these wounds is the use of immediate "free" muscle flaps. Godina and Bajec have demonstrated that "free" muscle flaps can be effective in the prevention of osteomyelitis in over four hundred cases of complex tibial fractures. Their reasons for choosing "free" flaps over "potentially" injured local muscle flaps is thought provoking. First, the survivability of "free" flaps, in their hands, is comparable to local muscle flaps — both 95%. Second, the size of the defect is a matter of little concern when the problem is approached with large "free" flaps such as the latissimus dorsi or rectus abdominis muscles. Third, the "zone of injury" is not further disturbed by additional dissection, which should preserve the remaining integrity of the "muscle-periosteal unit." Their final and weakest argument is that a successful "free" muscle flap never becomes ischemic while, in their opinion, a local muscle flap must always become ischemic. This line of reasoning is predicated on the differences in the terminal, end-artery vasculature of calf muscle flaps compared to the robust intramuscular vascular connections of freely transferred flat muscles — a factor which should mitigate against distal or peripheral muscle flap ischemia. This may be true, but it probably can never be proven. Whether their reasoning is correct or not, these authors have reconfirmed the fact that appropriate debridement and adequate muscle coverage can effectively prevent a vicious cycle; and the sooner this is done, the better. The ultimate nihilistic and defeatist argument against either early or late closure of infected bone with muscle flaps is that osteomyelitis will recur "if you wait long enough." We don't need dogs or pigs to refute this notion because we have already done these operations in humans.

CHOICE OF FLAPS

There are numerous factors which affect our decisions to use either a muscle, a musculocutaneous, or an axial flap. These considerations must be weighed in aggregate because no single factor is usually overriding in its importance. In the past we have been guided by the so-called *"reconstructive ladder"* as the primary determinate in choosing a logical surgical approach. In this scheme, simplicity of the procedure is emphasized, in that one is advised always to choose the simplest type of procedure first. For example, one progresses from a skin graft to a local flap and finally, to a distant flap. Unfortunately, this prefatory approach ignores all of the other attributes of a specific reconstruction which can contribute to its overall success. These important contributory factors obviously include durability, morbidity, and esthetic considerations. A skin graft may be simpler than a muscle flap, but it may be vastly inferior in other respects. There are also many times when a myocutaneous flap provides faster healing than a skin graft. The skin-grafted radical mastectomy defect is a good example of this. Although the latissimus dorsi myocutaneous flap is a more complex procedure, it provides an esthetic color match, a reconstitution of the contour deformity, and a durable and comfortable soft tissue surface. A "free" flap to the low-pretibial area may be more complex than a local muscle flap; but it may also prevent multiple re-operations, lessen the morbidity, and shorten the time of healing. In this instance, the criticism of prolonged operative time is an empty one.

Conversely, we can't be *extravagant in our choices*. A recto-vaginal fistula can be elegantly closed with an inferiorly based rectus abdominis muscle using an intra-abdominal approach. This same defect can also be repaired using a gracilis muscle which has an inconsequential donor site, or when the abdomen is already opened, an omental flap can easily be used. This approach obviates the need to rely on the extra abdominal "parts department." Most head and neck cancer defects can be corrected by using the "island" pectoralis paddle, but the surgeon who always chooses this method denigrates the value of the other helpful local flaps in the head and neck area. Surgical ignorance of all of the available options is forever inexcusable. "When your only tool is a hammer, the whole world looks like a nail" best describes such practices. Occasionally, we will want to use a less desirable choice in the first instance, in an effort to save our best flap for a recurrence or a later problem. Whether or not we use our best flap choice in the first instance, we must always be ready for its failure and have a backup flap in mind which will "dig us out of a hole."

SIZE AND ARC

Our foremost consideration is whether or not the proposed *flap will cover the defect*. This is primarily decided by the axis of the dominant vasculature and the expected size of the muscle or musculocutaneous flap. It is always imperative to know the exact extent of flap excursion since this is decided by immutable anatomical constants. This knowledge can only be gained through operative experience or through cadaver dissections.

VASCULATURE

The *location and relative dominance of the muscle vasculature* are the anatomic and physiologic keystones of muscle flap surgery. The deep vasculature of the muscles has been classified according to the various "Types" of vessel arrangements. Although this information is of critical importance, we tend to take a "lumper" rather than a "splitter" approach to the matter. It is not so important that one remembers which muscles are considered to be Type I or Type II, etc., for this is an almost impossible task. It is occasionally difficult even to remember the name of the dominant vessel supplying the muscle. Nevertheless, it is important to know the location and functional significance of each major muscular vessel. Most frequently transposed muscles are supplied by a dominant proximal vascular leash with a backup system of deep perforating vessels. A physiologic modifier of the vascular anatomy is the nature of the intramuscular vascular interconnections. Broad, flat muscles tend to have excellent intramuscular vascular connections while long, thin muscles more often have "segmental" vascular arrangements. The biceps femoris and sartorius muscles are the best examples of a "segmental" vasculature in which none of these deep vessels can be safely sacrificed. The rectus femoris muscle is a prime example of a dominant, proximal vasculature without any accompanying deep perforating system. The rectus abdominis muscle best exemplifies an equally dominant proximal and distal vasculature. The vascular anatomy of the gracilis muscle lies somewhere in between. The soleus and extensor digitorum communis muscles demonstrate balanced proximal, dominant, and distal deep perforating systems. Broad, flat muscles tend to have either a totally "segmental" vascular system, as is the case of the external oblique muscle, or a duplicate system, as seen in the arrangement of the pectoralis and latissimus muscle. The physiologic nature of these intramuscular vascular connections is the reason why numerous segmental vessels can be sacrificed in the case of the external oblique muscle and not in the case of the biceps femoris muscle.

ACCESSIBILITY

The ability to expose the flap through a *single operative field* is a mundane, but important consideration. Repositioning the patient is awkward, time-consuming, and precludes elevation of the flap at the time of the recreation of the deformity. This is the obvious reason why the "island" vertical trapezius myocutaneous flap is chosen less often for head and neck defects than is the pectoralis "paddle." The same criticism applies to the latissimus dorsi and pectoralis major myocutaneous flaps in the case of two operative fields. Even though the latissimus dorsi myocutaneous flap is just as useful as the pectoralis "paddle" flap for head and neck defects, it is less often chosen because of its lack of accessibility.

DONOR SITE

The *donor site considerations* are pivotal in the choice of a flap. The known problems range from the bothersome seroma of the latissimus dorsi flap donor site to the life-threatening carotid "blowout" potential of the sternomastoid flap donor site. Functional loss should always be considered, but it is usually a less important consideration than the donor site. These problems must be weighed in aggregate when choosing any muscle flap procedure.

SENSATION

Most muscle flaps maintain some pressure *sensibility,* but with rare exception, no surface sensibility. Most "island" myocutaneous flaps maintain neither deep nor superficial sensibility because the segmental nerves are distant from the "island" vessels and are sacrificed in the process of the flap elevation. Still, the deep pressure sensibility which persists in a muscle flap may be adequate to provide a durable surface for walking or for the protection of a skin graft. In the case of the gastrocnemius and soleus muscle flaps, surface tactile sensibility is somehow preserved. Restoration of the sensation to the major myocutaneous flaps is an awaiting horizon. This event could transform the highly desirable esthetic result of the rectus abdominis breast reconstruction into a sensate breast. The tensor fascia lata and external oblique myocutaneous flaps are unusual examples of flaps which sometimes maintain the integrity of their nerve supply following flap elevation.

FUNCTION

Because of the redundancy of muscle strength and actions, the *functional importance* of any given muscle is difficult to establish. It comes as a surprise that muscles which are as large as the latissimus, gastrocnemius, soleus, and rectus femoris can be sacrificed with little or no functional loss. One would think that the tensor fascia lata flap would be functionally less important than the rectus femoris myocutaneous flap, but this may not be the case. Conversely, hand and forearm muscle flaps are not included in this discussion because the use of any single muscle as a local flap in the hand or forearm may be difficult to justify. The gluteus maximus muscle is a functionally important muscle, and it is used judiciously in the walking patient. The tibialis anterior muscle is so important and unduplicated in foot dorsiflexion, as the peroneus longus and brevis muscles are in foot eversion, that these muscles are rarely considered as useful muscle flaps.

THE DEFECT

The size, location, depth, and *nature of the defect* ultimately determine which muscle flap will be applicable. Muscle is always chosen over other types of flaps when it is necessary to revascularize ischemic, irradiated, and infected wounds. A muscle flap alone is the standard choice for obliterating cavities. Fasciocutaneous flaps have virtually no place in either the eradication of an infection or in the obliteration of a contaminated cavity. The size and depth of the wound may also be the major factor in flap choices. For instance, the removal of a total hip prosthesis may give such a sizable wound that the TFL flap would have no effect in obliterating the defect. Further, the rectus femoris muscle flap may be too small to correct the resulting hip defect so that it may be necessary to use the larger vastus lateralis muscle flap to totally correct the problem. In the case of pretibial defects, failure to cover even one centimeter of the bone is tantamount to total failure. For this reason, one must always be prepared to use both the soleus and gastrocnemius muscle flaps to correct certain unanticipated pretibial problems. Most intrathoracic cavities are too sizable to completely obliterate even if all of the chest wall muscles were used in combination. Intrathoracic muscle transpositions are almost always employed as a "seal" and seldom as a sole means of cavitary obliteration.

The *types of exposed structures* must be dealt with individually. Exposed and dried bone is usually not infected nor a contributor to wound infections, and it can be safely debrided at the time of the definitive flap closure. Exposed or dried arteries are more perilous because such vessels can rupture at any time. This problem requires urgent coverage and total debridement of the surrounding ischemic wound with immediate and complete muscular coverage of the involved artery. The exposed or infected prosthetic arterial graft is even more difficult because a wider resection of the surrounding "pseudosheath" and ischemic marginal wound must be carried out, and the entire graft must be totally surrounded by muscle. Dried nerves may lose their epineural blood supply, which can lead to a significant functional nerve deficit. Drying of nerves should be avoided at all costs; but if it cannot, nerves may be partially revascularized with appropriate muscle flap coverage. Dried tendon is a less difficult situation to deal with because tendon can be covered with a vascularized flap and will completely reconstitute its sub-

stance even though the tendon is, in fact, dead and tanned. Conversely, the "soupy" tendon is autolyzed and must be excised. Metallic prostheses cannot always be removed, and removal is not always necessary. It may be necessary to remove metallic plates or intramedullary rods from long bones and replace them with an external fixation device when the infection extends into the screw hole sites or remains inaccessible to the muscle flap coverage. Exposed total knee and ankle joints have been successfully covered with muscle flaps even though the wound-healing logic of this event evades our explanation.

In the case of a bronchopleural fistula, the purpose of the flap is to seal the bronchopleural fistula. The transposed muscle is not intended to obliterate the remaining chest cavity which will obliterate itself. Neither will a muscle flap obliterate deeply imbedded infection in bone. This must always be surgically removed. One cannot expect even the most powerful antibiotics to have any curative effect on "undebrided" osteomyelitis. This is best exemplified by attempting to treat a tubular sequestrum of the tibia by removing the anterior cortex of the bone and covering it with a gastrocnemius and/or soleus muscle flap. Unless the entire sequestrum is removed, the muscle flaps will have no effect on the remaining infected bone, and neither will prolonged intravenous antibiotics. The nature of the defect requires us to consider factors other than which flaps will "reach" the defect. In the leg a skin-grafted soleus muscle flap is esthetically superior to the medical gastrocnemius myocutaneous flap because of the less attractive myocutaneous flap donor site skin graft. Although one can cite numerous disadvantages for the "island" vertical trapezius myocutaneous flap, it is the only local flap which will comfortably reach the occiput. The excellent color match achieved by the horizontal trapezius myocutaneous flap when it is used to replace anterior neck skin is also an important factor. This esthetic consideration alone would temper the usefulness of a skin grafted pectoralis muscle or a pectoralis "paddle" for the same problem. The nature of the defect is frequently the sole determinant for the choice of a flap. It is axiomatic that flaps transposed into irradiated wounds should carry their own blood supply. It must also be recognized that inadequate debridement of the surrounding irradiated tissue may lead to further necrosis of this tissue even though the muscle flap survives in the middle of a sea of dying irradiated skin. The volume of muscle bulk is probably a poor reason to choose a muscle to cover a pressure sore since this may or may not be protective against future ulcers. Contrary to the conventional wisdom, muscle flaps can be used in ischemic legs even when their primary vessels are not visualized on an arteriogram. If the muscle is not tender, has a good appearance, and is functioning well in situ, it may survive transposition. This would obviously not be our first choice, but it may be an option. A latissimus muscle flap may be desirable for a chest wall skeletal defect even when there is adequate overlying skin cover because it serves the purposes of both covering an artificial mesh and adding a second well vascularized layer to a potentially life-threatening wound. Primary skin closure of such a thoracic defect would be a simpler method in the "reconstructive ladder," but it would not afford the safety of a latissimus dorsi muscle flap closure, which is further up the "reconstructive ladder."

In summary, our decisions in regard to flap choices are multifaceted and complex. They must all lead toward solving the problem at hand in a balanced fashion. The proper design of a muscle flap procedure is the critical determinant in its success.

TEMPORALIS MUSCLE

ANATOMICAL CONSIDERATIONS

Surface Markings

The anterior margin of the temporalis muscle can be palpated by clenching the jaws. The superior margin of the muscle cannot be palpated, but it lies at a point halfway between the upper margin of the ear and the vertex of the skull. The insertion is palpable and visible near the mid-point of the zygomatic arch.

Origin and Insertion

The temporalis muscle originates from the temporal fossa and inserts into the coronoid process of the mandible. It functions in forceful posterior bite and in moments of extreme surgical anxiety. Because of the redundancy of the jaw muscles, it is a readily expendable muscle.

Adjacent Muscles

The temporalis muscle incorporates the pericranium on its deep surface and is surrounded by the galeal and frontalis fascia layers in its course to the coronoid process. The proximity of the galea is important because the galea has a completely independent vascular supply from the extracranial vessels. This prevents the temporalis muscle from forming a standard myocutaneous flap since there are no perforating vessels passing directly from the muscle to the scalp skin.

Vascular Pattern

The temporalis muscle is supplied by two deep temporal branches of the maxillary artery. These two vessels penetrate the under surface of the muscle just above its insertion and straddle the motor nerve to the muscle. The robust blood supply of the galea, which overlies the temporalis muscle, arises separately from the superficial temporal and occipital vessels. It is the dense arborization of these four extracranial vessels which usually allows the entire galeal layer to be raised on any single vessel and provides a consistent blood supply to the majority of the ipsilateral scalp skin. For this reason the temporalis muscle cannot be employed as a standard myocutaneous flap without the inclusion of the galea. This compound flap of scalp skin and temporalis muscle, in fact, represents a muscle flap and a separate fasciocutaneous flap.

Motor Nerve

Deep temporal nerve.

Sensory Nerve

Fifth cranial nerve.

USES

The temporalis muscle is an unusual muscle to employ only because it is overlooked. It is exceptionally useful for certain coverage problems contained within a radius of eight centimeters in any direction from the coronoid process. This includes the majority of the oropharynx, the mandible, and the mastoid area. The traditional application of the temporalis muscle flap has been for obliteration of the orbit. Its broader uses include the correction of mastoid, cheek, pharyngeal, and palatal defects because of its proximate rotation point. When it is necessary to correct massive intraoral defects, both temporalis muscles can be retrieved through a coronal incision. The two temporalis muscles can be used to reconstruct the palate, the entire floor of the mouth, or the posterior pharyngeal wall. This should not be surprising if it is recognized that the tonsillar fossa lies but a mere three centimeters away from the temporalis muscular insertion into the coronoid process. An even more obvious application is for coverage of the adjacent exposed dura or cranial bone. This broad range of applicability salvages the useful temporalis muscle flap from its present relegation to the rare need to obliterate an orbit.

REGIONAL FLAP COMPARISONS

This is certainly the most accessible muscle flap for ''high'' areas of coverage, extending from the body of the mandible and the mastoid bone inferiorly and to the orbit and forehead superiorly. Flap elevation is simple, and its transfer is certainly less complicated than that of the major chest wall flaps. Unlike the pectoralis and latissimus myocutaneous flaps, access to the neck is not required and bulk is not a problem. Because the intraoral muscle flap rapidly becomes re-epithelized, it is not necessary to skin graft a temporalis muscle flap which is transposed into the mouth. The temporalis muscle can also be used to transfer living ''split'' cranial bone to the middle and lower face.

DISADVANTAGES

There is no functional loss from the use of this muscle. However, if the muscle is left innervated, it will forcibly contract with chewing. This problem can be avoided by denervating the muscle at the time of its elevation. Because the pericranium is incorporated on the undersurface of the temporalis muscle flap, the exposed temporal bone must be covered with either galeal or scalp flaps. The donor site is generally good, but the loss of the temporalis muscle leaves an area of depression behind the lateral orbital rim.

ADVANTAGES

The temporalis muscle is simple to elevate and causes no functional loss. Its ability to replace the palate, the floor of the mouth, and the posterior pharynx is remarkable. One should not be surprised by this arc of rotation if the distance between the coronoid process and the upper margin of the muscle is "mentally" transposed to these inferior levels of inset. The great advantage of this muscle in intraoral applications is that it does not require skin grafting because it promptly reepithelizes with local epithelium. The temporalis muscle can also be combined with either a galeal fascial flap or a galeal fasciocutaneous scalp flap because of their distinct and separate blood supplies. This unusual combination of a temporalis muscle flap and a galeal fasciocutaneous flap adds significantly to the versatility of their individual coverage capabilities. Acland has recently clarified our generic understanding of the galea. He describes two fascial layers overlying the temporalis muscle. The deep temporal fascia is densely adherent to the temporalis muscle and is supplied by the deep temporal vessels. The dense fascial layer, which he designates as the superficial temporal fascia (A.K.A. galea), lies between the temporalis muscle and the scalp skin. This superficial layer of fascia is contiguous with the galeal and frontalis fascial layers and is supplied by the superficial temporal vessels.

COMPLICATIONS, PITFALLS, AND DONOR SITE

The viability of the temporalis muscle flap should never be questionable, providing the dominant vessels are not harmed. When it is desirable to include skin with the temporalis muscle flap, the extracranial vessels and the galea must be separately elevated. The limits of this galeal fasciocutaneous extension are not completely known at this point. It is obvious that the fasciocutaneous flap margins can be extended much further than the demonstrated case presentations.

The primary pitfall one encounters is to leave the motor innervation intact in a visible site of inset. In this case the muscle can cause an undesirable "twitch." Should this occur, it is difficult to return safely to the previous operative area and denervate the muscle, but it can be done. After a period of several weeks, the neurovascular bundle and the muscular insertion can be completely divided without causing necrosis of the muscle flap, provided it has an adequate bed of inset.

To protect the seventh nerve, the galeal and temporal fascial layers should be elevated separately. Although it would be difficult to injure, the main trunk of the fifth nerve lies just deep to the insertion of the temporalis muscle. Temporary removal and later replacement of the zygomatic arch facilitates a safe dissection of all of these neurovascular structures. Some contour deformity results from the loss of the temporalis muscle bulk beneath the scalp. It also creates a significant area of depression behind the lateral orbital rim and beneath the adjacent sideburn area.

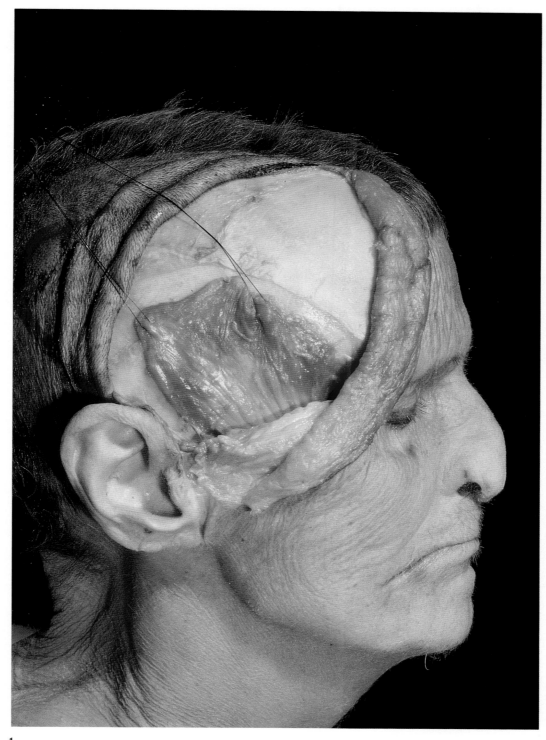

1

Temporalis muscle exposed through a coronal incision. The galea is retracted with the skin. Note the bony margins of the temporal fossa.

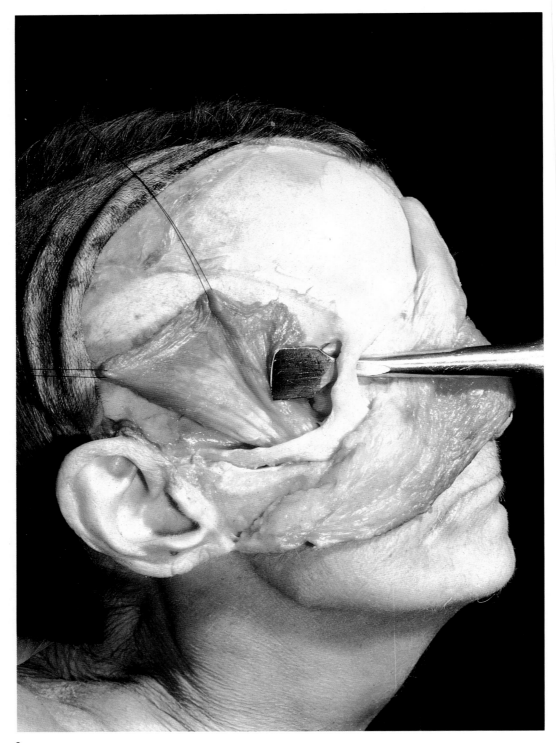

2

Exposure of the lateral orbital rim and the zygomatic arch.

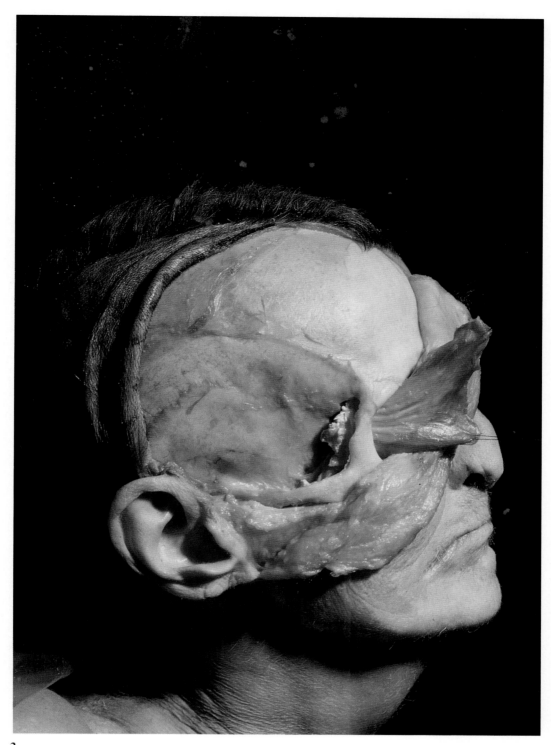

3

Temporalis muscle transposed into an orbital defect.

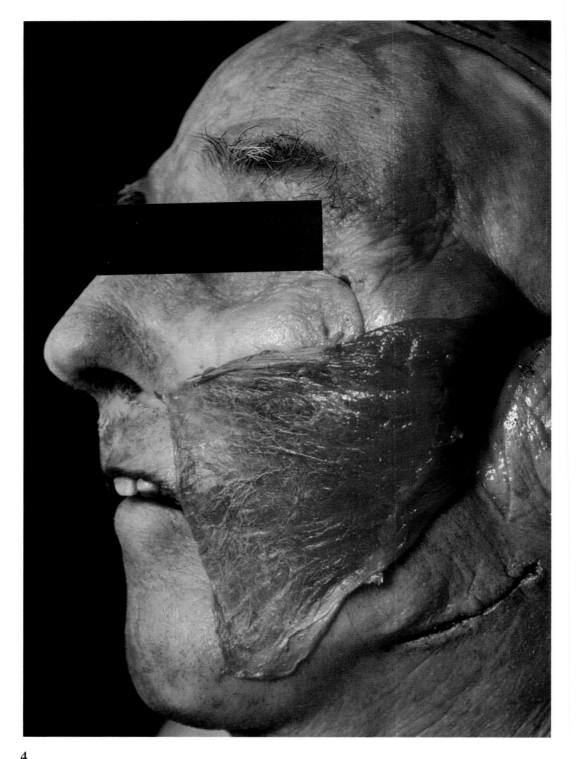

4

Temporalis muscle passed beneath the zygomatic arch. The proximity of the coronoid process allows the muscle to reach both the palate and the cheek.

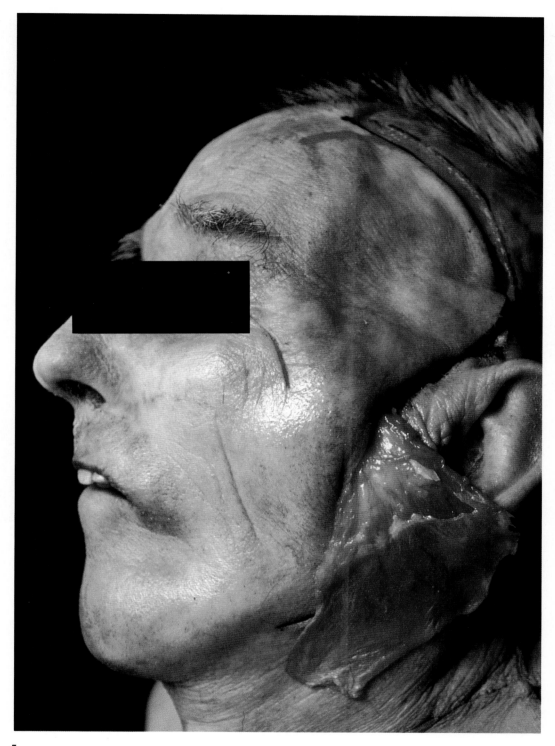

5

Downward extension of the temporalis muscle. Inferiorly, the muscle can be used to cover the mastoid process or the lateral pharyngeal wall.

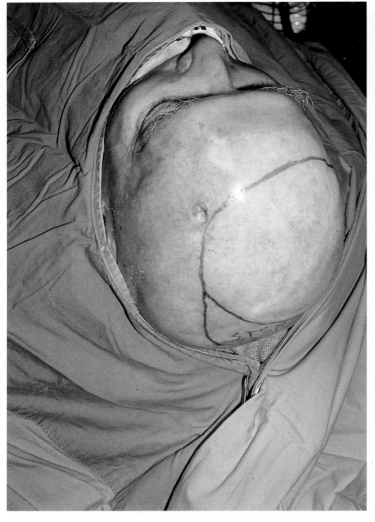

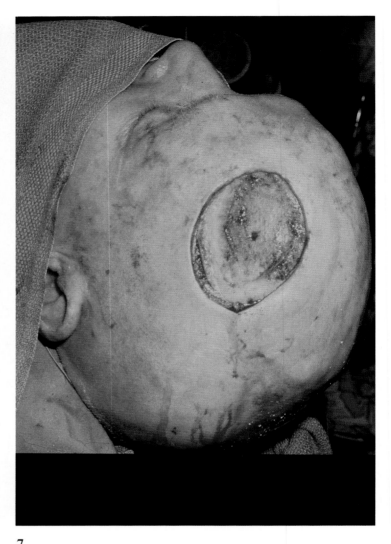

6

Seventy-four-year-old male with a recurrent basal cell carcinoma of the scalp. He had previously been treated with irradiation and later by a wide excision and a rotation scalp flap. (Case of P.G. Arnold)

7

The outer table of the skull is excised and sent for pathological examination.

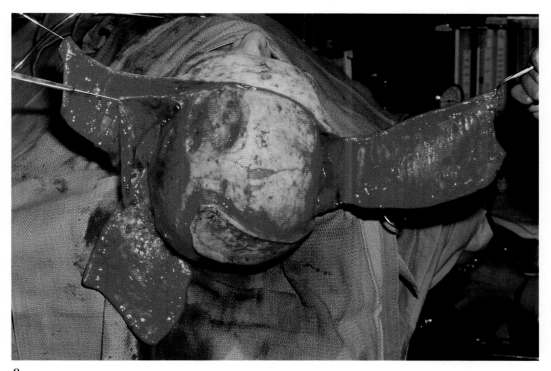

8

Three Orticochea flaps are elevated. The previous skin graft of the posterior scalp has not been disturbed.

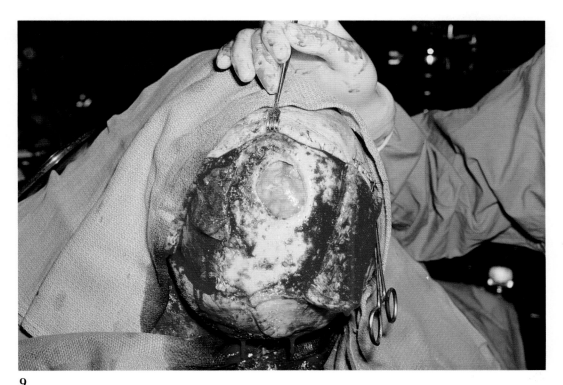

9

Pathological examination demonstrated tumor involvement of the inner table of the skull, but not the dura. Nevertheless, the dura was excised and replaced with cadaver homograft.

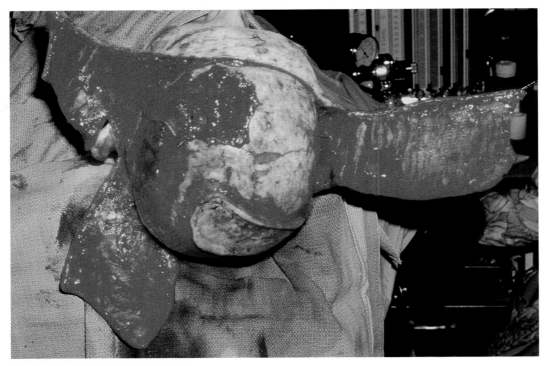

10

The dural homograft is covered with a temporalis muscle flap. The Orticochea flaps will be used for scalp closure.

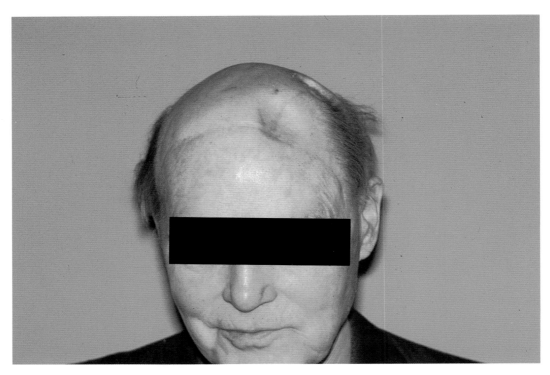

11

Postoperative appearance at four months. Bony reconstruction was temporarily deferred in the face of this aggressive tumor.

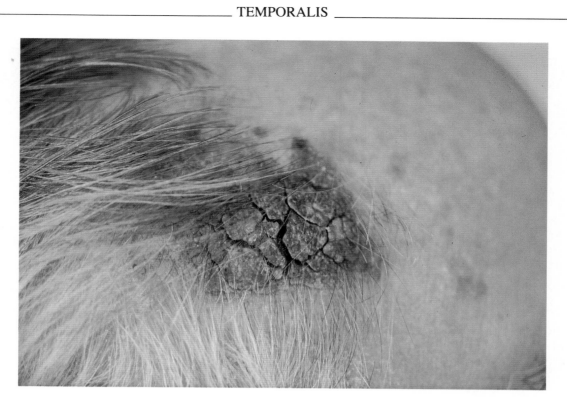

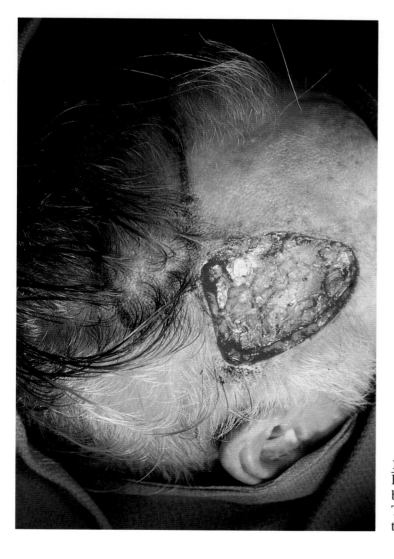

12, 13

Fifty-eight-year-old male with benign seborrheic keratoses of the temporal area. The confluent lesions were excised for esthetic reasons. (Case of J.B. McCraw)

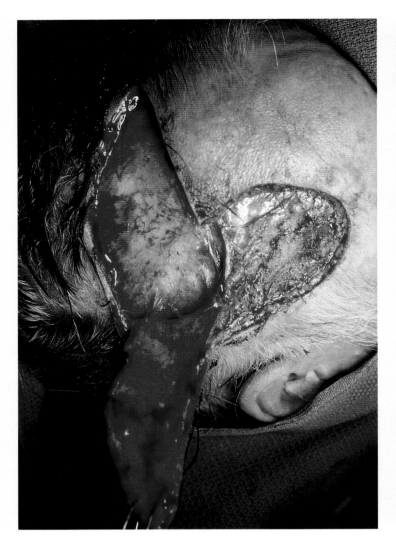 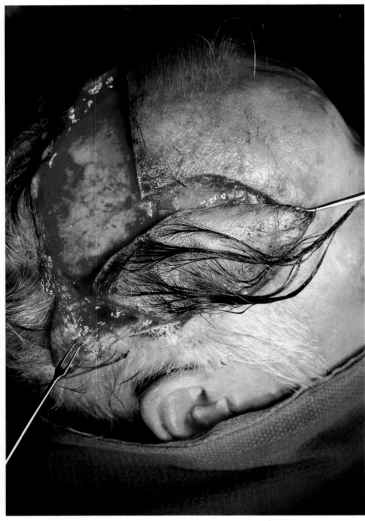

14, 15

Elevation and rotation of a galeal fascio-cutaneous flap from the central scalp. The temporalis muscle was not included with the flap.

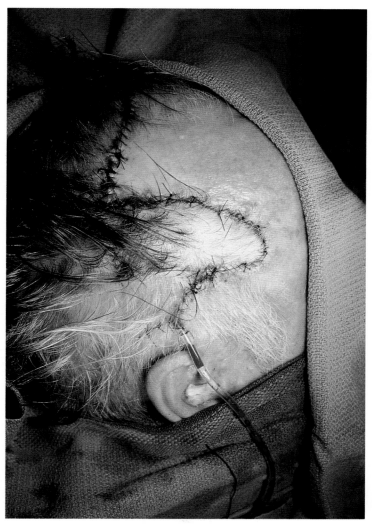

16

Ninety degree rotation of the flap and primary closure of the donor site.

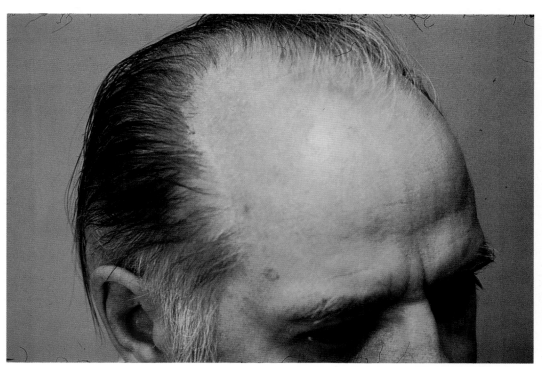

17

Postoperative result at six years. The hairline has been completely reconstituted.

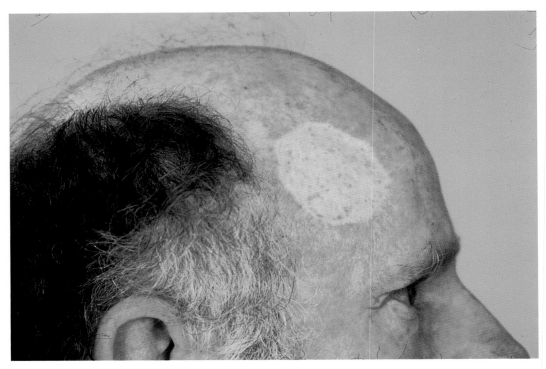

18

Fifty-three-year-old male with an unsightly skin graft taken from the thigh. A
level II melanoma had been excised ten
years earlier. (Case of J.B. McCraw)

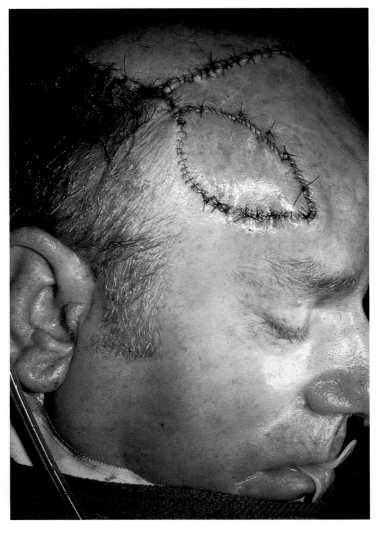

19

Rotation of a non-hairbearing galeal fasciocutaneous flap from the central scalp
to the forehead. Note the fluorescence of
the flap.

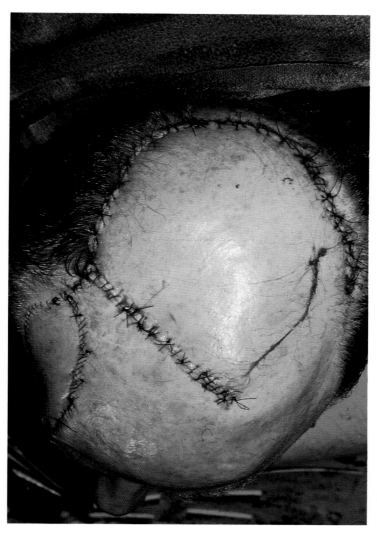

20

The scalp donor site was primarily closed
with a rotation scalp flap.

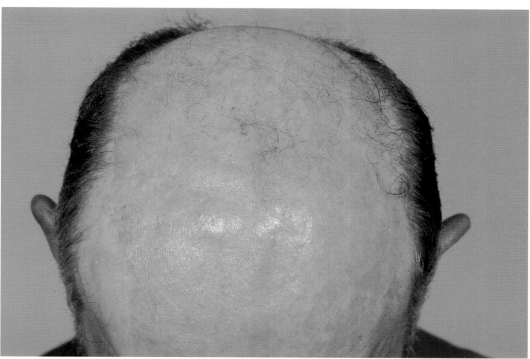

21

Healed scalp donor site at four years.

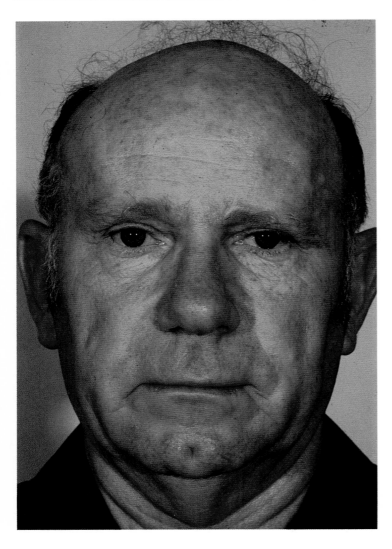

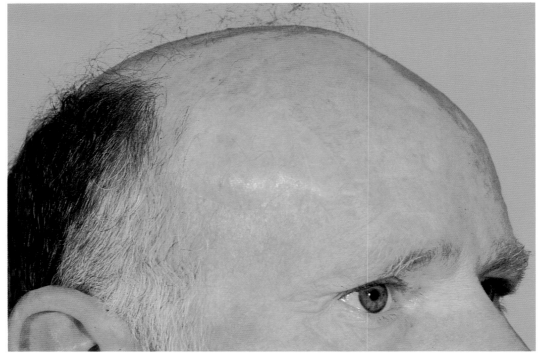

22, 23

The color match and contour of the forehead skin were nicely reconstructed by the fasciocutaneous flap.

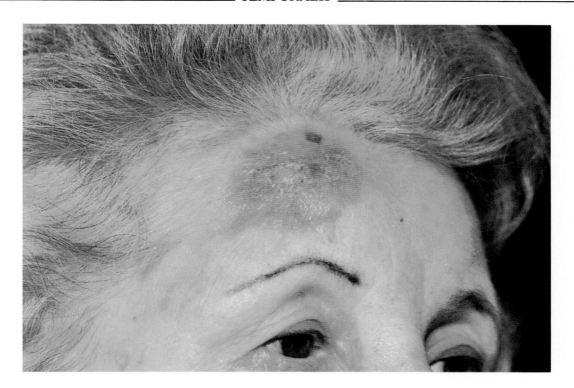

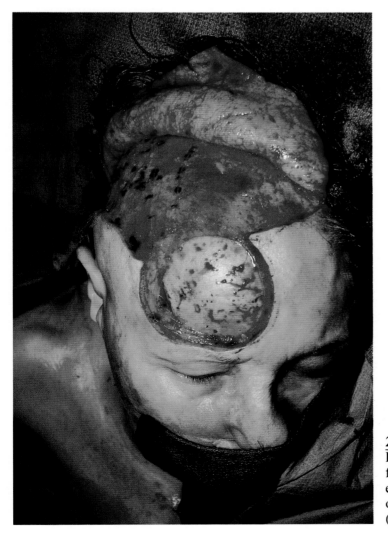

24, 25

Recurrent squamous cell carcinoma of the forehead in an elderly patient. The tumor excision was adequate with the removal of just the periosteum of the frontal bone. (Case of J.B. McCraw)

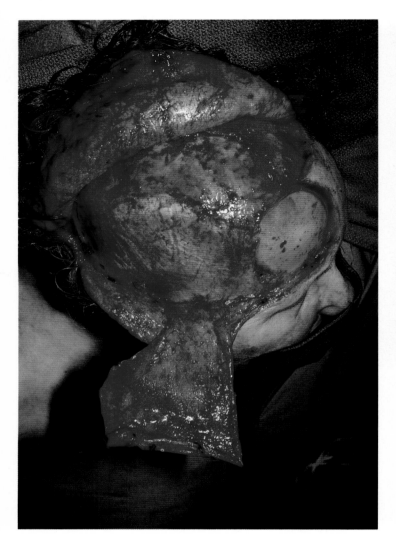
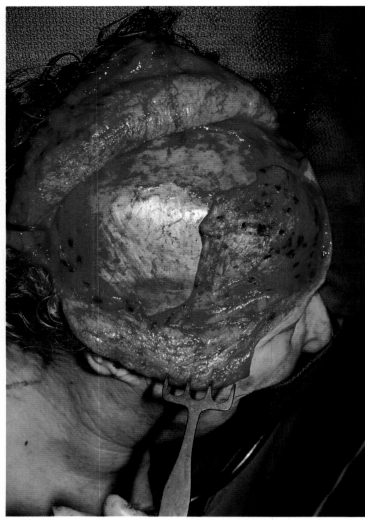

26, 27

A galeal flap is elevated on the superficial temporal vessels. Note the undisturbed temporalis muscle. The fascial flap is rotated onto the forehead to resurface the periosteal defect of the frontal bone.

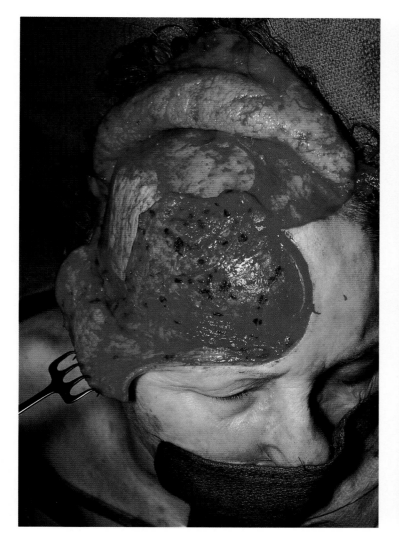
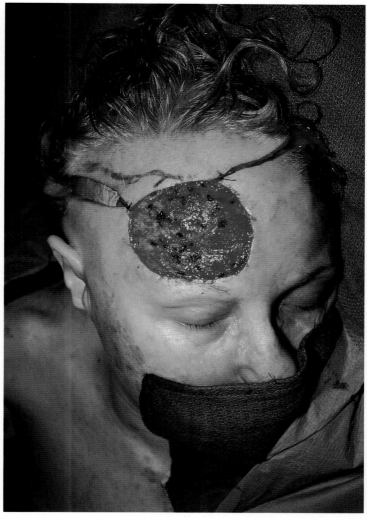

28, 29

Inset of the galeal flap into the forehead defect. The anterior margin of the remaining scalp flap did not fluoresce and was excised (blue mark). The extensive removal of the galea apparently devascularized this portion of the scalp.

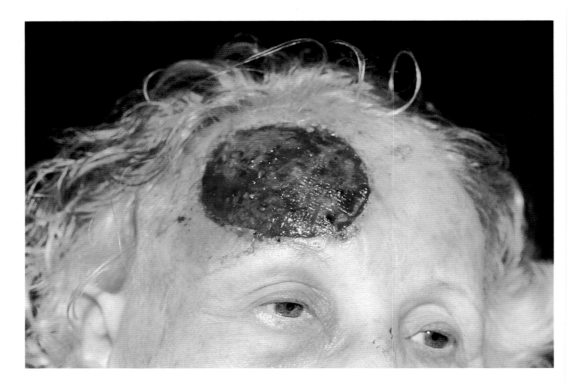

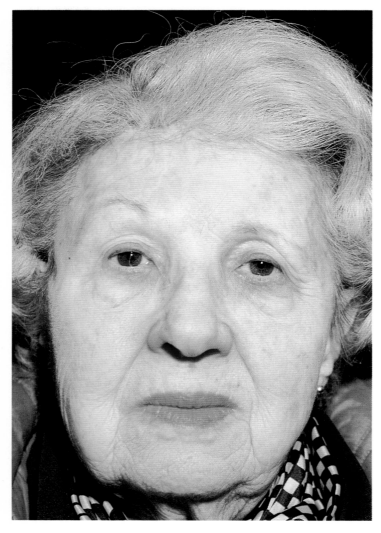

30, 31

Immediate skin grafting was not successful. A "delayed" skin graft is always recommended because of the paucity of small vessels in the galea. The eventual contour restoration of this difficult area was good.

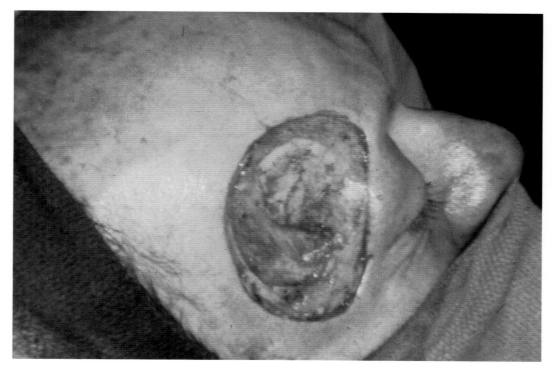

32

Wide excision of a recurrent, invasive squamous cell carcinoma of the right temple in a forty-three-year-old male.
(Case of G. Irons)

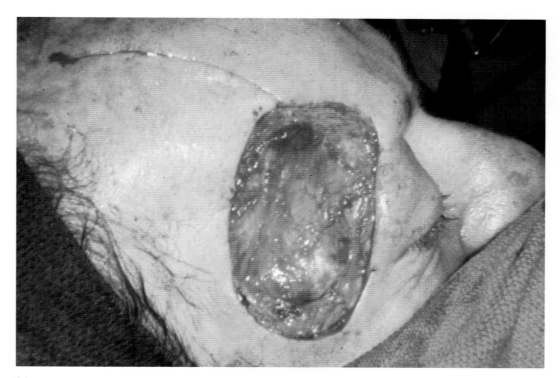

33

Anterior rotation of a temporalis muscle flap to cover the lateral orbital rim and the zygomatic arch.

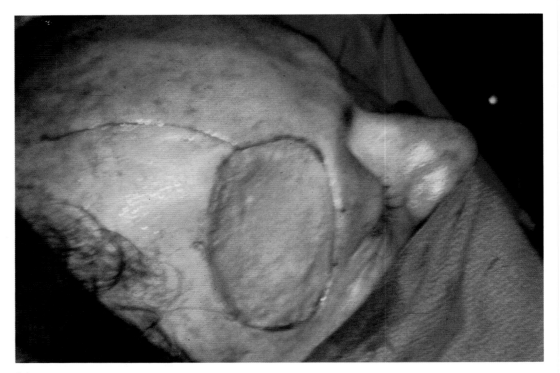

34

The temporalis muscle flap was immediately grafted.

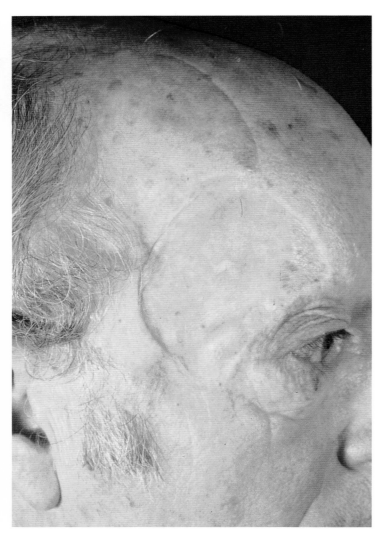

35

Appearance at five years.

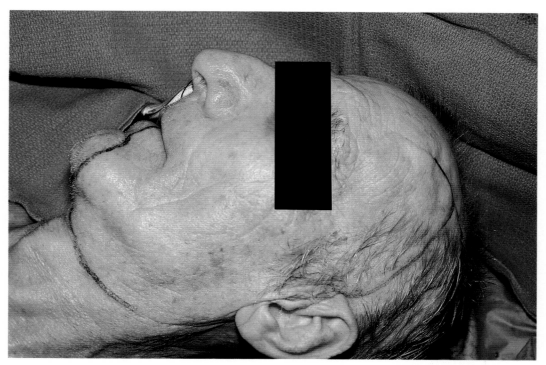

36

Low grade tonsillar carcinoma in a seventy-six-year-old man. Incisions are outlined for the retrieval of a temporalis muscle flap. (Case J.B. McCraw)

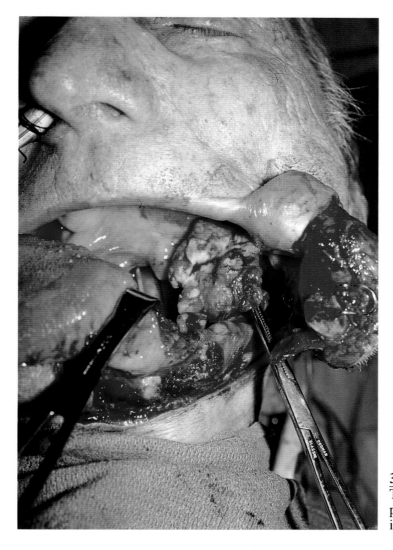

37

The massive tonsillar carcinoma is approached through a mandibular splitting incision.

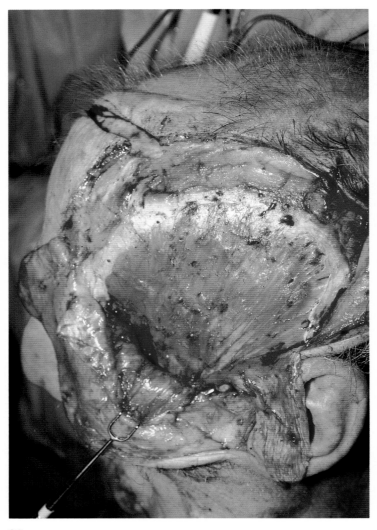

38

Exposure of the temporalis muscle. A rim of deep temporal fascia is left with the muscle for retention of sutures.

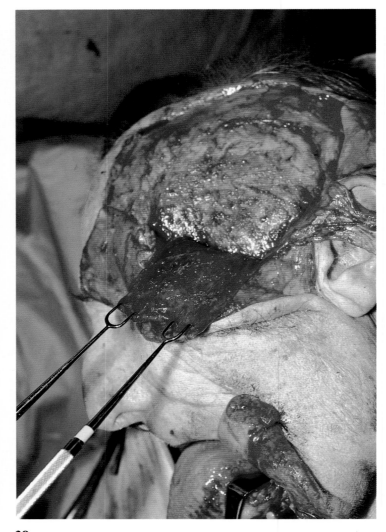

39

The temporalis muscle is passed beneath the zygomatic arch, which was temporarily removed and replaced.

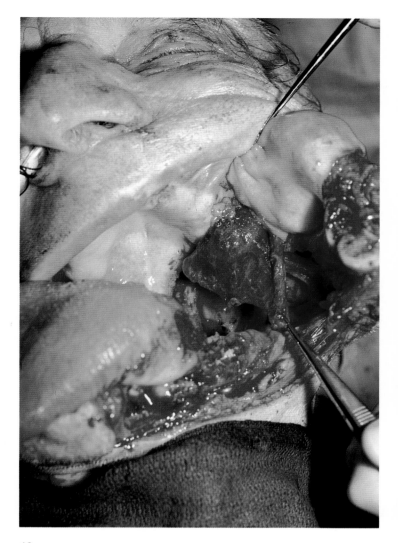

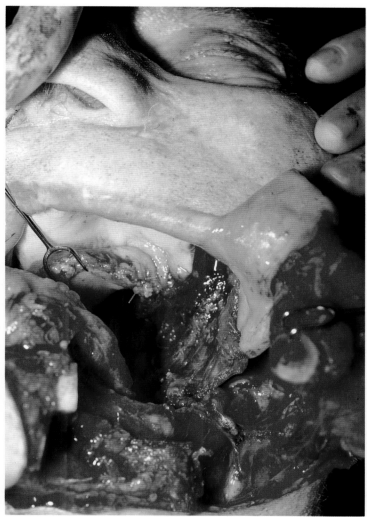

40

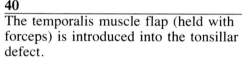

The temporalis muscle flap (held with forceps) is introduced into the tonsillar defect.

41

Flap inset. Skin grafting was not required. The flap was well healed three weeks following surgery when the patient died suddenly from a stroke.

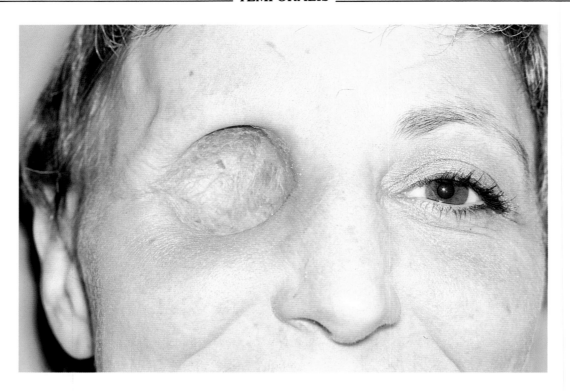

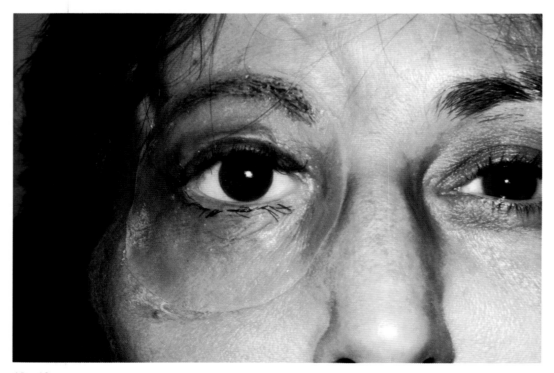

42, 43

Forty-year-old female two years following a temporalis flap to an orbital exenteration wound. The technique used in this case was identical to the cadaver dissection (fig 1-3). The wound has remained healed for five years. (Case of P.G. Arnold)

STERNOCLEIDOMASTOID

ANATOMICAL CONSIDERATIONS

Surface Markings

The surface markings are demonstrated by the course of the contracted sternocleidomastoid muscle, which can easily be palpated in the neck.

Origin and Insertion

The sternocleidomastoid muscle arises from two tendinous bands which straddle the head of the clavicle and the upper sternum. The muscle inserts over a broad area of the anterior and inferior surfaces of the mastoid process. The function of the sternocleidomastoid muscle is to tilt the head into the "his master's voice" (RCA® Radio) position.

Adjacent Muscles

Only the platysma muscle is superficial to the sternocleidomastoid muscle. The omohyoid and the other deep muscles of the neck lie subjacent to the sternocleidomastoid muscle. At its mastoid insertion the sternocleidomastoid muscle is appreciably fused with the trapezius muscle. No muscle runs parallel to the sternocleidomastoid muscle; hence, it splits the neck into anterior and posterior "halves."

Vascular Pattern

The sternocleidomastoid is a typical long thin muscle with a tripartite, segmental blood supply. The sternocleidomastoid muscle can be raised on either a superior or inferior vascular base, and it can carry a "paddle" of skin in either direction at the distal end of the muscle. The upper two-thirds of the muscle is independently supplied by the occipital artery. The lower two-thirds of the muscle is similarly supplied by the thyrocervical trunk. The superior thyroid vessels must be divided in the middle portion of the muscle whether the muscle is rotated superiorly or inferiorly.

Motor Nerve

Accessory nerve.

Sensory Nerve

Cervical plexus.

USES

Since the sternocleidomastoid flap can be raised on distinct inferior and superior pedicles, the muscle has different applications in its two separate arcs of rotation.

The inferiorly based flap, which is supplied by the thyrocervical trunk, provides a "paddle" of skin attached to the upper portion of the sternocleidomastoid muscle that will reach the larynx, the trachea, and the jugular notch. The superiorly based flap is generally used for intraoral problems which include small defects (i.e. five by five cm) in the anterior floor of the mouth, the sulcus, and the tonsillar fossa. It is almost never used for cheek skin replacement because of the associated donor site deformity.

REGIONAL FLAP COMPARISONS

The sternocleidomastoid flap is a reasonably reliable and readily accessible flap. It has generally fallen into disfavor because of the usefulness of the other local flaps. For instance, the galeal fascia flap and the temporalis muscle flap both offer much less donor deformity. Unlike the sternocleidomastoid flap, each of these flaps will reach the forehead and the orbit. The temporalis muscle flap provides more than comparable intraoral coverage. Further, small intraoral and cheek defects can be repaired just as effectively with the platysma myocutaneous flap but at a much smaller price. The pectoralis "paddle" is the most common distant flap chosen for major intraoral defects because it is larger and more reliable than the sternocleidomastoid flap. When a sternocleidomastoid flap is seriously considered for an intraoral defect, it is also logical to consider a "free" jejunal flap. In this special instance a radical departure from the "reconstructive ladder" method of thinking is reasonable.

DISADVANTAGES

The use of the sternocleidomastoid flap is virtually never recommended in the irradiated neck. It is discouraged not because it won't survive but rather because the vertical closure of the irradiated neck skin may place the carotid vessels in jeopardy. Should one have to use a secondary flap to resurface the neck, the sternocleidomastoid flap becomes superfluous because the other major flaps, e.g. the latissimus and the pectoralis musculocutaneous flaps, can simultaneously resurface the neck and repair an intraoral defect.

The reliability of the sternocleidomastoid flap is very good unless the skin "paddle" is extended past the point where there are good sternomastoid muscular connections to the skin. This specifically applies to the skin "paddle" distal to the clavicle, which preferably should be delayed. Occasionally, the vascular pedicle is not well visualized in its superior location because of the surrounding perivascular fatty tissue.

The functional loss with the use of this muscle is only noticed with forcible activities. It does leave a major contour deformity which is comparable to the defect of a standard radical neck dissection. Elevation of the sternocleidomastoid muscle also disrupts the majority of the sensory nerves to the ear and to the ipsilateral neck skin.

Its use is contraindicated in the clinically "positive" neck. It also should not be used when the palpable lymph nodes impinge upon any surface of the sternocleidomastoid muscle. This is particularly true in the upper neck where adequate excision of the lymphatic tissue necessitates the resection of a portion of the upper sternocleidomastoid muscle or its supplying vessels. In the "conservative" neck dissection, which spares the jugular vein, theoretically the use of this flap should not hamper the lymphatic dissection in the lower two-thirds of the neck.

ADVANTAGES

The sternocleidomastoid myocutaneous flap is easily elevated and readily accessible for small intraoral or upper pharyngeal defects. The inferiorly based flap can offer straightforward solutions to some difficult postirradiation healing problems in the laryngeal and upper tracheal areas. Although the sternocleidomastoid flap has several commendable features, the disadvantages related to the donor site often outweigh its recognized advantages.

COMPLICATIONS, PITFALLS, AND DONOR SITE

When the sternocleidomastoid myocutaneous flap is used for intraoral coverage, there is always concern about a watertight closure. This encourages the operator to constrict the muscle as it enters the oral cavity. Any muscular compression should be avoided because the ensuing muscular swelling can compromise the vascularity of the muscle and lead to flap necrosis.

The primary pitfalls are related to identification and protection of the dominant vasculature during flap elevation. This is particularly true of the upper vessels which are surrounded by fat and difficult to identify. One may be confused as to what is the highest "safe" point of dissection because the two superior vessels enter the muscle from the occipital artery without any singular dominance between them. One should always fluoresce this flap to assess its viability. This is especially important when it is used in the critical intraoral and pharyngeal areas. Although total flap loss has not occurred, minimal losses have been sustained in the distal cutaneous "paddle" of the superiorly based flap.

This is not a particularly cold sensitive flap, nor is it one in which we have noted vascular "spasm." Both the donor site contour deformity and the potentially fragile skin closure over the carotid vessels offer quite major disadvantages.

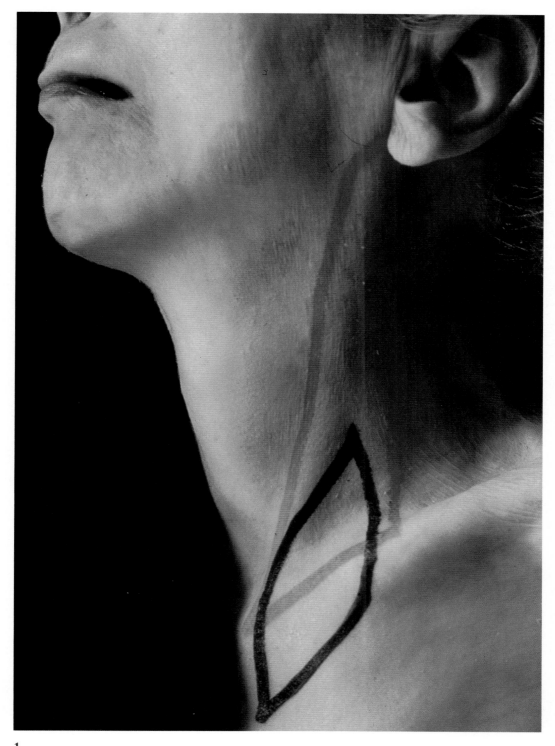

1

The red markings outline the sternoclei-domastoid muscle. All of the skin overlying the muscle can be included with the compound flap. The cutaneous segment distal to the clavicle (outlined in black) should be "delayed" to ensure its viability.

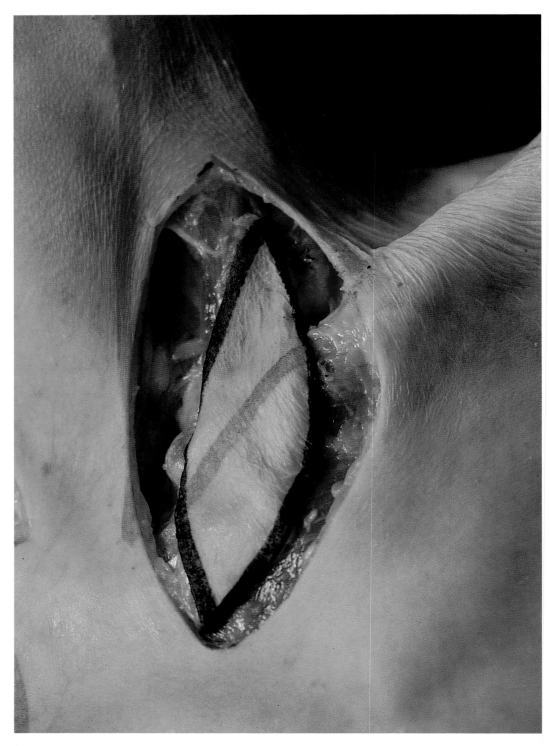

2

The distal skin "paddle" is outlined. The sternocleidomastoid muscle is exposed by first dividing the platysma muscle which is always carried with the compound flap.

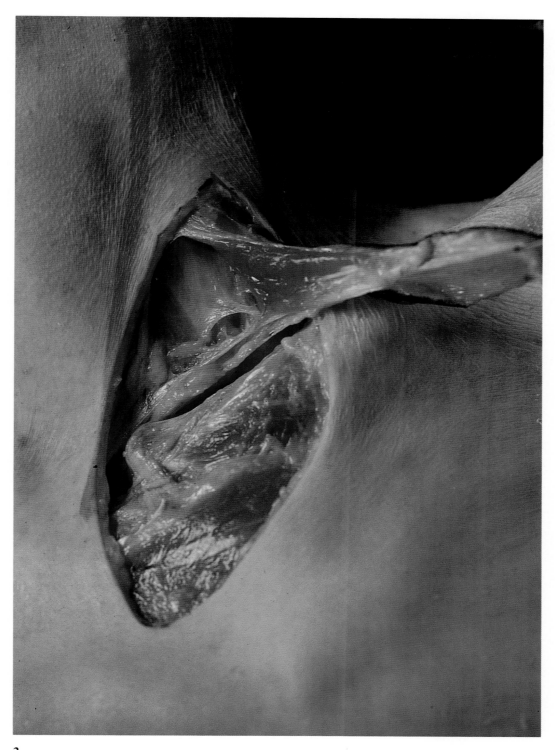

3

The inferior blood supply from the thyrocervical trunk is seen just above the clavicle in this fatty areolar layer.

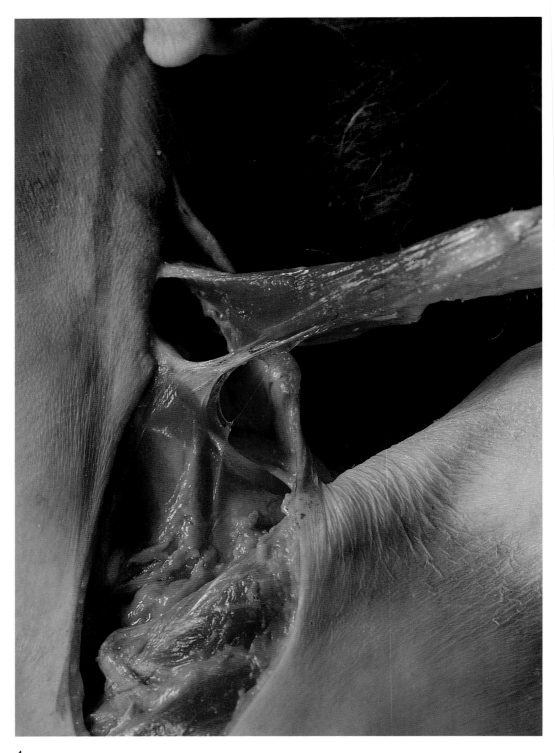

4

The middle blood supply from the superior thyroid vessel is seen entering the mid-portion of the sternomastoid muscle above the omohyoid muscle.

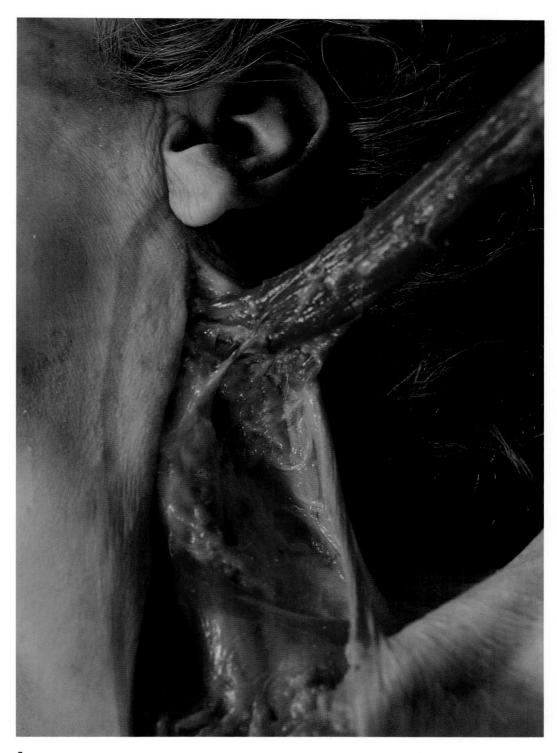

5

The superior blood supply from the occipital artery passes laterally from the external carotid artery. Isolation of these vessels can be difficult because of the surrounding perivascular fat.

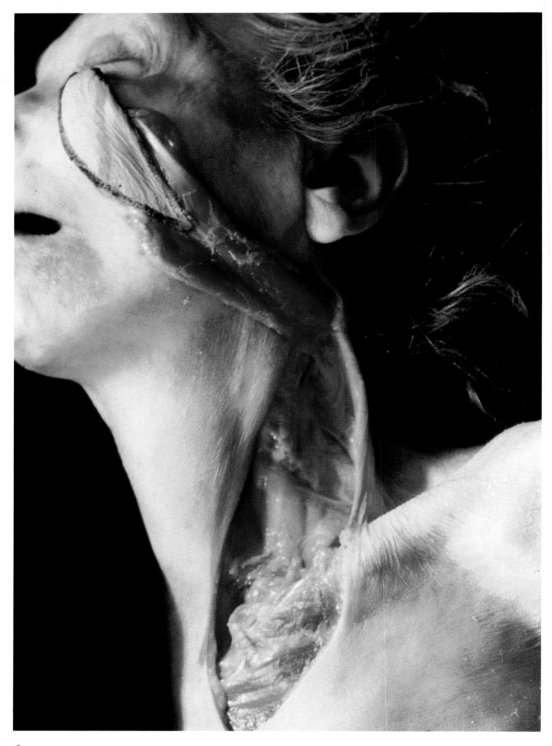

6
The arc of the superiorly based flap extends from the zygoma to the mastoid area.

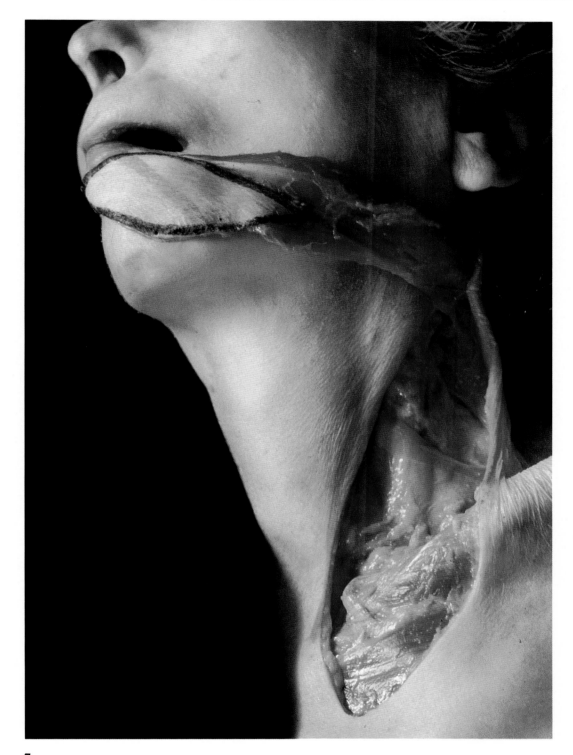

7

The distal skin "paddle" reaches the chin
and the floor of the mouth. Only the neck
skin which is directly attached to the sternocleidomastoid muscle can be expected
to survive without a "delay."

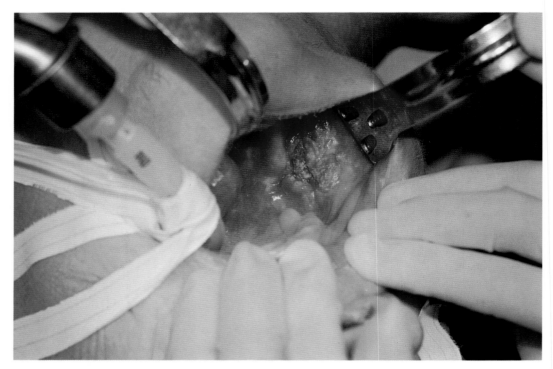

8

Fifty-six-year-old female with a well differentiated squamous cell carcinoma of the buccal mucosa in the area of Stensen's duct. The tumor involved both the mandible and the hard palate. (Case of J.B. McCraw)

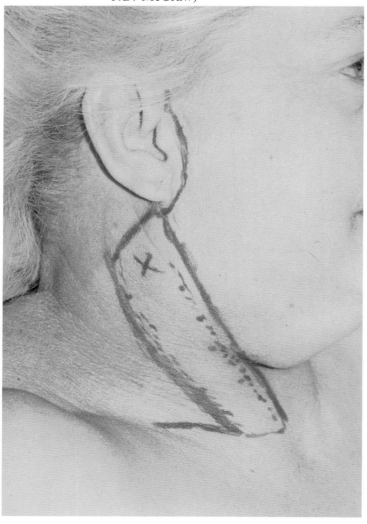

9

Outlined sternocleidomastoid flap. The tumor and the clinically "negative" neck were treated with preoperative irradiation.

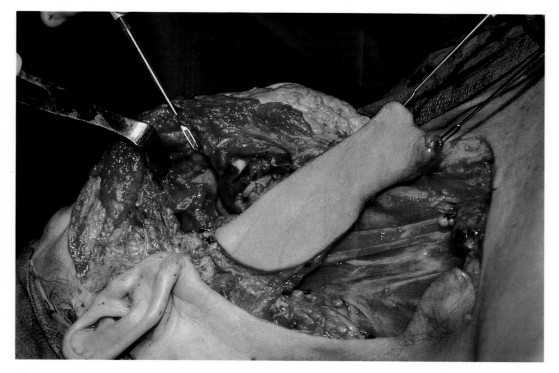

10

Elevated sternocleidomastoid flap adjacent to the resected body of the mandible. The margin of the hard palate resection is retracted. A total parotidectomy was also done to protect the facial nerve in the deep dissection of the tumor.

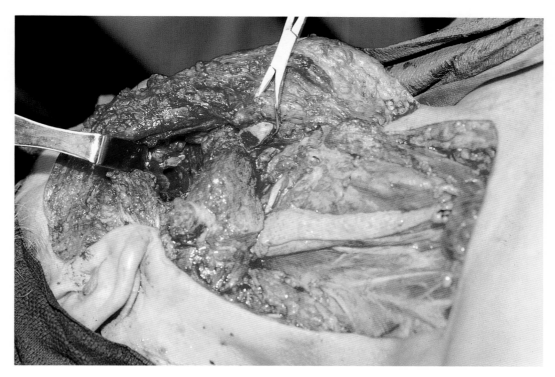

11

Flap inset beneath the resected body of the mandible which is retracted. A dermis graft was used to cover the carotid artery.

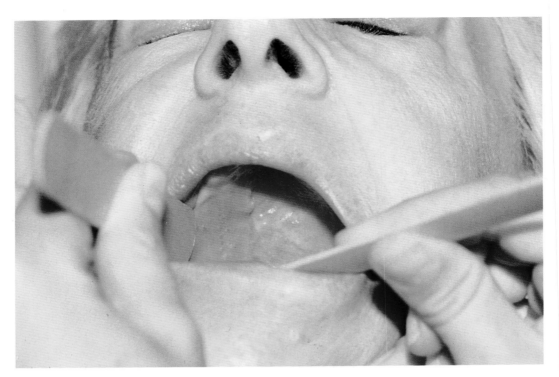

12

The sternocleidomastoid flap resurfaced half of the hard palate and the buccal mucosa.

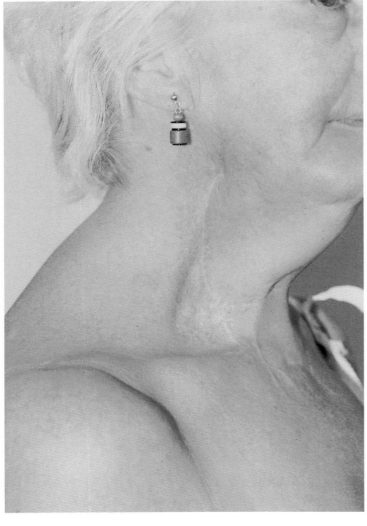

13

Appearance at two years. The donor site deformity is significant.

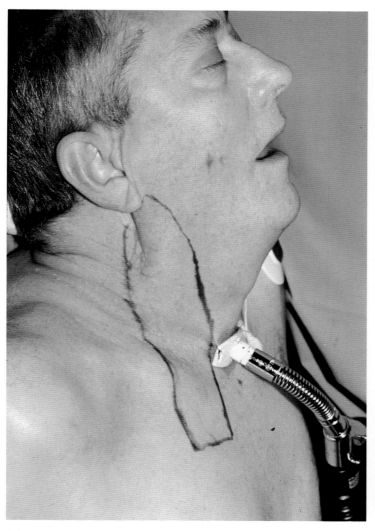

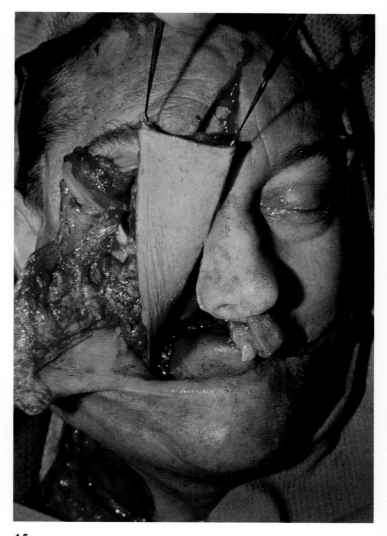

14

Outline of an "extended" sternocleido-mastoid flap in a patient with an invasive adenocarcinoma of the maxillary antrum. (Case of J.B. McCraw and W.P. Magee)

15

Upward excursion of the sternocleidomas-toid flap. The resection included the max-illa, the orbit, the sphenoid sinus, and half of the septum and hard palate.

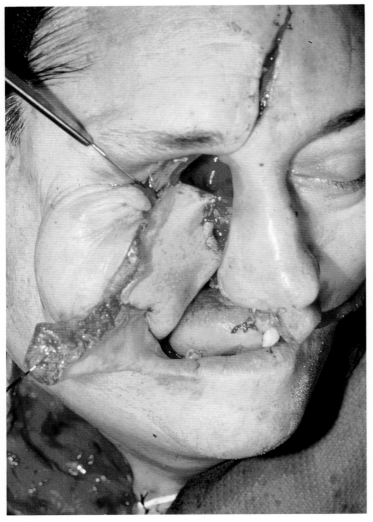

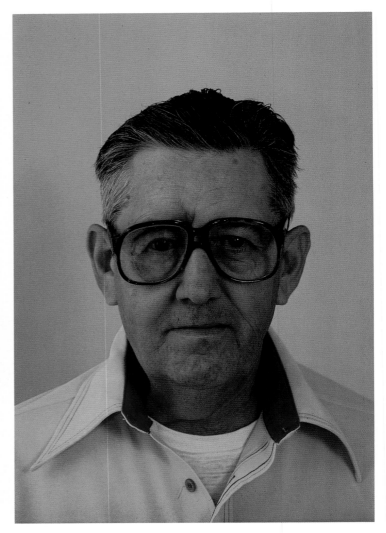

16

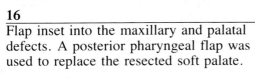

Flap inset into the maxillary and palatal defects. A posterior pharyngeal flap was used to replace the resected soft palate.

17

Seven years following the procedure. The orbital exenteration deformity is camouflaged with a prosthesis.

PLATYSMA

ANATOMICAL CONSIDERATIONS

Surface Markings

The platysma muscle extends from a point near the anterior midline of the neck to the border of the trapezius muscle posteriorly. This very wide and thin muscle overlaps both the clavicle and the mandible. The muscular expanse is best demonstrated by an exaggerated "grizzly bear" grimace.

Origin and Insertion

The muscular origin extends in a broad front from the manubrium to the acromion. The insertion covers the lower margin of the mandible and is connected to the risorius and angular depressor muscles of the lower lip. Through these connections the platysma muscle contributes to lower lip depression in the process of its surface contraction of the neck skin. Its functional loss in the neck is not replaced by other muscles, but this loss is seldom noticed.

Adjacent Muscles

The platysma muscle is densely adherent to the anterior neck skin and overlies all of the deep structures of the neck. Above the mandible it coalesces with the superficial muscular aponeurotic system (S.M.A.S.) of the cheek.

Vascular Pattern

The vascular pattern is variable and diffuse, but the predominant vessels supplying the muscle enter its undersurface at the lower mandibular border in the area of the facial artery. The secondary blood supply enters the muscle from the superior thyroid vessels. Both sets of vessels contribute numerous small, deep perforating vessels to the muscle. The vascular connections between the platysma muscle and the overlying neck skin are best described as "delicate."

Motor Nerve

Facial nerve.

Sensory Nerve

Cervical plexus.

USES

The platysma myocutaneous flap is one which is commonly overlooked. Nonetheless, it is very useful for limited intraoral or surface coverage problems in an arc extending eight to ten centimeters from the level of the facial artery at the mandible. This arc includes the lower cheek, the lower lip, the floor of the mouth, and the mastoid area.

REGIONAL FLAP COMPARISONS

The platysma myocutaneous flap is best compared to the temporalis muscle flap because of the similar ease of elevation and the lack of functional loss. This should make it a reasonable consideration for limited coverage problems in the general area around the facial artery. The donor site is much less deforming than that of the sternocleidomastoid myocutaneous flap, and it is obviously less complicated to elevate than the other major chest, back, or neck flaps. Its thinness is unmatched by any other myocutaneous flap.

DISADVANTAGES

The primary disadvantage of this interesting flap is that the dominant vasculature is seldom visualized; therefore, any unusual vascular location could compromise the viability of the most distal portion of the flap. Unless one carefully unfolds the flap as it passes over the mandible, a bulge will be evident. After the flap is in place for several weeks, this bulge can be resected without harming the viability of the flap. Like any muscle flap, constriction of the muscle beneath a tight subcutaneous tunnel is verboten. It does not have the disadvantage of the temporalis muscle in twitching since it is denervated by its elevation. This flap should not be used at the time of a neck dissection since the removal of the platysma muscle will harm the blood supply to the remaining neck flaps.

ADVANTAGES

The platysma myocutaneous flap is simple to use and causes very little harm to the neck contour. The color match of the skin is relatively favorable for lower cheek and lateral chin coverage, and its appearance is vastly superior to a full-thickness skin graft in these areas. In men the cutaneous segment can be designed to carry either hair-bearing or non-hair-bearing skin, depending on the elected location of the skin "island" in the neck. The skin "island" can be made quite small because the flap skin receives its blood supply directly from multiple, minute muscular perforating vessels. This also allows one to close the donor defect primarily.

COMPLICATIONS, PITFALLS, AND DONOR SITE

The number of platysma cases done to date is so small that the full spectrum of complications is indeterminate. We have not experienced a flap failure, but the flap has not been used in an irradiated field. To this point all dissections have been stopped below the level of the facial artery. The flap has not been used as a pure "island" flap on skeletonized facial vessels; rather it has only been used as a cutaneous "paddle" on a broad surface of platysma muscle. The primary pitfall is to rotate the muscle timidly, thereby leaving a muscular bulge at the point where the muscle crosses the mandible. It is possible to injure the marginal mandibular nerve if the dissection is carried above the facial vessels, but this is easily avoided.

The primarily closed donor site leaves little deformity even when a vertical closure is required. A skin graft may be needed for a large platysma myocutaneous flap because extreme neck movements require considerable elasticity in the remaining neck skin. Every attempt should be made to keep the donor site within the "neck collar" area since this acts as a "camouflage" and also increases the arc of flap rotation.

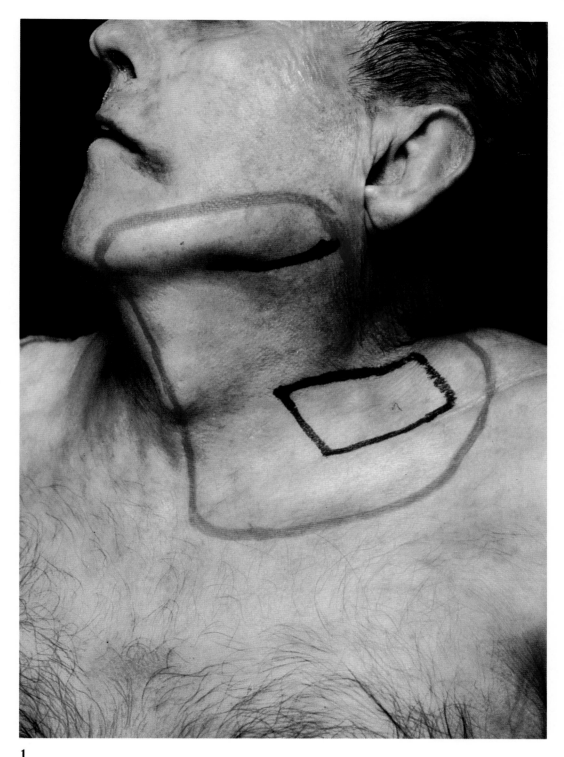

1

The platysma muscle is outlined in red with its extensions onto the cheek and the area below the clavicle. The location of the skin island (outlined in black) is chosen because it overlies the most prominent platysmal ''band.'' This lateral location also improves the arc of rotation of the flap. The upper black line, adjacent to the mandible, is a proposed counterincision which can be used to facilitate the dissection of the facial vessels.

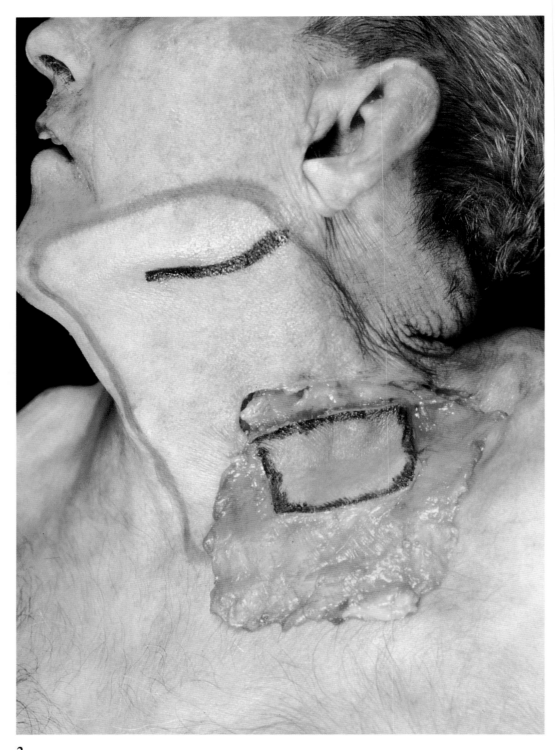

2

The infraclavicular portion of the muscle is elevated to demonstrate its extensive origin. The skin ''island'' is placed just lateral to the sternocleidomastoid muscle in a hairless area.

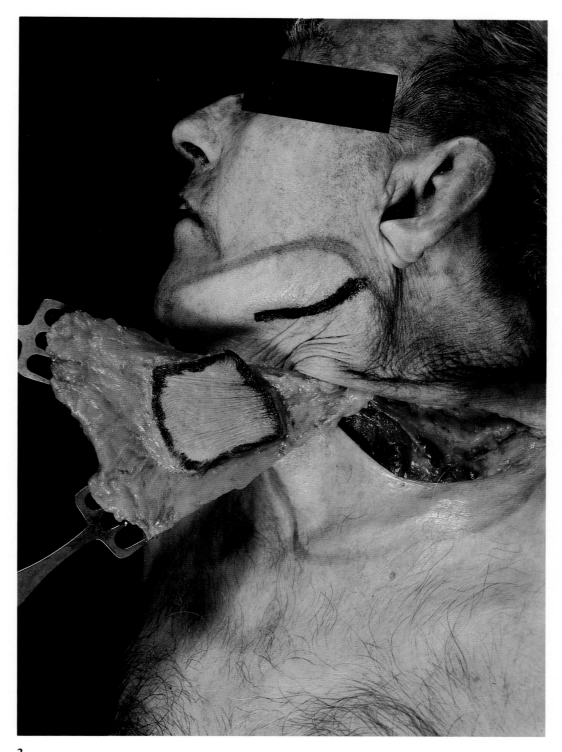

3

If the muscle is elevated only to the level of the facial artery the primary blood supply from the facial artery should not be harmed. This will provide a muscle flap which will cover the larynx, the lower cheek, and the mastoid process.

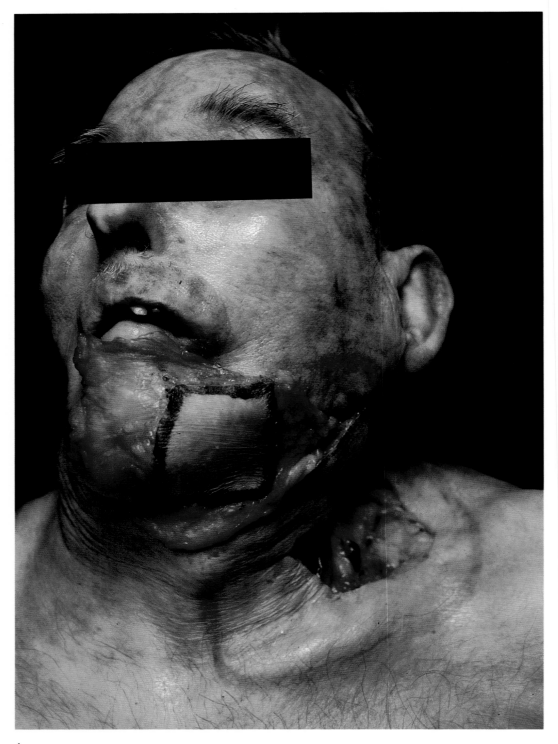

4

Anteriorly, the skin "paddle" reaches the
chin as well as the floor of the mouth.
The portion of the muscle seen covering
the chin is not always viable because the
blood supply to the distal muscle from
the facial artery is variable.

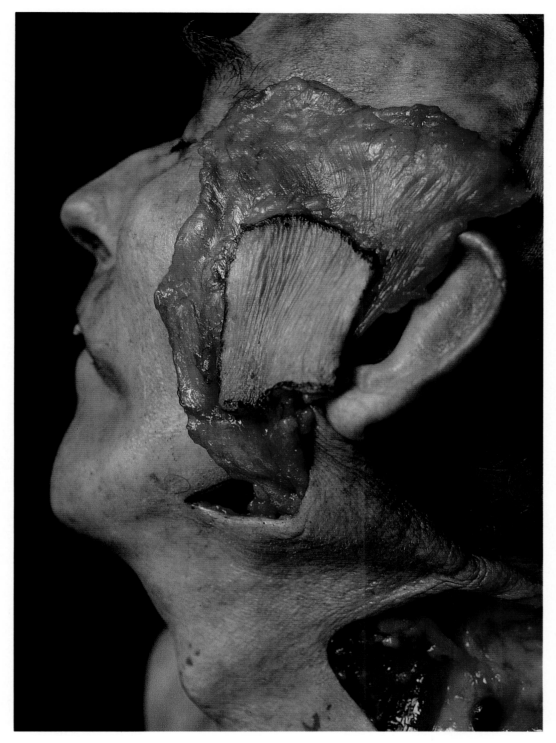

5

Upward extension of the flap onto the
cheek. The platysma flap will also reach
the posterior sulcus and the tonsillar area.

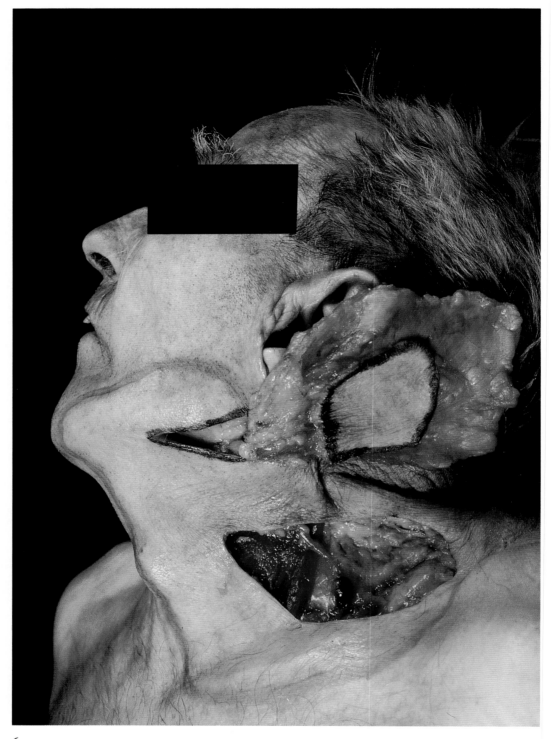

6

Posterior flap rotation into the mastoid area.

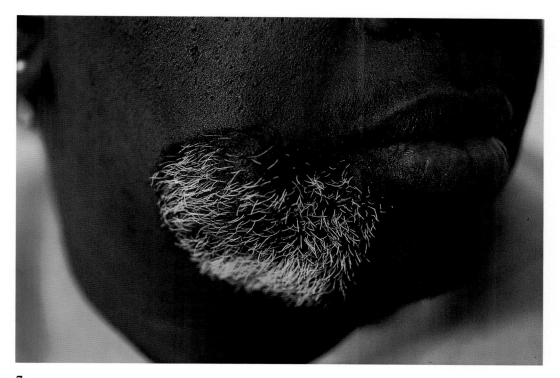

7

Thirty-five-year-old female with a benign congenital hairy nevus of the cheek.
(Case of J.B. McCraw)

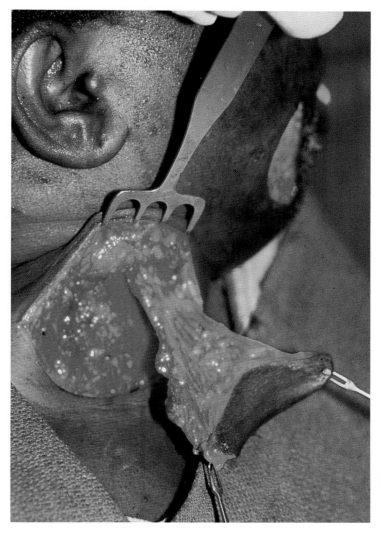

8

The platysma muscle is elevated to the level of the facial vessels. A skin "island" is carried from the lower neck.

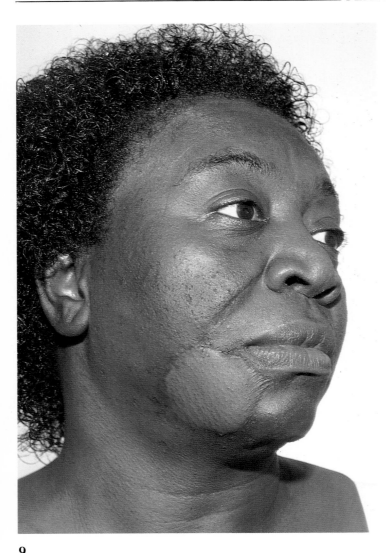

9

Appearance at six years. The platysma myocutaneous flap provides an acceptable contour restoration and a fair color match.

TRAPEZIUS

ANATOMICAL CONSIDERATIONS

Surface Markings

The trapezius is a sail-shaped muscle which originates from the midline of the back and the base of the skull and then sweeps in a lateral fashion toward the spine of the scapula and the tip of the clavicle. It is palpable throughout its course in the muscular person.

Origin and Insertion

The muscle originates from a broad aponeurosis, which extends from the twelfth thoracic spine to the cervical vertebrae and to the occiput of the cranium. The muscle has a broad insertion extending from the spine of the scapula to the tip of the clavicle. This important muscle offers multiple functions which elevate and retract the scapula and shoulder, tilt the head laterally and posteriorly, and assist in abduction of the arm.

Adjacent Muscles

Along its cervical origin the trapezius muscle overlies the deep muscles of the neck, including the semispinalis and the splenius capitis muscles. Inferiorly, both rhomboid muscles are deep to the trapezius muscle. Laterally, it covers a small portion of the latissimus dorsi muscle. As it sweeps to its insertion into the spine of the scapula and the acromion, the trapezius muscle covers both the supraspinatus and infraspinatus muscles.

Vascular Pattern

The dominant blood supply to the trapezius muscle is from the transverse cervical artery. This branch of the thyrocervical trunk passes from the anterior neck to the posterior neck and divides into an ascending and a descending branch at the border of the trapezius muscle. The ascending branch parallels the anterior border of the trapezius muscle in the shoulder and supplies the portion of the muscle which overlies the spine of the scapula. The descending branch passes beneath the trapezius muscle at the base of the neck and runs parallel to the vertebral column. In its longitudinal course the descending branch supplies the entire thoracic portion of the trapezius muscle. This distinct division of the transverse cervical artery supports separate and independent vascular territories of the lateral (shoulder) portion and the vertical (thoracic) portion of the trapezius muscle. This is the reason that both territories can also be raised as "island" myocutaneous flaps. In addition to the dominant longitudinal blood supply, there are numerous deep perforating vessels from the intercostal system which penetrate the paraspinous portion of the trapezius muscle. Because of the diffuse vascular connections within the trapezius muscle, the majority of the thoracic portion of the muscle can be raised on the deep perforating system to supply a "turnover" muscle flap. This vascular system is similar to the situations of the pectoralis major and latissimus dorsi muscles.

The upper trapezius muscle in the neck is supplied by branches of the occipital artery. This independent vascular arrangement allows the cervical portion of the trapezius muscle to form a separate myocutaneous flap, which can be extended onto the lateral shoulder as a fasciocutaneous flap. This horizontal trapezius myocutaneous flap is similar in outline to the Mütter flap (1842) except that it includes the cervical portion of the trapezius muscle to enhance the mobility and viability of the attached fasciocutaneous flap.

Motor Nerve

Spinal accessory nerve.

Sensory Nerve

Cervical and intercostal nerves.

USES

The trapezius muscle is seldom transposed as a pure muscle flap except for applications in the mid-thoracic spine. Even in this situation, a V to Y myocutaneous flap has the advantages of primary closure of the donor site and a more durable surface cover.

The trapezius unit is usually employed either as a horizontal shoulder fasciocutaneous flap or as a vertical "island" myocutaneous flap. The horizontal trapezius myocutaneous flap is used primarily for surface coverage problems of the ipsilateral neck, but it will easily reach the posterior occiput and can be extended onto the opposite neck. The excellent color match and similar replacement of neck skin are the commending features of this simple transposition flap.

The vertical trapezius myocutaneous flap is generally employed as an "island" flap and is the most accessible chest wall flap to the occiput. Because of its lack of proximity, it is a secondary choice for intraoral problems. It does serve as a reliable "second" flap for complex facial reconstructions. When the supplying transverse cervical artery is elevated to the level of the subclavian artery, the anterior arc of rotation of the vertical "island" flap includes the temporal area, the opposite neck, the inframammary fold, and the axilla.

The ascending branch of the transverse cervical artery can be used to carry the spine of the scapula and its overlying trapezius muscle as an ''island'' flap. This composite flap is seldom used because of its unfavorable donor site, but it will introduce living bone into the areas of the zygoma and mandible. In the case of complex facial reconstructions, the transverse cervical artery branches (ascending and descending) can be used to simultaneously carry the osteomyocutaneous flap from the scapula and the ''island'' vertical myocutaneous flap from the back.

REGIONAL FLAP COMPARISONS

The thoracic portion of the trapezius muscle can be advanced directly over the thoracic spine in a fashion similar to the bilateral latissimus dorsi advancement closure of the meningomyelocele defect. A unilateral trapezius muscle can also be rotated over the thoracic spine without harming its function since this only redirects the muscular origin. Rotation of the trapezius muscle onto the neck requires complete detachment of the muscular insertion from the scapula. Although the severity of a neck or an occipital defect may justify this maneuver, detachment of the muscle from the scapula may result in shoulder pain and inability to stabilize the shoulder in an overhead position. Unfortunately, this function is irreplaceable. It is better to consider first an ''island'' latissimus dorsi muscle flap for these defects. The latissimus muscle flap will usually reach the posterior neck and lower occiput, but if it does not, no bridges are burned, and the vertical trapezius muscle rotation flap can still be used. The same criticism or worse can be leveled against the ''island'' trapezius osteomyocutaneous flap. The benefits of transposing living muscle and bone to the face must be carefully weighed against the disadvantages of a ghastly donor site and a certain shoulder disability. An extensive ''island'' dissection of this type does qualify for the ''gee whiz'' category, but one case is enough for almost anybody's collection.

The horizontal (shoulder) fasciocutaneous flap is unmatched in its ability to introduce skin of similar color and texture to the anterior and lateral neck. By comparison, transposed skin from the back (latissimus and trapezius myocutaneous flaps) is too dark for the neck, and transposed skin from the anterior chest (pectoralis ''paddle'' and medial deltopectoral flaps) is too pale for the neck. The location of this skin-grafted donor site is far superior to the location of the skin-grafted pectoralis ''paddle'' or deltopectoral donor sites.

It should be emphasized that the horizontal trapezius flap includes only the trapezius muscle in the neck, not the shoulder or the back. Inclusion of the cervical portion of the trapezius muscle in the shoulder fasciocutaneous flap enhances the flap mobility into the areas of the chin and the anterior neck. This was an important consideration at a time when the deltopectoral, total forehead, and sternomastoid flaps were the only other choices in the ''axial'' flap reconstruction of head and neck cancer defects. Once other reliable flaps were developed, the horizontal trapezius flap was seldom used for oral cancer defects, in part because of its donor site, but more specifically because of the obligatory orocutaneous fistula. The horizontal trapezius flap is more often rotated posteriorly to cover difficult defects of the occiput and temporal areas as well as to reconstruct certain cervical and thoracic spine defects. Like the vertical trapezius myocutaneous flap, it makes an excellent flap of second election and a serviceable ''duplicate'' flap in situations which necessitate two major flaps. It also has the advantage of a separate blood supply from the occipital artery.

The ''island'' vertical trapezius myocutaneous flap finds its greatest usefulness in the correction of high occipital and temporal scalp defects which are not accessible to the other major flaps. Only the latissimus flap warrants a comparison in this regard. Even though the latissimus muscle is much longer than the trapezius muscle, its lateral rotation point limits its coverage to the lower neck and occiput. Although the ''island'' vertical trapezius myocutaneous flap will reach the midface and the oropharyngeal area, its lack of proximity and its donor site considerations have inhibited its applications in many defects of the head and neck area. The proximity of the pectoralis ''paddle'' and the reliability of the latissimus myocutaneous flap continue to commend their utility in the head and neck area. The arc of the ''island'' vertical trapezius myocutaneous flap also includes the axilla, the inframammary fold, and the upper half of the sternum when its supplying vessels are dissected to the level of the thyrocervical trunk. Nevertheless, this flap is rarely considered for anterior chest defects unless the pectoralis, latissimus, and rectus abdominis muscles are all congenitally absent or have recently died.

DISADVANTAGES

The primary disadvantage of the horizontal trapezius myocutaneous flap is the donor defect if a skin graft is required. This is particularly objectionable when the flap is extended onto the area of the shoulder because the lateral shoulder has the same propensity for dense scarring as the deltoid area. The potential sacrifice of the spinal accessory nerve has been suggested as a disadvantage, but neither branch of the spinal accessory nerve is necessarily lost in the elevation of either the vertical or horizontal trapezius flaps.

The primary disadvantage of the vertical trapezius flap is that it is located on the back. This creates positioning problems when it is used for intraoral defects or surface problems of the neck. This criticism obviously does not apply when the flap is used for coverage problems of the occiput and of the upper spine. The donor site considerations are even more serious in nature. The donor site scar and closure are acceptable if the cutaneous segment is no more than five centimeters in width. When the donor site is wider than this, closure of the back wound can be difficult, and tightly closed donor sites can impair the normal "stretchability" of the back skin in forward movements of the shoulder. Even a five centimeter defect is hard to close and may result in a wide scar. It probably is not possible to close a defect greater than nine centimeters primarily. When a skin graft is required for the closure of the donor defect, the appearance is remarkably bad. It is also a difficult area to skin graft because of the obligatory back movements. Disruption of this back wound must be a recognized possibility. It is a disastrous complication when it occurs because one may be asked to skin graft three sides of a prolapsing scapula. Early secondary closure following multiple operative debridements is the only acceptable conclusion to such a dire saga.

ADVANTAGES

The horizontal trapezius fasciocutaneous flap is an excellent choice for major coverage problems of the neck because of its proximity and favorable color match. As a simple transposition flap, it is more easily manipulated than either the pectoralis "paddle" or the latissimus myocutaneous flap. A trapezius muscle or musculocutaneous flap provides unique coverage of the upper thoracic spine, and the donor site of the transposition of one or both muscles is inconsequential unless it is necessary to separate the trapezius muscle from the scapula.

The "island" vertical trapezius flap serves as a reliable alternative to the other major chest flaps for problems of the head and neck area. Were it not for the donor site and positioning problems, it would be routinely considered. It can be directly transposed to the upper posterior chest, and its arc of rotation onto the occiput is unmatched by even the latissimus myocutaneous flap.

PITFALLS, COMPLICATIONS, AND DONOR SITE

Although it is possible to injure the spinal accessory nerve, it is rarely necessary to sacrifice this nerve in the mobilization of any of the trapezius flaps. The cervical (neck) portion of the trapezius muscle, which is included with the horizontal flap, is divided medial to the spinal accessory nerve while the vertical flap dissection is carried only to the level of the branches of the spinal accessory nerve. However, if the nerve is injured, it will cause the same drooping, painful shoulder disability which is associated with the resection of this nerve in a radical neck dissection. The horizontal flap can readily be used at the time of a radical neck dissection since its blood supply is gained from the occipital artery, which is above the area of the dissection. It is possible to use the vertical flap at the time of a neck dissection, but this adds a significant amount of tedium to the extirpation through the process of protecting the transverse cervical vessels. If a radical neck dissection has been done at an earlier time, one should expect that the transverse cervical artery will have been sacrificed. In this case, one may presume that the vertical flap would be unusable.

The most significant problems with both the transverse and vertical flaps involve their donor site defects. Whether the donor site is skin-grafted or primarily closed, it is sometimes difficult to obtain early primary healing because of back motion. Hypertrophic scarring is common when either donor defect is closed under tension. Disruption of the vertical trapezius flap donor site is a dreaded complication which may result in significant shoulder disability. The "salvage" closure of this disruption defect may even require the use of a secondary latissimus flap because of the magnitude of the resulting cavity.

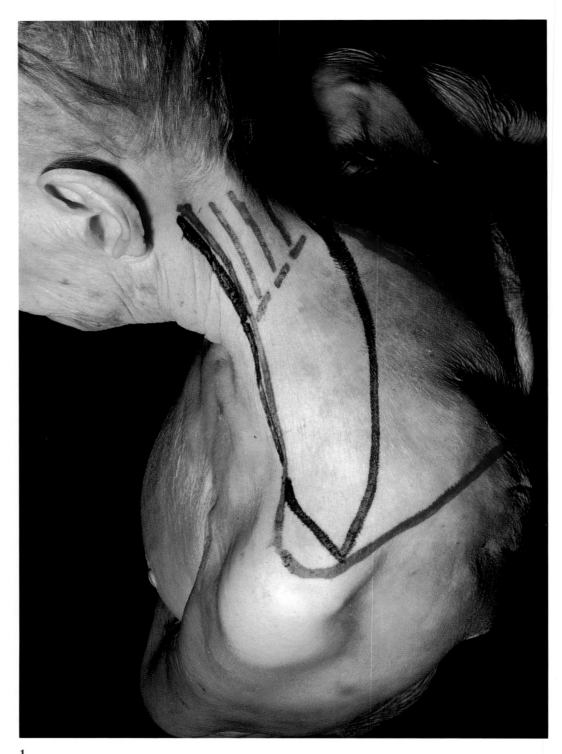

1

Outline of the extended horizontal trape-zius myocutaneous flap. The trapezius muscle is shown in red. Only the trape-zius muscle in the neck is carried with the flap.

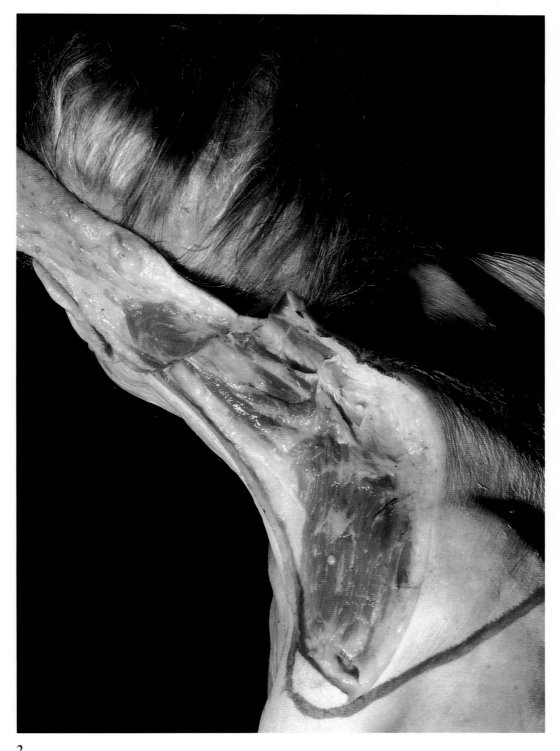

2

Elevated flap. The cervical portion of the trapezius muscle is included with the compound flap. The horizontal portion of the trapezius muscle is undisturbed. The distal skin of the flap is supplied by the perifascial perforators as a fasciocutaneous flap.

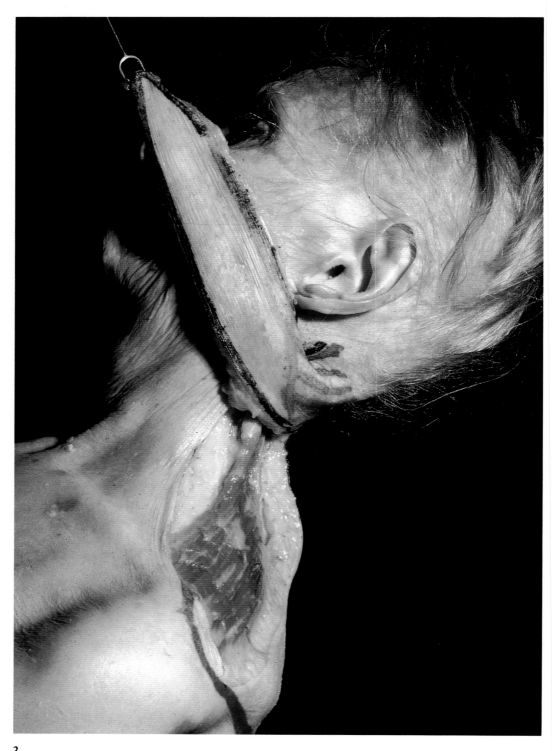

3

Upward excursion onto the cheek.

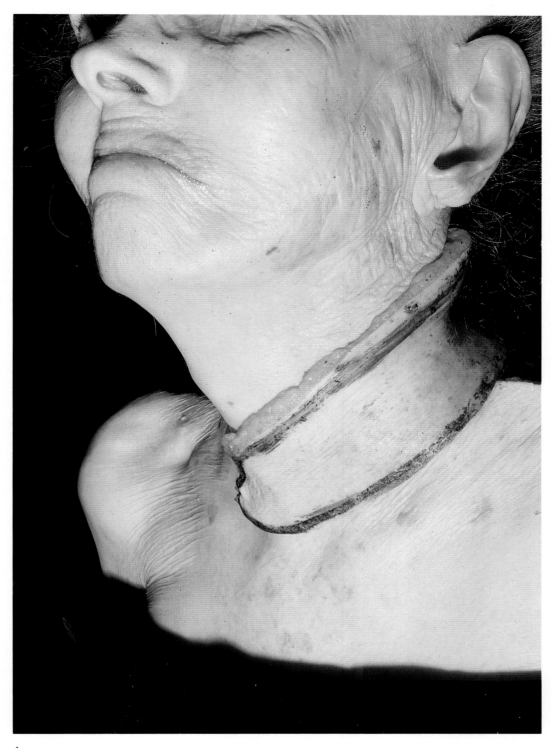

4

Anterior neck coverage.

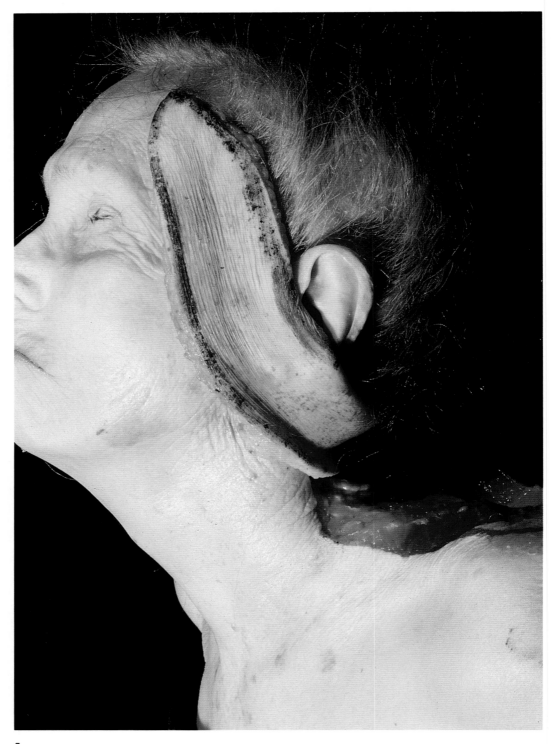

5

Temporal coverage.

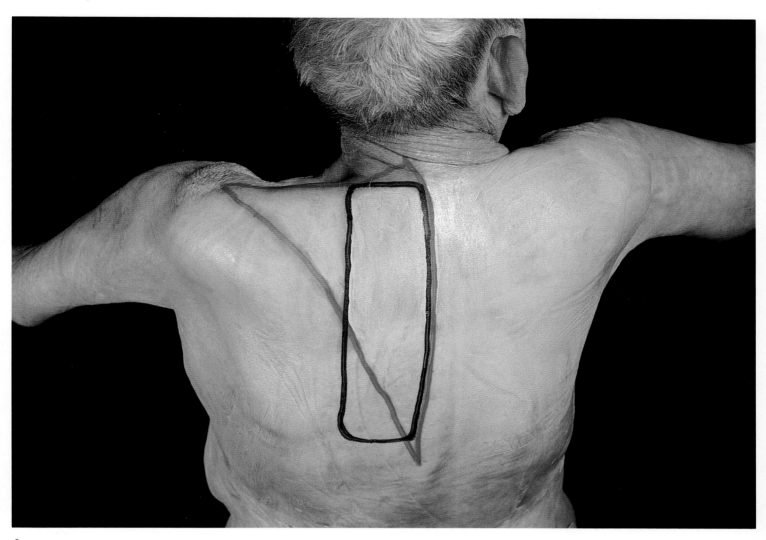

6

Outline of the ''island'' vertical trapezius myocutaneous flap. The trapezius muscle is outlined in red. A wider flap, i.e. more than nine centimeters, is difficult to close primarily.

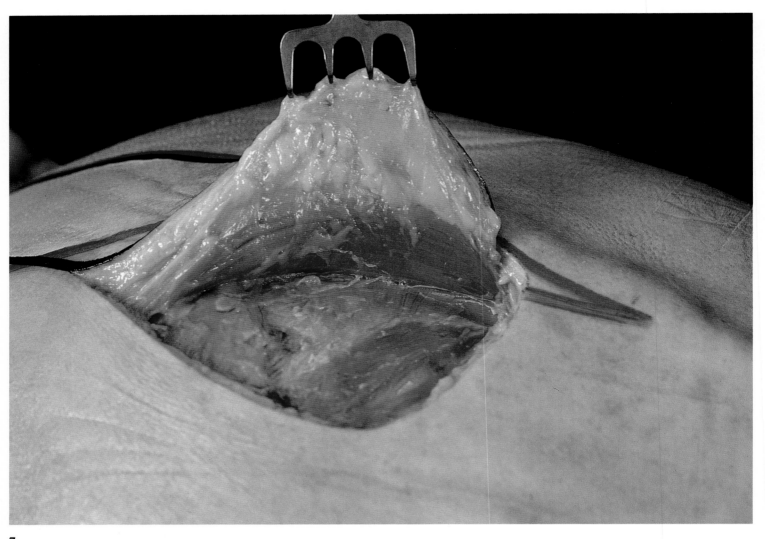

7

The trapezius muscle is first identified at its lower lateral margin. The medial margin of the trapezius muscle is then separated from the thoracolumbar fascia.

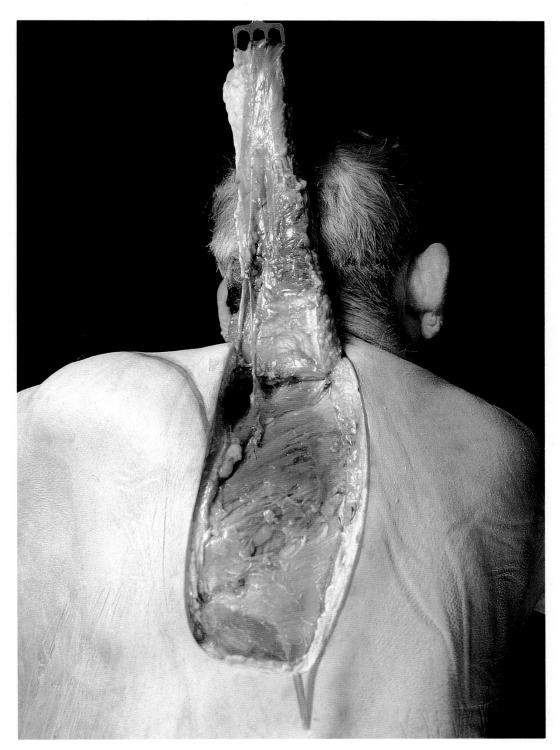

8

Only the vertical portion of the trapezius muscle is carried with the flap. The spinal accessory nerve must be protected as the cervical portion of the trapezius muscle is divided.

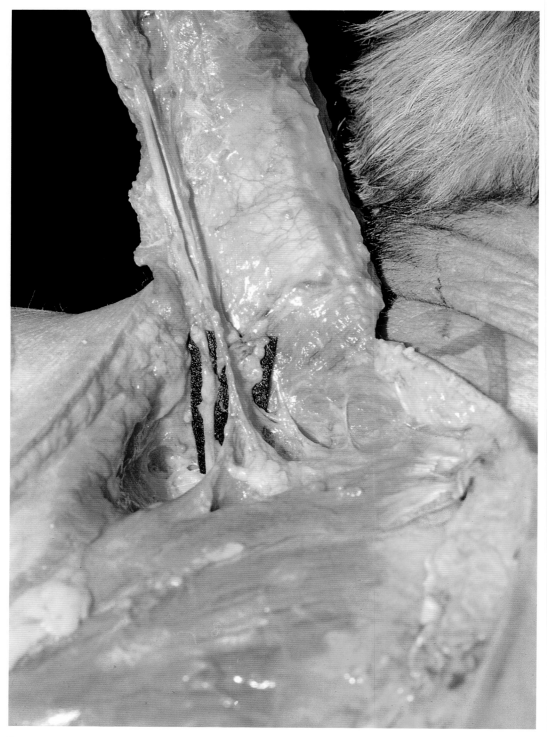

9

The transverse cervical vessels are seen on the undersurface of the flap (outlined with black felt). If these vessels are traced to the thyrocervical trunk, the flap will reach the inframmary fold, anteriorly. The creation of a pure (dangling vessel) "island" flap is not necessary for most applications.

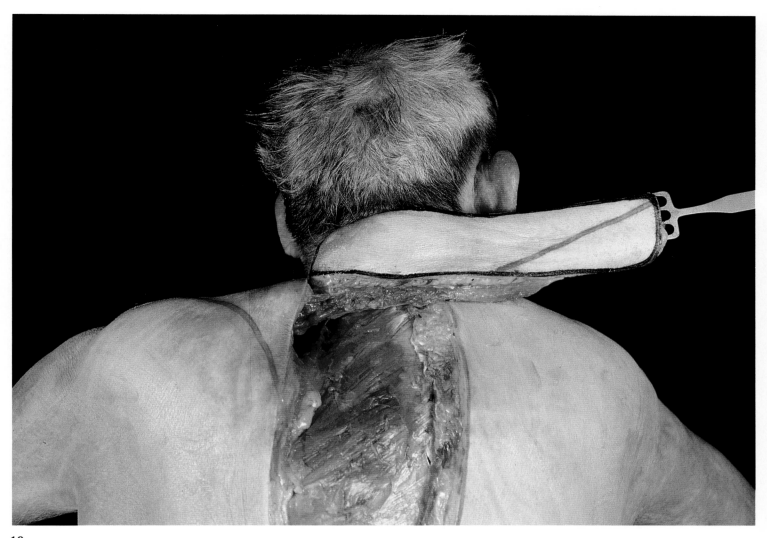

10

Flap excursion onto the opposite
shoulder.

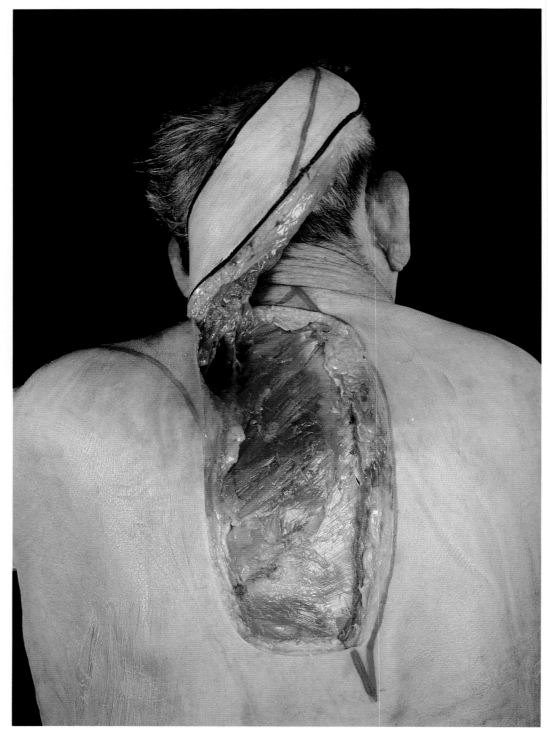

11

Unique occipital coverage provided by the
vertical trapezius flap.

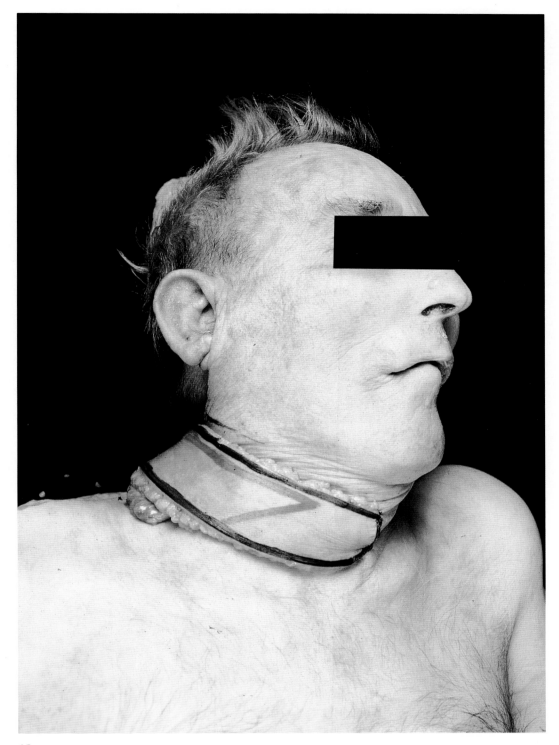

12

Anterior coverage of the opposite neck.

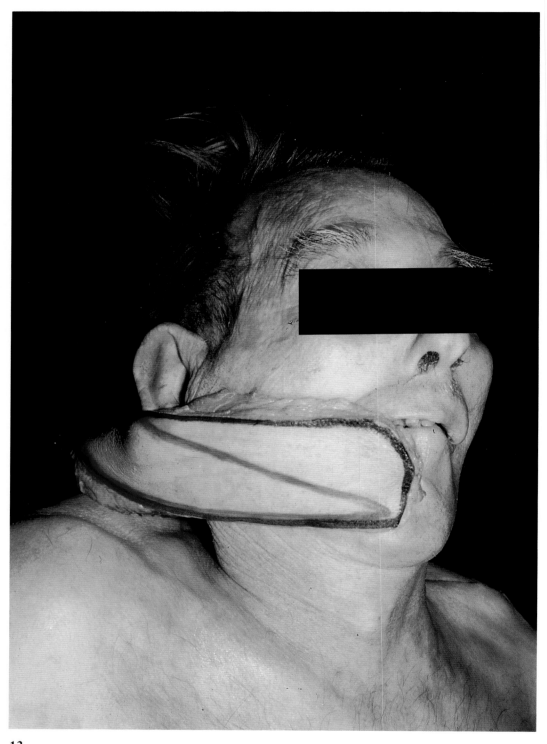

13

Coverage of the opposite cheek. The flap is seldom used for intraoral problems because of its lack of proximity and positioning considerations.

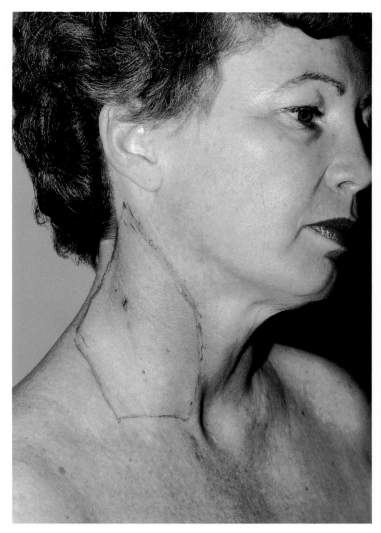

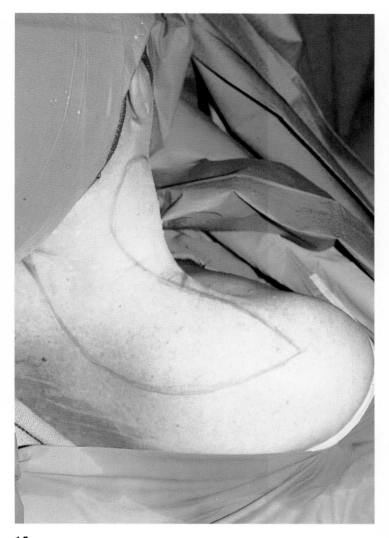

14

A young patient with a level III melanoma of the right neck. The area of skin excision is outlined. (Case of J.B. McCraw)

15

The standard transverse or horizontal trapezius flap can be transposed without a delay. The trapezius muscle is divided at the angle between the neck and shoulder. The flap distal to the neck is a fasciocutaneous flap. One cannot expect to primarily close a donor defect of this magnitude.

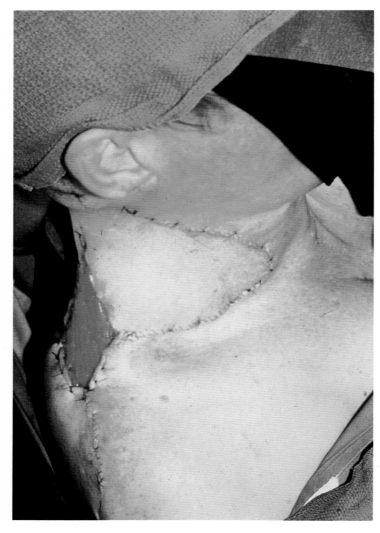

16

Following the neck dissection, the flap is immediately transposed to replace the resected neck skin. The donor defect is partially closed. The remaining trapezius muscle is visible on the donor site and will be skin grafted.

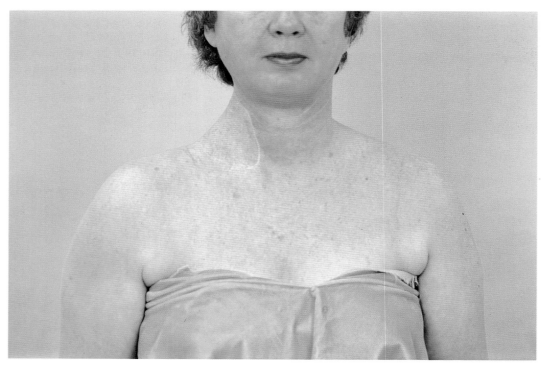

17

The lateral neck "bulk" is caused by levator hypertrophy. This "bulk" is never related to the trapezius muscle, since muscle is not transposed into the anterior neck.

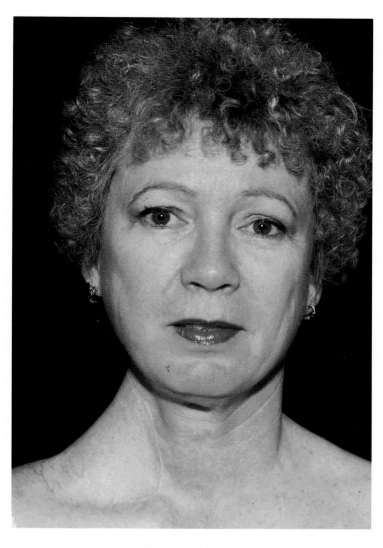

18

The patient is alive and well ten years following the surgery. Note the excellent flap color match with the neck skin.

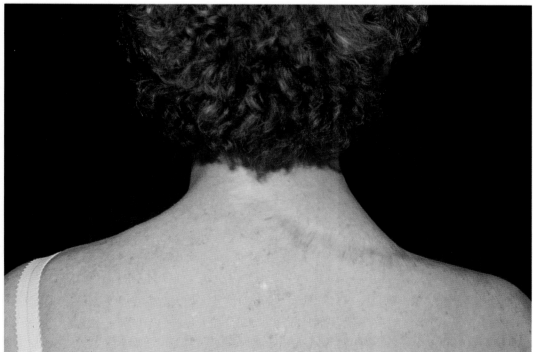

19

View of the donor site after secondary removal of the donor site skin graft.

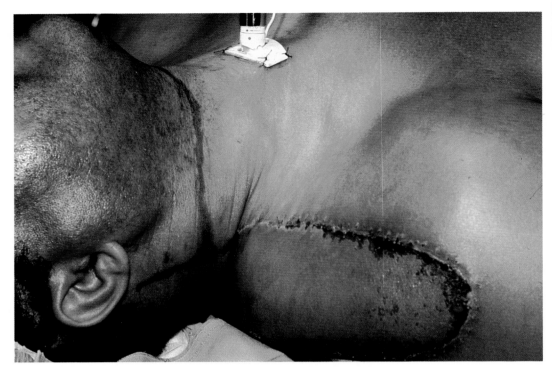

20

"Delayed" horizontal trapezius myocutaneous flap for an extensive intraoral reconstruction. The "delay" was effected by elevating the distal half of the flap and resulted in some superficial loss of the distal flap. (Case of J.B. McCraw)

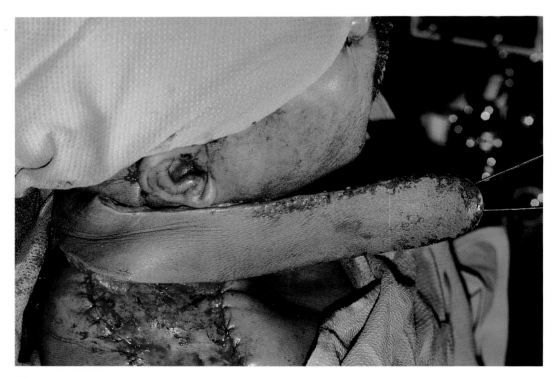

21

Anterior excursion of the "delayed" horizontal trapezius flap. The donor site had been grafted at the time of the flap "delay."

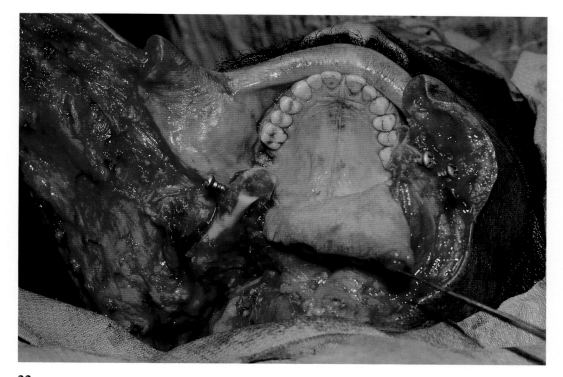

22

The tumor resection included the central mandible, the floor of the mouth, and one-half of the tongue.

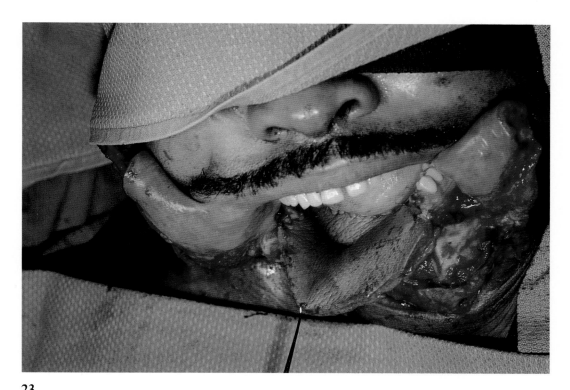

23

The trapezius flap was used to provide intraoral lining as well as coverage for a mandibular bone graft.

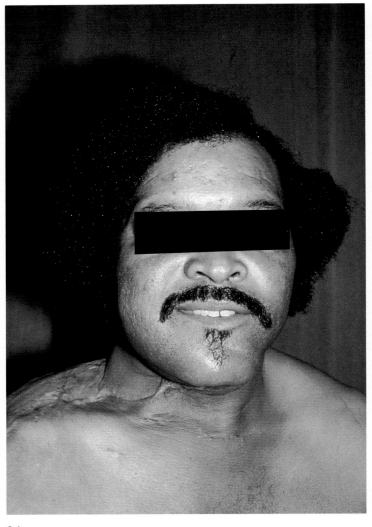

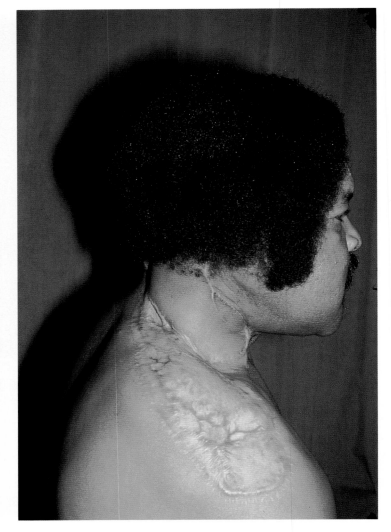

24

Anterior view of the mandibular contour.

25

The proximal portion of the trapezius flap was returned to the neck to cover an exposed carotid vessel. Note the unsatisfactory donor site appearance.

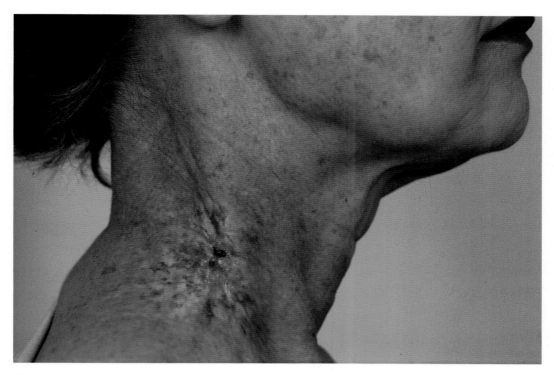

26

Malignant transformation of a long-standing irradiation ulcer of the neck. (Case of J.B. McCraw)

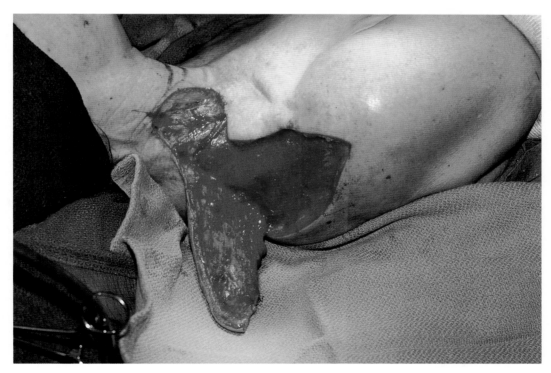

27

Deformity following tumor resection and elevated horizontal trapezius flap. Note that the distal flap is only a fasciocutaneous flap and does not include the underlying trapezius muscle of the shoulder.

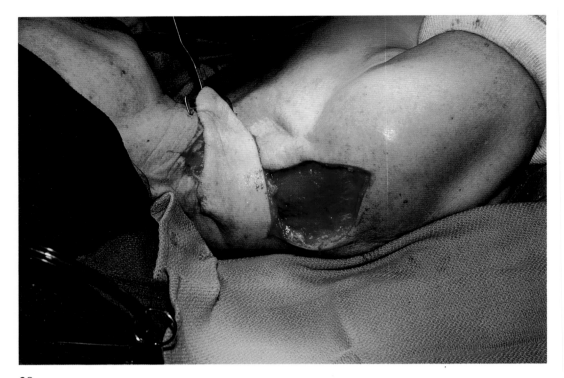

28

The fasciocutaneous portion of the flap is rotated into the neck defect. It was not necessary to either elevate or divide the trapezius muscle in the neck to obtain an adequate flap rotation.

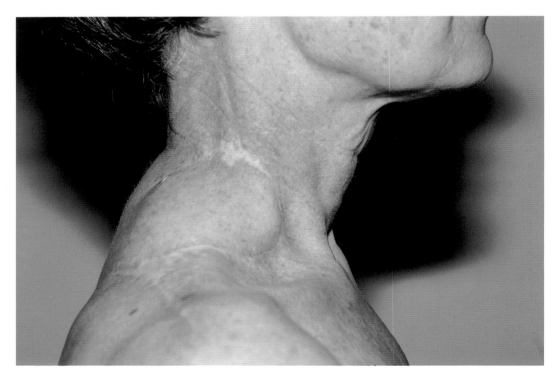

29

Healed flap at six years. The donor site was primarily closed.

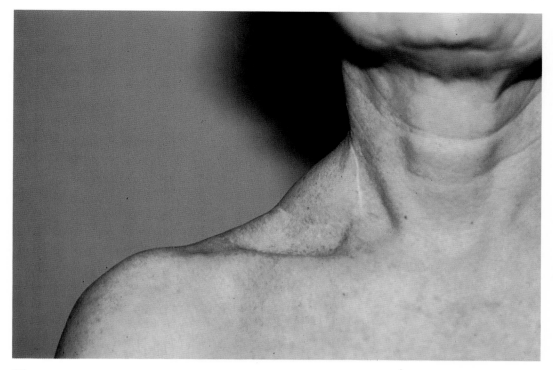

30

The color match of the flap skin and neck skin is excellent. Shoulder function is unaffected by the use of this fasciocutaneous flap.

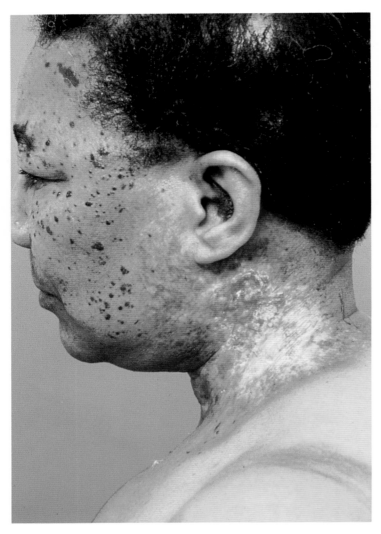

31

Invasive squamous cell carcinoma of the left neck arising in an irradiation ulcer. The patient was treated for Hodgkin's disease thirty years earlier. This 1975 case predated our present capabilities with the pectoralis and latissimus myocutaneous flaps. (Case of J.B. McCraw)

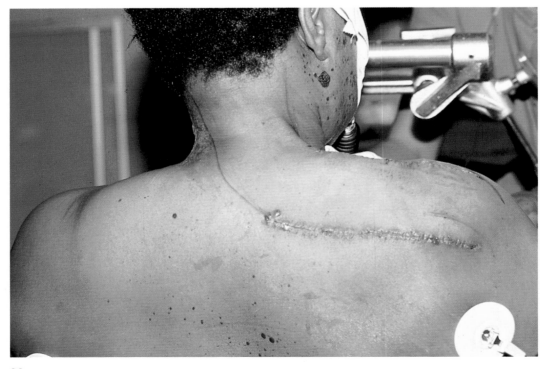

32

An extended "opposite" horizontal trapezius flap was "delayed" by making parallel incisions and undermining the mid-portion of the flap. A neurosurgical head-frame was used to simultaneously gain access to both the right neck and the left neck areas.

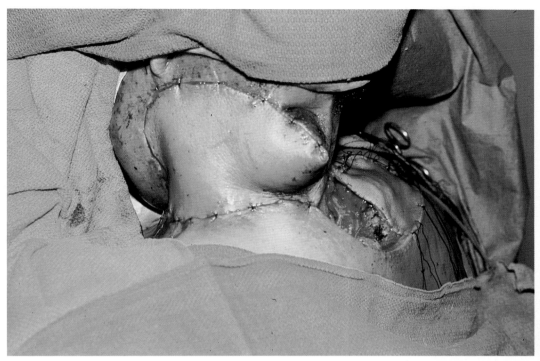

33

The flap was rotated from the right shoulder to the left neck to cover the area of the tumor excision and the radical neck dissection. It was not necessary to use the "random" portion of the flap. It can be seen on the donor defect as a full thickness graft.

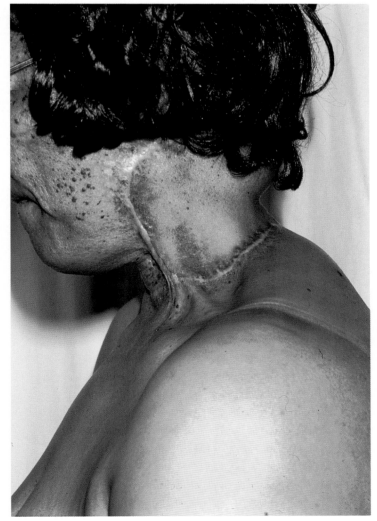

34

Seven years following the surgery. It was possible to resurface the majority of the neck with this "opposite" trapezius flap. The "dog ear" was never removed at the patient's request.

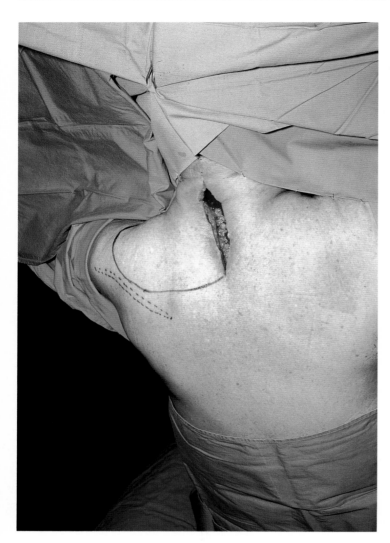

35

Seventy-six-year-old male with a chronically infected cervical laminectomy wound. Two previous attempts at direct closure had been unsuccessful. A combined horizontal and vertical trapezius myocutaneous flap is outlined on the left shoulder. (Case of P.G. Arnold)

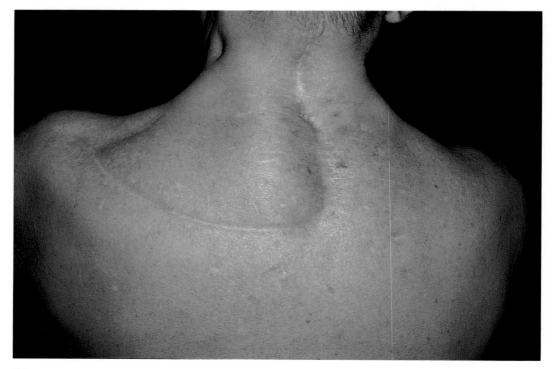

36

Two years following the V-Y closure which advanced the flap from the left shoulder to the upper back. The trapezius muscle provided good coverage of the thoracic spine.

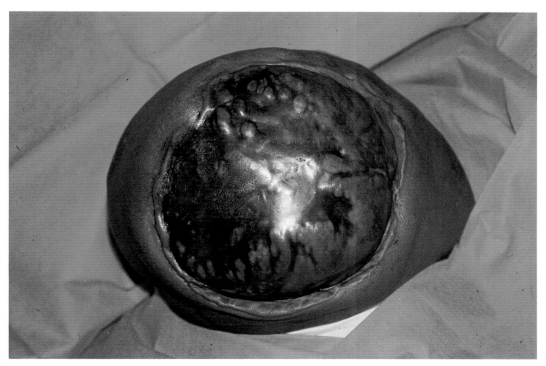

37

Sixteen-year-old female who presented with congenital absence of the skull that had been previously covered with split-thickness skin grafts. (Case of T. Arganese, R. Albin, and R. O'Donnell)

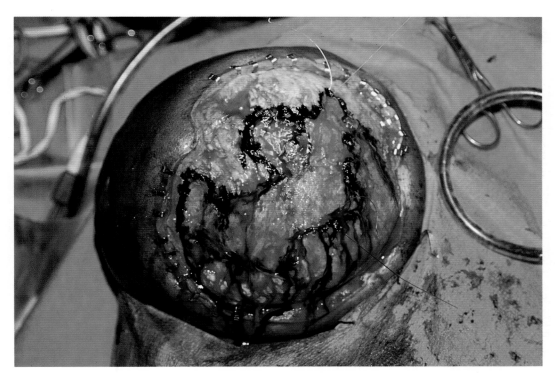

38

Appearance following removal of the skin grafts.

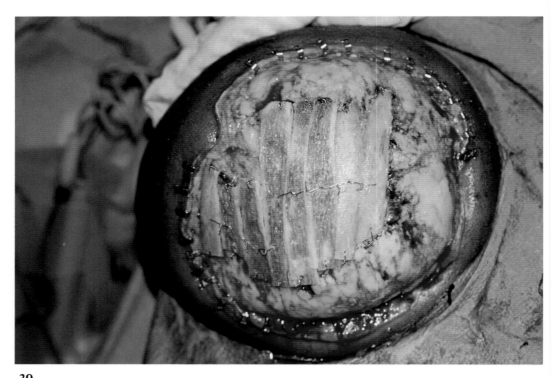

39

The skull was reconstructed with a split rib cranioplasty.

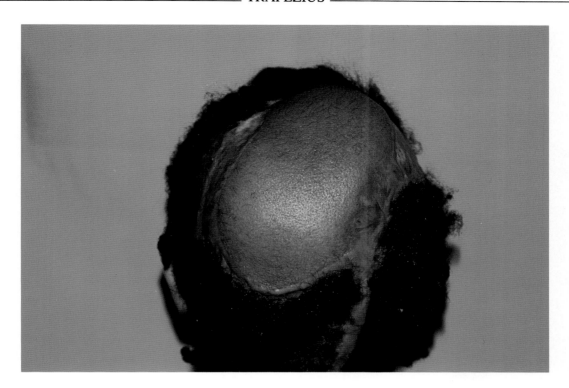

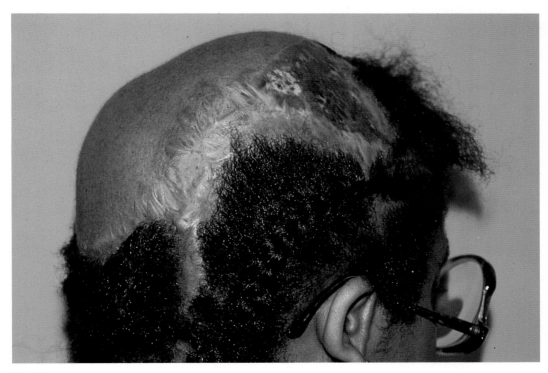

40, 41
Appearance six months following a vertical trapezius myocutaneous flap reconstruction.

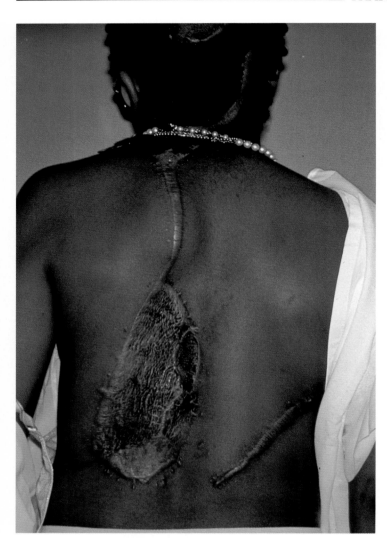

42

Skin-grafted donor site at six months.

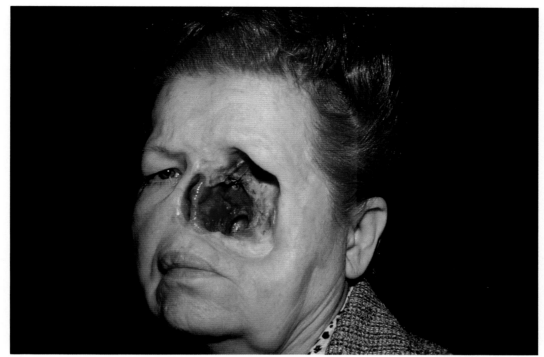

43

A sixty-nine-year-old female with a large orbitomaxillary nasal defect following resection of a recurrent basal cell carcinoma five years previously. Five thousand rads of irradiation were given in the postoperative period. (Case of H. Rosen)

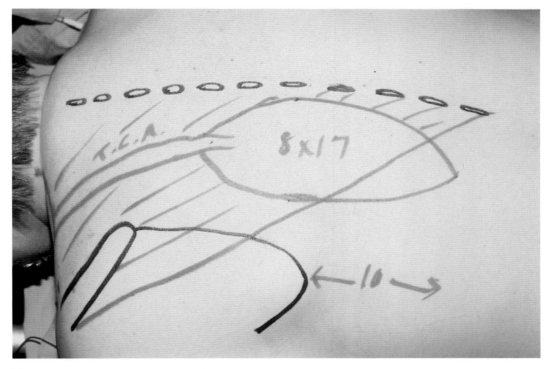

44

Standard design of an extended vertical trapezius myocutaneous flap. The long axis of the flap lies midway between the vertebral spine and the medial border of the scapula. The distal margin of the flap extends ten centimeters below the tip scapula.

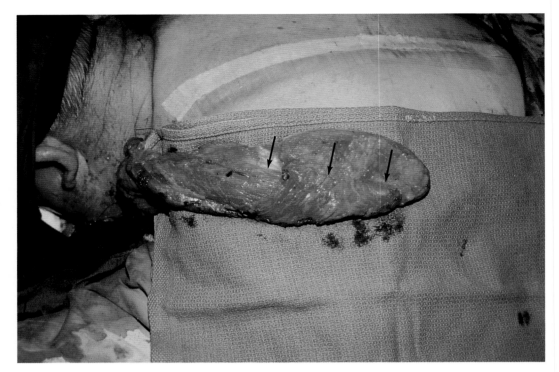

45

The donor site is closed primarily. The vascular pedicle is rotated 180 degrees demonstrating the ''random'' portion of the flap. Arrows point to the border of the trapezius muscle.

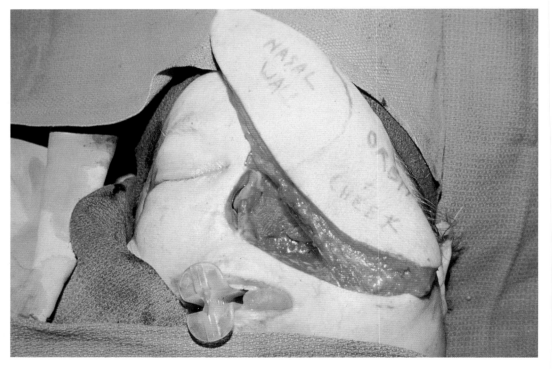

46

The flap is tunneled subcutaneously onto the cheek and orbit. The distal half is used to reconstruct the lateral nasal wall and the nasopharynx in preparation for a nasal reconstruction.

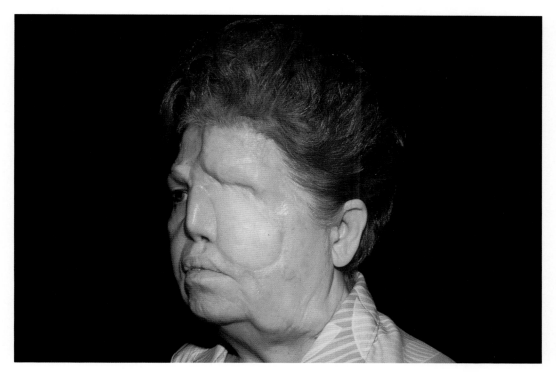

47

Appearance eighteen months following inset of the trapezius flap and eight months following a forehead flap nasal reconstruction.

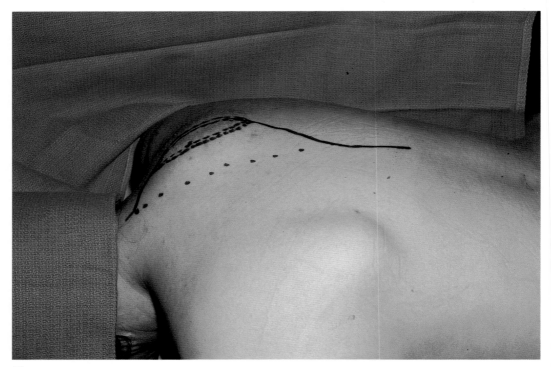

48

Forty-six-year-old woman with a hemangiopericytoma of the right paraspinous musculature in the upper thoracic area.
(Case of P.G. Arnold)

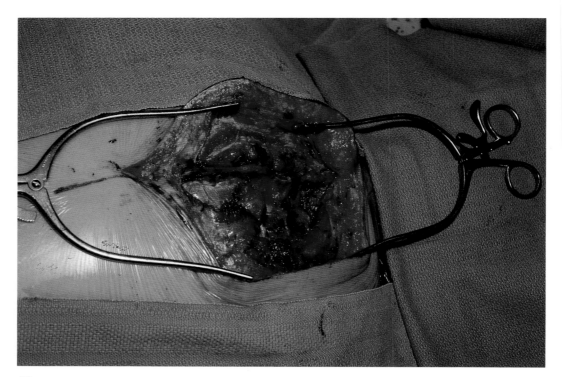

49

The wide excision of the tumor, as well as the right trapezius and paraspinous musculature, resulted in a large dead space and exposure of the thoracic vertebrae.

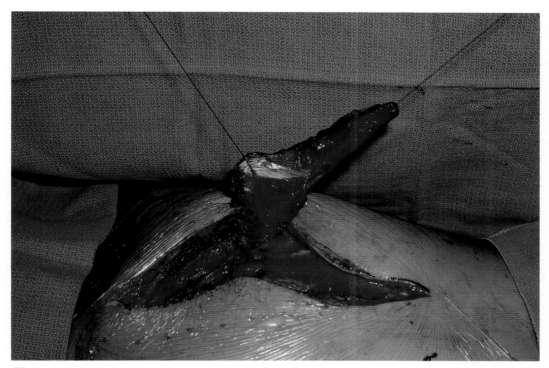

50

The left trapezius muscle was elevated as
an "island" flap on the proximal
vasculature.

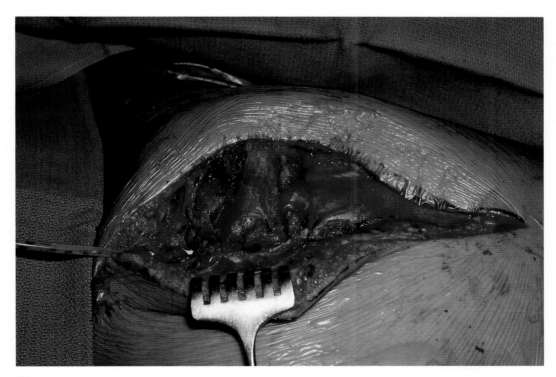

51

Transposition of the "island" trapezius
muscle flap to cover the bony defect.

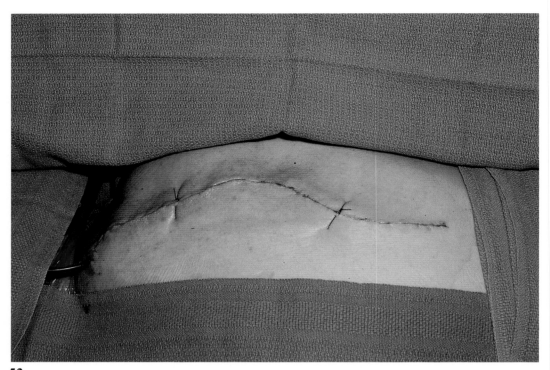

52

Primary closure of the skin. Note the bulk provided by the left trapezius muscle flap.

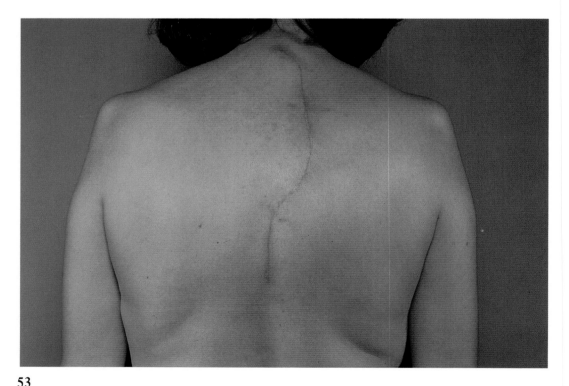

53

Healed wound at two months.

PECTORALIS MUSCLE

ANATOMICAL CONSIDERATIONS

Surface Markings

The pectoralis muscle parallels the clavicle superiorly and the sternum, medially. The lateral border is palpable as the anterior axillary fold which extends from the lower margin of the deltoid muscle to slightly below the nipple. The inferior border of the muscle partially covers the fifth rib and the superior extent of the rectus abdominis and serratus anterior fascia attachments to the chest wall.

Origin and Insertion

The muscle originates over a broad front which encompasses the sternum, the clavicle, and the first five ribs. Inferiorly, the origin of the pectoralis major muscle extends approximately five centimeters beyond the limits of the pectoralis minor muscle. The pectoralis major muscle can be considered to have a secondary clavicular "head" which originates from the upper three ribs and the full length of the clavicle. The muscle inserts into the intertubercular groove of the humerus just lateral to the insertion of the latissimus dorsi muscle. If the other eighteen shoulder girdle muscles are still intact, the functional loss of the pectoralis muscle is seldom detectable.

Adjacent Muscles

The bulk of the pectoralis major muscle overlies the anterior aspects of the first five intercostal muscles and completely covers the pectoralis minor muscle. Inferiorly and laterally, the pectoralis muscle abuts upon the multipennate origin of the serratus anterior muscle and the upper margin of the rectus abdominis muscle.

Vascular Pattern

The pectoralis major muscle is a classic example of a broad, flat muscle with an abundant intramuscular arborization between the two separate vascular systems. The primary blood supply is from the thoracoacromial vessels, and the secondary vascular supply is from the numerous deep perforating branches of the internal mammary artery which lie adjacent to the sternum. These parasternal perforating vessels finally perforate the skin to form the vascular basis for the medial deltopectoral flap.

The *thoracoacromial artery* is a short branch from the second part of the axillary artery. This artery passes on the medial border of the pectoralis minor muscle and pierces the clavipectoral fascia to divide into four arterial branches: pectoral, acromial, clavicular, and deltoid. The *pectoral branch* is the largest of these vessels and enters both the pectoralis major and minor muscles at the level of the mid-clavicle. It is this branch which supplies the standard pectoralis major "island" flap. The pectoral branch is easily seen on the undersurface of the pectoralis major muscle above the level of the third rib, but it is not well identified in the distal half of the muscle. The intramuscular course of this vessel parallels the fibers of the muscle, after splitting in the mid-portion of the muscle. This vessel is a significant contributor to the blood supply of the breast. It also has extensive anastomoses with the perforating branches of the internal mammary artery and the lateral thoracic artery. The *acromial branch* runs laterally over the coracoid process in its course to the deltoid muscle, where it anastomoses with the branches of the suprascapular artery. The *deltoid branch* arises near the acromial branch. Terminally, it parallels the cephalic vein in the interval between the pectoralis major and the deltoid muscles. The *clavicular branch* runs medially in the clavicular portion of the pectoralis major and provides branches to the sternoclavicular joint and the subclavius muscle.

In raising an "island" pectoralis major or pectoralis minor muscle flap, only the *pectoral branch* is normally preserved. The *acromial branch* can be quite large and may require ligation, but it should not be confused with the dominant blood supply. Because of the extensive intramuscular collateralization, one can also use only the acromial branch to supply a pectoralis muscle "island" flap when it is necessary to do so for a lateral defect.

Motor Nerve

The upper half of the pectoralis major muscle is innervated by the *lateral pectoral nerve*, and the lower or lateral half of the muscle is innervated by the *medial pectoral nerve*. This nerve is designated as *medial or lateral* because of its exit point from the brachial plexus rather than because of its relationship to the coracoid process or the pectoralis minor muscle.

Sensory Nerve

Intercostal nerves.

USES

The pectoralis major muscle offers a wide variety of surface applications in the area of the sternum, the anterior chest, and the shoulder. Because of the large number of median sternotomies performed for coronary artery bypass procedures, one of the most common uses is for chronic sternotomy infections. When a chest wall or sternal reconstruction requires stabilization with either autogeneous bone or an artificial mesh, the pectoralis major muscle provides an excellent source for both coverage and revascularization. For intrathoracic purposes the pectoralis major muscle will reach virtually any site within the upper chest and mediastinum. In unusual circumstances of irradiation or chronic infection, the pectoralis muscle can be transposed to the neck, shoulder, arm, and axilla. It is also a secondary source of functional muscle replacement for the biceps and triceps muscle of the arm.

REGIONAL FLAP COMPARISONS

Basically, the pectoralis major muscle is the mirror image of its counterpart on the back — the latissimus dorsi muscle. Both muscles are used essentially for the same types of problems in different locations. When the pectoralis major and latissimus muscles are not available, the serratus muscle is equally as useful, particularly for intrathoracic defects. The latissimus dorsi muscle is used more often than the pectoralis major muscle for the restoration of elbow flexion because of its relative strength and lesser donor site deformity.

DISADVANTAGES

The disadvantage of using the pectoralis major muscle is primarily cosmetic in nature, particularly in men. The prominent visibility of the ribs cannot be camouflaged, but an attempt should be made to preserve the contour of the anterior axillary fold. This is done by leaving the lateral margin of the pectoralis muscle as a static band between the chest wall and the humerus. Although the pectoralis major muscle would seem to be a functionally important muscle, it is not.

ADVANTAGES

The advantages of the pectoralis major muscle flap are readily apparent. The vertical length of the muscle measures at least twenty centimeters so that the expected muscle coverage can be estimated by measuring twenty centimeters from its axis of rotation at the midclavicle. The expected arc of rotation easily encompasses the neck, the upper two-thirds of the sternal area, and the upper anterior chest as well as the shoulder and the axilla. The muscle can also be passed directly into the chest and the mediastinum. The pectoralis major muscle is particularly helpful in avascular situations caused by irradiation or infection. The two pectoralis muscles am-

ply provide complete muscle coverage of the infected sternotomy wound. This complete muscle coverage is absolutely necessary to eradicate the residual infection whether the sternum is partially or totally excised. The pectoralis major muscle will also provide good revascularization for rib grafts or artificial mesh grafts which are used to replace the sternum or the chest wall.

COMPLICATIONS, PITFALLS, AND DONOR SITE

Because numerous vessels are encountered during the flap elevation, the procedure should be done under direct vision to prevent an unrecognized hematoma. For the same reason the large area of dissection should always be adequately decompressed with suction drains. When the humeral insertion is divided, bleeding can be expected from the acromial branch of the thoracoacromial axis. Care must also be taken to protect the axillary and cephalic veins which pass along side the pectoralis major muscular insertion.

The pectoralis fascia should be meticulously preserved in the flap elevation because this provides a dense fascial layer which will hold sutures. If this is not done, one may be left with a frayed and ragged muscle and need to use large suture bites which can devascularize the muscle. The donor site does result in a significant contour deformity, but this obvious disadvantage is mitigated by the reconstructive benefits obtained from the use of this versatile muscle flap.

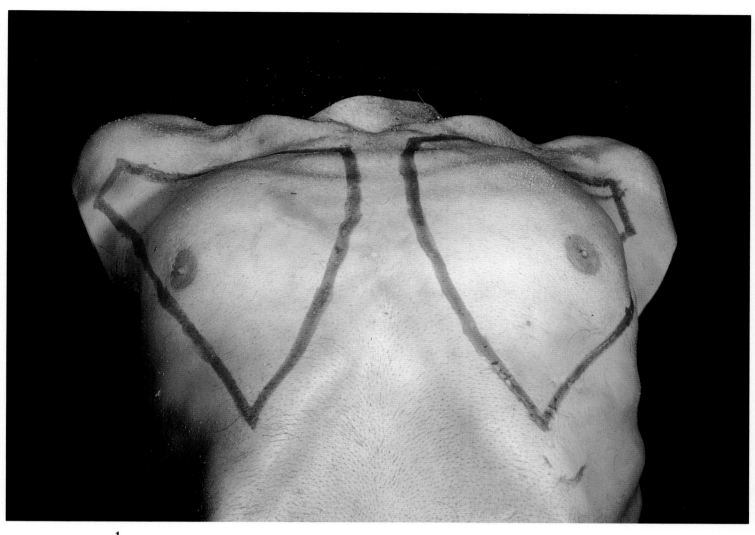

1

Surface markings of the pectoralis major
muscles.

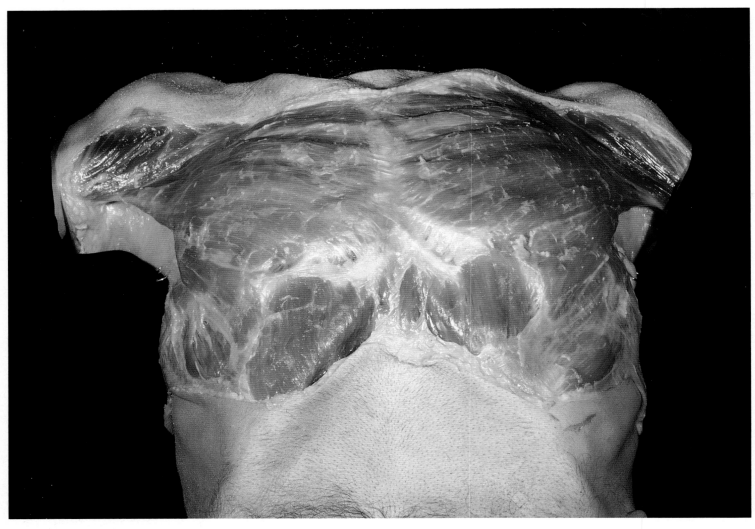

2

Full view of the pectoralis major muscles.
Note the relationships of the deltoid muscle superiorly and the rectus abdominis
and serratus anterior muscles inferiorly.

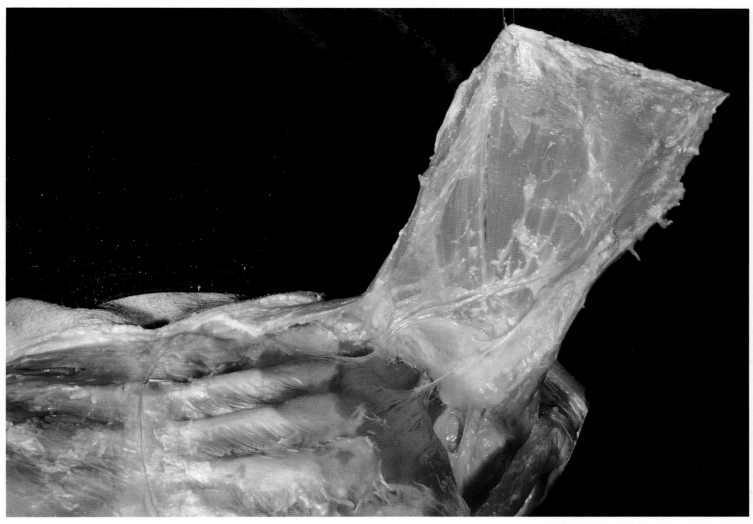

3

Completely elevated left pectoralis major
muscle. The thoracoacromial vessels are
seen on the undersurface of the muscle.
The muscular insertion has been divided.
A three centimeter ''strip'' of the pectoralis muscle has been left in place laterally
in order to maintain some of the contour
of the anterior axillary fold.

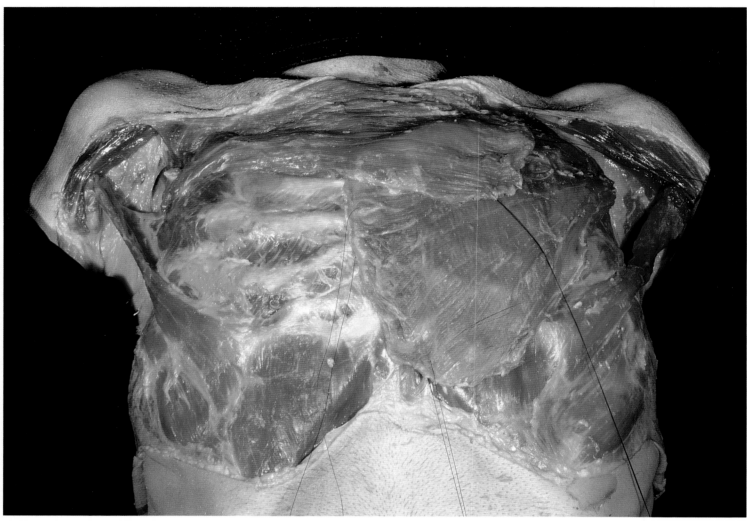

4

The left pectoralis muscle is advanced
over the lower sternum after dividing the
muscular insertion. The right muscle is
rotated onto the upper chest wall after re-
leasing its insertion. Note that a static
band of the right pectoralis muscle has
been left to simulate the anterior axillary
fold.

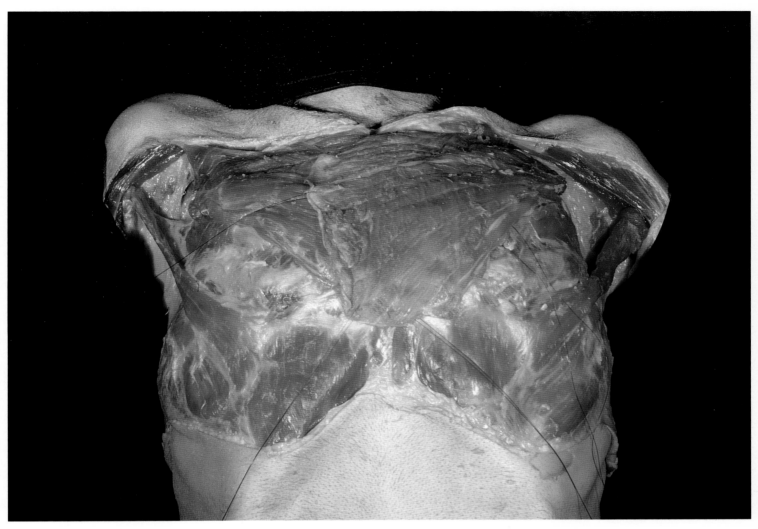

5

Crossing pectoralis muscles with the right
muscle passed behind the left muscle.
Both muscular insertions have been
divided.

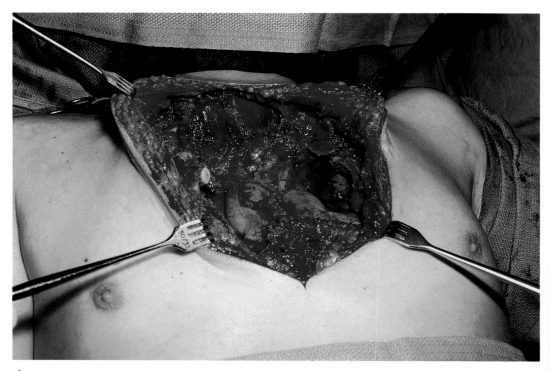

6

Chondrosarcoma of the manubrium in a young patient. The resection included the upper two-thirds of the sternum and the adjacent ribs. (Case of P.G. Arnold)

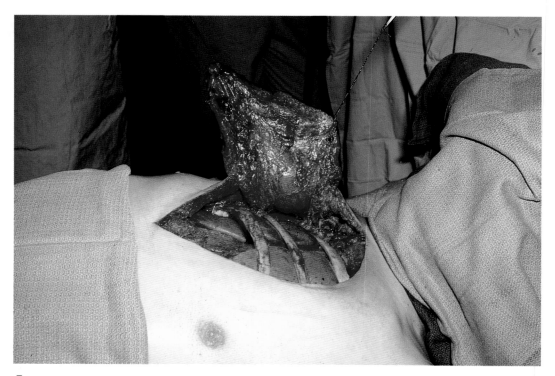

7

The large structural defect has been reconstituted with rib grafts. A right pectoralis major muscle flap is elevated to cover the rib grafts.

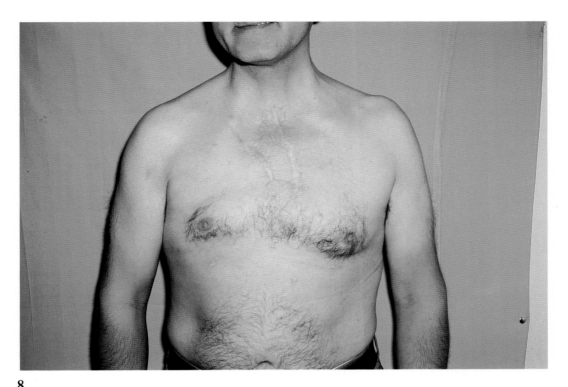

8

Anterior view at three years. Note the
"weakened" right anterior axillary fold.
The patient has survived for eight years.

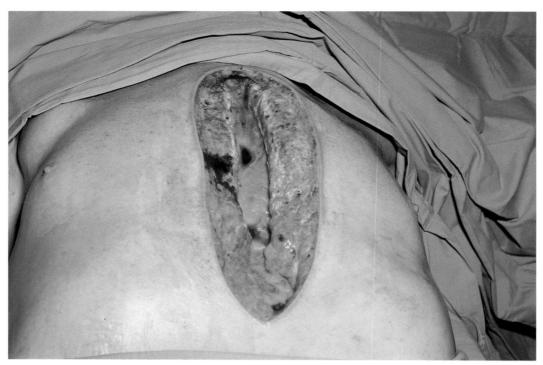

9

Seventy-five-year-old male with an infected median sternotomy following a coronary artery bypass. The open wound was treated with frequent dressing changes and showers until there was no further drainage. (Case of P.G. Arnold)

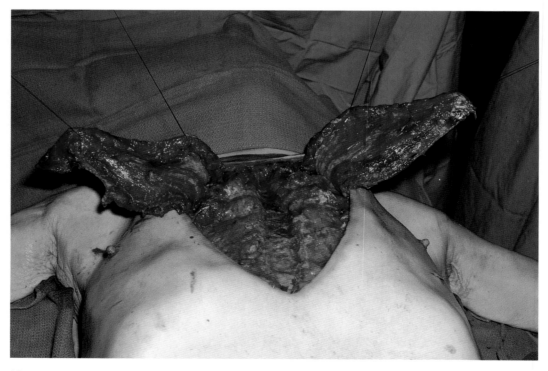

10

Elevation of the pectoralis major muscles at the time of the initial operative debridement.

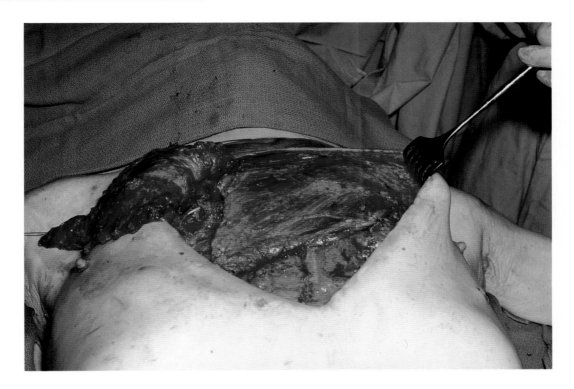

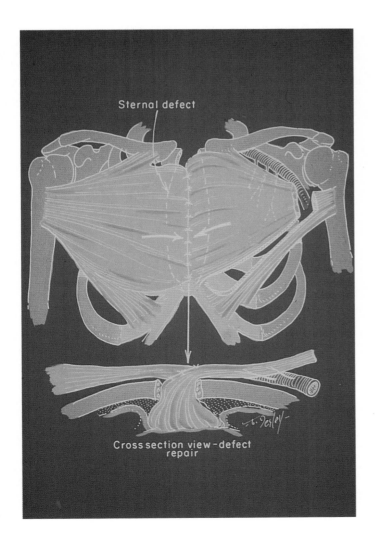

Sternal defect

Cross section view - defect repair

11, 12
The humeral insertion of the left (non-dominant) pectoralis muscle was divided. This facilitated the movement of the left pectoralis muscle into a mediastinal position (see illustration) to fill in the sternal defect.

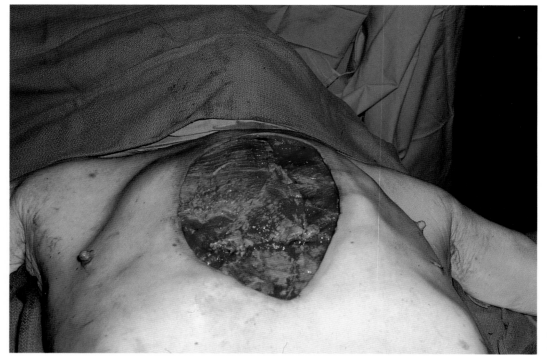

13

The right pectoralis muscle was brought completely over the sternal defect and approximated to the opposite muscle. Both muscular insertions were eventually divided in this case, but it is not always necessary to divide the insertion of the second muscle.

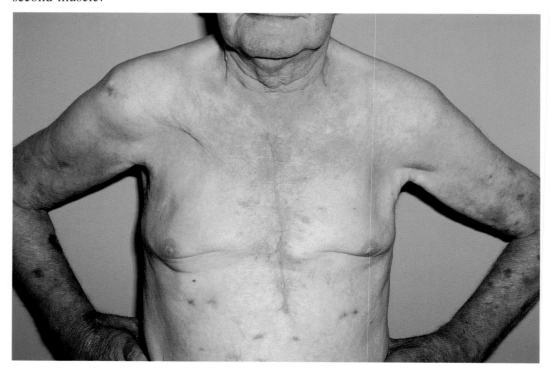

14

Appearance one year following closure. The skin was directly approximated without buried sutures. The contour deformity of the anterior axillary folds is a small price to pay for such a complex wound closure.

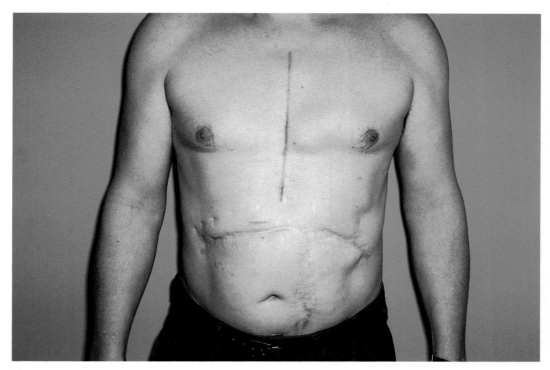

15

Forty-one-year-old man with a recurrent fibrosarcoma of the sternal area. The abdominal scarring is unrelated to the previous sarcoma resection. (Case of P.G. Arnold)

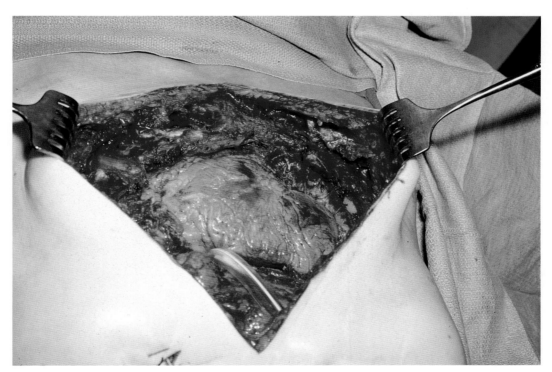

16

The tumor resection included the lower two-thirds of the sternum along with the adjacent costal cartilages and pericardium.

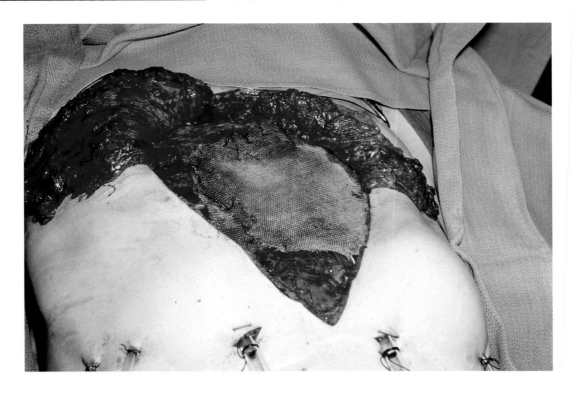

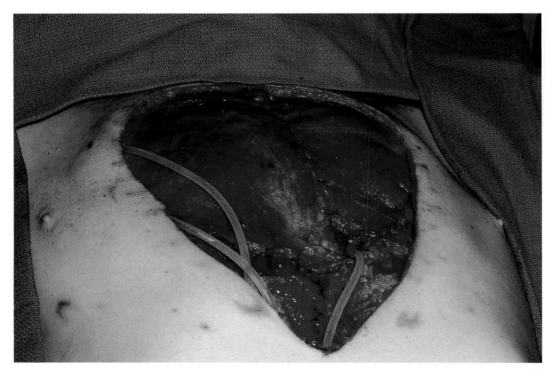

17, 18

Prolene® mesh has been used to stabilize the sternal defect. Both pectoralis major muscles are elevated to cover the artificial mesh.

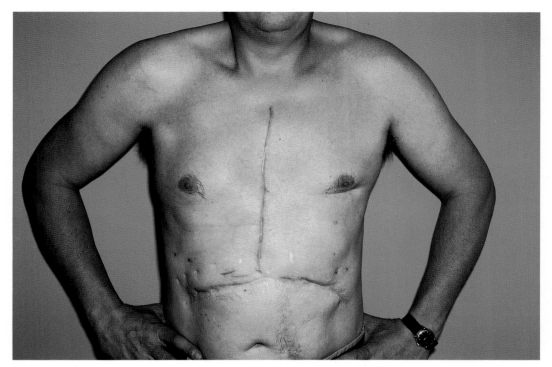

19

Healed wound at six months. The loss of the pectoralis major muscles does not contribute to a significant contour deformity in this patient.

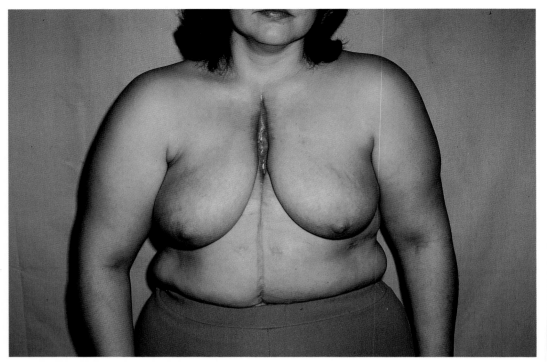

20

Thirty-five-year-old female following mediastinal irradiation for Hodgkin's disease fifteen years earlier. Two years prior to this photograph a pericardiectomy was done and the wound never healed. She presents with a persistent osteomyelitis and suppurative mediastinitis with constant drainage. (Case of P.G. Arnold)

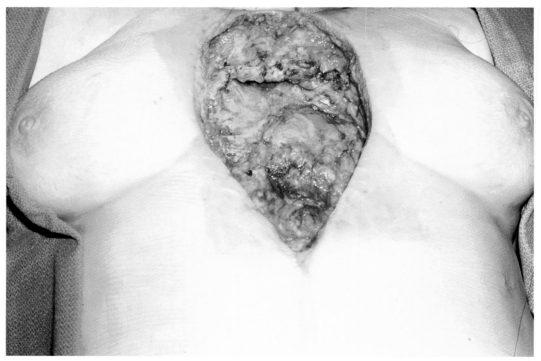

21

The sternum was completely resected at the initial debridement. The suppurative infection diffusely involved the mediastinal structures. The epicardium is exposed and dessicating in spite of constant moist dressings.

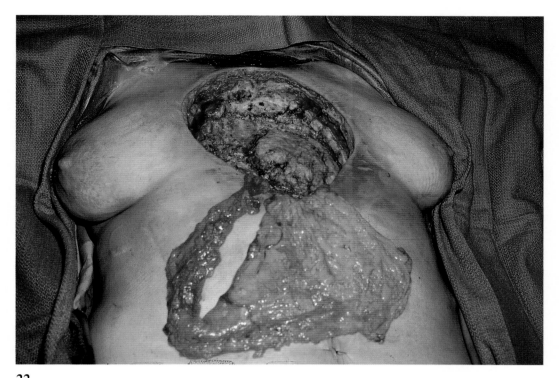

22

The omentum was mobilized to cover the exposed heart.

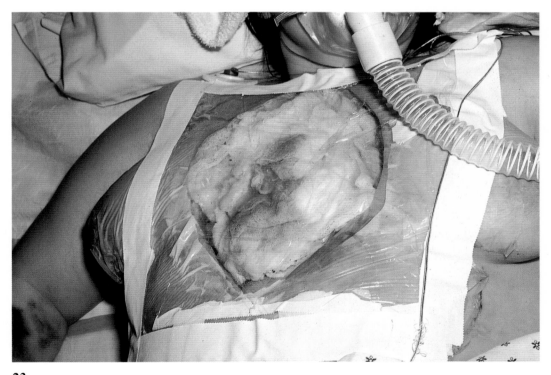

23

Moist gauze dressing changes were continued for a week following the omental transposition to control the mediastinal sepsis.

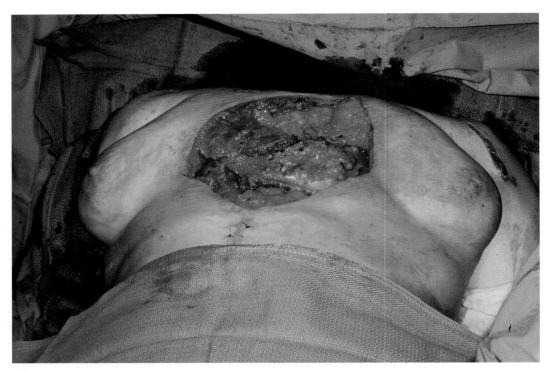

24

Both pectoralis major muscles were transposed over the omentum to complete the sternal coverage.

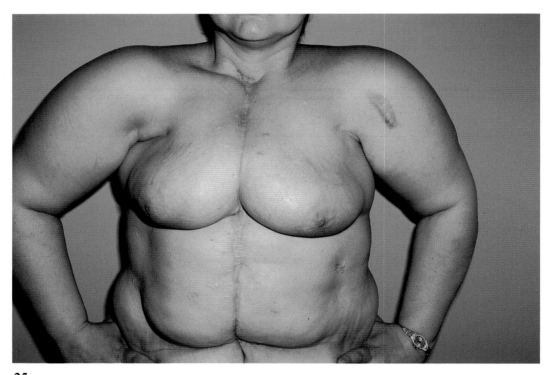

25

A midline skin closure was achieved. The wound has remained healed for five years.

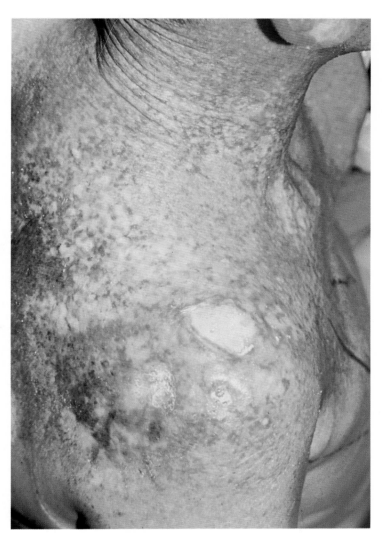

26
Fifty-seven-year-old male with suppurative osteoradionecrosis of the shoulder. The neck was irradiated thirty years earlier for Hodgkin's disease. (Case of J.B. McCraw and R. Neff)

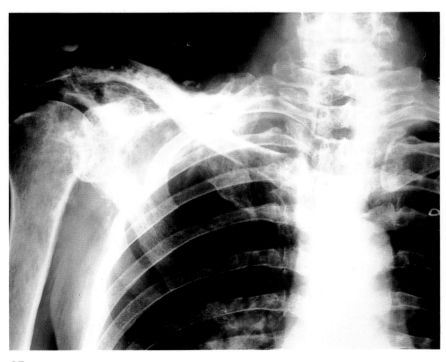

27
The entire shoulder girdle is affected by the irradiation damage.

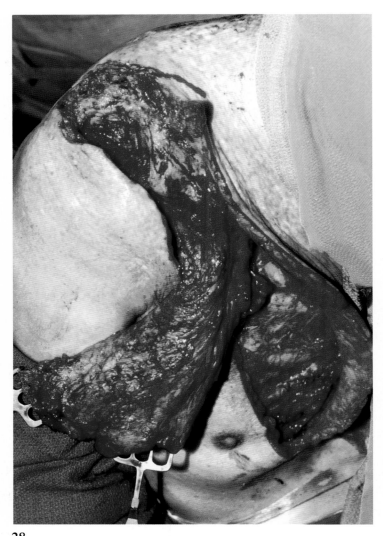

28

Resection of the humeral head and the glenoid fossa. The intense irradiation fibrosis made elevation of the pectoralis muscle flap difficult.

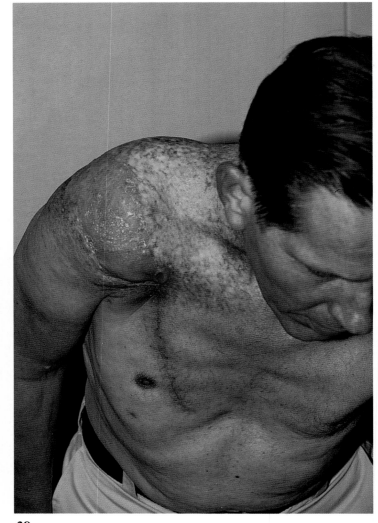

29

Healed skin graft on the pectoralis major muscle. The osteomyelitis was obliterated and shoulder motion was slightly improved. Note the donor site deformity in a thin male.

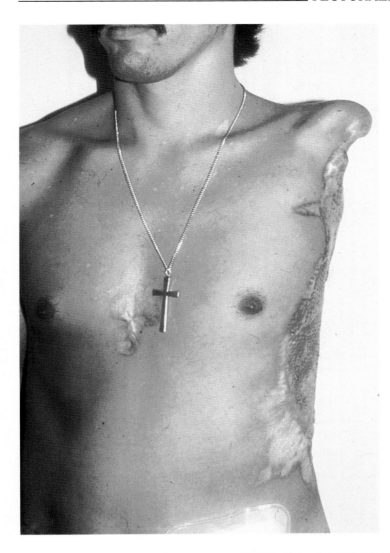

30
Twenty-four-year-old male who lost his left arm, scapula, and latissimus muscle in a high voltage injury. The skin-grafted clavicle was painful. (Case of J.B. McCraw)

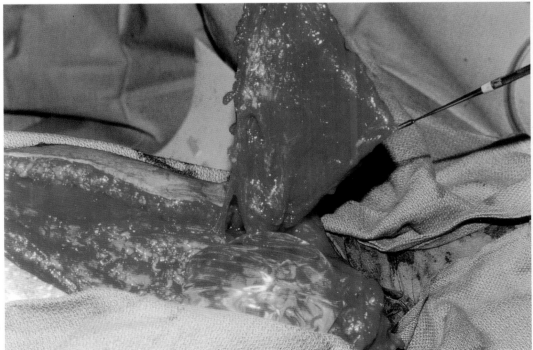

31
A silicone gel breast prosthesis is used to correct the contour deformity. The elevated pectoralis major muscle will cover the implant which is seen below the clavicle.

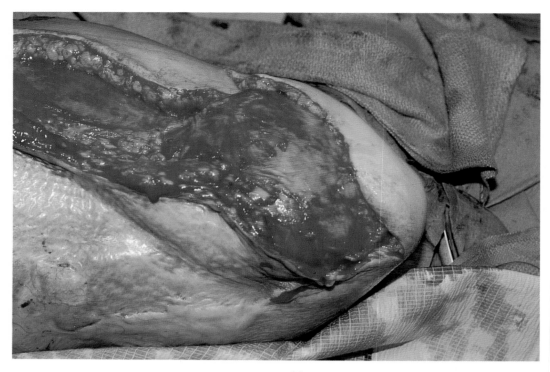

32

Lateral view of the shoulder demonstrating the pectoralis muscle covering the silicone implant. The pectoralis muscle was skin grafted.

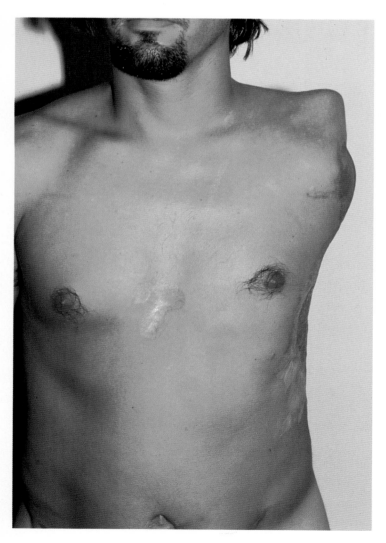

33

Healed muscle flap and skin graft at six months. The improved soft tissue cover relieved the bone pain and improved his ability to wear normal clothes. As expected, the implant developed a capsule.

PECTORALIS MYOCUTANEOUS FLAP

ANATOMICAL CONSIDERATIONS

See Pectoralis muscle.

USES

The pectoralis major myocutaneous flap is almost always designed as a "paddle." The term "paddle" was coined to denote the cutaneous segment which is supplied more by an extension of the muscle fascia, rather than by direct attachment to the muscle itself. A "cookie cutter" segment of skin which is directly attached to a muscle is usually termed a skin "island." This term must also be contrasted with the term "pure island flap" which refers to the isolated or "dangling" supplying vessels rather than to the design of the cutaneous segment.

The pectoralis "paddle" finds its primary applications in intraoral and pharyngeal defects which warrant a major chest flap rather than a smaller local flap. Although it is possible for the pectoralis muscle to carry all of the skin of the breast area, the resulting skin-grafted donor site is comparable to the radical mastectomy deformity. For this reason every attempt should be made to close the donor site primarily without any distortion of the nipple or breast. When a large myocutaneous flap is required for major chest wall or sternal problems, the esthetic deformity is a secondary consideration. However, this considerable donor site deformity does encourage us to choose a skin-grafted pectoralis muscle flap rather than a pectoralis musculocutaneous flap for adjacent chest wall defects.

REGIONAL FLAP COMPARISONS

Even though the medially based deltopectoral flap is just as useful for surface problems of the neck, the pectoralis "paddle" is preferred for intraoral or pharyngeal problems because of its reliability and versatility. "Free" jejunal transfers offer an excellent substitute for oral mucosa and appear to provide better swallowing in the replacement of the cervical esophagus. Unfortunately, the potential for abdominal donor site morbidity and mortality has tempered its use, probably unfairly. The "what if you lost the flap" mentality also presents a psychological road block which necessitates a justification for using the jejunal "free" flap. Now that the survivability of this "free" flap is comparable to the pectoralis "paddle" transfer, the magnitude of certain defects provides adequate justification for its routine consideration. For example, if the "free" jejunal flap can not only replace the cervical esophagus but also provide normal swallowing and prevent a laryngectomy, it is almost illogical to ask where the flap came from. In the case of smaller, non-crippling intraoral defects, the pectoralis "paddle" probably is still the standard against which other flaps are judged. The pectoralis myocutaneous "paddle" also supplies muscle coverage to the vascular structures of the neck, which may be lifesaving in the case of a major wound breakdown or an infection. The superior flap mobility for temporal and cheek reconstructions is comparable to the latissimus dorsi myocutaneous flap. Both of these flaps can provide massive amounts of skin, but the compound latissimus dorsi flap is usually preferred for very large defects because a skin-grafted donor site is better placed on the back rather than on the anterior chest. For extremely large defects it is preferable to skin graft the transposed pectoralis or latissimus muscle flap and to leave the donor site skin intact. One advantage of the pectoralis "paddle" is that the muscle can be employed to carry the fourth rib as a vascularized unit for mandibular reconstruction. The vertical trapezius "island" myocutaneous flap covers areas of the posterior neck and occiput which are not reached by the pectoralis "paddle," but it is seldom used for intraoral defects because of its lack of proximity and its troublesome donor site closure. The horizontal trapezius myocutaneous flap is more accessible for anterior and lateral neck coverage, and it gives a better color match than any of the other locally available myocutaneous flaps. When compared to the excellent color match of the horizontal trapezius myocutaneous flap, transferred back skin is too dark and anterior chest skin is too pale. While the sternocleidomastoid myocutaneous flap is acceptable for certain small areas of intraoral coverage, it results in a significant neck deformity and a worrisome vertical closure in the line of the carotid vessels.

DISADVANTAGES

The pectoralis major is an esthetically important muscle, and its total loss is highly visible. The frequent undesirability of the pectoralis "paddle" donor site is rationalized against the even worse donor site deformities of the forehead and deltopectoral flaps. The passivity and sufferability of head and neck cancer patients also serve to distract our attention away from the pectoralis "paddle" donor site. These combined deformities of visible ribs, distorted nipple position, and the loss of the anterior axillary fold contour would be viewed more critically by a small-breasted twenty-year-old female without a cancer of the mouth. To lessen the donor site deformity, the muscle should be elevated as a pure "island" flap, and the contour of the anterior axillary fold should be left undisturbed. Although all of the skin directly attached to the pectoralis muscle can routinely be expected to survive, the pectoralis "paddle" will not survive without adequate attachments to the muscle and the muscular fascia. These limitations of flap design ultimately determine the size and the location of a viable pectoralis "paddle." The pectoralis "paddle" is a moderately "cold sensitive" flap which should be protected during elevation and inset.

ADVANTAGES

The broad arc of rotation of the pectoralis "paddle" extends for a distance of twenty centimeters from the center of the clavicle. This distance can be accurately measured to predict the proper preoperative location of the "paddle." The cutaneous segment can be centered over the inframammary fold or extended onto the lateral chest wall or sternum. This versatility of flap design facilitates a primary closure of the donor site without distortion of the nipple. The lower chest wall skin is usually less hairy than back or upper chest wall skin, which is advantageous for intraoral or pharyngeal lining.

COMPLICATIONS, PITFALLS, AND DONOR SITE

The primary pitfalls are related to inadequate identification of the thoracoacromial vessels on the undersur-

face of the muscle. When one is elevating this muscle, the vessels will initially be seen at a point approximately eight centimeters below the mid clavicle. The vessels pass near the coracoid process and are densely adherent to the undersurface of the muscle and surrounded by areolar tissue. If the thoracoacromial vessels are approached from the anterior surface of the muscle near the clavicle, they can be injured in this "blind" dissection. The upward rotation of the flap can be improved either by creating a pure "island" flap or by partially dividing the humeral insertion. The lateral portion of the humeral insertion should be left intact to maintain the contour of the anterior axillary fold. When the muscle is passed over the clavicle, it should be appropriately thinned so that an unsightly bulge is not created. If bulk is a problem in using this muscle, the muscle can be denervated at the time of the flap elevation. In executing the rotation of the flap, it is possible to twist the pedicle into a 360 degree arc and occlude the blood flow. This should not happen if the proper orientation is maintained. The muscle is useful to recreate the bulk of an excised sternocleidomastoid muscle, but it may also form a "band" as it transverses the neck. If a "band" is created, it can be divided after a few weeks even though the thoracoacromial vessels may be included as part of the "band." If a skin graft is used for the donor site, the resulting appearance is as bad as the radical mastectomy deformity.

For some reason seroma formation has not been as common as it has been with the latissimus dorsi flap. Neither has the remaining skin of the chest wall necrosed from the loss of the underlying pectoralis perforators. However, if a significant number of internal mammary perforators are removed, the medially based deltopectoral flap is probably converted into a "random" flap, but we have not had the occasion to test this notion.

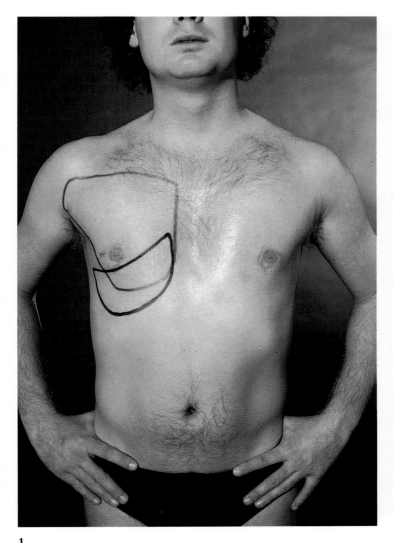

1

Outline of the pectoralis major muscle in red and a pectoralis "paddle" in black.

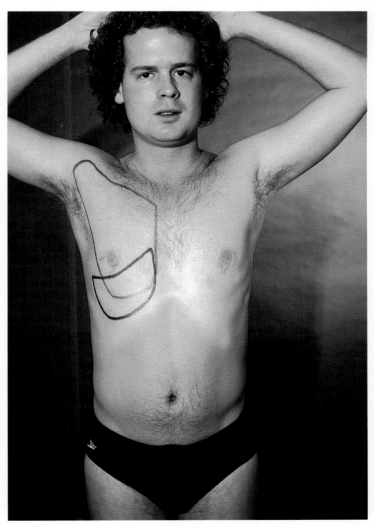

2

Demonstration of the "extensibility" of the chest wall skin which facilitates a primary closure of the donor defect.

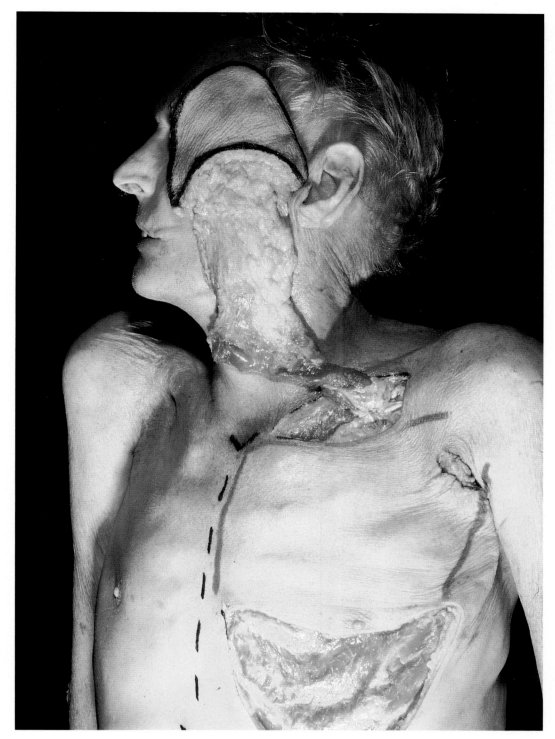

12

The superior excursion of the "island" pectoralis "paddle" is demonstrated. The flap will also reach the periorbital area and the occiput.

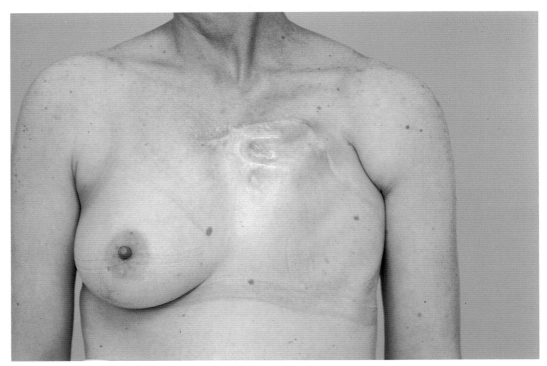

13

Thirty-eight-year-old female who had undergone a radical mastectomy and irradiation. The patient sought relief from the painful skin graft. The left latissimus dorsi muscle was devascularized. A breast reconstruction was not anticipated. (Case of J.B. McCraw)

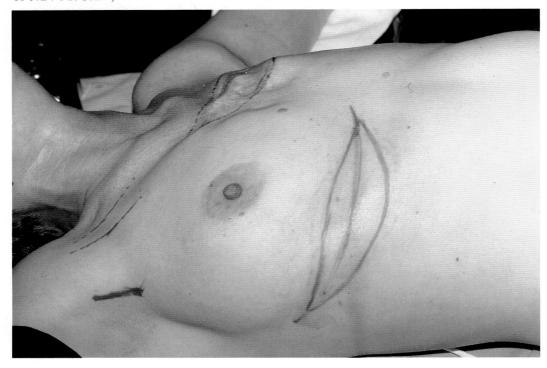

14

Outline of the pectoralis ''paddle'' overlying the inframammary fold. This procedure was designed before the term ''paddle'' was coined. This was our first attempt to ''carry'' this remotely attached skin with the pectoralis muscle.

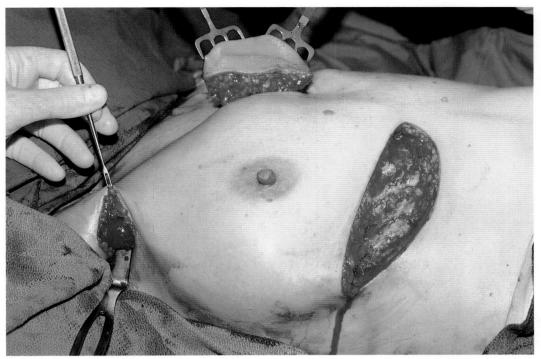

15

The pectoralis "paddle" is passed beneath the breast. The humeral insertion is retracted. It was not necessary to divide the insertion in order to facilitate the flap mobility.

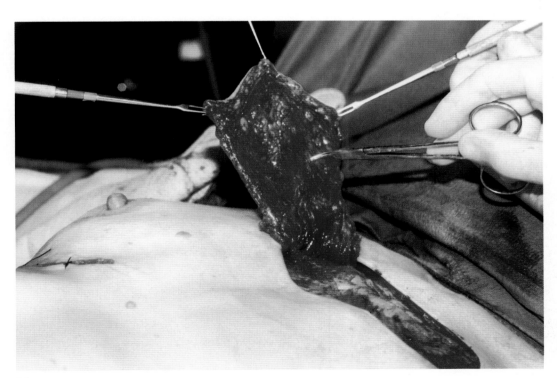

16

The clamp denotes the distal extent of the muscular attachments to the skin "paddle." It was presumed that the fascial extensions of the pectoralis muscle would "carry" the inframmary fold skin. Had this not been the case, it was known that the pectoralis muscle alone could have been used to correct the defect.

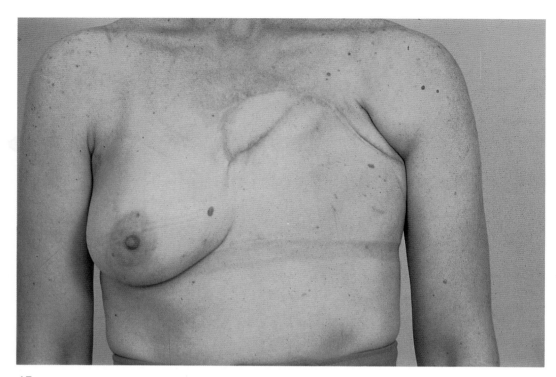

17

Healed pectoralis ''paddle.'' The right
breast contour is essentially unchanged.

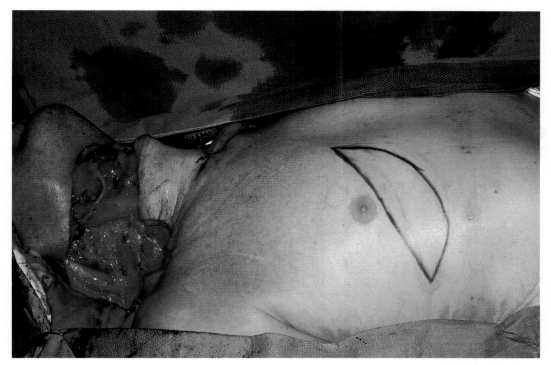

18

Fifty-six-year-old man with a squamous cell carcinoma of the floor of the mouth which did not involve the mandible. The patient had undergone preoperative irradiation to the lesion and the neck. An in-continuity neck dissection was done at the time of the tumor excision. A pectoralis ''paddle'' is outlined. (Case of J.B. Mc-Craw and D. Sly)

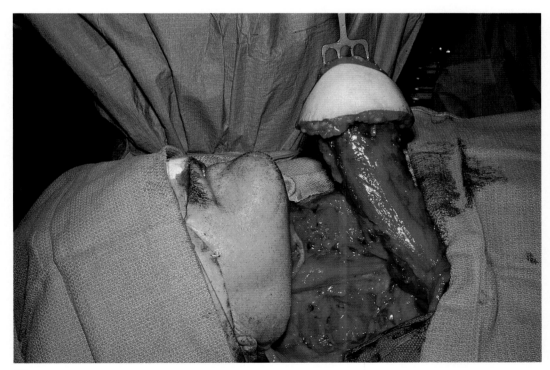

19

Elevated pectoralis ''paddle.'' The pectoralis muscle provides a protective layer for the carotid artery at the time of the neck dissection.

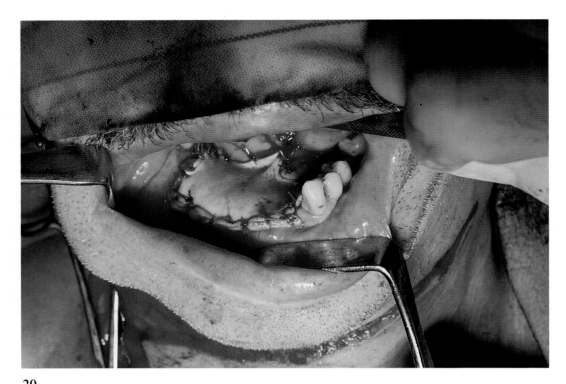

20

Inset flap. Only the inner half of the
mandible was excised.

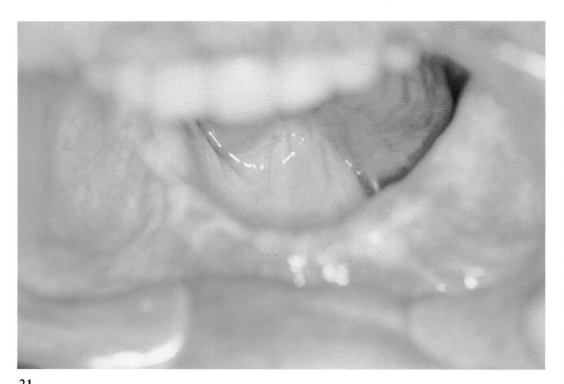

21

Healed flap at two years.

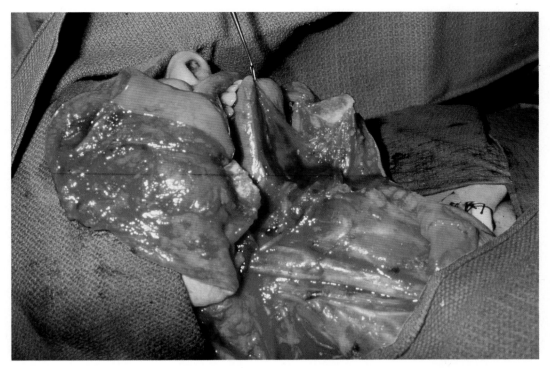

22

Fifty-six-year-old female with an aggressive squamous carcinoma of the floor of the mouth. The resection included the central mandible and a portion of the tongue. (Case of W.P. Magee)

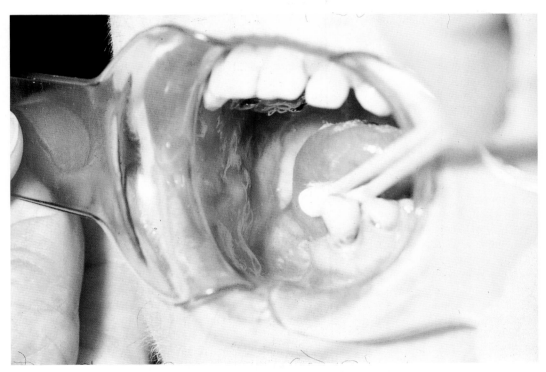

23

Healed pectoralis "paddle." The fourth rib was carried with the flap to reconstruct the central mandible.

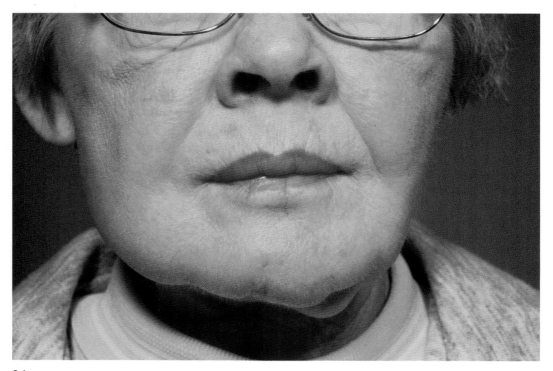

24

Six months following the hemimandibular
replacement.

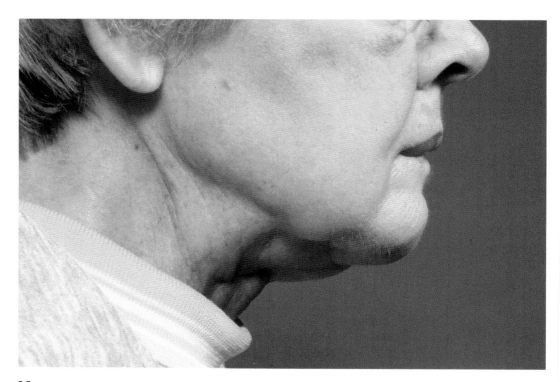

25

Lateral view of the mandibular contour at
six months.

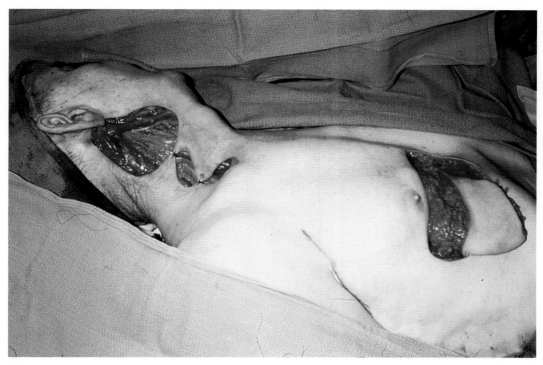

26

Resection of a malignant spindle cell tumor of the neck in a sixty-seven-year-old male. (Case of J.B. McCraw)

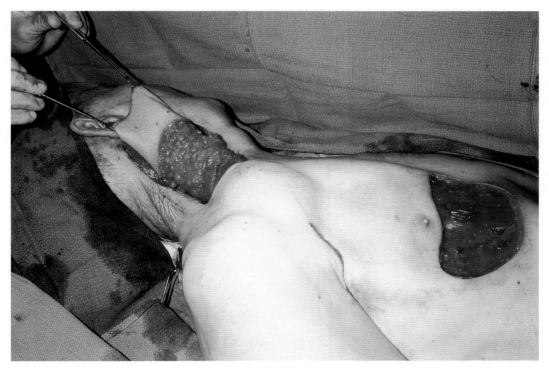

27

Pectoralis ''paddle'' brought into the neck for skin replacement.

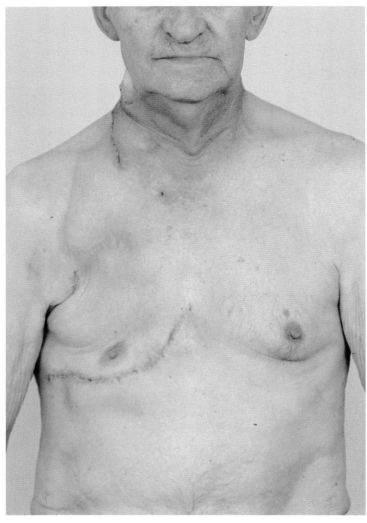

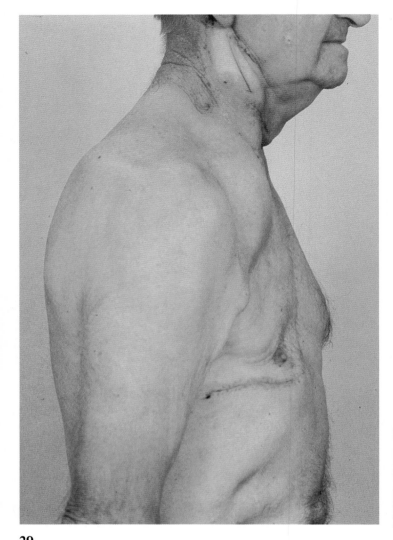

28

Healed donor site. Note the unnecessary muscle bulk in the upper chest which accentuates the lower chest concavity.

29

Healed flap at two weeks when irradiation treatments were begun. The pale color of the flap persisted.

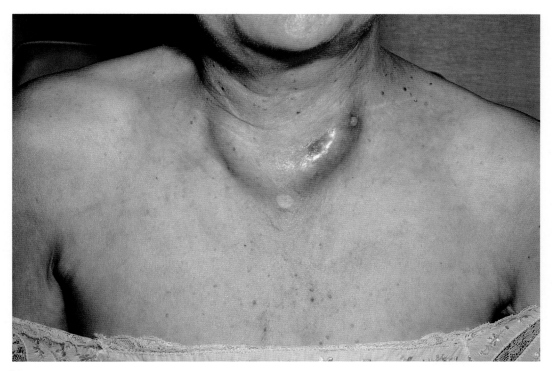

30

Infected Dacron® prosthesis from the right subclavian artery to the left carotid artery. The right carotid and vertebral arteries were occluded. The Dacron® graft was critical to survival. (Case of P.G. Arnold)

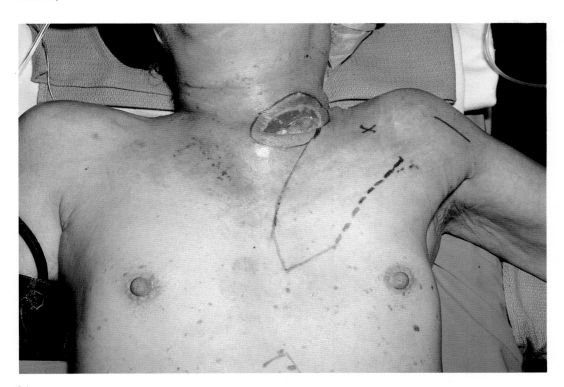

31

Open wound and exposed vessels. A pectoralis myocutaneous flap is outlined.

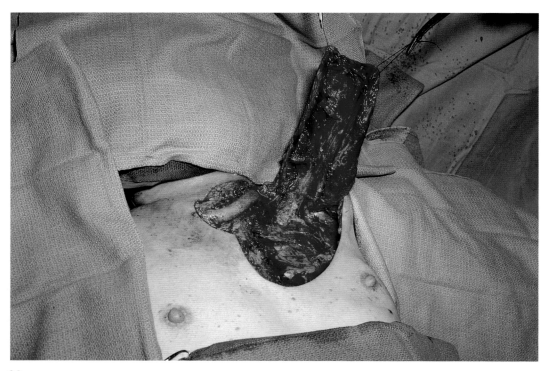

32

Elevated pectoralis major myocutaneous flap. The debrided Dacron® graft is visible in the neck wound. Dilute Betadine® irrigation was used for two weeks.

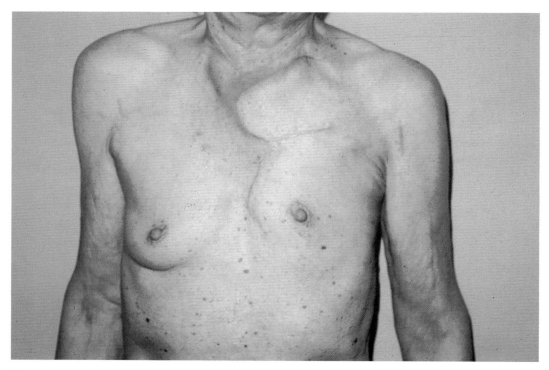

33

Healed flap at six weeks. The patient succumbed to a heart attack after seven months. The vascular graft was found to be uninfected at the time of the postmortum examination.

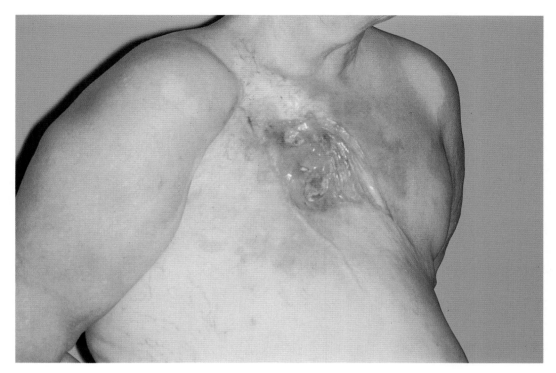

34
Sixty-year-old female with extensive osteoradionecrosis of the right upper chest wall. The patient had previously undergone a right radical mastectomy and a left modified mastectomy. (Case of P.G. Arnold)

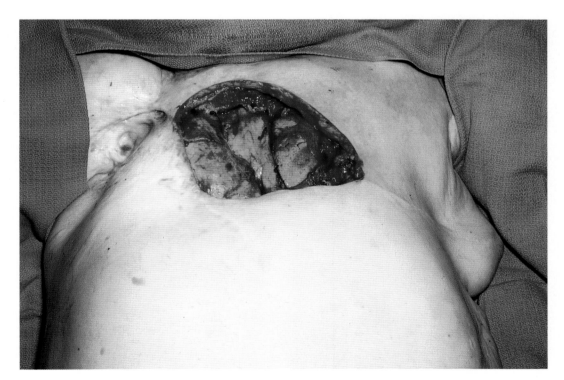

35
The chest wall resection included four ribs and the sternum. Note the transverse left mastectomy scar.

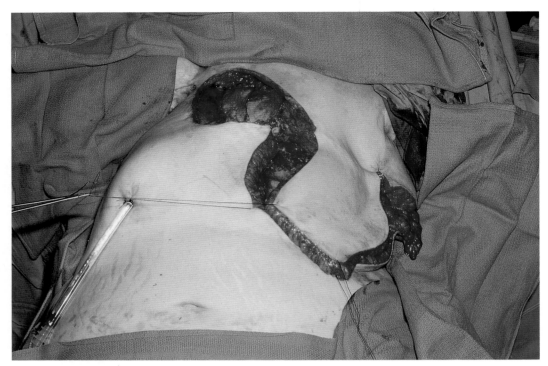

36

Elevated left pectoralis myocutaneous flap with the transverse mastectomy scar at the "base" of the flap. The pectoralis muscle was left attached to the skin distal to the mastectomy scar.

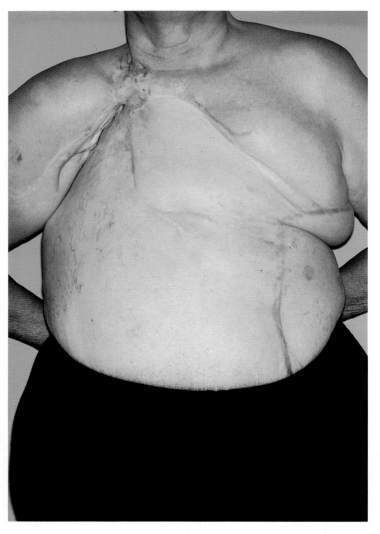

37

Stable chest wall at two years. Note that the skin "island" is supplied by pectoralis muscle attachments which developed after the mastectomy.

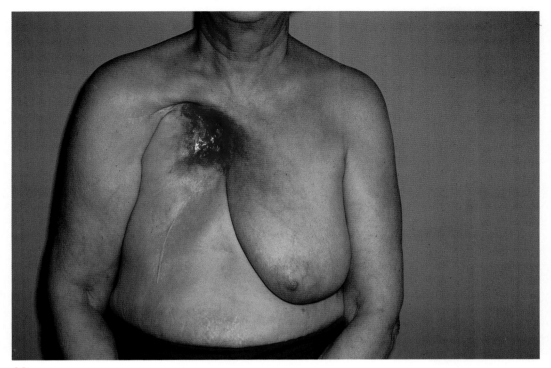

38

Sixty-five-year-old female with painful osteoradionecrosis eight years following a right radical mastectomy. A chest wall recurrence had been treated with irradiation three years earlier. (Case of P.G. Arnold)

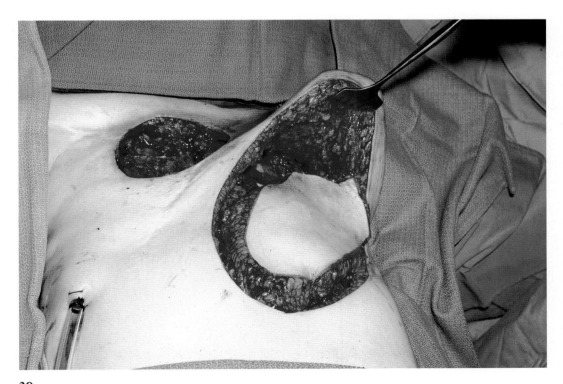

39

Large pectoralis ''paddle'' elevated. The full-thickness chest wall defect is seen above.

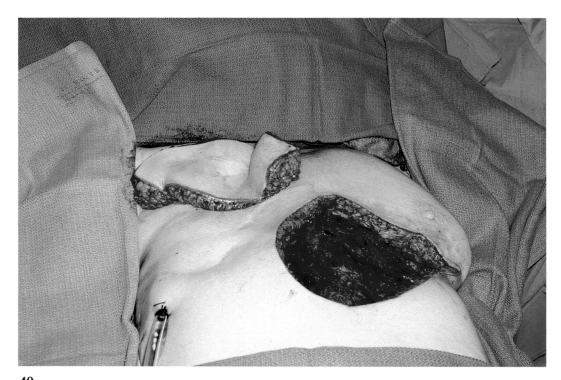

40

Transposed pectoralis flap. The large donor defect will be closed primarily.

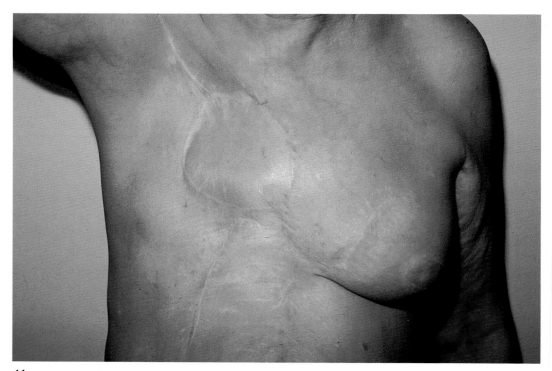

41

Healed flap at two years. The patient continues to do well six years postoperatively.

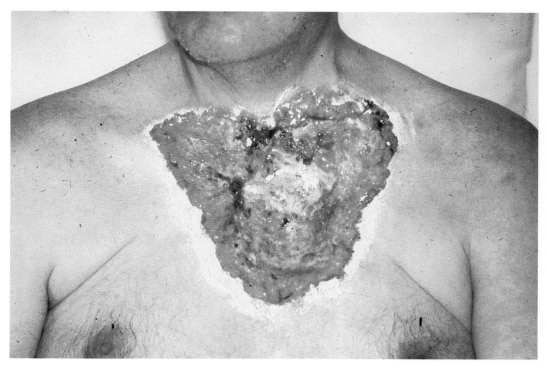

42

Neglected basal cell carcinoma of the anterior chest in a fifty-seven-year-old male. (Case of P.G. Arnold and J. Masson)

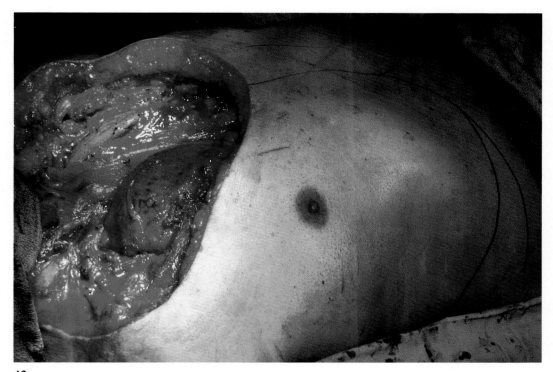

43

This massive resection of the sternum and the adjacent ribs extended laterally to the thoracoacromial vessels. Bilateral pectoralis myocutaneous rotation flaps are outlined.

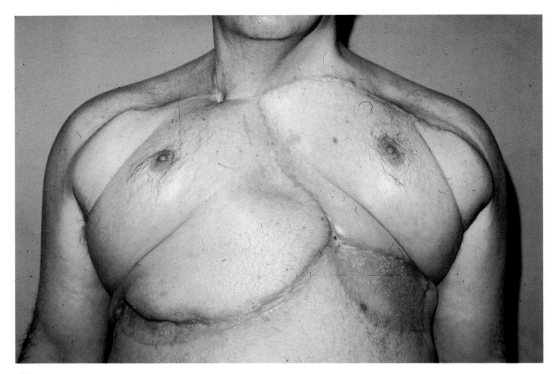

44

Healed pectoralis myocutaneous flaps. No additional skeletal reconstruction was required. Although the closure is unattractive, it solved an extremely difficult problem.

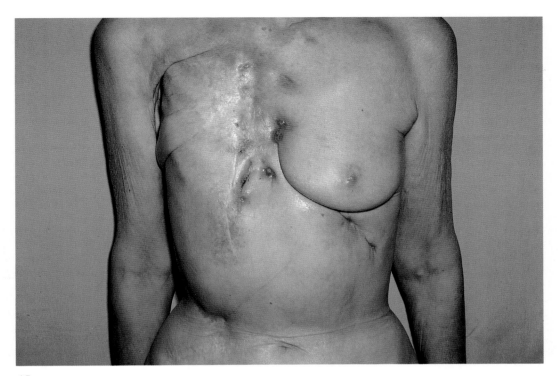

45

Sixty-seven-year-old female with osteoradionecrosis of the sternum and costal cartilages. A right radical mastectomy had
been done twenty-five years earlier. Three
years of intensive antibiotic therapy had
not changed the nature of the infection.
(Case of P.G. Arnold)

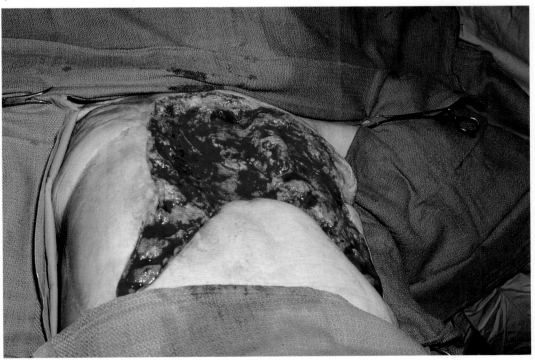

46

The massive resection included the entire
sternum and all of the costal cartilages.

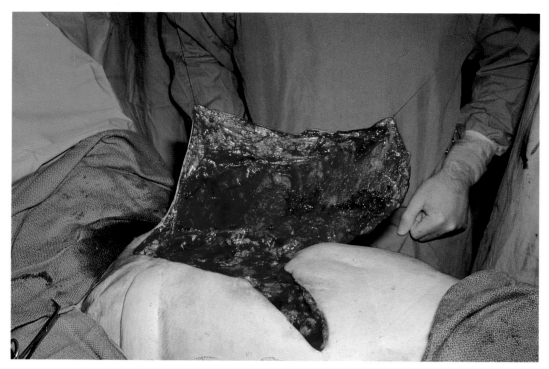

47

The left pectoralis and latissimus muscles were used to carry a large compound chest wall flap.

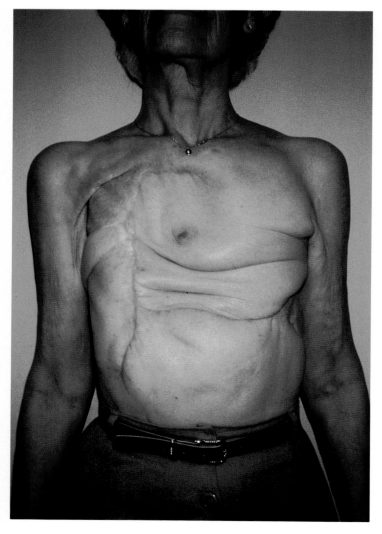

48

Healed wound at one year. The donor defect was partially closed with a "reversed" abdominoplasty. The centralized breast was an acceptable price to pay for relief from the recalcitrant infection.

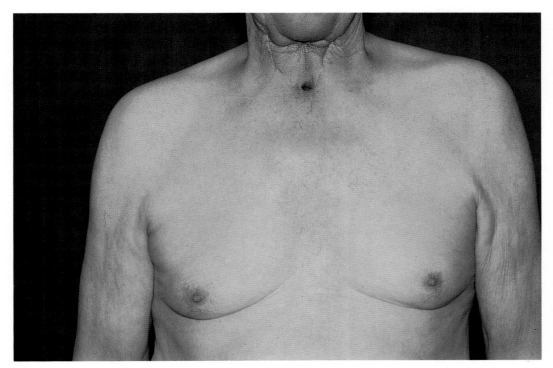

49

Fifty-seven-year-old man following a laryngectomy and irradiation to both necks. The tumor was locally recurrent at the tracheal stoma and in the pharynx. The patient was unable to swallow saliva. (Case of J.B. McCraw and G. Meredith)

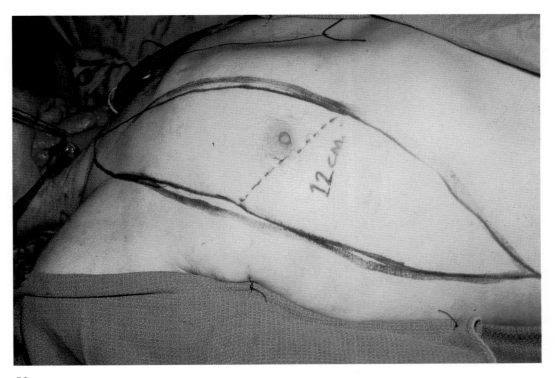

50

Pectoralis major myocutaneous flap outlined. The lower margin of the pectoralis muscle is marked at the level of the nipple. The distal flap extends well below the margin of the rib cage.

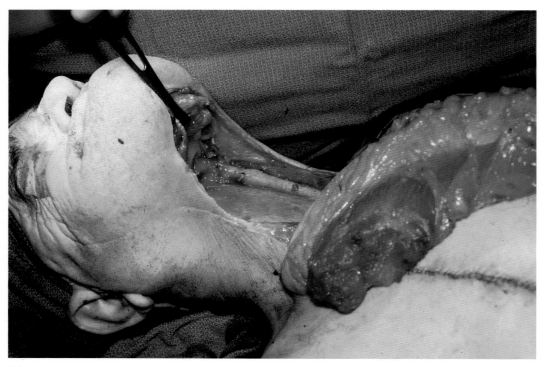

51

Completed pharyngectomy and bilateral neck dissections which included the majority of the anterior neck skin.

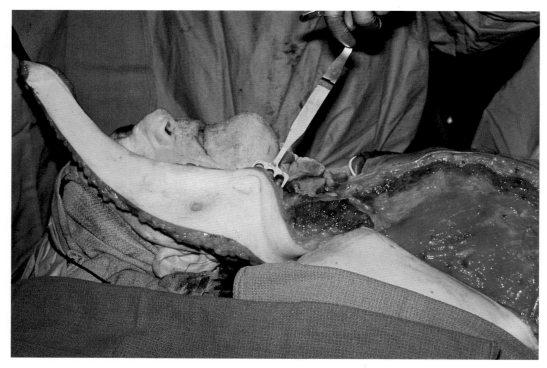

52

Superiorly elevated flap with the transposed nipple at the level of the ear. The flap skin fluoresced completely.

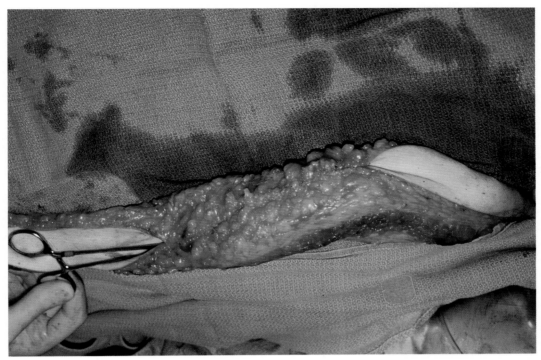

53

The cutaneous segment was tubed for the total pharyngeal reconstruction. The muscular surface of the flap will be skin grafted.

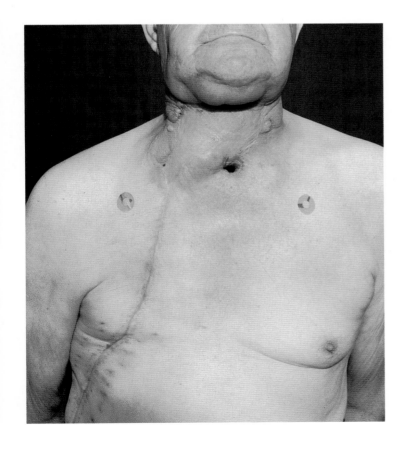

54

Healed flap and donor site. The patient was able to swallow immediately, but the tumor recurred in a matter of weeks.

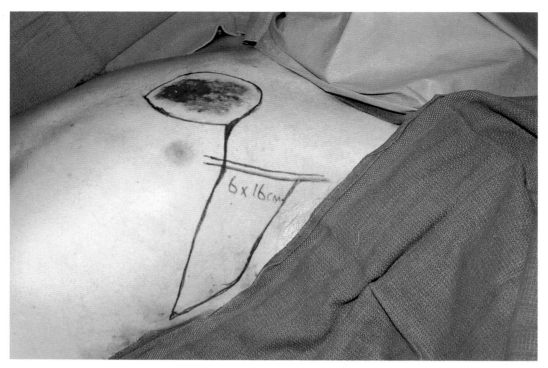

55

Neglected, ulcerated basal cell carcinoma
of the sternal area in a fifty-two-year-old
man. (Case of J.B. McCraw)

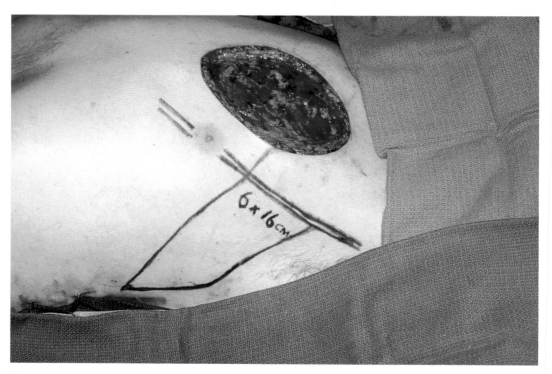

56

Operative defect and proposed pectoralis
myocutaneous flap. The lateral margin of
the pectoralis major muscle is outlined in
blue. Distal to this line, the flap skin is
not attached to the muscle.

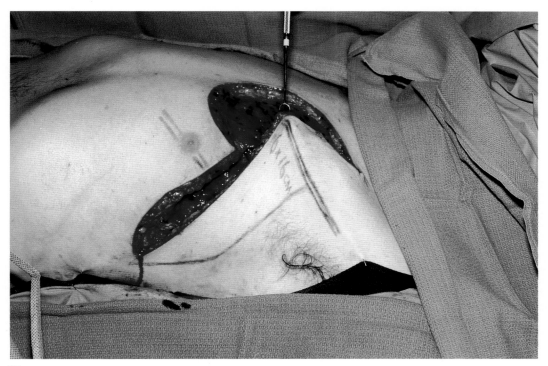

57

Advancement of the skin from any direction would have distorted the nipple position.

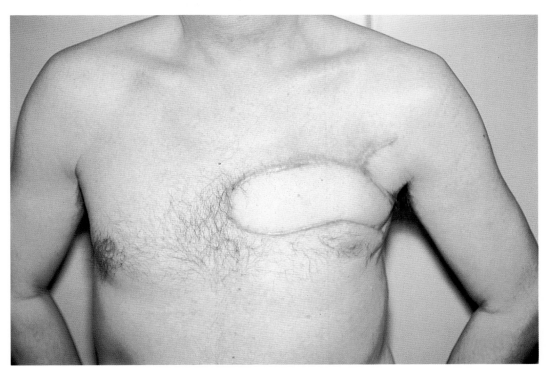

58

Healed transposition flap from the lateral chest at three months. The contour restoration is superior to a skin graft and the nipple position is unchanged.

LATISSIMUS DORSI

ANATOMICAL CONSIDERATIONS

Surface Markings

The margins of the latissimus dorsi muscle extend from the tip of the scapula to the midline of the back posteriorly and to the iliac crest inferiorly. The anterior border of the muscle passes on an oblique line from the midpoint of the iliac crest to the axilla. This prominent border forms the posterior axillary fold with the teres major muscle.

Origin and Insertion

The muscle originates from a broad front, extending from the iliac crest and the surface of the external oblique muscle inferiorly to the thoracolumbar fascia and the spines of the lower six vertebrae posteriorly. In the midportion of the latissimus muscle there is a significant attachment to the surface of the serratus anterior muscle and the lower four ribs. Superiorly it is densely adherent to the surface of the teres major muscle. The latissimus muscle inserts into the lesser tubercle and the intertubercular groove of the humerus in front of the teres major muscle. Although there are numerous important functions of the latissimus dorsi muscle, the only one which is unduplicated by other muscles is best described by the terminal action of "pushing off" with a ski pole. Otherwise, it primarily acts as an adductor and medial rotator of the arm.

Adjacent Muscles

The latissimus dorsi muscle covers a portion of the paraspinous muscles and the majority of the serratus anterior muscle. Inferiorly it is fused with the external oblique muscle. Superiorly it is firmly attached to the inferior border of the teres major muscle.

Vascular Pattern

The latissimus dorsi muscle has a dual blood supply from the subscapular artery and the posterior paraspinous perforators. Both circulatory systems are diffusely interconnected in the classic fashion of a broad, flat muscle. The thoracodorsal branch of the subscapular artery, measuring approximately 2.5 millimeters in diameter, is the dominant blood supply. When this vessel has been sacrificed, the muscle can still be carried on the highest branch of the circumflex scapular artery. Though somewhat smaller, this vessel usually provides a reliable blood supply. Either of these proximal vessels can supply the entire muscle with the exception of the most distal aspects of the latissimus muscle. The distal muscle is predominantly supplied by the posterior perforating vessels, which are seen as two rows of segmental vessels respectively lying five to ten centimeters from the midline of the back. There are usually four to five vessels in each segmental row, and their individual size approximates 1.5 millimeters in diameter.

Motor Nerve

Thoracodorsal nerve.

Sensory Nerve

Dorsal cutaneous rami (D six through twelve).

USES

In addition to its frequent use for breast reconstructions, the latissimus dorsi flap is applicable to many anterior and posterior chest wall defects as well as major coverage problems of the axilla, shoulder, and neck. It is used less often than the pectoralis major myocutaneous flap for intra-oral defects, but the latissimus flap will more easily cover massive defects of the temporal area. The latissimus muscle flap will always reach the upper sternum, but it cannot be relied upon to cover the lower one-third of the sternum. The latissimus muscle serves as an excellent functional replacement for the biceps muscle or, less commonly, the triceps muscle. It also can be used to correct surface coverage problems of the upper arm extending to the elbow. The proximally based latissimus muscle is the obvious flap of choice for major upper back and scapular defects.

The latissimus muscle has occasionally been used as a "reversed" flap for defects of the lower thoracic and lumbar areas, but the muscle is almost always employed as a bilateral myocutaneous advancement flap for these defects. This bilateral latissimus dorsi advancement flap has revolutionized the soft tissue coverage in spina bifida patients because of its simplicity and reliability. In these cases the release of the anterior fascial attachments of the latissimus muscle to the chest wall and chest skin facilitates an adequate posterior advancement without the need for a counterincision or a skin graft in the flank. This uncomplicated maneuver significantly decreases the morbidity, blood loss, and operative time in these critical newborn neurosurgical closures. Unlike the "reversed" latissimus flap, bilateral advancement flaps do not defunctionalize the latissimus muscle in paraplegic spina bifida patients.

REGIONAL FLAP COMPARISONS

The pectoralis and latissimus muscles have comparable capabilities for their respective anterior and posterior chest wall applications. The latissimus myocutaneous flap is preferred for posterior back, posterior neck, and temporal defects which are not reached by the pectoralis major flap. Conversely, the pectoralis flap is more accessible for defects of the sternum, anterior chest, neck, and the intra-oral area. Both flaps can be used for replacement of the upper arm skin and for elbow flexion, but the latissimus dorsi muscle is usually chosen because of its muscular strength, its size, and its less significant donor site deformity. The latissimus muscle flap is useful for defects of the posterior neck, but the occiput can be covered more easily by either the horizontal or the vertical trapezius myocutaneous flaps. For defects of the posterior spine, bilateral advancement latissimus dorsi myocutaneous flaps provide unique coverage for spina bifida defects or complicated laminectomy wounds. Although the latissimus muscle can be used as a "reversed" flap, bilateral latissimus dorsi myocutaneous advancement flaps are simpler to elevate and are much more reliable.

For purposes of breast reconstruction the latissimus dorsi flap is best compared to the transverse rectus abdominis myocutaneous (TRAM) flap. The TRAM (Hartrampf) flap is always preferred for an extensive radical mastectomy defect or for reconstructing a very large breast when necessary for symmetry. Because of its inherent softness and superb contour restoration capabilities, the TRAM flap has supplanted the use of the latissimus flap in most cases of breast reconstruction. The latissimus flap is still commonly used for the modified or simple mastectomy defect, but our enthusiasm has been tempered recently because we have identified an extremely high incidence of deforming capsular contractures. While the latissimus breast reconstruction has the advantages of improved implant coverage and a more natural "tear-drop" shape when compared to a subpectoral reconstruction, it also has the same implant-related imperfections found in the simpler subpectoral reconstruction. Elimination of implants in breast reconstruction has emerged as a more critical determinant of success than any other factor. We have abandoned the notion that simply giving the implants better muscular coverage could solve the "implant dilemma." For this reason, the TRAM procedure virtually always gives a better result than the latissimus procedure especially for patients with larger deformities. This change in attitude toward the latissimus reconstruction is remarkable when one considers that until 1981 the latissimus breast reconstruction was the unparalled standard method.

DISADVANTAGES

If all of the other muscles of the shoulder girdle are intact, the loss of the latissimus dorsi muscular function is rarely noticeable in normal activities, including tennis and golf. It has even been used in athletes who later returned to such activities as rope climbing, push-ups, and special military forces activities. Occasionally, the use of this muscle will result in some winging of the scapula. It can also compromise the motion of the posterior "push off," where the hand is directed behind the back. Because this is an important function in snow skiing, it must be considered in certain patients. For this reason the latissimus dorsi flap is not always championed by plastic surgeons in the ski areas of Europe.

The primary disadvantages are related to donor site complications. Unfortunately donor site pain and seroma formation are the rule rather than the exception. If the width of the skin removal exceeds five centimeters, one can expect a widened scar. When it is necessary to skin graft the donor site, poor graft "take" in this mobile area and an unsightly contour depression should be anticipated. In the event that the muscle is denervated, the muscle will still "carry" skin, but it does not contribute any appreciable bulk to the recipient site. No flap losses have been encountered when the thoracodorsal vessels have been intact in nonirradiated tissue. Minimal flap loss has occurred when the proximal flap was supplied by only the circumflex scapular vessels. If the latissimus muscle has been totally transected by a prior posterolateral thoracotomy, the latissimus muscle absolutely will not survive elevation in the area distal to the muscular scar.

ADVANTAGES

The robust viability of this magnanimous muscle flap constitutes its major commending feature even when it is only vascularized by the circumflex scapular vessels. It is certainly one of the most versatile flaps for reconstructive problems of the chest wall and the upper arm. The muscle flap alone will also supply unique coverage for massive defects of the temporal area, the neck, and the shoulder. Overall, the usefulness of this remarkable flap far overshadows its recognized disadvantages.

COMPLICATIONS, PITFALLS, AND DONOR SITE

Major complications have almost always been related to the extremely rare flap loss which has been caused by the absence of the thoracodorsal vessels or by massive amounts of irradiation to the axilla. If the donor vessels are appropriately mobilized, the flap does not appear to be subject to vascular "spasm." Neither is cold a recognized threat to the flap.

Generally, the pitfalls of flap dissection are related to minor technicalities. While the dissection is straightforward, one must be sure to detach the upper border of the muscle from the teres major muscle so this attachment does not leave a "lump" in the axilla in the process of anterior transposition. It is also easy to elevate the serratus anterior muscle accidentally in the posterior flap dissection. The serratus anterior muscle should be carefully identified, and if it is raised with the latissimus muscle, it should be resutured to its site of origin. Following a radical mastectomy, the anterior border of the latissimus muscle may be so densely scarred that it is fused with the serratus anterior muscle. It is imperative to identify the latissimus dorsi muscle precisely; otherwise one can injure the thoracodorsal vessels which lie close to the anterior border of the muscle. In the case of a scarred muscle, the safest approach is to identify the latissimus muscle posteriorly and superiorly. This can easily be done by entering the submuscular plane at the thoracolumbar fascia, separating the latissimus and teres major muscles, and then finally identifying the vascular leash and the anterior border of the latissimus muscle in the axilla.

One should take care to protect the long thoracic nerve during the dissection even though it has not been injured in our cases. It is important to maintain a relaxed position of the arm during the flap dissection to prevent a stretch of the brachial plexus. Abduction of the neck and external rotation of the shoulder accentuate this stretch because this position produces the maximal tension on the brachial plexus. A few temporary ulnar nerve palsies have occurred, which suggest that precautionary measures are warranted. For this reason the arm should be draped "free" and observed directly.

The donor site has contributed the biggest disadvantage of this flap because of the high incidence of seroma formation which occurs even with adequate suction drainage. These seromas are occasionally difficult to eradicate and can result in the formation of a bursa. If this happens, it is usually possible to collapse the cavity with a Penrose drain. After four to six weeks this becomes an intractable problem, and it may be necessary to abrade or excise the two surfaces of the "bursa" to obtain healing.

The donor site itself does not create any significant surface depression nor any excessive prominence of the ribs, but if more than five centimeters of skin is carried with the muscle, a widened scar can be expected. If a skin graft is required for the donor site, the resulting contour deformity can be remarkably unattractive, particularly in the obese patient.

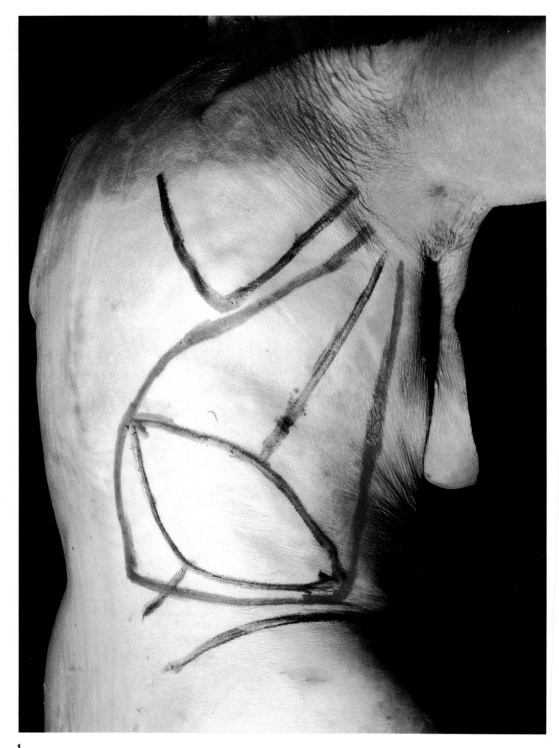

1

Transversely oriented skin "island" on
the lower portion of the latissimus muscle
in a fresh cadaver. The scapula and iliac
crest are outlined in black.

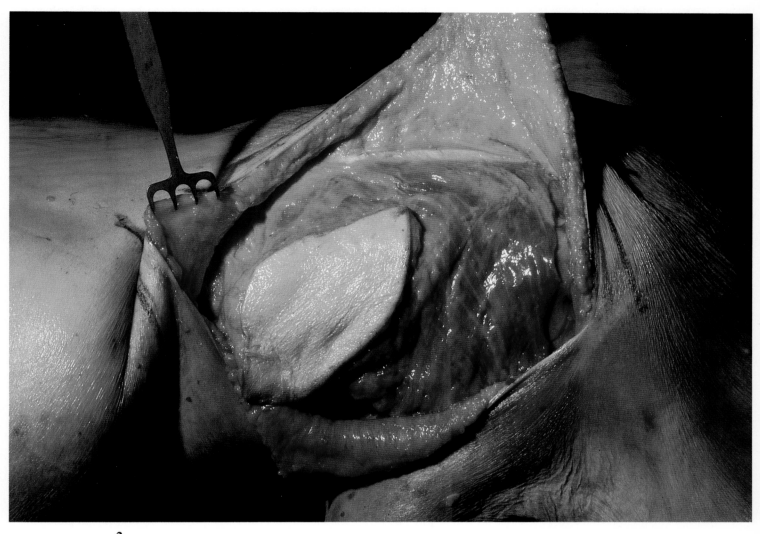

2

Latissimus muscle exposed through a vertical incision. The thoracolumbar fascia is visible superiorly.

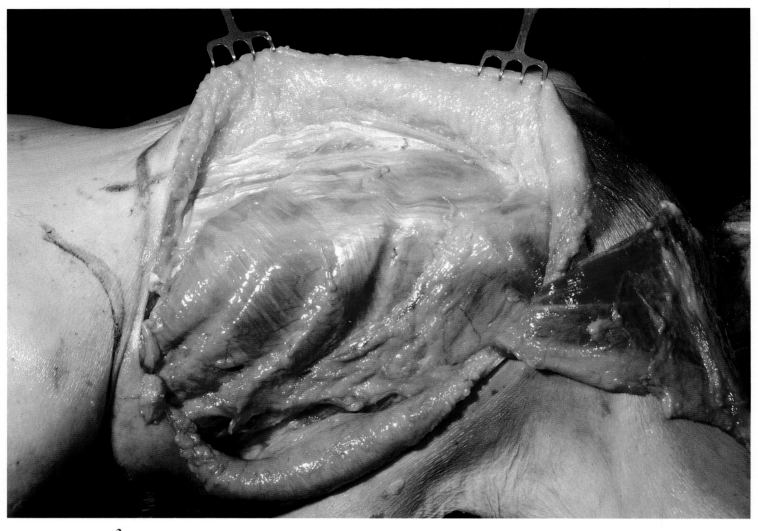

3

Transposed latissimus muscle. The serratus anterior and external oblique muscles are seen on the chest wall.

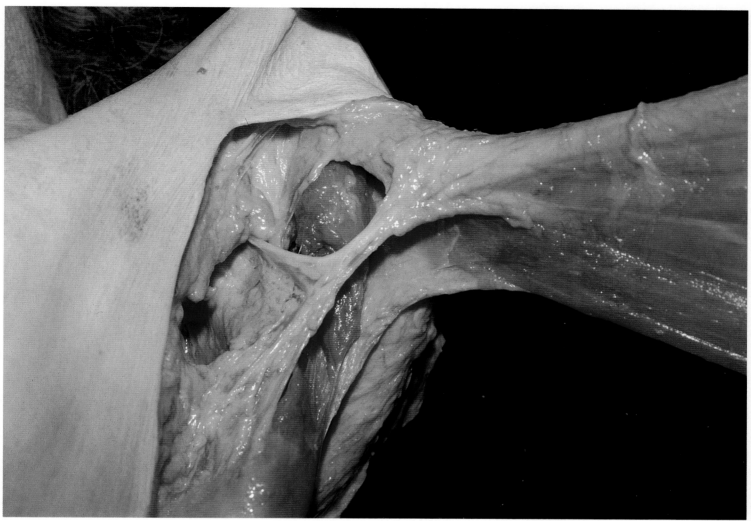

4

This left axillary dissection demonstrates
the subscapular artery with its major
branches which pass superiorly to the latissimus dorsi muscle and inferiorly to the
serratus anterior muscle. The thoracodorsal artery is seen crossing the surface of
the teres major muscle and entering the
undersurface of the latissimus muscle approximately two centimeters from its anterior border.

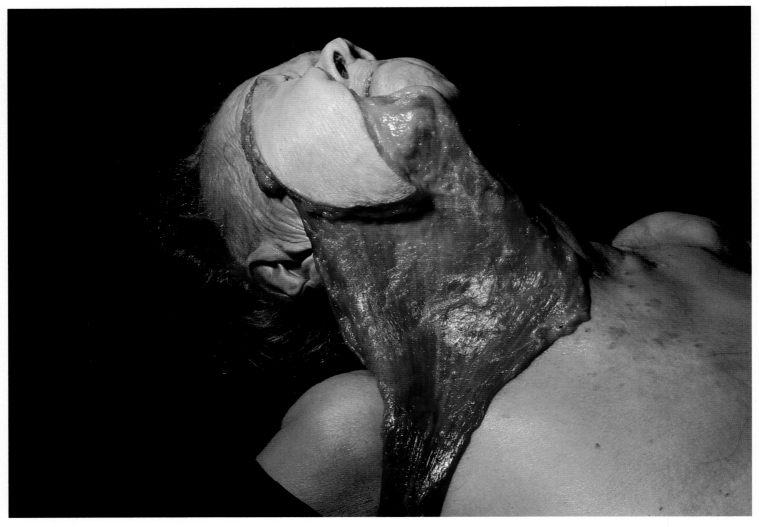

5

Upward rotation of the low transverse
skin "island" to the face. The posterior
portion of the latissimus muscle covers
the lower neck.

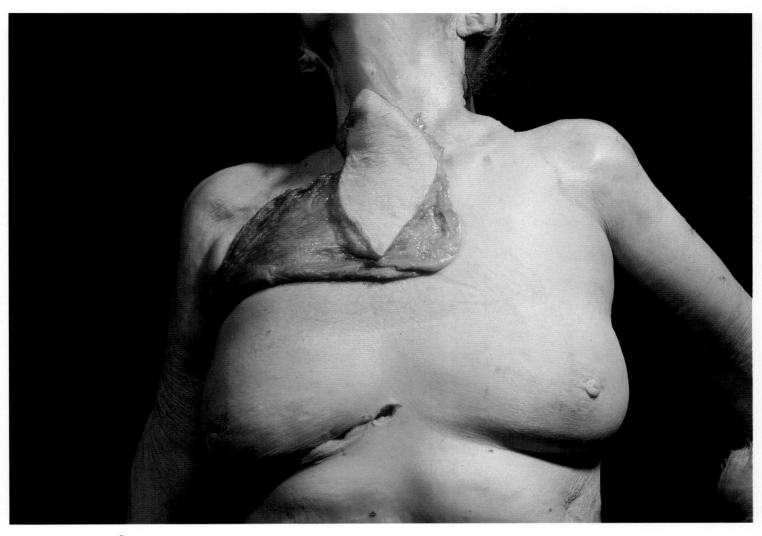

6

Coverage of the upper sternum by the
low, transverse skin "island."

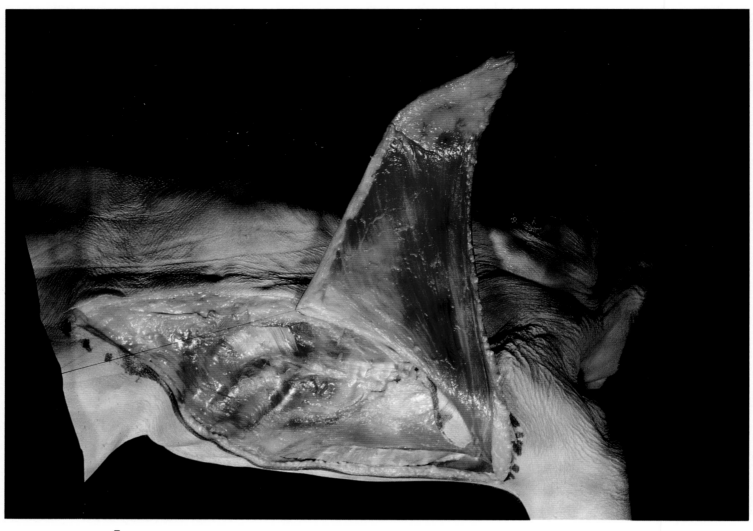

7

Total elevation of the latissimus muscle
and its overlying skin in a fresh cadaver.

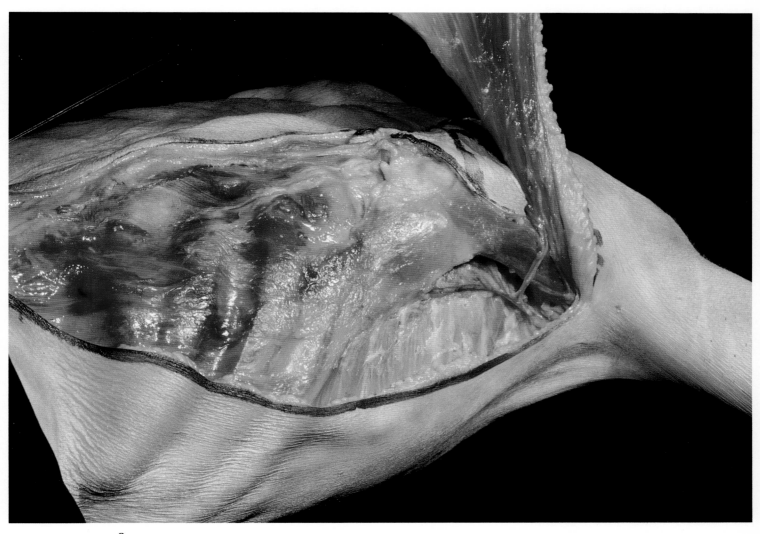

8

Elevation of the latissimus flap exposes
the thoracodorsal artery and the serratus
anterior branch.

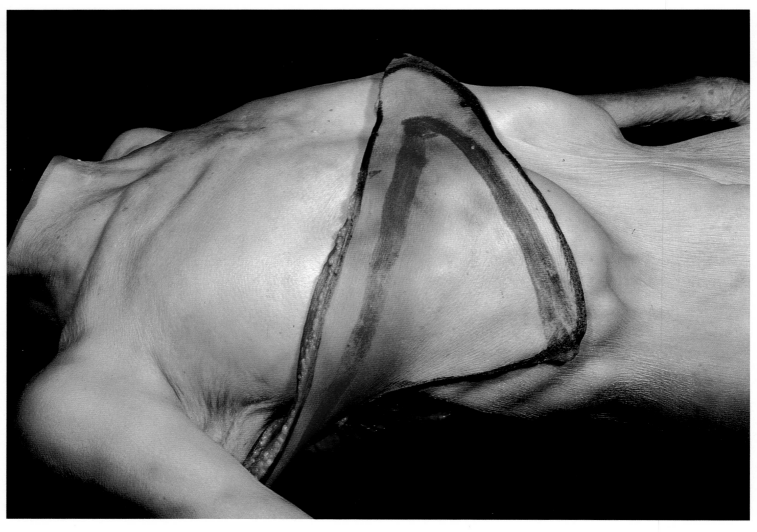

9

Transposition of the entire latissimus
muscle and all of its overlying skin to the
lower chest wall and sternum.

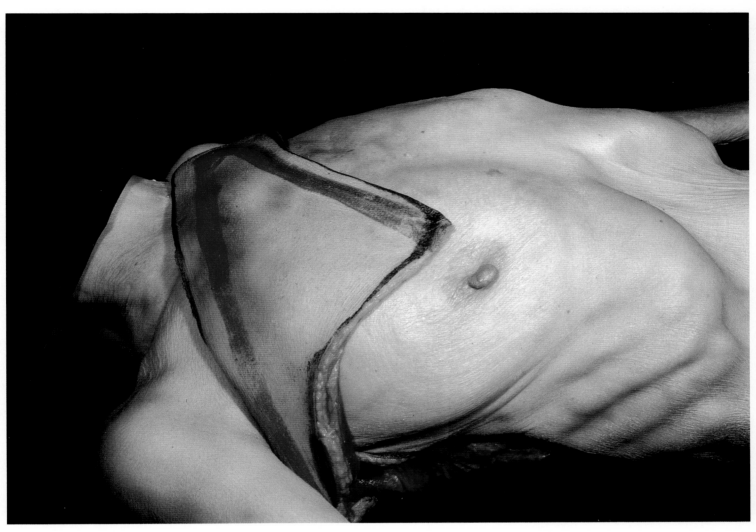

10

Transposition of the complete latissimus myocutaneous unit to the upper chest wall.

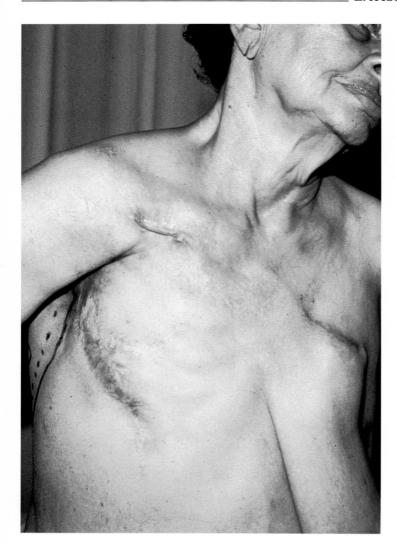

11

Fifty-nine-year-old patient with an exposed cardiac pacemaker wire adjacent to the clavicle. The patient had previously had a radical mastectomy and the surrounding skin had been heavily irradiated. The pacemaker wire was not infected from a technical standpoint. It was important to salvage this pacemaker since all previous implantations had failed. This 1974 case is included for historical interest since it is apparently the first latissimus dorsi myocutaneous flap done in the United States. (Case of J.B. McCraw)

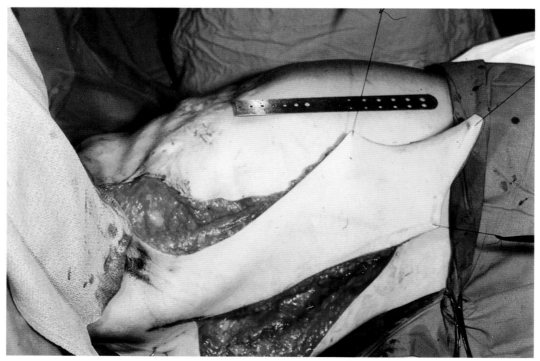

12

As a precautionary measure, the thoracodorsal vessels were identified prior to flap elevation. The anterior half of the latissimus muscle and its overlying skin were elevated without a "delay." It is interesting to note that this is precisely the same operation performed by Professor Tansini seventy-five years earlier.

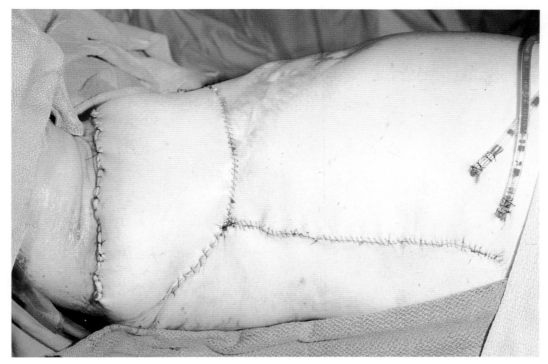

13

The latissimus muscle was used to sur-
round the pacemaker wire following a
wide debridement. An "island" skin flap
was not created since it was not known at
the time whether this would harm the viability of the distal flap skin.

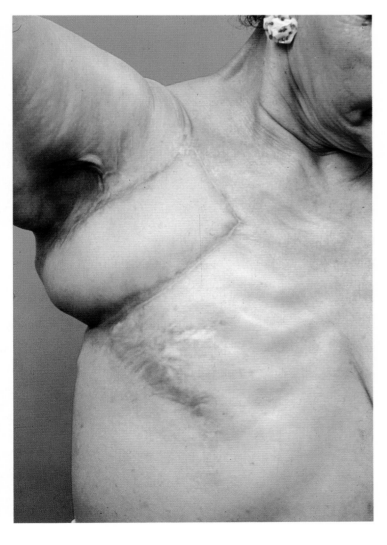

14

Healed latissimus myocutaneous flap with
salvage of the pacemaker.

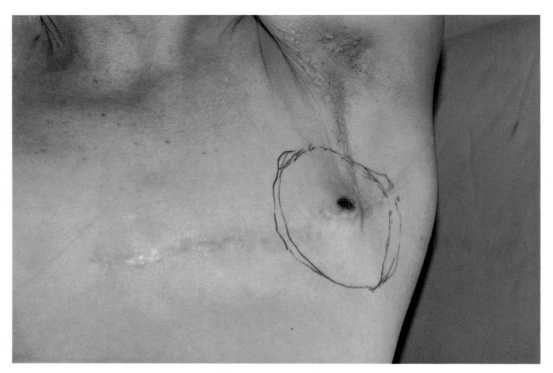

15

Sixty-year-old patient with what was thought to be "persistent" tumor in a three-month-old mastectomy scar. (Case of J.B. McCraw and J.W. Baker)

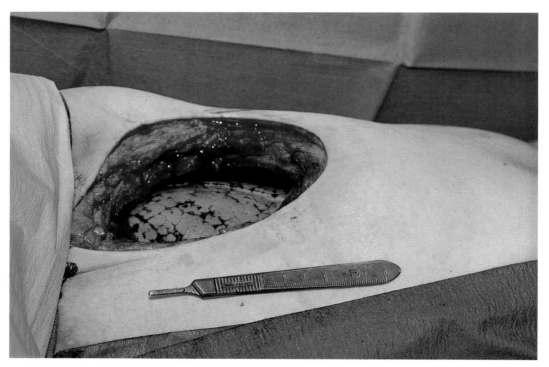

16

The tumor excision included the full thickness of the chest wall. Even though the metastatic survey was unremarkable, a small, recurrent tumor nodule was found on the surface of the lung.

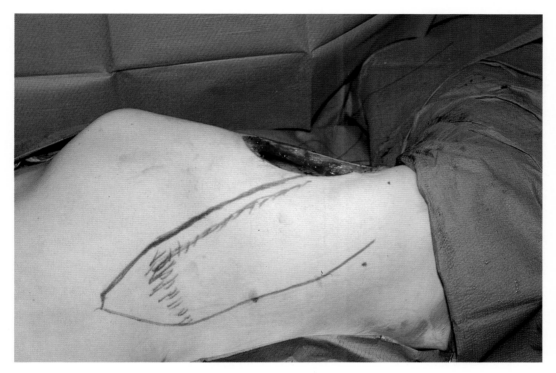

17

Outline of the latissimus dorsi musculocutaneous flap which includes the anterior
half of the muscle.

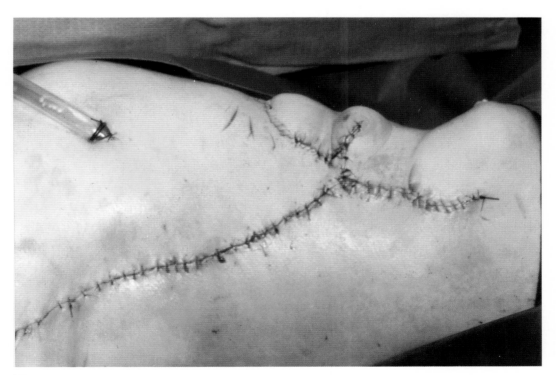

18

The latissimus dorsi muscle was first approximated to the chest wall defect. The
skin was then forcibly contoured to accommodate the muscle closure.

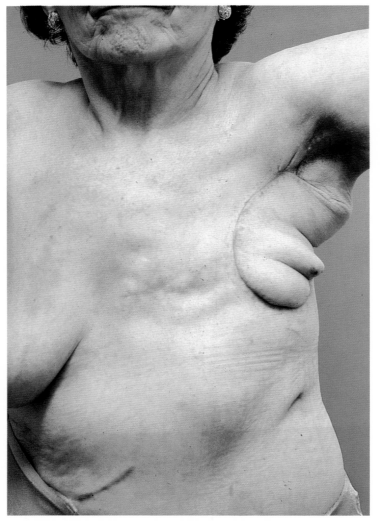

19

Healed myocutaneous flap at one year. This case is of interest because it is the first reported latissimus dorsi myocutaneous flap used for a full-thickness chest wall defect. The ability of the flap to withstand the convoluted closure confirmed the impression that the myocutaneous flap skin is directly supplied by the underlying muscle rather than by longitudinal cutaneous vessels. This simple principle had not been established at that time.

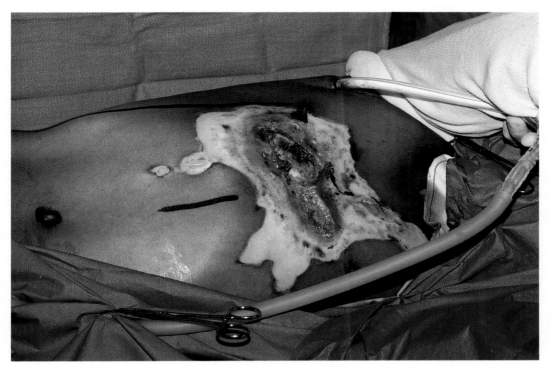

20

Thirty-six-year-old male who sustained a high voltage electrical injury with full-thickness destruction of the chest wall. A chest tube was placed in the axilla to control the sucking chest wound, and the patient was immediately brought to the operating room. (Case of J.B. McCraw and J.W. Baker)

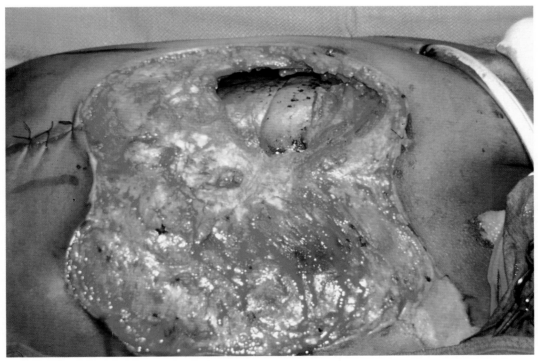

21

Four ribs were excised from the right anterior chest wall. The lower half of the sternum was later removed. The middle lobe of the right lung was also injured by the high voltage injury and a partial lobectomy was necessary.

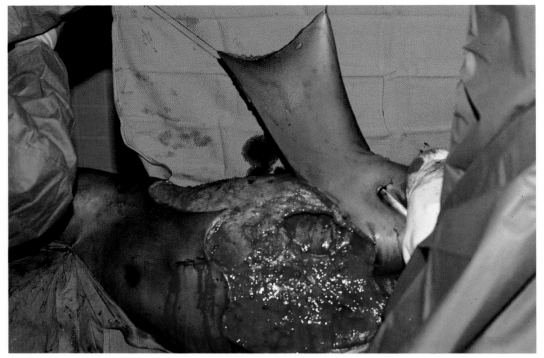

22

The entire latissimus muscle was elevated with a massive amount of skin which extended from the level of the nipple to the iliac crest and to the midline of the back posteriorly.

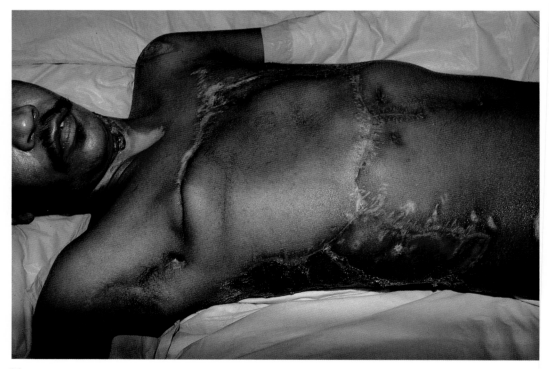

23

Healed flap and donor site at six weeks. The patient eventually returned to his previous employment. The coverage of potentially lethal chest wounds is now a routine matter. In 1976 we were unsure whether such a large myocutaneous flap would survive.

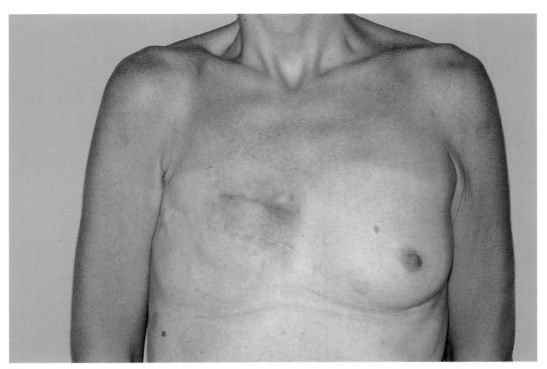

24

Forty-five-year-old woman following a modified radical mastectomy with a chest wall recurrence of breast cancer. (Case of P.G. Arnold)

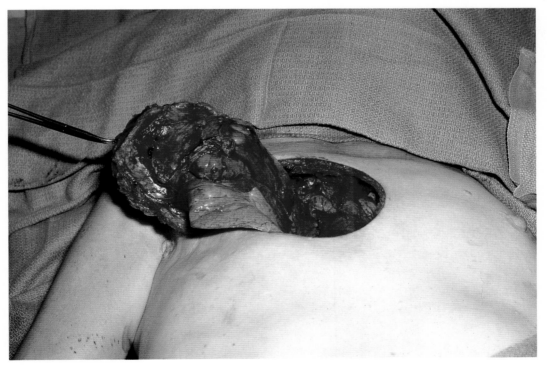

25

The full-thickness chest wall resection includes a portion of the underlying lung which is attached to the tumor.

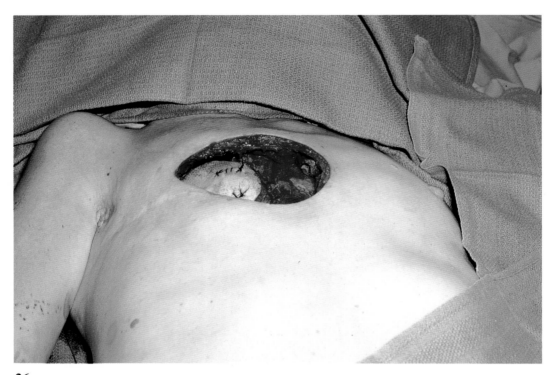

26

Chest wall defect. Gortex® was used to
replace the thoracic skeleton.

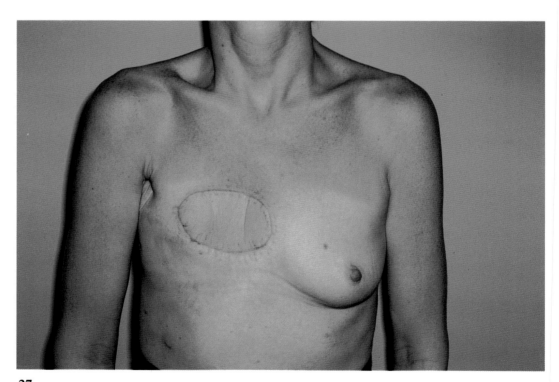

27

A latissimus dorsi myocutaneous flap was
used to correct the soft tissue defect.

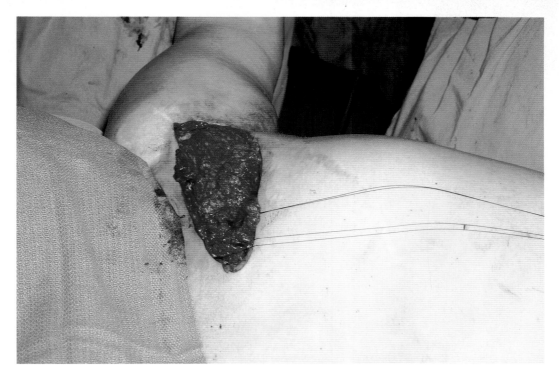

40

The latissimus muscle was transposed over the subclavian vessels and prepared for a delayed skin graft.

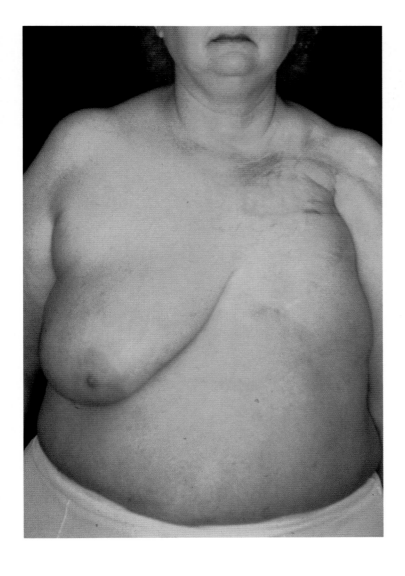

41

Postoperative result at seven months. The wound has remained soundly healed.

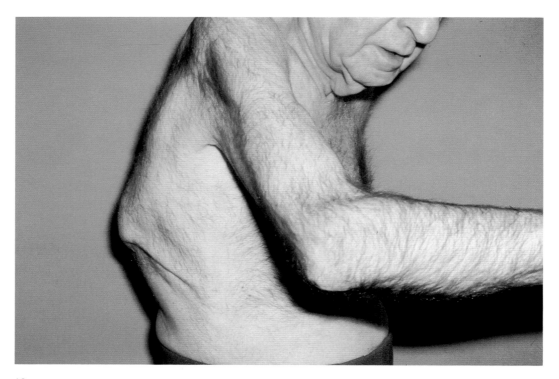

42

Seventy-eight-year-old man with a recurrent sarcoma of the posterior chest. The tumor recurred a few months following a limited local resection. (Case of P.G. Arnold)

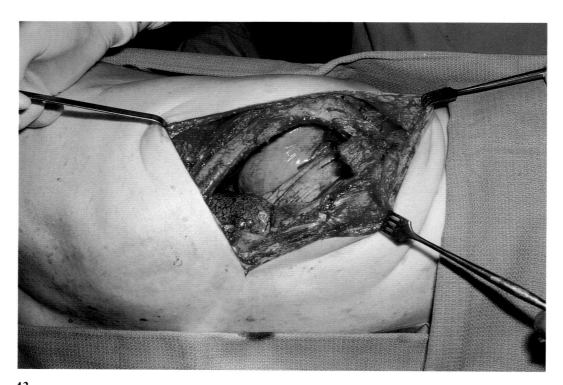

43

The tumor excision included three ribs.

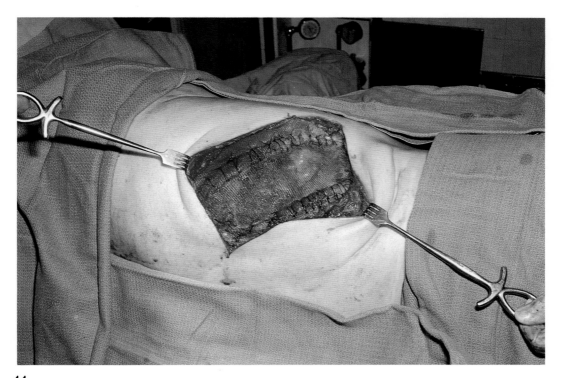

44

The skeletal defect was closed with Prolene® mesh.

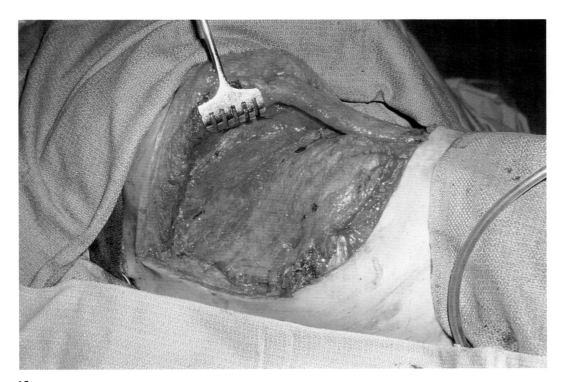

45

A latissimus muscle flap was rotated inferiorly to cover the Prolene® mesh. The skin was closed primarily over the chest wall repair.

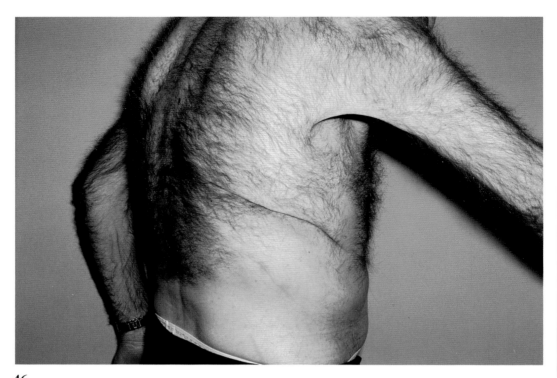

46

Healed wound at two years. The tumor
has not recurred.

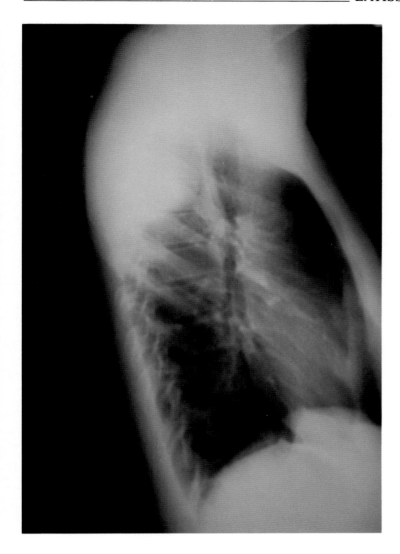

47

Recurrent osteoblastoma of the upper back in a thirty-year-old female, six months following a limited resection. (Case of P.G. Arnold)

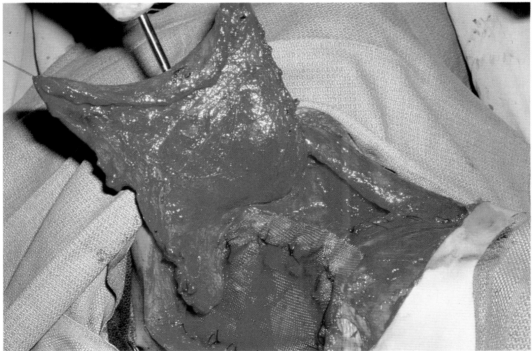

48

The full-thickness chest wall resection included five ribs and the paraspinous muscles. The skeletal defect was repaired with Prolene® mesh.

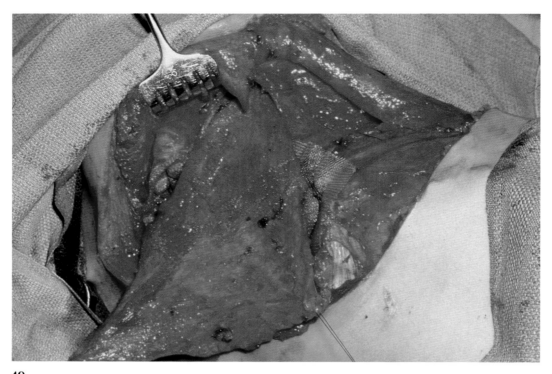

49

Latissimus dorsi muscle flap elevated to cover the Prolene® mesh.

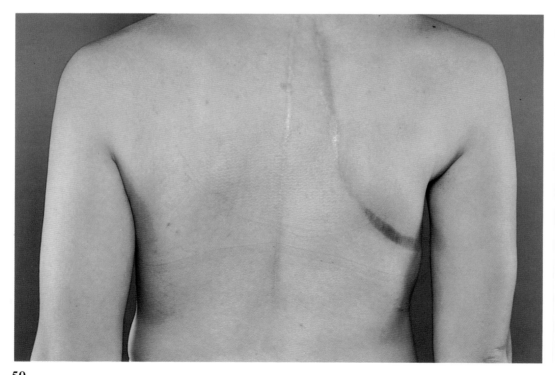

50

Appearance at two years. Note the winging of the scapula which resulted from the removal of the paraspinous muscles.

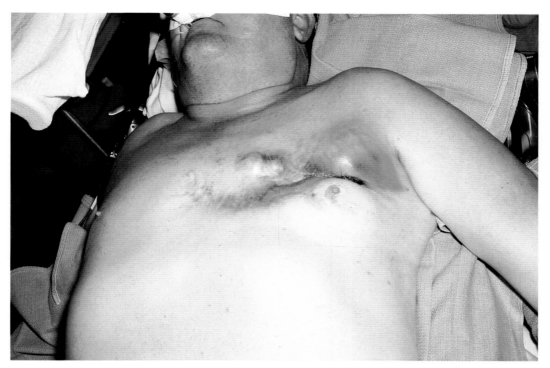

51

Recurrent osteosarcoma of the anterior chest wall in a fifty-six-year-old male. (Case of P.G. Arnold)

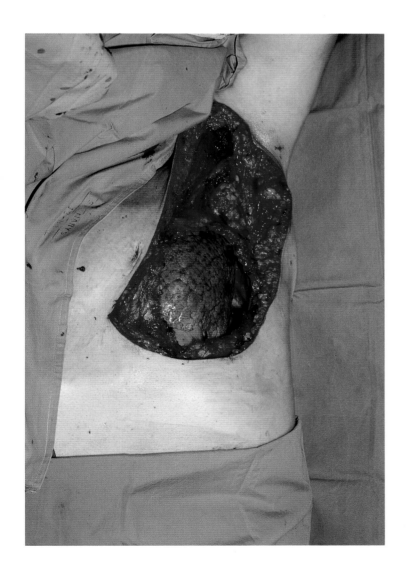

52

The full thickness resection of the tumor included four ribs.

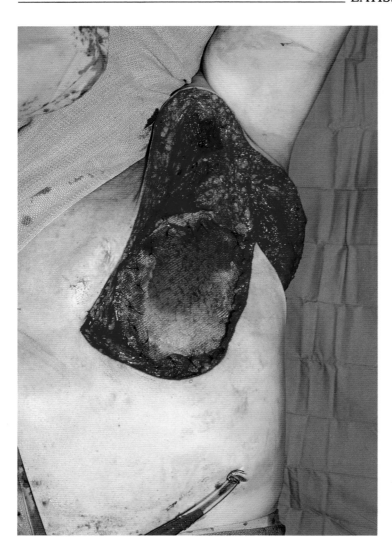

Prolene® mesh stabilization of the chest wall.

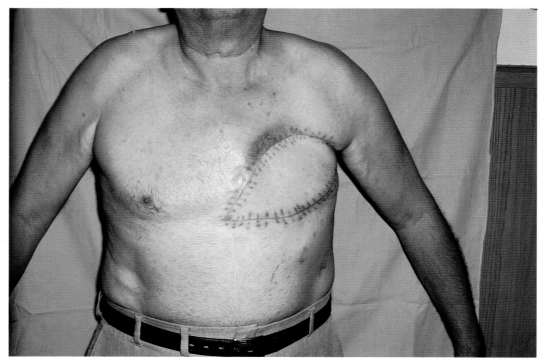

54
Healed latissimus myocutaneous flap at six weeks. The patient has survived nine years.

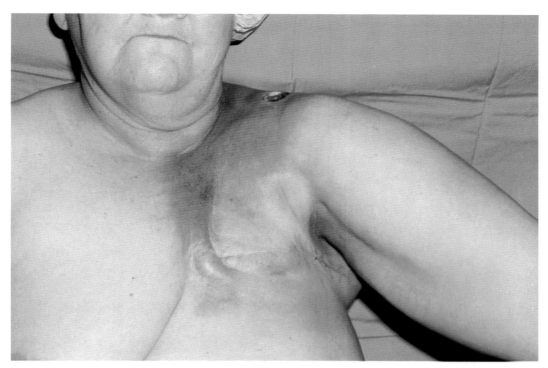

55

Painful osteoradionecrosis of the shoulder ten years following a radical mastectomy and massive irradiation. (Case of P.G. Arnold)

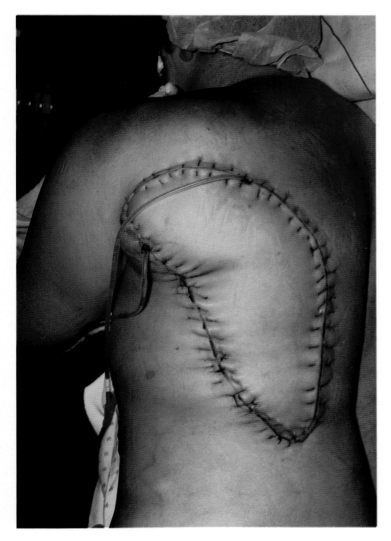

56

Because the thoracodorsal vessels had been heavily irradiated, the cutaneous segment of the flap was "delayed" in this very early case.

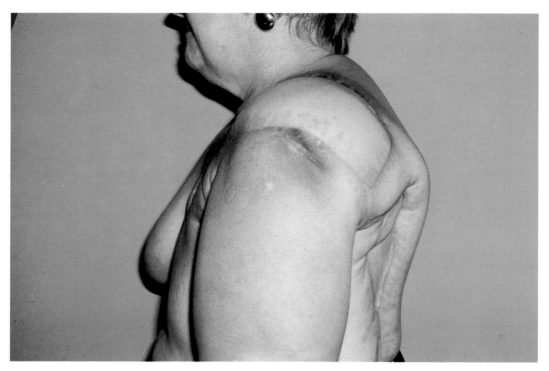

57

Latissimus flap transferred to the shoulder. A skin graft was necessary for the donor site closure. The resulting deformity is significant in this obese patient.

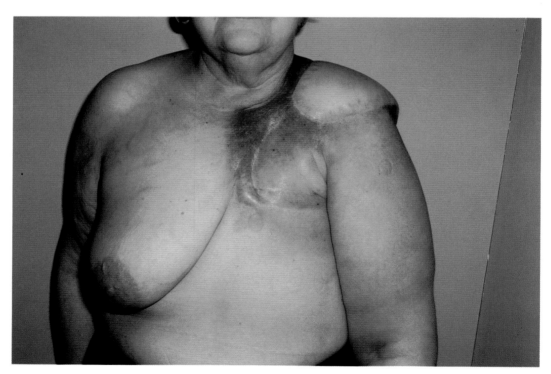

58

Healed flap six months following surgery.

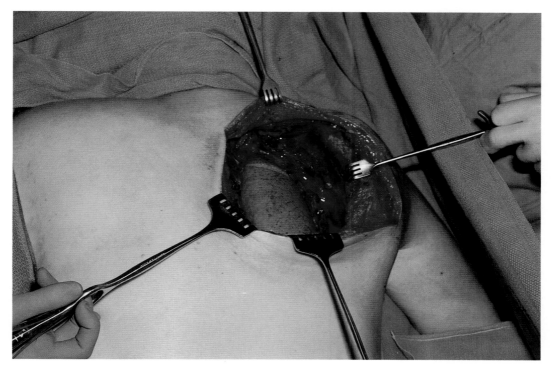

59

Fifty-one-year-old man with a recurrent malignant fibrous histiocytoma of the upper back following a local resection. A wider resection included four ribs and the paravertebral and medial scapular muscles. (Case of P.G. Arnold)

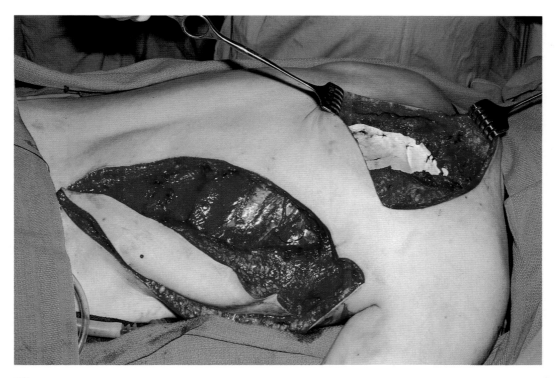

60

Elevated latissimus myocutaneous flap. A Gortex® patch was used for the skeletal defect.

195

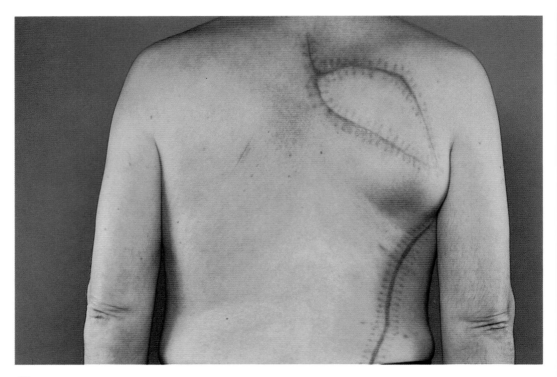

61

Healed flap at six months. The winging of the scapula was caused by the resection of its stablizing musculature.

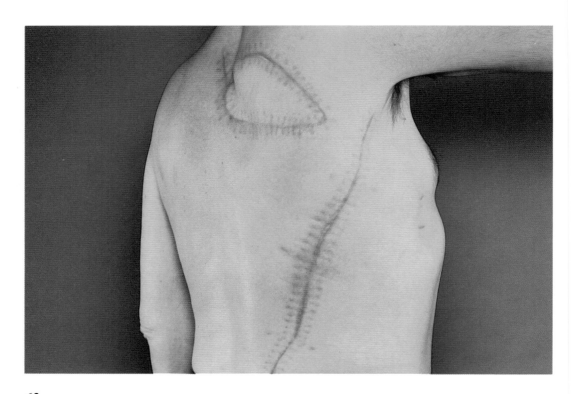

62

The postoperative shoulder motion is acceptable.

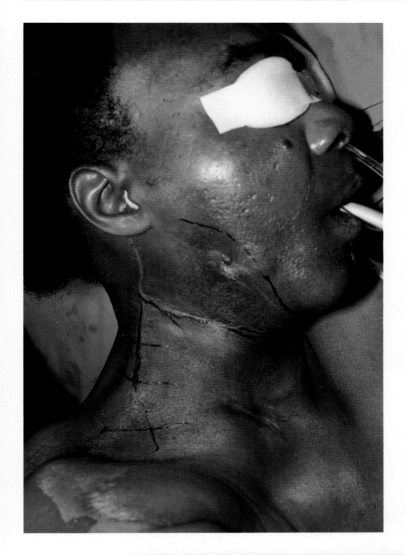

63

Fifty-five-year-old male following a composite resection and irradiation for a tonsillar carcinoma. The reconstructed mandible was grossly infected. A pectoralis "paddle" had previously been used.
(Case of J.B. McCraw and W.P. Magee)

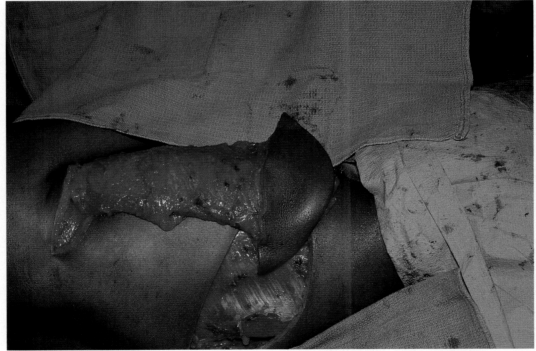

64

A low transverse latissimus dorsi skin "island" was chosen for the mandibular defect. An axillary counterincision was used to retrieve the latissimus muscle from beneath the intervening skin bridge.

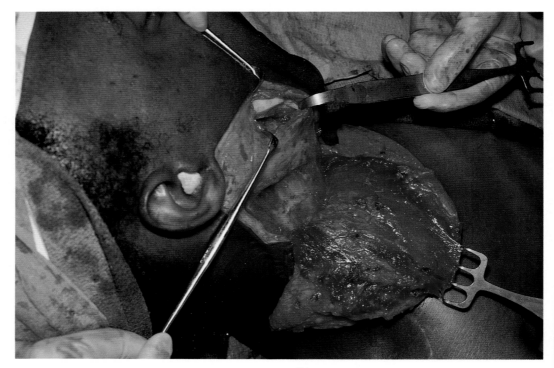

65

Exposure of the infected mandible with the latissimus flap ready for inset.

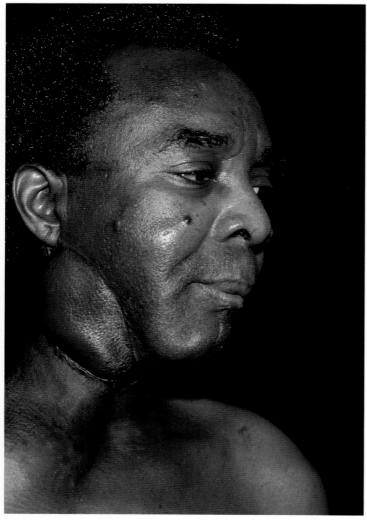

66

Postoperative view of the inset flap at one year.

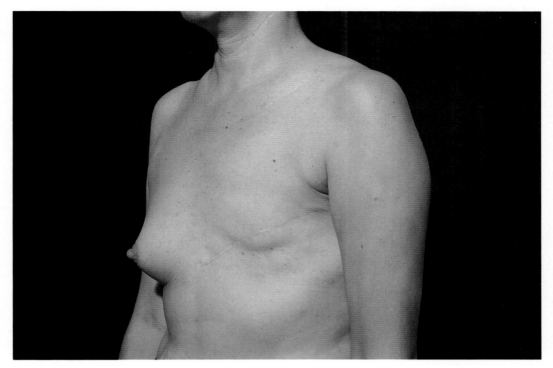

67

Thirty-six-year-old female six months following a modified mastectomy for a poorly differentiated inner quadrant adenocarcinoma. Pathological examination demonstrated seven of ten involved axillary nodes as well as positive internal mammary nodes. The patient insisted on an early reconstruction because of the poor prognosis. (Case of J.B. McCraw)

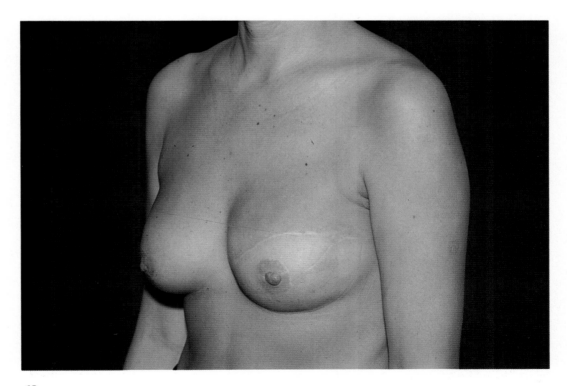

68

A left latissimus breast reconstruction and a right subpectoral augmentation were done seven months following the mastectomy. The nipple-areolar reconstruction was completed one month later.

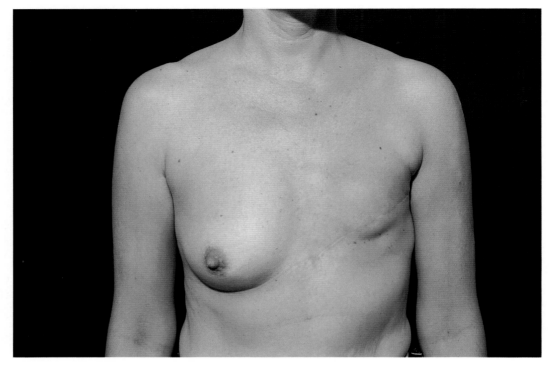

69

Preoperative frontal view. The excellent skin cover and the low and oblique incision were favorable for a latissimus breast reconstruction. The pectoralis muscle was intact and innervated.

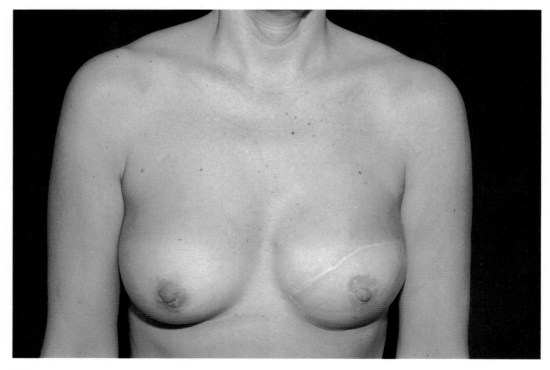

70

Postoperative view at two and one-half years. Both breasts have remained soft. The patient has survived for five years.

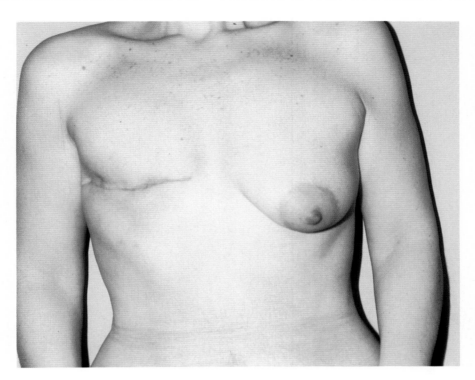

71

Forty-eight-year-old female who had undergone a right modified mastectomy for lobular carcinoma. A ''mirror image'' biopsy of the opposite breast was positive for in situ disease. (Case of P.G. Arnold)

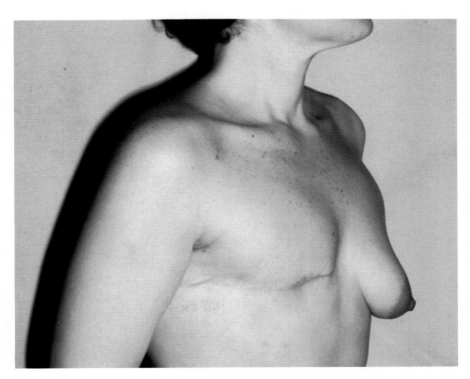

72

The lower half of the pectoralis major was denervated by the dissection of the pectoralis minor.

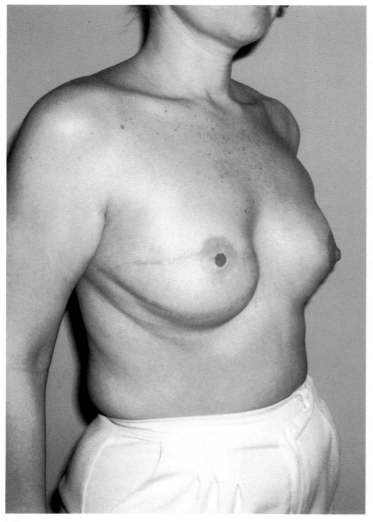

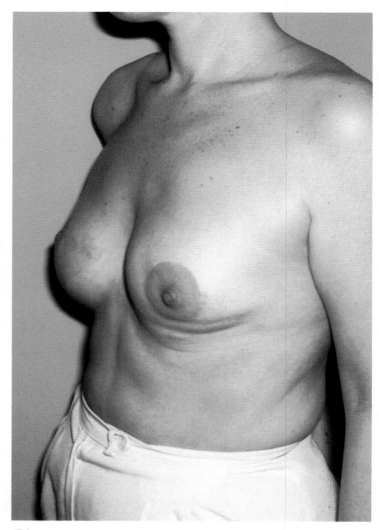

73

One year following a right latissimus dorsi breast reconstruction and a left prophylactic mastectomy and immediate subpectoral reconstruction.

74

The contour and shape of the right latissimus breast reconstruction is better than the left subpectoral breast reconstruction.

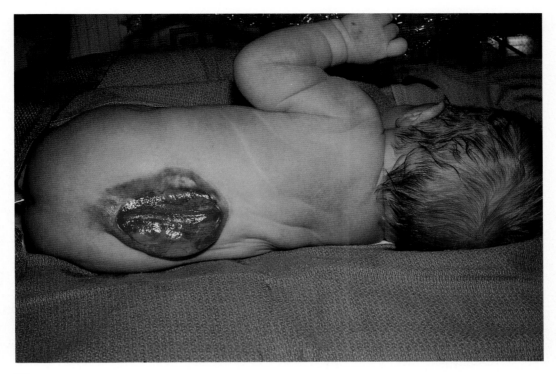

75

This six-hour-old infant was born with a large meningomyelocele. (Case of J.B. McCraw and J. Penix)

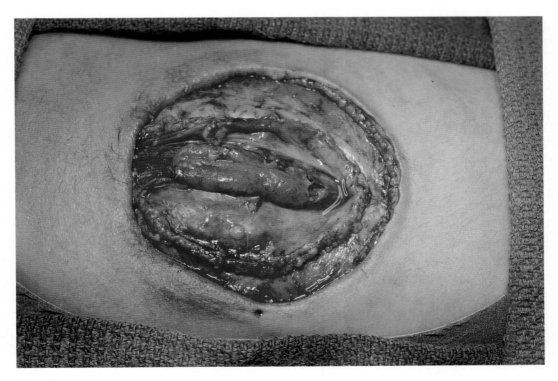

76

Defect remaining following the dural dissection.

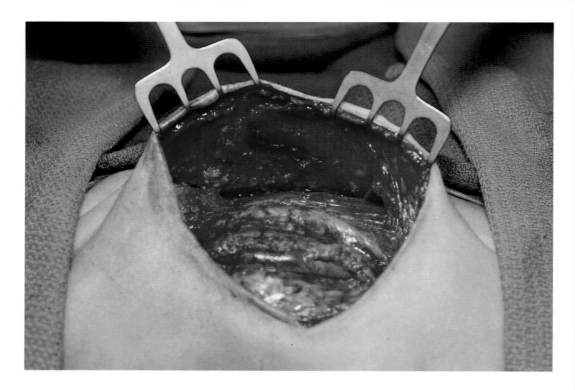

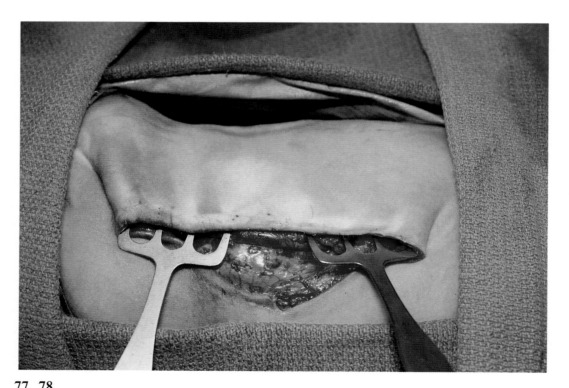

77, 78

Following the dural closure, both latissimus dorsi muscles were elevated as composite flaps. Division of the fascial attachments of the latissimus muscle to the anterior chest wall allows the composite flaps to advance to the posterior midline.

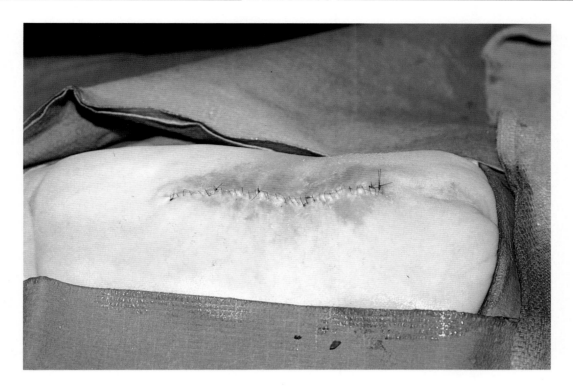

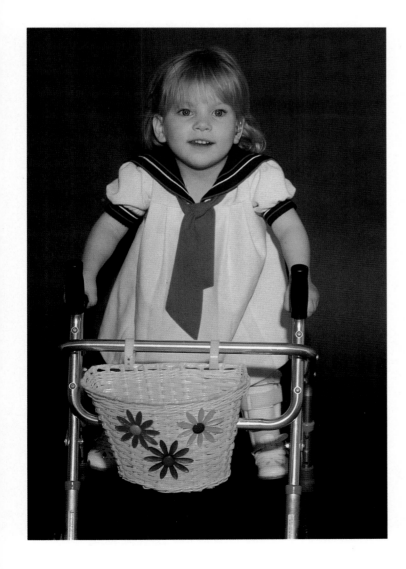

79, 80

The latissimus muscles and the overlying skin of the flaps were closed in separate layers. The patient is able to walk with braces.

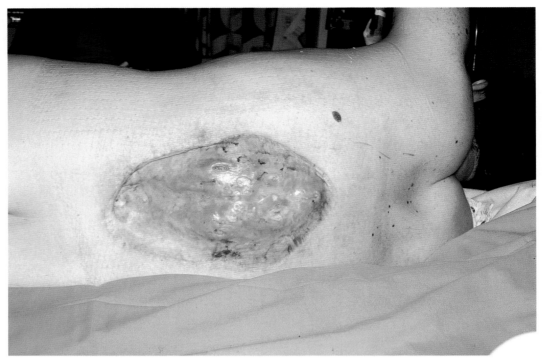

81

This forty-seven-year-old man had previously undergone a resection of a massive spinal cord tumor. The dural defect was skin grafted and heavily irradiated. He was being treated for meningitis which was the result of multiple CSF fistulas in the skin graft. (Case of P.G. Arnold)

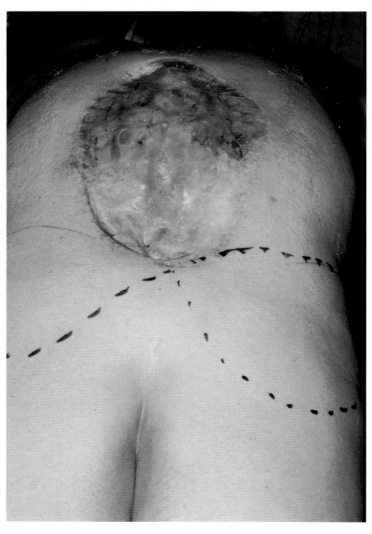

82

Posterior view of the dural skin grafts. Bilateral latissimus dorsi myocutaneous flaps are outlined.

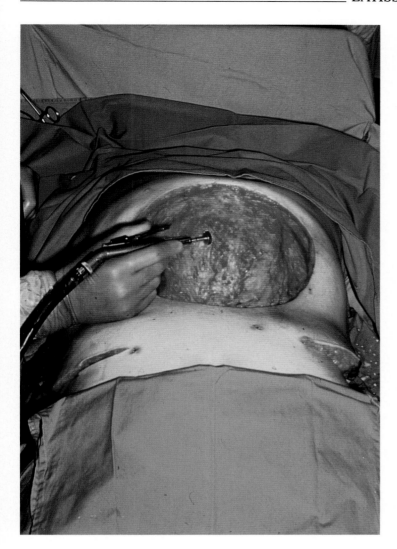

83

The dural skin graft was removed with a motorized wire brush following the elevation of the bilateral latissimus myocutaneous flaps.

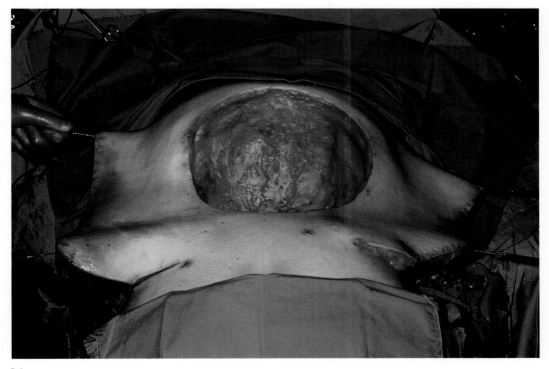

84

The latissimus dorsi myocutaneous flaps are demonstrated with the inferior "backcuts." The flaps were elevated two days earlier at the time of the initial debridement. Neither humeral insertion was divided.

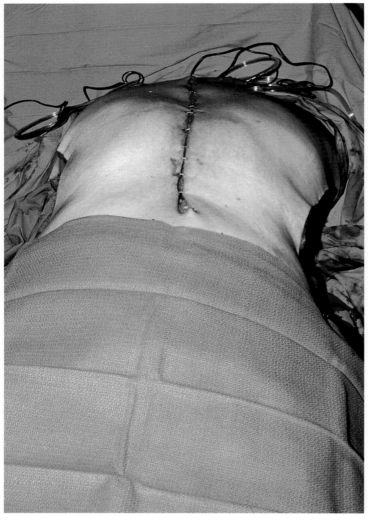

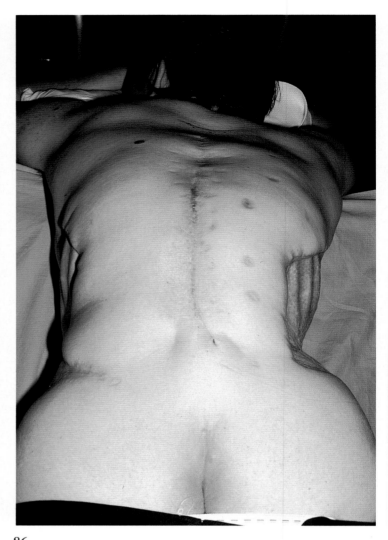

85

The latissimus flaps were approximated in the midline to provide complete muscle coverage of the dura. The flanks were grafted in a delayed fashion.

86

Three years following surgery. The muscular closure accomplished a resolution of the CSF leaks and may have saved the patient from a lethal course of meningitis.

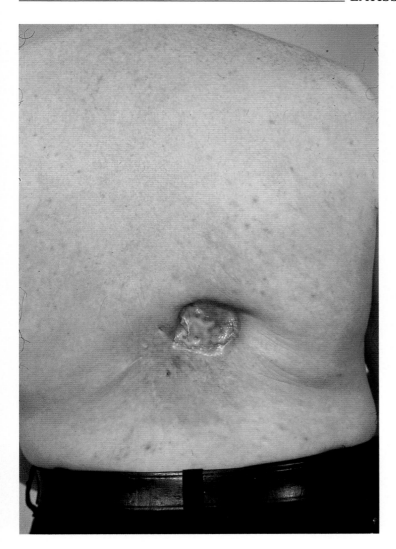

87

Fifty-five-year-old man with a liposarcoma which had been treated with a wide excision and seven thousand rads of external beam irradiation. The irradiation ulcer was caused by a breakdown of recurrent tumor. (Case of J.B. McCraw and J. Penix)

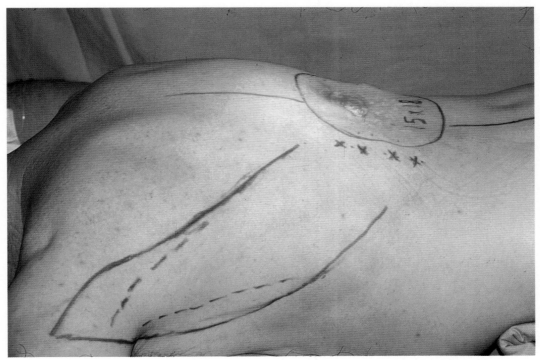

88

Outline of a "reversed" latissimus myocutaneous flap. The posterior perforators are marked with X's. A fifteen by eighteen centimeter tumor resection is planned.

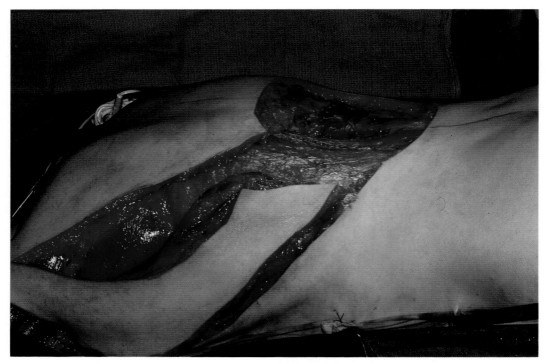

89

The "reversed" latissimus dorsi flap is elevated to the margin of the left paraspinous muscles. The thoracodorsal vessels and the latissimus dorsi muscular insertion have already been divided.

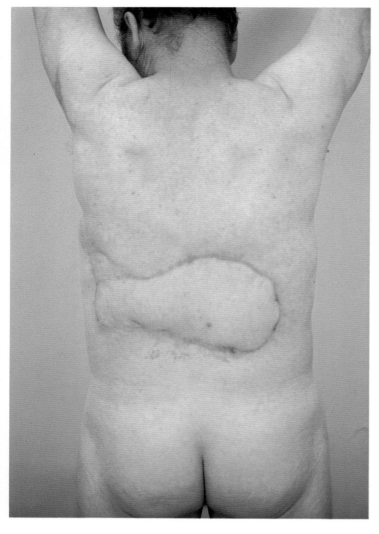

90

The flap was rotated over a 130 degree arc on the posterior perforators. A small split-thickness skin graft was placed on the serratus anterior muscle just above the base of the flap. The patient has been free of disease and ulceration for the eight years following this operation.

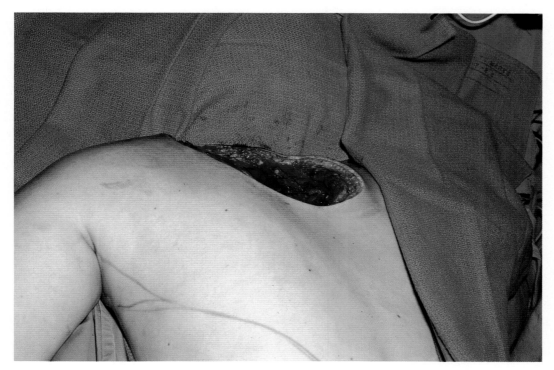

91

Twelve-year-old female with rhabdomyosarcoma of the interscapular region. The wide excision included skin and the underlying paravertebral muscles. (Case of P.G. Arnold)

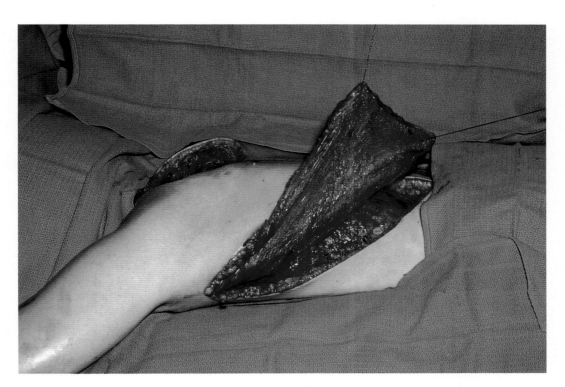

92

The left latissimus dorsi muscle is elevated on its thoracodorsal vessels to cover the exposed thoracic spine.

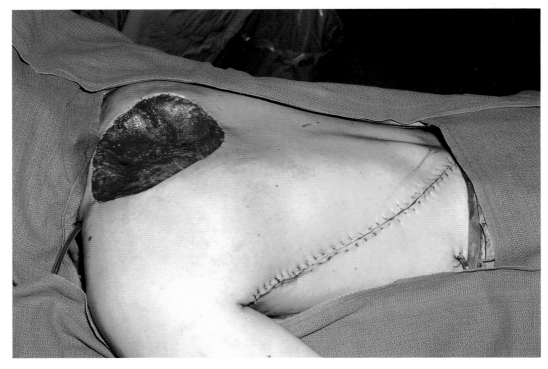

93

The latissimus muscle flap has been tunneled beneath the upper back skin. The donor site was closed directly.

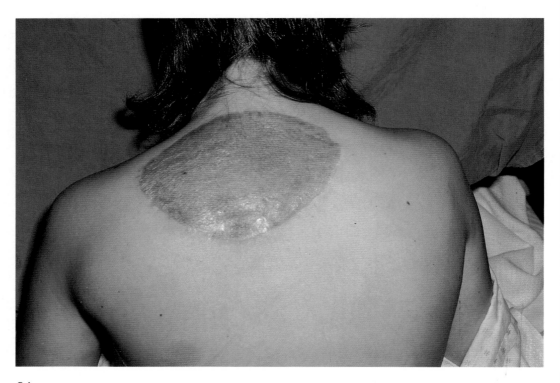

94

Appearance six weeks following the reconstruction.

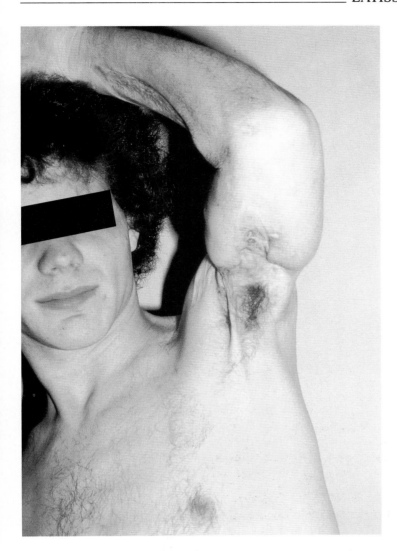

95

This twenty-year-old male presented one year following a complete amputation of the arm at the shoulder and a successful replantation. A latissimus myocutaneous flap will be used to provide surface replacement of the lost axillary and arm skin, functional reconstitution of the lost biceps muscle, and vascularized coverage of nerve grafts to the hand. (Case of P.G. Arnold)

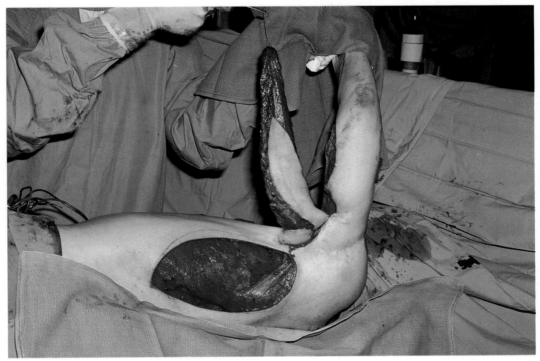

96

The latissimus flap is readied for transfer into the arm.

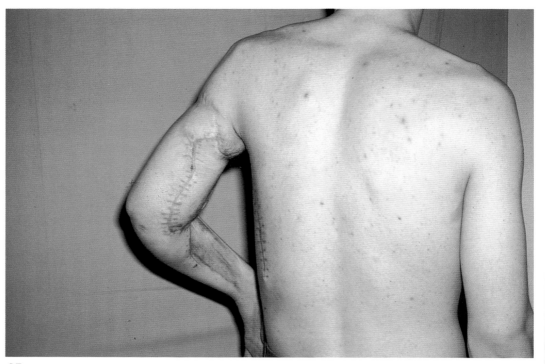

97
Nerve grafting was completed at the time of the latissimus muscle flap transfer to the biceps muscle.

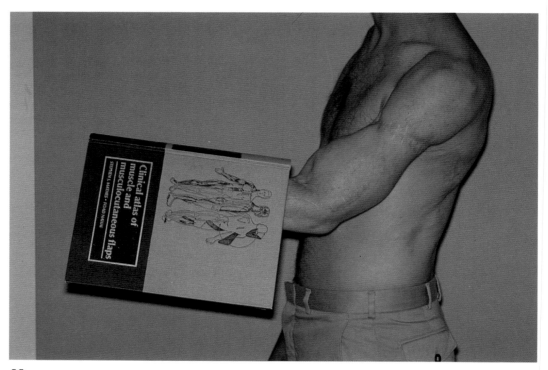

98
The forcefulness of elbow flexion is demonstrated eighteen months following the latissimus muscle transfer to the biceps brachii. He is able to lift the fine book of our friends Steve and Foad.

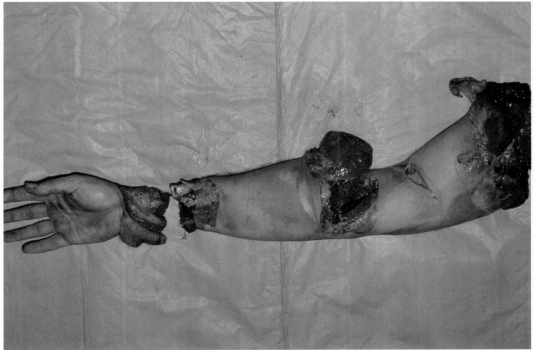

99

Twenty-five-year-old male with a massive avulsion injury of his right arm from an industrial windlass. A replantation was only briefly considered. (Case of J.B. McCraw)

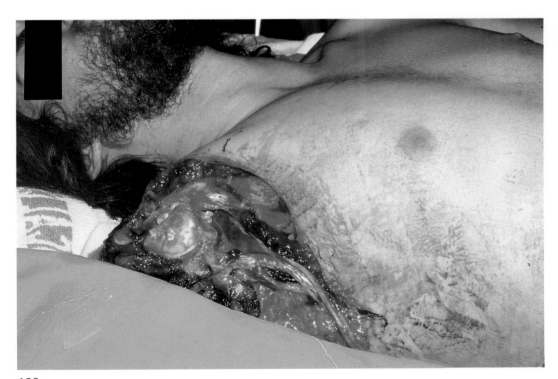

100

The amputation site became grossly infected and the clavicle and glenoid fossa were exposed.

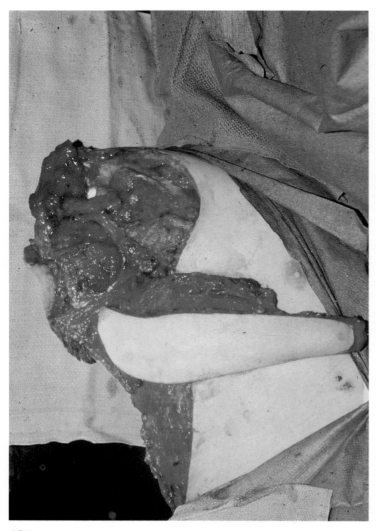

101

A latissimus myocutaneous flap was designed to provide total muscle coverage of the infected shoulder wound.

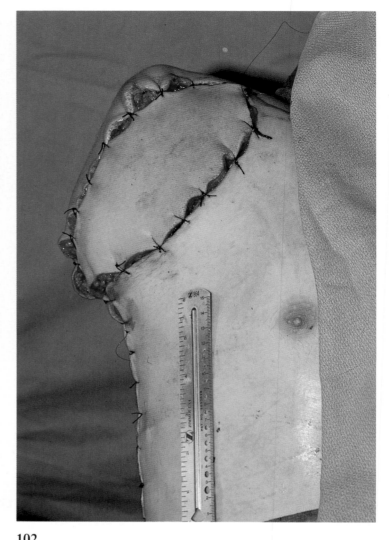

102

This early case demonstrated that the latissimus myocutaneous flap could withstand the significant "crossing tension" which was produced by these temporary 2-0 silk sutures.

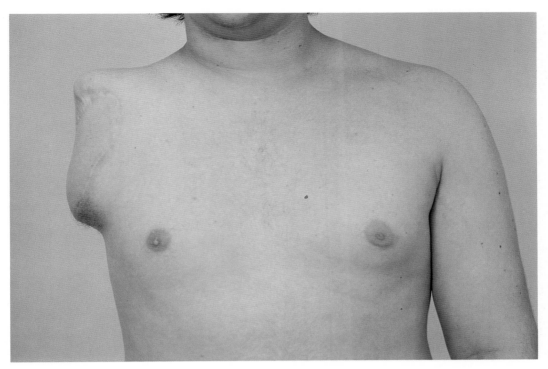

103

The wound healed primarily and the patient was discharged from the hospital on the fifth postoperative day. Had a skin graft been used, approximately three inches of the clavicle would have protruded from the chest wall.

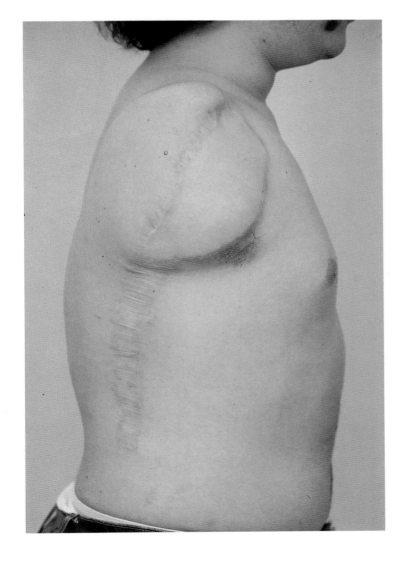

104

The excellent soft tissue coverage enabled the patient to tolerate a heavy arm prosthesis.

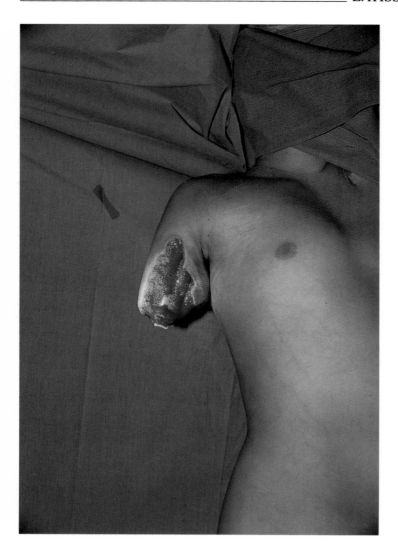

105

Young man with a high amputation from a grain auger injury. Maintenance of stump length was important for the use of an above-elbow prosthesis. A reamputation near the axilla would have been required to cover the exposed bone. (Case of P.G. Arnold)

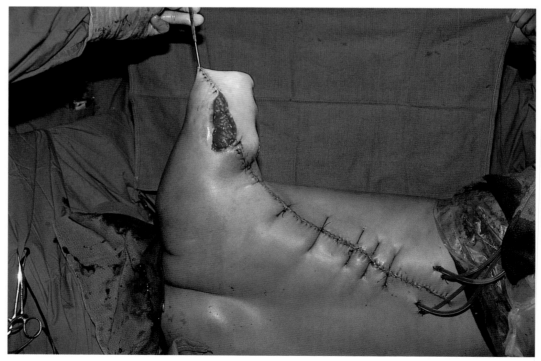

106

Latissimus dorsi myocutaneous flap coverage of the exposed humerus.

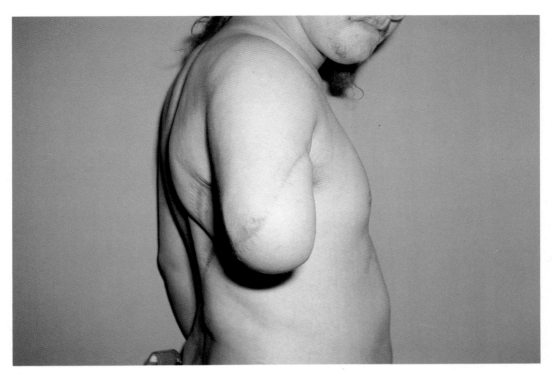

107

Postoperative view at five months. The
full length of the stump was maintained.

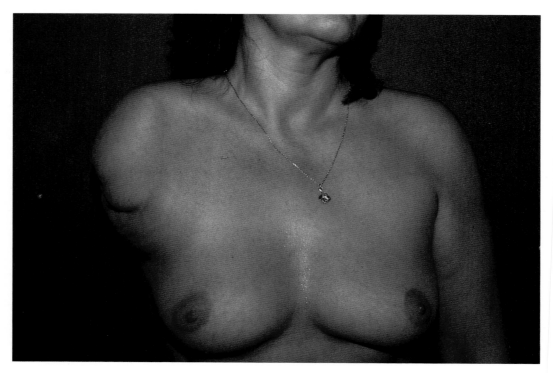

108

Austrian woman with a short above-elbow amputation stump following an auto accident. The patient had no use of the right upper extremity. (Case of C. Papp)

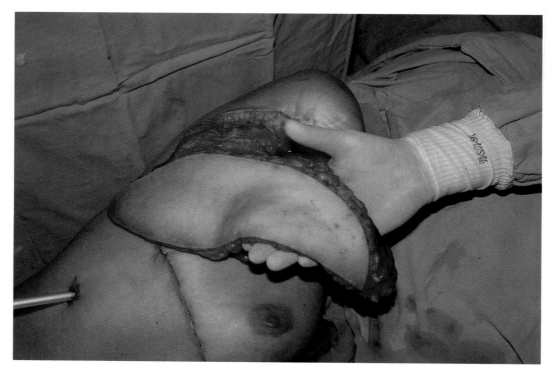

109

Combined latissimus and serratus myocutaneous flap which also contained the sixth and seventh ribs and intercostal muscles.

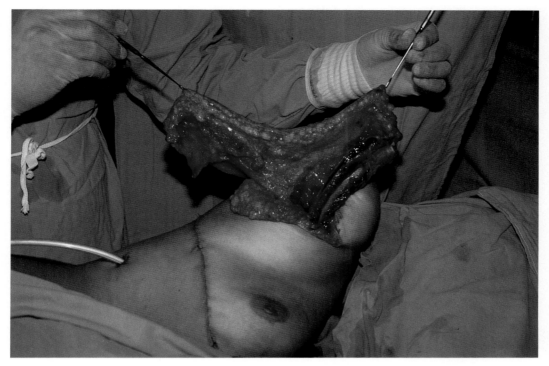

110

The excursion of the composite flap was tethered by the intercostal vessels which were divided. The blood supply to the intercostal muscles and ribs was sustained by the attached chest wall muscles. To maintain the integrity of the intercostal vessels the fourth and fifth ribs could have been used instead of the sixth and seventh ribs.

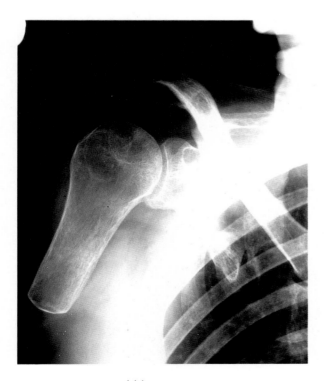

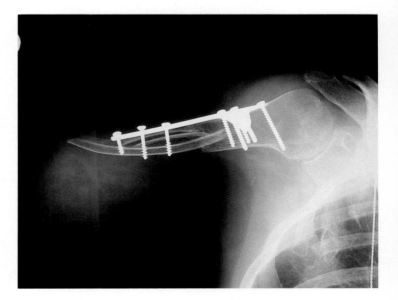

111

X-ray comparison of the preoperative and postoperative amputation stump.

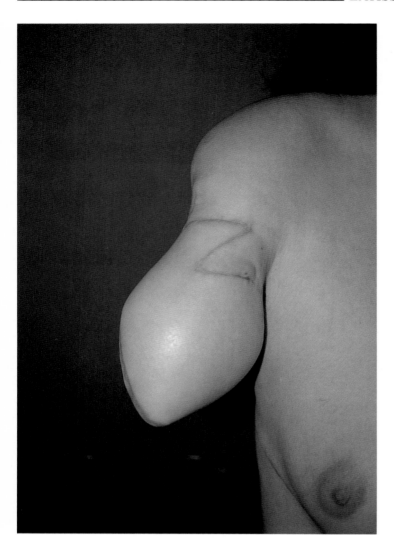

112

Three months following the first procedure, a Z-plasty was performed to reduce lymphadema.

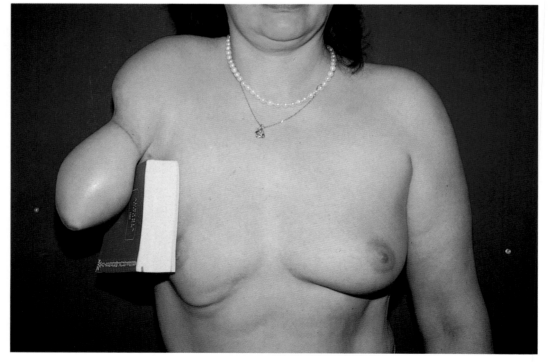

113

The patient is able to hold large objects with the stump and can comfortably wear a prosthesis.

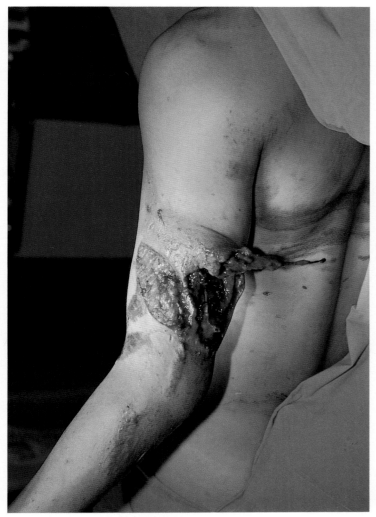
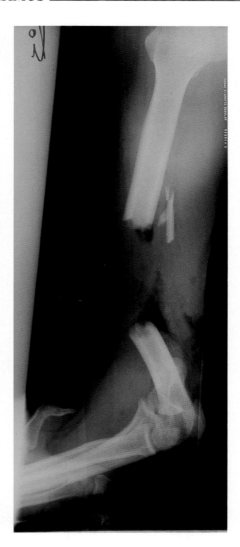

114, 115

Complex injury to the triceps muscle with avulsion of the radial nerve. A 7.5 centimeter segmental loss of the humerus is seen on the x-ray. (Case of C. Papp)

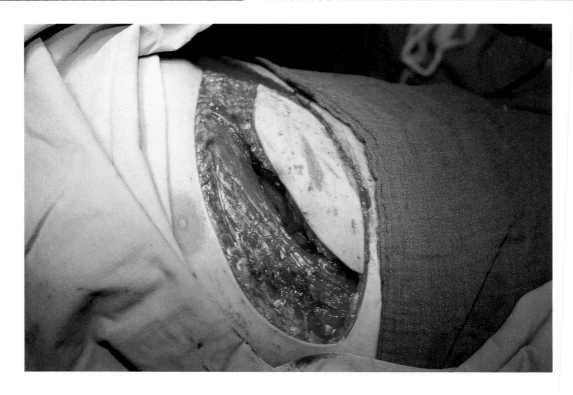

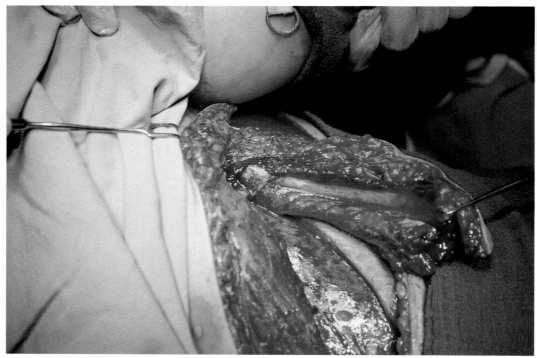

116, 117
Elevated fourth rib with its adjacent intercostal muscles. The overlying skin was
carried with the intercostal flap to replace
the lost arm skin.

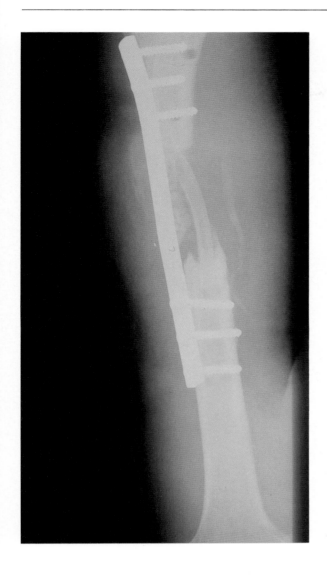

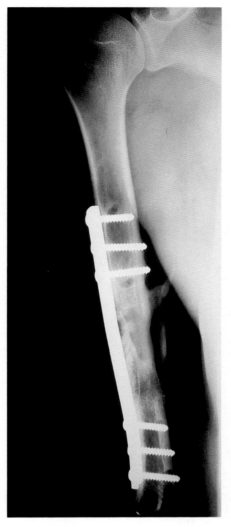

118, 119
X-ray comparison of the healing rib inter-position flap at two months and at two years.

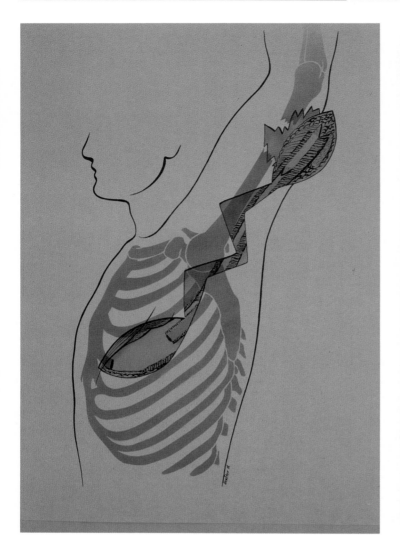

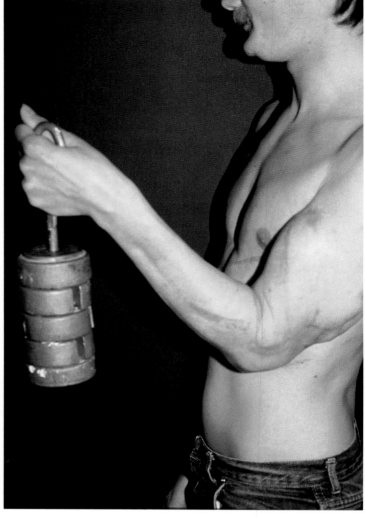

120, 121

Illustration of the route of the "island" intercostal myocutaneous flap. The successful repair of the segmental defect of the radial nerve and the humerus enabled the patient to return to normal activities. He is shown lifting five kilograms.

SERRATUS ANTERIOR

ANATOMICAL CONSIDERATIONS

Surface Markings

Only the anterior border of the serratus anterior muscle can be palpated as it passes from the lower aspect of the anterior axillary line to the medial border of the scapula. The posterior border of the muscle is covered by the larger latissimus muscle and is not palpable. The average size of the serratus anterior muscle is ten by twenty centimeters.

Origin and Insertion

The serratus anterior muscle originates from the anterior surface of the seventh through the tenth ribs and inserts on the costal surface of the vertebral border of the scapula.

Adjacent Muscles

The multipinnate origin of the muscle lies just inferior and lateral to the pectoralis major muscle. In its course toward the scapula the serratus anterior muscle is covered by the latissimus dorsi muscle. The bulk of the serratus anterior muscle is located between the latissimus dorsi and the pectoralis major muscles, where the muscle resides in the hollow between the anterior and posterior axillary folds. In the axillary hollow, the upper part of the serratus anterior muscle is surrounded by the musculature of the shoulder girdle.

Vascular Pattern

The serratus anterior muscle is supplied by two proximal, dominant pedicles which arise in the axilla. The lateral thoracic artery is visible on the lateral surface of the muscle. A branch of the thoracodorsal artery enters the posterior aspect of the serratus muscle before it terminates in the latissimus dorsi muscle. The thoracodorsal branch is the more dominant of the two vessels and consistently arises three to six centimeters cephalad to the vascular leash of the latissimus dorsi muscle.

Motor Nerve

Long thoracic nerve.

Sensory Nerve

Intercostal and long thoracic nerves.

USES

The serratus anterior can be used as a muscle, musculocutaneous, or osteomyocutaneous flap. The muscle flap alone is applicable to chest wall reconstructions which lie within the twenty centimeter arc around the vascular axis in the axilla. The muscle is most often used to vascularize an autogenous rib graft or to cover a foreign body placement such as Prolene® mesh. It can be transposed intrathoracically to reach most areas of the tracheobronchial tree and the heart. Its most common intrathoracic application is in the reinforcement of secondary airway closures such as a bronchopleural fistula, but it also can be used for primary reconstructions of the trachea and the bronchi.

The serratus anterior muscle can also be used to carry its overlying skin as a musculocutaneous flap. This composite flap is most commonly employed in conjunction with the pectoralis major muscle. In this application both of these muscles are elevated with a large amount of skin from the anterior and lateral chest and moved centrally. As an osteomyocutaneous flap, the primary applications have been as ''free'' microvascular transfers. The serratus anterior muscle is recognized as one of the most versatile ''free'' tissue donor sites because of its advantageous features of size and vascular capabilities. Its versatility is expanded by the direct attachment of the muscle to both the underlying ribs and the overlying skin.

REGIONAL FLAP COMPARISONS

Although the serratus anterior muscle is not as large as either the pectoralis major or the latissimus dorsi muscles, it has a similar, robust blood supply and is ideally suited for both intrathoracic and extrathoracic uses. For this reason, it is primarily compared to the latissimus and pectoralis muscles for intrathoracic and extrathoracic reconstructions. The serratus anterior is distinguished from these other two muscles by being more difficult to dissect and by having a more limited arc of rotation. The left pectoralis major muscle is more often used as a reinforcing layer for the ventricular myocardium because it is more accessible. The latissimus muscle is larger but it is usually transected by the standard posterolateral thoracotomy. It is unusual to employ the serratus anterior as a myocutaneous flap since skin is seldom needed in the common chest wall and intrathoracic applications of the muscle flap. The direct adherence of the serratus anterior muscle to the underlying intercostal muscle provides a unique rib-carrying capability which is not offered by the pectoralis major or the latissimus dorsi muscle flaps.

DISADVANTAGES

The primary disadvantage of transposing the entire serratus anterior muscle is the resulting winging of the scapula. The muscle is important for scapular stabilization in overhead arm movements such as the tennis serve. This unique muscular function alone limits the elective application of the serratus anterior muscle flap in certain individuals. It is also less anatomically distinct and more difficult to dissect than either the pectoralis major or the latissimus dorsi muscles. For reasons of convenience the serratus anterior muscle flap is generally not used if one of the other major chest wall muscles is available.

ADVANTAGES

When compared to the latissimus dorsi muscle, the smaller size of the serratus anterior muscle is an advantage in reinforcing a tracheal or bronchial stump. A very large and bulky muscle flap is more a disadvantage than an advantage in this application. The distinct advantage of the serratus muscle is found in situations involving intrathoracic defects following a thoracotomy. The latissimus muscle is usually divided in a standard posterolateral thoracotomy and cannot be transposed as a complete muscle, while the serratus anterior muscle is not divided. The dominant vasculature is found high in the axilla, which facilitates the use of this muscle for both intrathoracic and extrathoracic problems of the upper chest.

COMPLICATIONS, PITFALLS, AND DONOR SITE

The complications involved with this muscle are much the same as its two extrathoracic neighbors, the pectoralis and latissimus muscles. The two dominant vessels of the serratus muscle can be difficult to dissect in their high axillary location, but this feature does allow the muscle to reach most of the superior intrathoracic structures. This excursion of the muscle flap, however, must be facilitated by a second thoracotomy in the region of the dominant vessels. Adequate exposure through retraction of the latissimus dorsi and the pectoralis major muscles is required for the safe removal of the muscle from its origination on the chest wall and its attachment to the scapula. Since this is a dissection over a large area, hematoma and seroma collections must be avoided by meticulous hemostasis and adequate suction drainage.

The donor site is not a significant problem unless a full-thickness chest wall defect is created in the process of elevating an osteomyocutaneous flap. This defect is correctable by the transposition of the latissimus dorsi muscle and should not present a problem with appropriate planning. Winging of the scapula is usually not noticed by the patient, but it can create a problem in the athletic person. Winging of the scapula is a particular concern in elective "free" flap applications when compared to the relative merits of the other available donor sites. For intrathoracic applications this minor functional "trade off" is an inconsequential consideration when compared to the benefits of this muscle flap. Given the choice between the correction of a difficult or life-threatening intrathoracic problem and this functional deficit, the decision is an easy one.

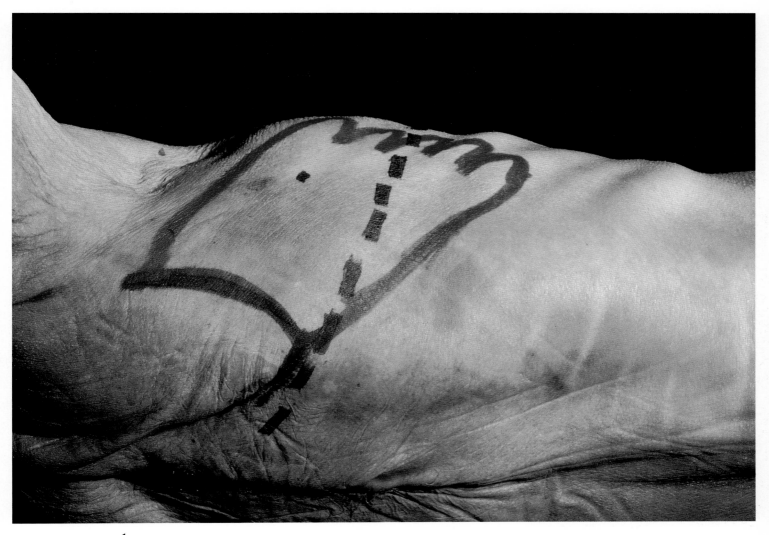

1
The general anatomical location of the serratus anterior muscle is depicted on the back. The scapula is outlined in black.

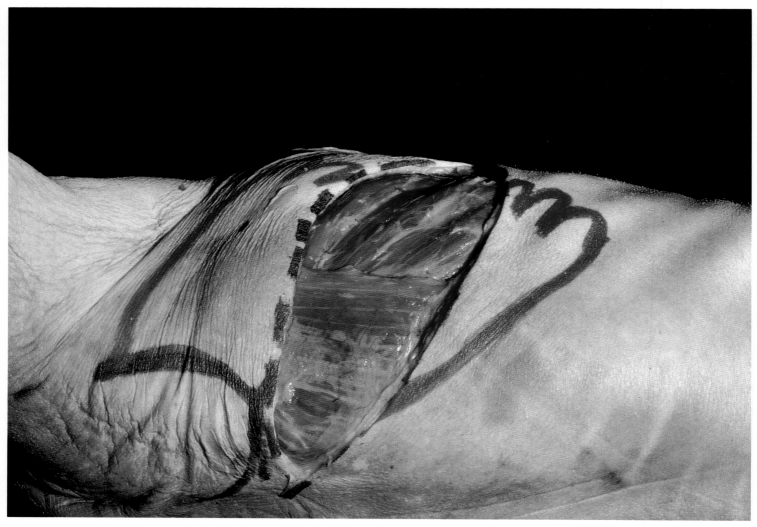

2

The skin incision is made at the level of a standard thoracotomy exposing the latissimus dorsi muscle posteriorly and the "fingers" of the serratus anterior muscular origin.

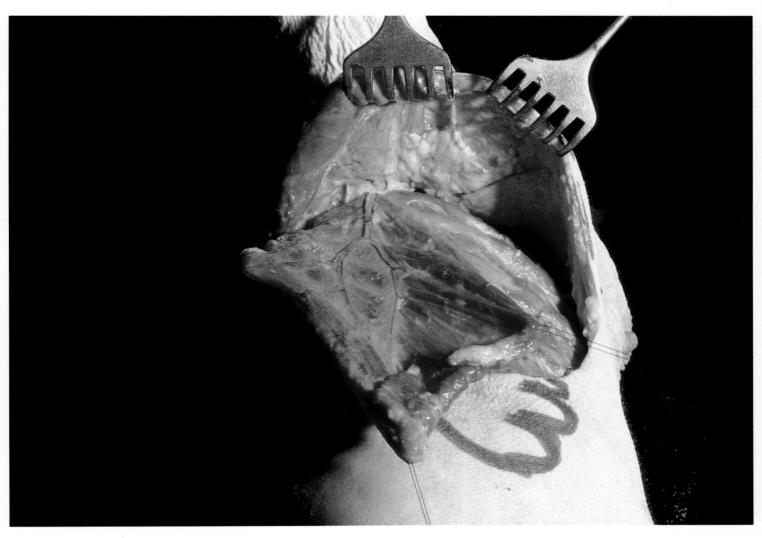

3

The serratus anterior muscle is exposed by dividing and elevating the latissimus muscle. One can readily appreciate the generous blood supply provided by the subscapular artery.

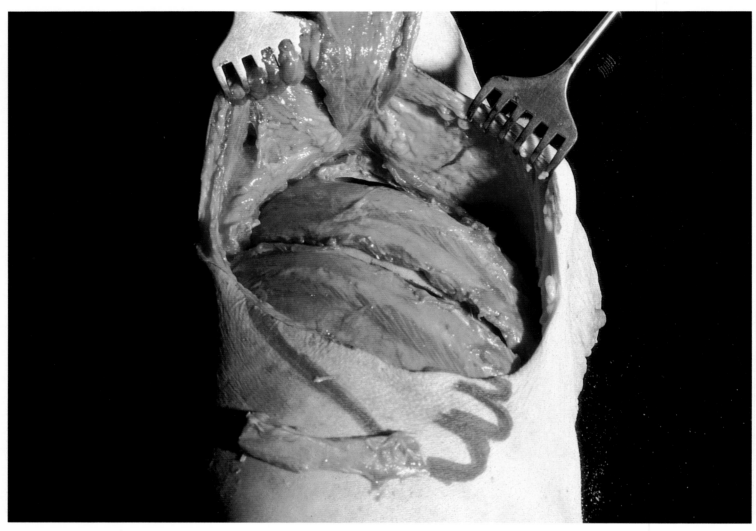

4

The serratus anterior muscle is elevated as an "island" flap and retracted. Thoracotomies have been placed in the second and fifth interspaces. The "second" thoracotomy is created by removing approximately a nine centimeter segment of the second rib near the vascular axis.

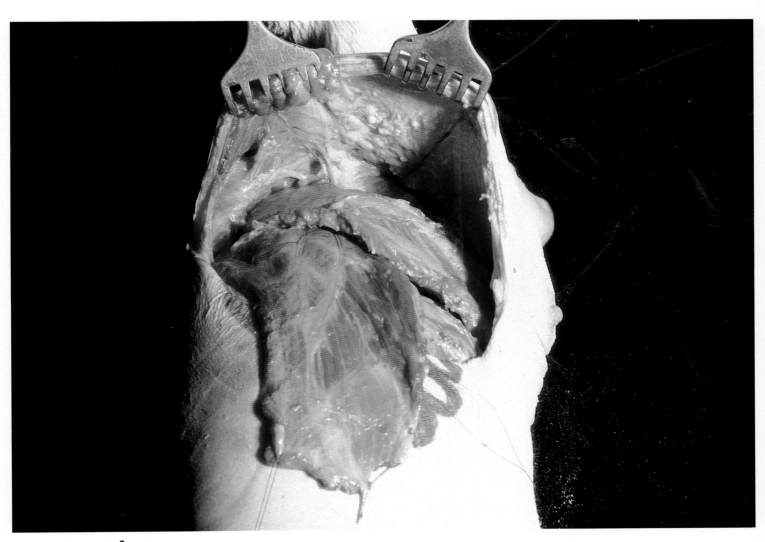

5

The "island" serratus muscle flap is passed into the chest through the second interspace and out of the chest through the fifth interspace to demonstrate the amount of muscle available for intrathoracic transposition.

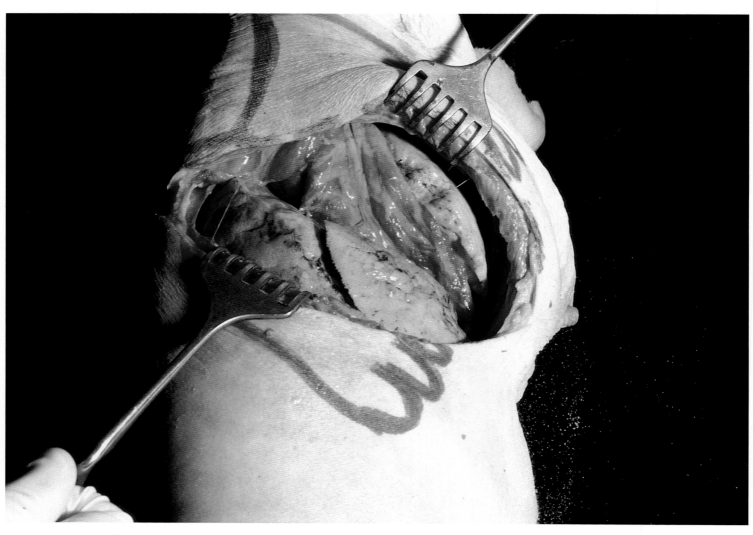

6

The serratus anterior muscle is then passed into the chest through the new thoracotomy at the level of the second interspace. The flap easily reaches all of the mediastinal structures.

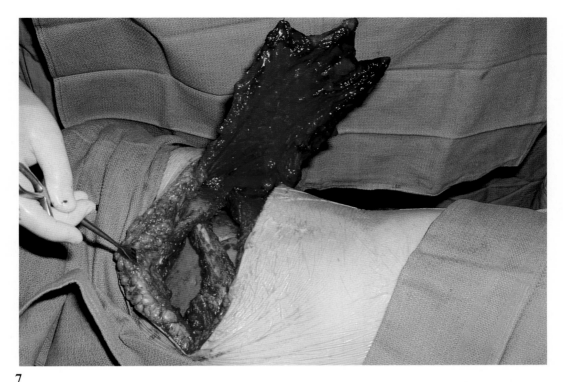

7

This sixty-nine-year-old man presented with a carcinoma of the lung which had invaded the posterior chest wall. A combined resection of the lung and a three rib incontinuity chest wall resection has been completed. The serratus anterior muscle is elevated and readied for transposition over the chest wall defect. (Case of P.G. Arnold)

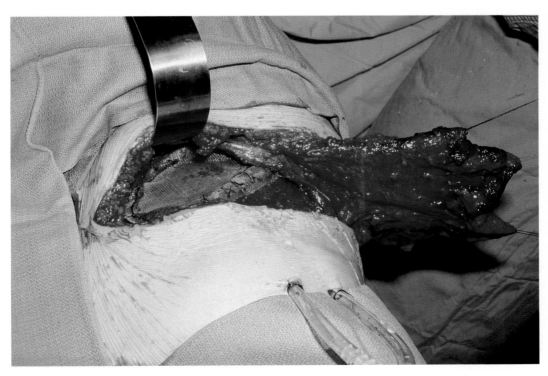

8

The posterior thoracic wall defect has been reconstructed with Prolene® mesh. The large serratus muscle is retracted.

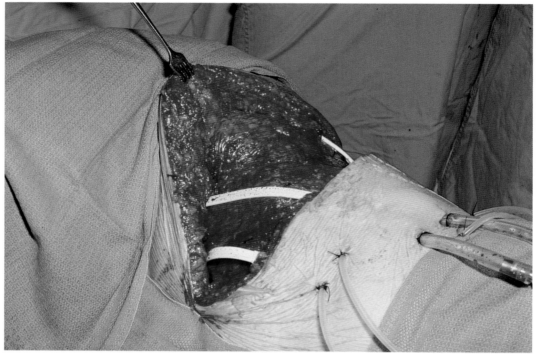

9

The serratus muscle flap is transposed over the Prolene® mesh. Multiple drains have been placed. The overlying skin will be closed primarily.

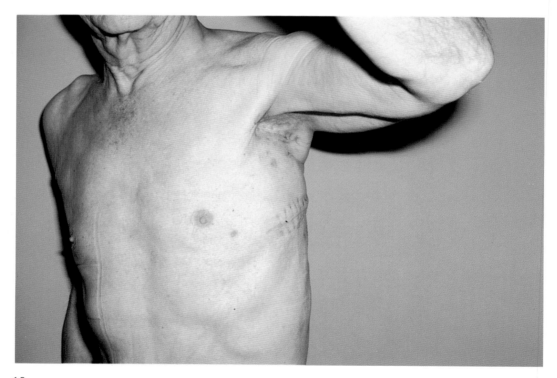

10

Appearance of the patient six months following the surgery.

INTRATHORACIC MUSCLE FLAPS

INTRODUCTION

The use of an intrathoracic muscle transposition to correct a bronchopleural fistula was first described in the early Twentieth Century by Abrashanoff (1911) and later by Kanavel (1921). Since that time intrathoracic muscle flaps have been used to reinforce bronchial stump closures, obliterate empyema cavities, and bolster problem suture lines of the trachea, esophagus, heart, and great vessels. When compared to open and infected wounds of the extremity and trunk, the same problems within the chest cavity can be precipitous and life-threatening. Because of the unusual nature of these procedures, the special technical considerations are reviewed in this chapter.

GENERAL CONSIDERATIONS

The most commonly used muscles in these types of procedures have been the serratus anterior, the pectoralis major, the latissimus dorsi, and the rectus abdominis muscles. The first three muscles are always transposed into the intrathoracic position through a separate thoracotomy to improve their arc of rotation. This access is gained by removing five to ten centimeters of one or more ribs. The pectoralis major muscle flap is usually introduced through the second rib bed in the midaxillary line. The latissimus dorsi muscle flap is passed into the chest through a second rib thoracotomy in the posterior axillary line. The serratus anterior muscle is introduced at approximately the same level in the midaxillary line. All of these "second" thoracotomies are placed near the axis of rotation of the muscle flap so the dominant vasculature will not tether a "straight shot" into the thorax. The most direct passage for the rectus abdominis muscle flap is through the anterior leaf of the diaphram, which is a harmless maneuver. The superiorly based rectus abdominis muscle flap is a distant choice for intrathoracic problems because of its remote location and its inability to reach the upper thorax.

CHOICE OF MUSCLE FLAPS

When the intrathoracic problem is isolated, such as a "clean" reinforcement of a tracheal suture line or a bronchial stump closure, a small, malleable, and accessible muscle is ideal. The fourth and fifth intercostal muscles do produce a major chest wall donor defect, but they do fill these criteria and have excellent suture

retention capabilities. The rectus abdominis muscle flap is unusual to consider because of its remoteness. One of the three major extrathoracic muscle flaps — latissimus, pectoralis, or serratus — is usually chosen, even for isolated defects, because of its reliability and accessibility. The location of the existing thoracotomy is the most important factor in this choice of muscle flap since it is easier to use a muscle which lies nearest to the existing thoracotomy.

A previous standard posterolateral thoracotomy is the most common reason for not using the latissimus muscle flap. The previously divided latissimus muscle will survive in situ on its respective proximal and distal blood supplies, but the total muscle will not survive elevation as a proximally based muscle flap. The remaining "stump" of the latissimus can be used to provide bulk even though its full length is not serviceable as a standard muscle flap. Although the latissimus muscle is criticized because of its bulk, the anterior portion of the muscle can be skeletonized on the dominant vascular bundle to provide a long, thin flap. More often, its bulk is an advantage.

The pectoralis major muscle is usually not injured during a standard thoracotomy, and this is a common reason to choose it instead of the latissimus muscle flap. It is a large muscle, and the mobilization requires a significant amount of dissection. The accessibility of the pectoralis muscle flap to the upper chest and mediastinum is its major commending feature. The donor site deformity of this reliable flap is its most detractive feature. When transposed to the intrathoracic position, the large pectoralis muscle occupies a considerable space. This is of great benefit when obliterating an upper lobe empyema cavity, wrapping the aortic arch, reinforcing the anterior surface of the heart, or repairing a fistula between the trachea and the great vessels. Like the latissimus muscle flap, the pectoralis major muscle can be skeletonized along the distribution of its dominant vasculature. Both of these muscles are known for their poor suture retention capabilities.

The serratus anterior muscle is ideally located for intrathoracic transposition. It is relatively thin and quite malleable. Its dual proximal blood supply is consistent and durable. The muscle can be transposed comfortably around the mediastinal structures, including the carina, the esophagus, and the trachea. The serratus muscle is usually available since it is seldom transected in the standard thoracotomy. It is our first choice for reinforcement of bronchial stumps, tracheal closures, and other hilar structures.

The rectus abdominis muscle can be used when the previously described muscles have already been used or are absent for some other reason. Other muscles have been utilized as "free" microvascular transfers inside the chest in the rare circumstance in which the latissimus, pectoralis, serratus, and rectus abdominis muscles are not available.

CLINICAL SITUATIONS

Bronchopleural fistula

Bronchopleural fistula with empyema is a dreaded but fortunately an uncommon complication following lobectomy or pneumonectomy. It is even more problematic when previous radiation therapy has been employed. Radiation therapy alone with "cavitation" of the pulmonary parenchyma can also be a cause of empyema.

The first step in wound management is to control the empyema cavity by removing the appropriate number of ribs in a dependent drainage area. This extensive exposure not only allows the cavity to drain but also gives complete access to the infected chest cavity itself for wound care. Irrigation and dressing changes over a variable period of time (days to months) may be necessary before a surgically "clean" wound can be obtained. Ideally it is desirable to wait until the wound is clean before an extrathoracic muscle is transposed into the area of the leak either to plug the leak or to reinforce a direct secondary closure. Once the extrathoracic muscle is transposed over the leaking bronchus, it is simply dressed with an occlusive dressing. The thoracic "window" provides access for pleural drainage and further dressing changes. The dressing is usually changed every twenty-four to forty-eight hours or until the muscle has become firmly "stuck" and sealed the bronchial leak. Once the bronchopleural fistula is under control, consideration can be given to the closure of the chest wall itself. This is usually done by instilling an antibiotic solution and closing the skin directly. Occasionally a thoracoplasty may be necessary to collapse the stiffened chest wall. The authors personally prefer the Clagett procedure, which is a direct skin closure over the antibiotic-filled chest cavity. Before this closure can be successful, the empyema cavity must be controlled, and the bronchopleural fistula must be sealed by the muscle flap closure.

Threatened bronchopleural fistula

When a patient has undergone radiation therapy for a malignancy and a so-called "completion pneumonectomy" is indicated, it is helpful to reinforce the bronchial stump closure with a muscle flap transposition. In a clean wound without an empyema it is reasonable to transpose the muscle over the bronchus and to close the thorax directly as in any other pneumonectomy. If there is any question we would tend to dress the thoracic cavity with an occlusive dressing and close it only when the wound is surgically "clean" and the bronchial stump closure has been secured by a healed muscle flap. This tentative approach is taken in view of the relative ischemia of radiated bronchial stumps and the possible sequelae of a bronchial leak.

Empyema

Occasionally a small tuberculous empyema may be present in the upper lobe region and occupy only a small percentage of the overall thorax. In this situation decortication procedures may not allow the lung to expand adequately and obliterate the thoracic space. It is possible to transpose either the pectoralis major or the latissimus dorsi to obliterate such a small space. It is impossible to fill the entire hemithorax with the extrathoracic muscles since their mass does not nearly approximate the volume of the normal hemithorax.

Reinforcement of suture lines of the heart and great vessels

The pectoralis major muscle has been the most commonly used muscle in this particular situation because of its accessibility. If the suture line in the heart or great vessels is somewhat precarious because of previous irradiation or active infection, it seems reasonable to reinforce these closures with a well-vascularized muscle flap.

Esophageal repair

Complicated esophageal repairs are known to be associated with disastrous complications related to failures of wound healing. If it is necessary to mobilize the esophagus extensively so a direct esophageal repair can be accomplished, it seems reasonable to reinforce this repair with transposed, healthy muscle. A muscle flap does not harm the esophageal motility, and it can prevent a suture line leak and a possibly fatal mediastinitis in this single layer closure.

SUMMARY

Intrathoracic infections, which eventually result in a residual pleural space and a bronchopleural fistula, have been consistent and dreaded complications of pulmonary surgery. Intrathoracic infections and irradiation in association with cardiovascular reconstructive procedures have been equally perplexing. Treatment of these life-threatening infections has included antibiotic irrigations, pulmonary resections, and extensive thoracoplasty. All of these methods have had some success, but failure is usually the result of a persistent pleural space which leads to an empyema and eventual breakdown of the intrathoracic repair.

Muscle appears to be the ideal tissue to place in the contaminated or infected intrathoracic wound. The ability of the muscle to combat local contamination has been clearly demonstrated experimentally by Chang and Mathes and confirmed clinically by all of us who have performed muscle flaps under these circumstances. Elsewhere in the body, excellent results have been obtained in reconstructive operations using muscle flaps to close soft tissue defects which are the result of radiation necrosis, trauma, or infection. It follows that an intrathoracic problem with the same origin can be treated similarly.

This is not to say that muscle transpositions are indicated in all patients with chronic intrathoracic infections. Many patients with pleural space infections can be adequately managed with tube thoracostomy drainage, decortication, and systemic antibiotics. Those patients who do not respond to this conservative regimen can often be successfully managed by decortication of the lung, by advancement of the diaphragm, by creation of a pleural tent, or by a limited thoracoplasty. When these methods are unsuccessful or seem likely to fail, an intrathoracic muscle transposition becomes a reasonable alternative. It is certainly applicable in patients with a chronic bronchopleural fistula, especially in association with irradiation or destructive lung disease. In these patients conventional pulmonary resection is difficult because the remaining lung often has restrictive lung disease, which prevents postoperative expansion. Muscle transposition has been most helpful in patients with postpneumonectomy empyema. We feel that intrathoracic transposition of extrathoracic skeletal muscles is an excellent method of treatment for certain persistent, life-threatening intrathoracic infections.

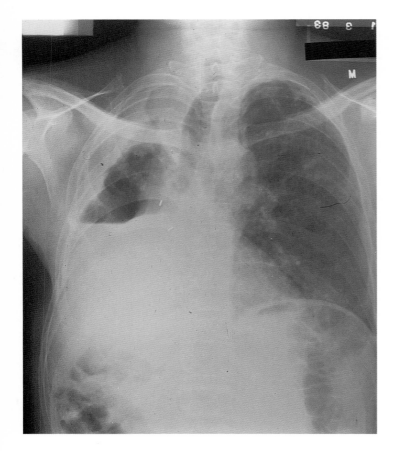

1

Fifty-five-year-old man several months following a right pneumonectomy which was complicated by an empyema and a bronchopleural fistula. A longer than average stump of main stem bronchus was left at the time of the initial resection. (Case of P.G. Arnold)

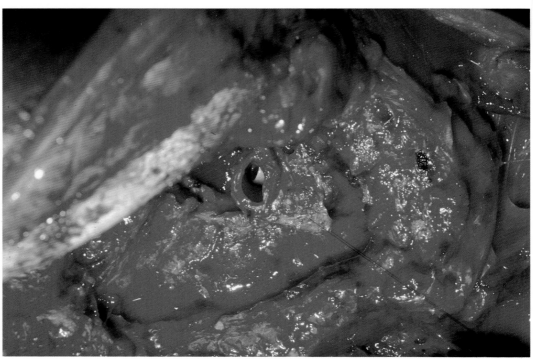

2

The pleural cavity was reopened and the right main stem bronchus was mobilized. Tip of the endotracheal tube can be seen through the cut end of the right main stem bronchus.

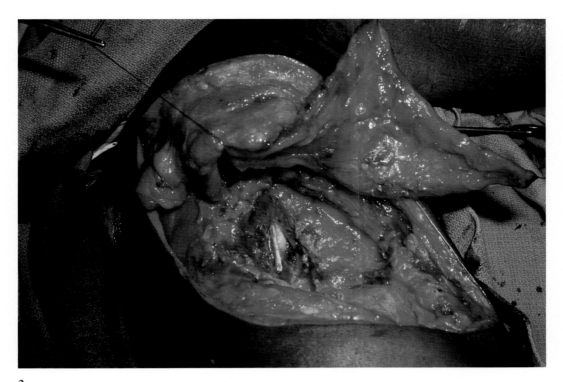

3

The serratus anterior muscle is elevated as an "island" muscle flap on the thoracodorsal and long thoracic vessels.

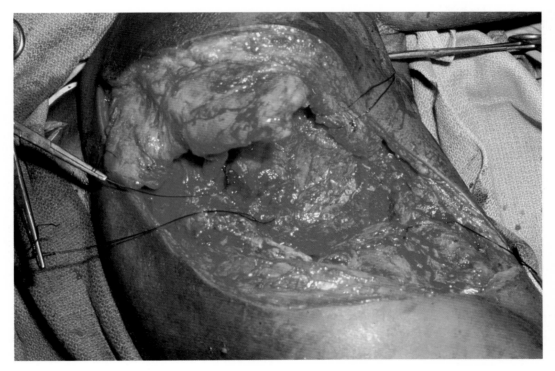

4

Ribs three through seven have been excised. The serratus muscle has been placed directly into the chest to form a "seal" for the repaired bronchus.

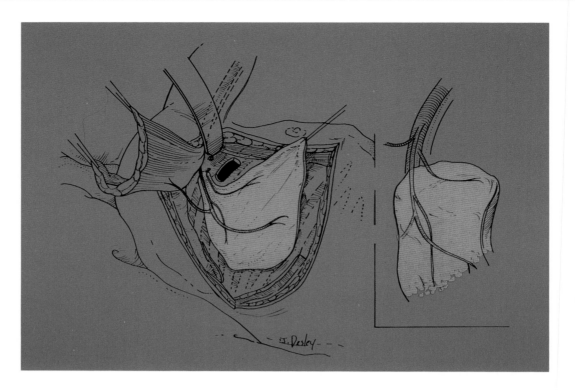

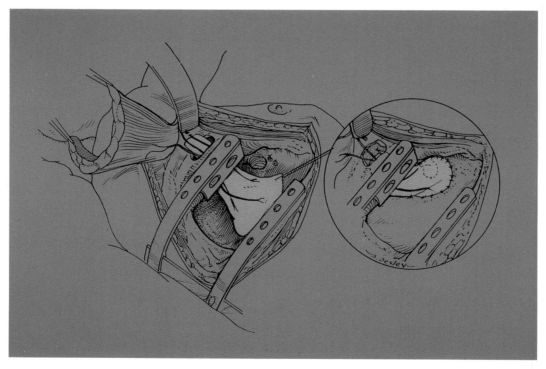

5, 6

Demonstration of the surgical technique showing the "island" serratus anterior muscle, which is supplied by the thoracodorsal and long thoracic vessels. The serratus anterior muscle flap is introduced into the chest through a second thoracotomy. The inset muscle is used to bolster the closure of the right mainstem bronchus.

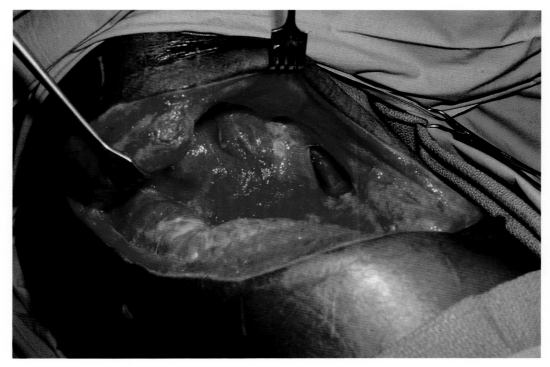

7

Appearance of the wound two weeks following muscle transposition. The wound is "clean" and the serratus muscle is firmly adherent to the secondarily closed bronchus. The entire chest cavity had been treated with frequent changes of moist gauze soaked with diluted Betadine®.

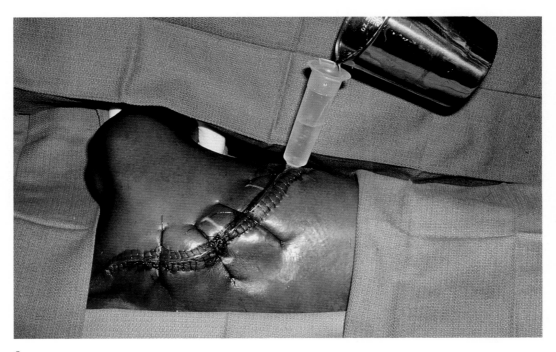

8

The surface wound was then closed directly. The chest cavity was filled with antibiotic solution at the termination of the procedure.

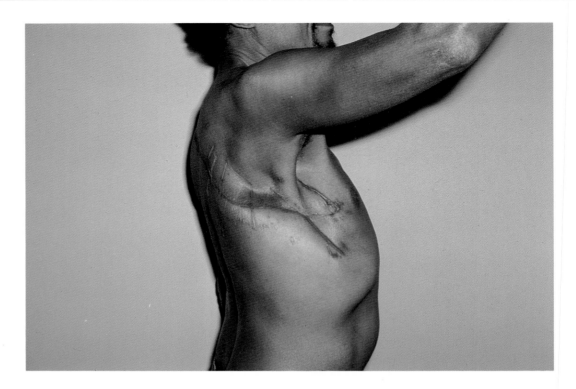

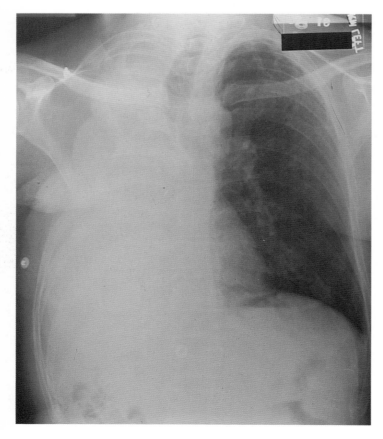

9, 10

Appearance of the surface closure and x-ray one year following the procedure. The Clagett method of obliterating a ''clean'' thoracic cavity is still an effective procedure. Note the relatively midline position of the air-filled trachea.

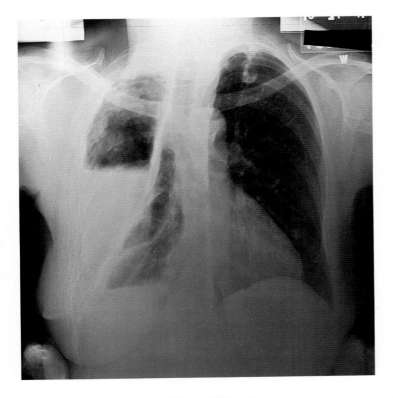

11

Sixty-five-year-old female with arrested tuberculosis which was treated with a therapeutic pneumothorax. Twelve years later she developed an empyema and a bronchopleural fistula. (Case of P.G. Arnold)

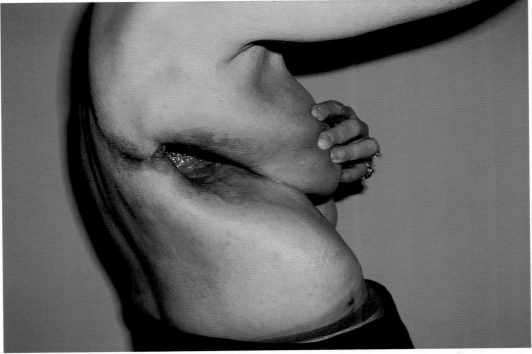

12

The empyema was drained with an "open thoracic window" technique which provided complete access to the chest wound. The bronchopleural fistula persists.

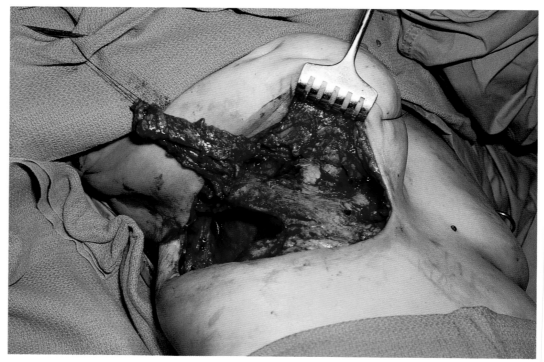

13

A completion pneumonectomy was performed. The latissimus dorsi muscle was mobilized for intrathoracic transposition to reinforce the bronchial stump closure. Approximately seven centimeters of the second rib was resected to allow direct transposition of the latissimus muscle. This "second" thoracotomy prevents kinking of the muscle flap and allows it to reach the main stem bronchus.

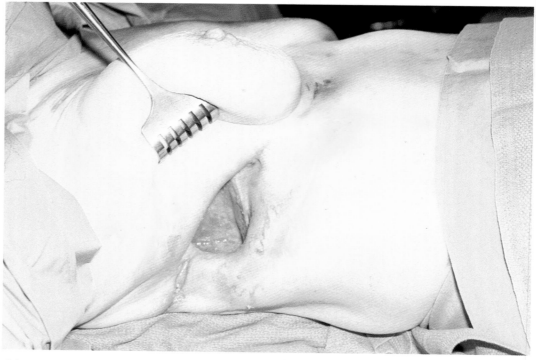

14

Following the closure of the broncho-pleural fistula with the latissimus muscle flap, the wound was dressed in an open fashion for several weeks, until the healing of the bronchus was assured and the wound was clean. Once this was accomplished the entire thoracic cavity was filled with an antibiotic solution and the surface wound was closed primarily.

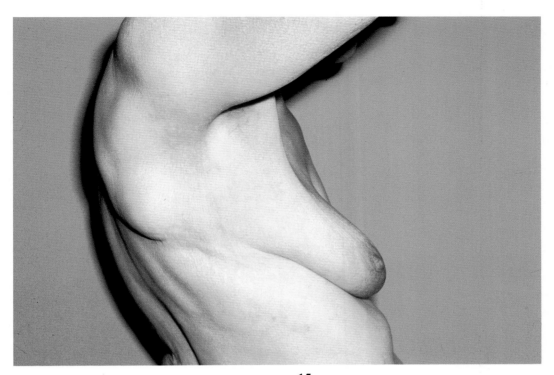

15

Appearance of the chest wall closure at one year.

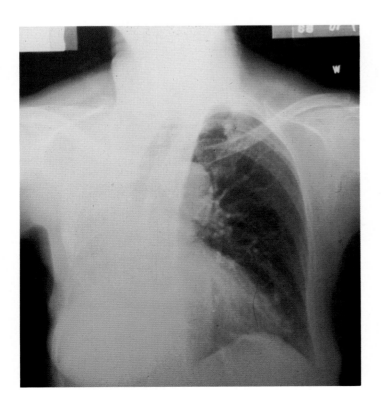

16

This standard chest x-ray demonstrates the healed right main stem bronchus and the obliterated right thoracic cavity at two years.

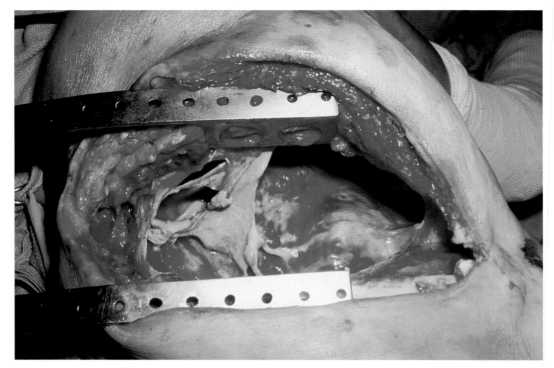

17

Fifty-seven-year-old man with a post pneumonectomy empyema secondary to a bronchial stump failure. Appearance at the time of empyema drainage and closure of the bronchus. (Case of P.G. Arnold)

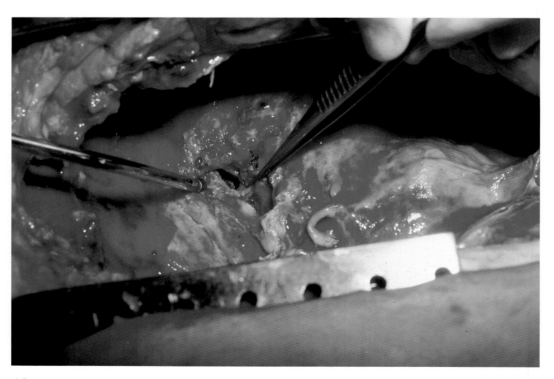

18

The bronchial stump failure is demonstrated. During this procedure the chest wound was debrided and the bronchial stump was reclosed and reinforced with a latissimus dorsi muscle flap.

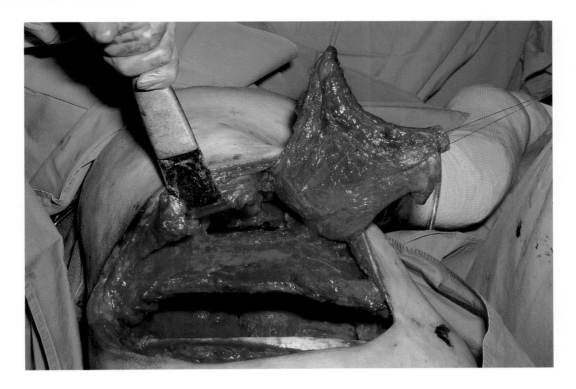

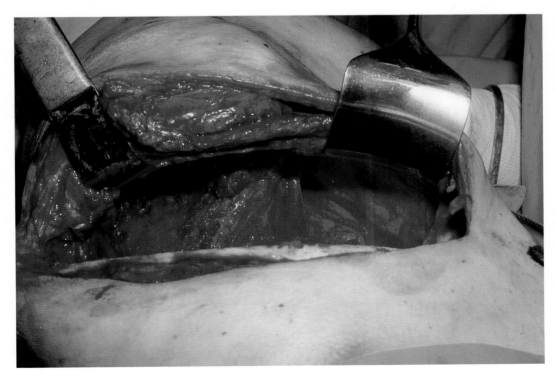

19, 20

Only the proximal portion of the latissimus dorsi muscle could be mobilized because the muscle had been previously divided at the initial thoracotomy. A small secondary thoracotomy was made in the midaxillary line by removing ten centimeters of the third rib. This allowed a "direct" transposition of the shortened latissimus muscle into the chest for closure of the bronchopleural fistula.

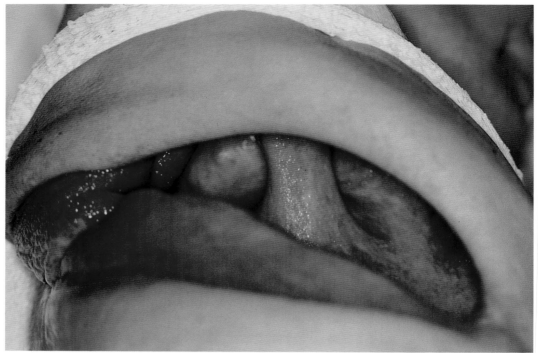

21

The wound was then left open for dressing changes. Note the granulating muscle flap. Once the wound was surgically "clean," the skin edges were closed and the chest cavity was filled with an antibiotic solution. The secondary surface closure is usually done after several weeks, depending on the condition of the chest wound. No attempt is made to obliterate the remaining chest cavity. It is simply closed and filled with an antibiotic solution.

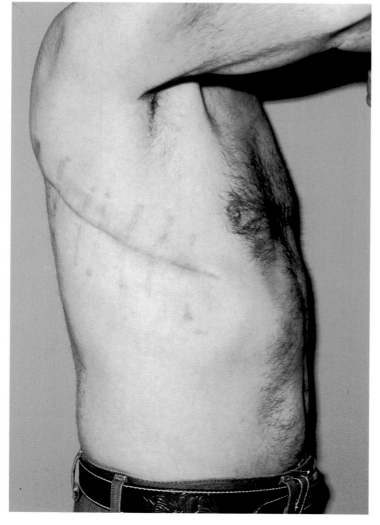

22

Healed chest closure at nine months.

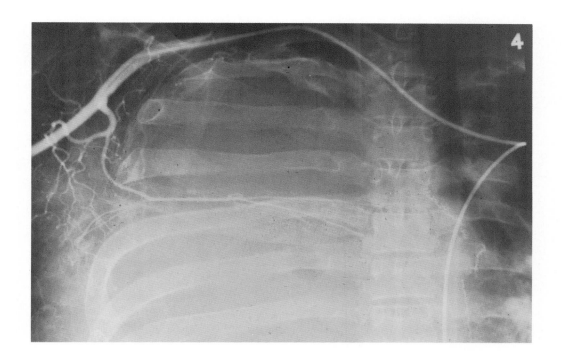

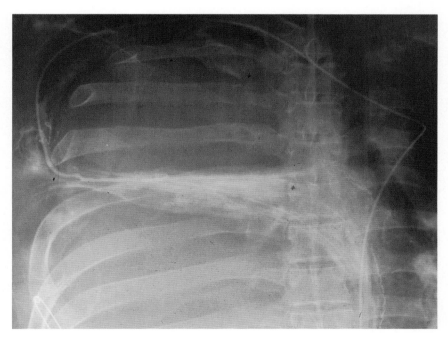

23, 24

Angiogram of the thoracodorsal artery
one week following transposition of the
latissimus muscle into the chest. Venous
phase of the same angiogram.

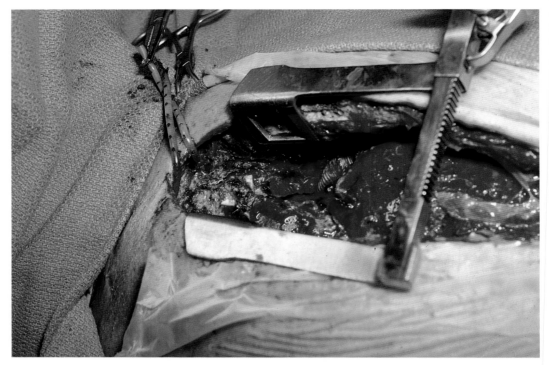

25

Thirty-year-old female who had undergone four major cardiac procedures over a six year period including the correction of a V.S.D., pulmonary artery atresia, and aortic insufficiency. In the most recent procedure a Dacron® conduit was inserted between the right ventricle and the pulmonary artery. It was complicated by an infected false aneurysm of the ascending aorta. The Dacron® conduit is visible in the base of the wound. (Case of P.G. Arnold)

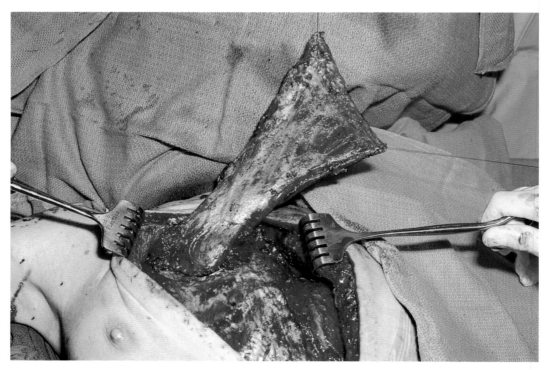

26

The right pectoralis major muscle was raised as an "island" flap to cover the Dacron® prosthesis and the aorta.

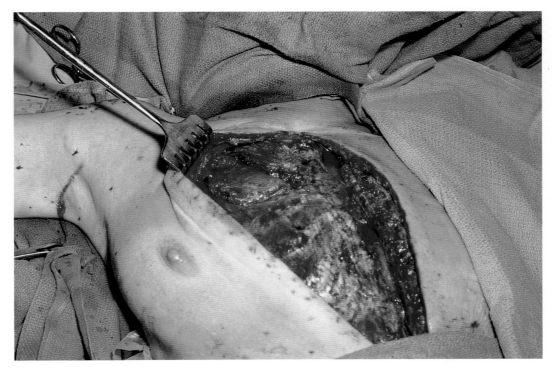

27

The second and third ribs were excised to allow the pectoralis muscle to reach both the infected aorta and the right ventricle.

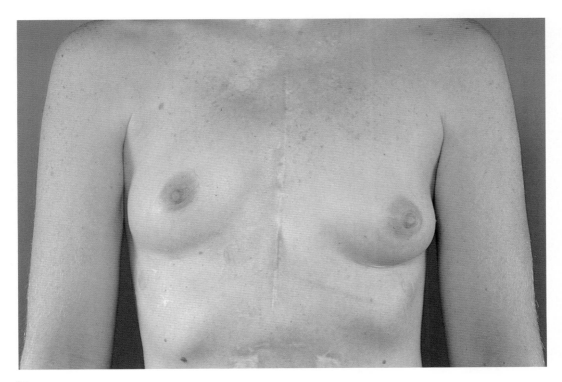

28

Appearance at five years. The wound has remained healed and the patient has been asymptomatic following this closure.

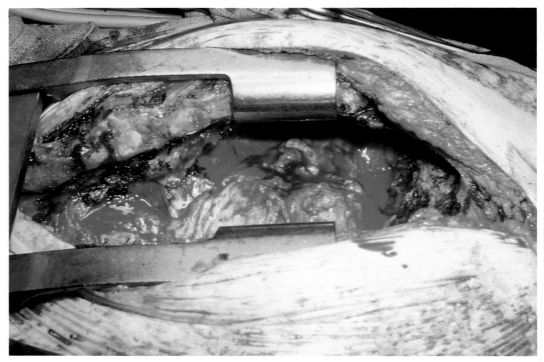

29

This fifty-four-year-old man had undergone a ventricular aneurysmectomy three years and six years earlier. At this exploration for a left ventricular pseudoaneurysm an abscess was found surrounding the heart. This was apparently related to the Teflon® felt reinforcement pads. No bacteria were found on the gram stain, but the culture was positive for Klebsiella pneumoniae. (Case of P.G. Arnold and H. Schaff)

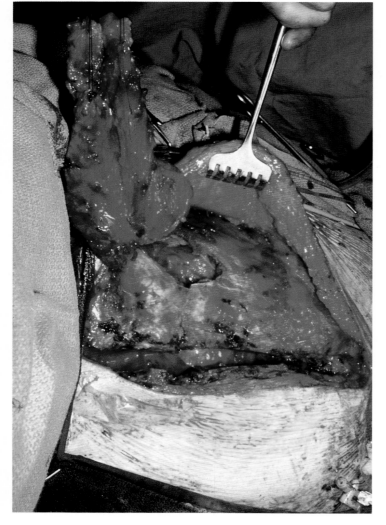

30

An "island" pectoralis major muscle flap was elevated, at the time of the secondary ventricular closure. The muscle was divided from its humeral insertion and passed into the chest by removing a twelve centimeter segment of the third rib.

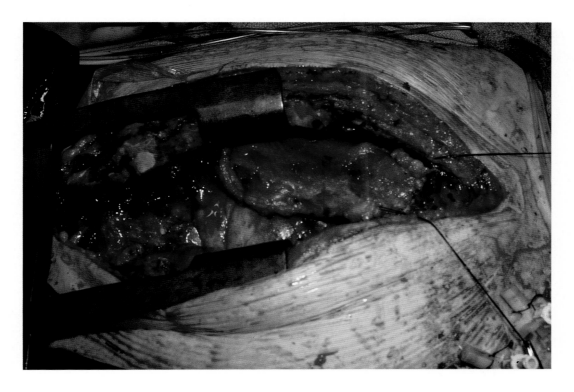

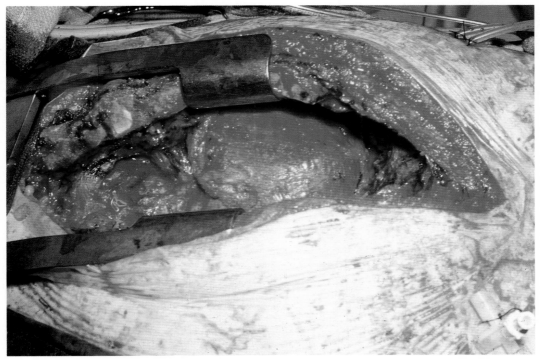

31, 32

Pectoralis muscle passed to its intrathoracic location and sutured over the heart to reinforce the ventricular repair.

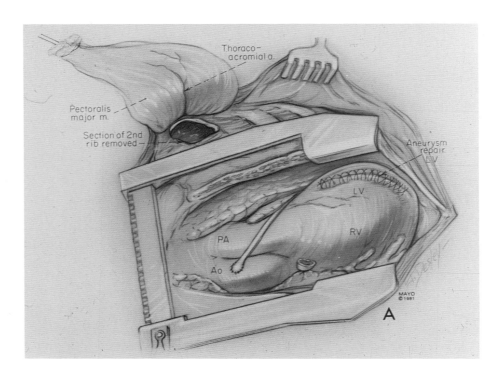

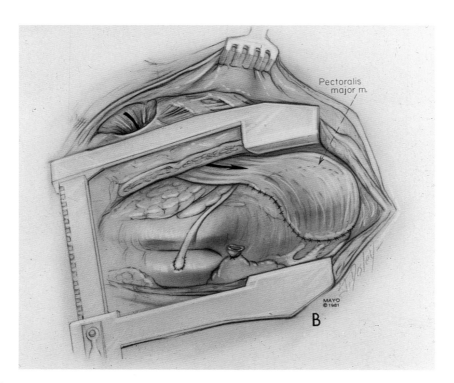

33, 34

Illustrations of the procedure. After a right atriofemoral artery bypass was established the aneurysm was opened and resected along with the previously placed Teflon® felt pads. The fibrous edges of the left ventricle were then closed with multiple layers of 0 Prolene® without using felt pads. The pectoralis muscle was used to reinforce the left ventricular closure.

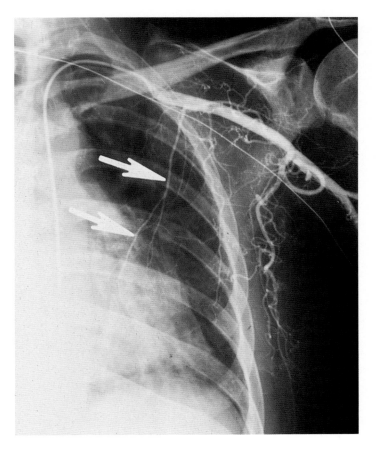

35

Arteriogram demonstrating the patency of the thoracoacromial vessels and the intrathoracic location of the pectoralis major muscle.

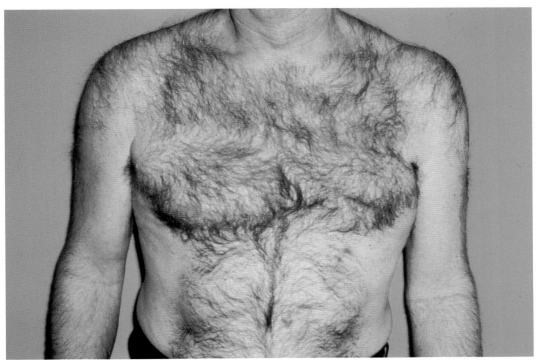

36

Appearance two years following surgery. The patient's chest pain was completely relieved and he returned to full activity. A two dimensional echocardiogram demonstrated no evidence of a recurrent pseudoaneurysm.

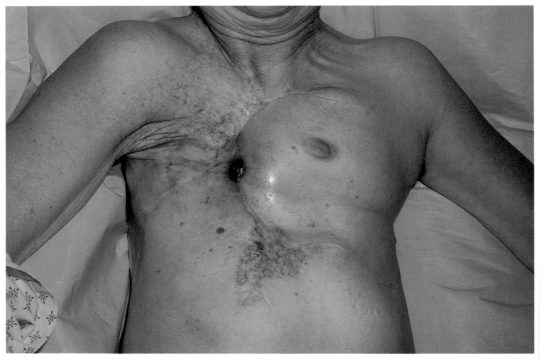

37

Forty-five-year-old woman who had previously undergone a right radical mastectomy and closure of an irradiation ulcer by centralizing the remaining left breast. When the patient was first seen she gave a history of "bleeding a lot" from the "blood blister" at the margin of the left breast flap. (Case of P.G. Arnold)

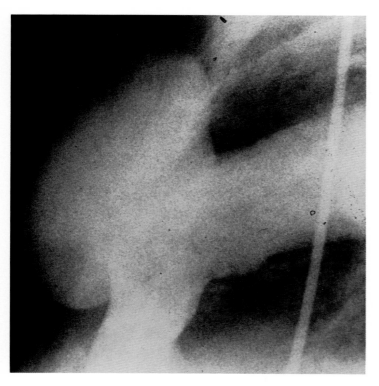

38

Lateral view of an angiogram demonstrating a large aneurysm of the pulmonary outflow tract. The aneurysm had eroded through the irradiated and infected sternum. The "blood blister" proved to be the surface of the pulmonary artery aneurysm.

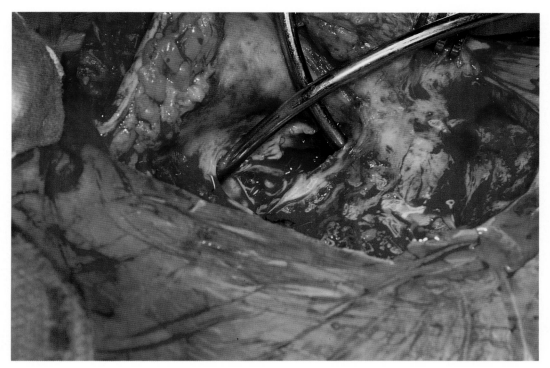

39

Opened aneurysm with the aspirators in the base of the pulmonary outflow tract. The aneurysm wall is reflected superiorly.

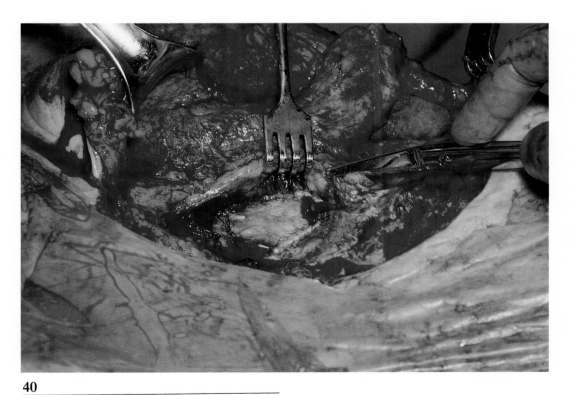

40

The anterior wall of the aneurysm was resected and repaired with a fascia lata graft. The adjacent infected sternum was also resected.

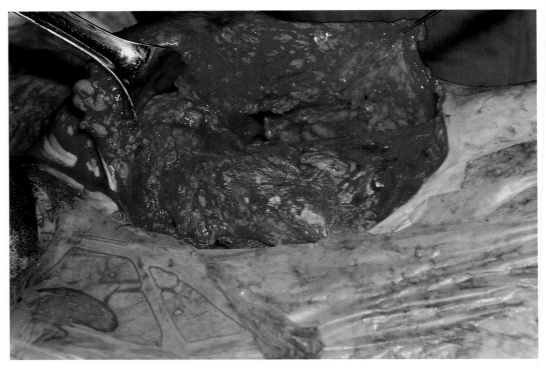

41

The pectoralis muscle was transposed into the chest to reinforce the vascular repair and vascularize the fascia lata graft.

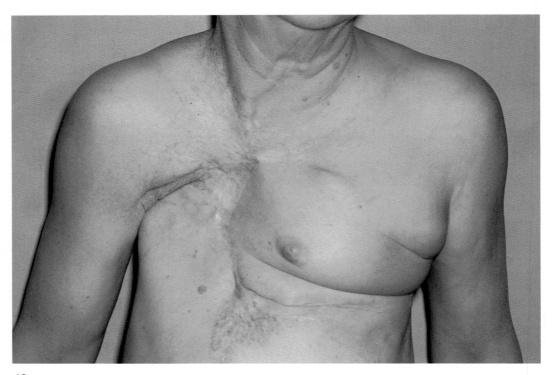

42

Appearance of the closure at two years. Neither the infection or the aneurysm has recurred.

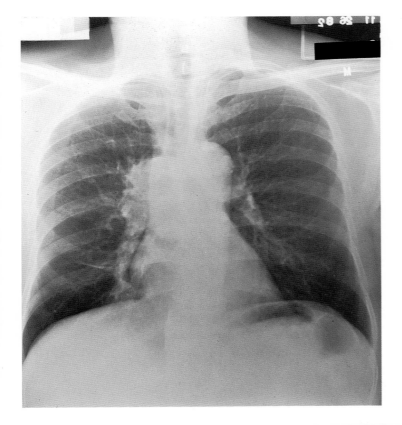

43

Chest x-ray of a forty-nine-year-old man with a squamous cell carcinoma of the right main stem bronchus extending onto the trachea. (Case of P.G. Arnold and P. Pairolero)

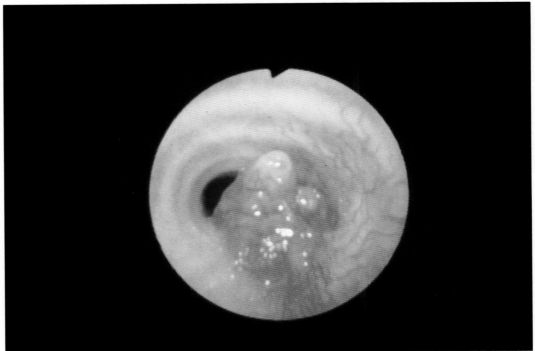

44

Endoscopic appearance of the large tumor which virtually occludes the right mainstem bronchus and partially fills the trachea. The left mainstem bronchus is barely visible.

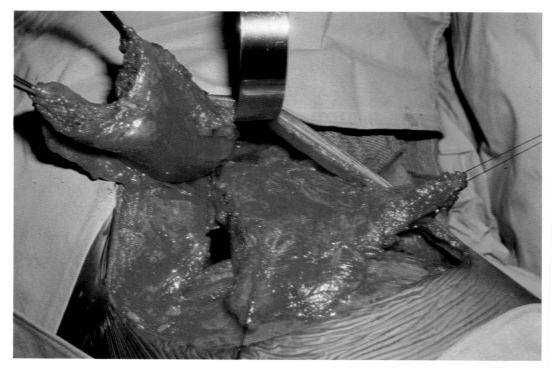

45

Mobilization of the transected latissimus dorsi muscle and the entire serratus anterior muscle at the time of the right posterolateral thoracotomy.

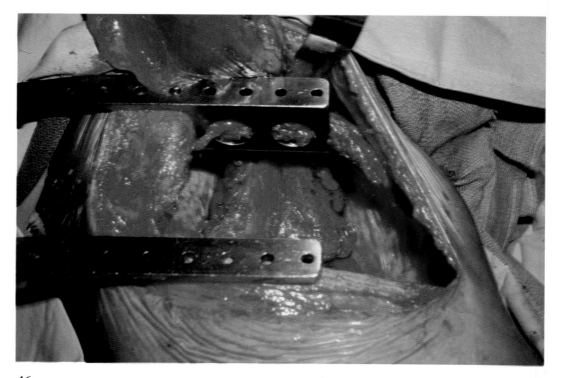

46

A "sleeve" pneumonectomy has been completed. The serratus anterior muscle has been transposed intrathoracically to reconstruct the ten centimeter tracheal wall defect.

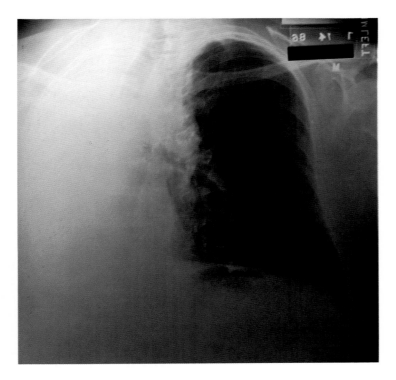

47

Chest x-ray four years postoperatively. The serratus muscle flap covering the tracheal defect was completely reepithelialized with columnar epithelium.

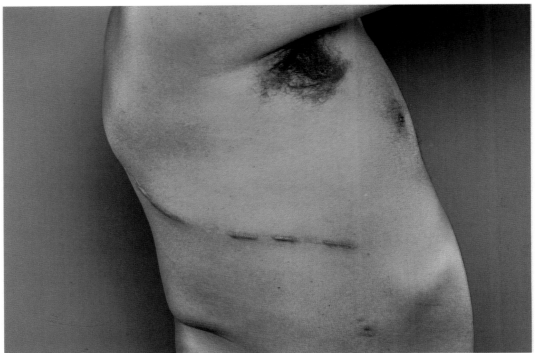

48

Appearance of the patient four years postoperatively.

VERTICAL RECTUS

ANATOMICAL CONSIDERATIONS

Surface Markings

The lateral margins of the two rectus abdominis muscles are easily palpated in a thin person. This is best done by having the patient simultaneously raise the legs and forcibly flex the neck while in a supine position. Only the portion of the muscle which extends onto the chest wall is difficult to palpate.

Origin and Insertion

The rectus abdominis muscle inserts into the pubic tubercle and the pubic crest. It originates over a broad area of the chest wall which encompasses the cartilages of the sixth, seventh, and eighth ribs. Laterally the muscle has an important relationship to the fascial confluence of the anterior and lateral abdominal wall musculature at the semilunaris ligament. Medially the muscle is loosely attached to the linea alba. The primary function of the rectus abdominis muscle is in assisting torso flexion. The loss of one muscle is seldom functionally detectable, but the loss of both muscles can result in some weakness of "pelvic tilt" in the supine position.

Adjacent muscles

The paired rectus abdominis muscles are the major vertically oriented muscles of the abdominal wall. They are partially fused to the origins of the pectoralis major and serratus anterior muscles superiorly. They share fascial attachments with the external and internal oblique muscles laterally and are contiguous with the puborectalis muscles inferiorly.

Vascular Pattern

The deep inferior epigastric artery arises from the common femoral artery and obliquely transverses the posterior undersurface of the rectus abdominis muscle. This is the dominant vessel of the rectus muscle and it will reliably supply the entire muscle. Although there is a vascular "watershed" between the superior and inferior epigastric systems, these vascular connections are seldom visible on the posterior surface of the muscle.

The superior epigastric artery branches from the internal mammary artery and passes between the xiphoid and the eighth rib cartilage on the undersurface of the rectus abdominis muscle. The superior vessels will reliably supply the upper two-thirds of the muscle, extending to a point approximately halfway between the pubis and umbilicus. The "watershed" between the superior and inferior deep epigastric systems occurs in the central portion of the muscle at a point near the umbilicus. The deep inferior epigastric vessels are easily visualized on the undersurface of the muscle throughout its course, while the smaller superior epigastric vessels are seen only for a distance of approximately five centimeters distal to the chest wall margin. Although the deep inferior epigastric artery is clearly the dominant vascular system, a significant secondary contribution is made by the posterior perforating vessels which accompany the eighth through the twelfth sensory and motor nerves to the rectus abdominis muscle. These deep perforating vessels penetrate the posterior fascial sheathe and enter the rectus abdominis muscle in its posterior midline. Even though these posterior perforating vessels are viewed as a minor system, they can maintain the viability of the entire muscle in the absence of both the superior epigastric and the deep inferior epigastric vessels. For this reason the muscle cannot necessarily be considered to have been "delayed" if only one or the other of these major systems has been interrupted. There is also a minor contribution made by perforating vessels which pass directly from the internal mammary artery into the proximal portion of the rectus abdominis muscle on the chest wall. The viability of the superiorly based flap is probably enhanced by leaving the rectus abdominis muscle attached to the chest wall because of these direct thoracic branches from the internal mammary vessels. For this reason it is safer simply to divide the medial and lateral fascial attachments of the muscle to the chest wall to improve upward mobility rather than to elevate the muscle totally away from the chest wall. The lower costal cartilages can also be removed for this same purpose, but this has been employed only on a few occasions.

Motor Nerve

Intercostal nerves five through twelve.

Sensory Nerves

Intercostal nerves five through twelve.

USES

The superiorly based vertical rectus abdominis myocutaneous flap is generally considered as a secondary option for lower chest wall and sternal defects and for reconstruction of the breast following mastectomy. Since its rotation point is near the midline, comparable coverage is provided for either the ipsilateral or the contralateral lower chest wall. The standard vertical myocutaneous flap will reach the jugular notch and a point approximately five centimeters from the apex of the axilla. The standard Hartrampf flap has a similar arc of rotation, but it provides a significantly larger volume of tissue.

The inferiorly based rectus abdominis myocutaneous flap is most commonly used for large defects of the lateral abdomen, groin, and hip. It also has certain applications in massive surface defects of the perineum and in total vaginal defects. Ian Taylor has recently described a long inferiorly based "island" flap with a cutaneous segment which extends obliquely onto the chest wall. This radial extension further improves the arc of the inferior rectus abdominis flap and allows it to reach the midthigh.

REGIONAL FLAP COMPARISONS

Reconstruction of the upper two-thirds of the sternum and the central chest wall is usually accomplished by using the pectoralis major muscles either as "island" muscle flaps or as bilateral myocutaneous advancement flaps. The pectoralis major muscle is usually preferred over the vertical rectus abdominis flap for sternal defects because of its reliability, its ease of dissection, and its lesser donor site morbidity.

The lower one-third of the sternum and the adjacent chest wall is not always reached by either the pectoralis major or the latissimus dorsi muscles, even though both muscles may extend to the lower sternum. This is the usual reason for considering the vertical rectus abdominis flap for central chest defects. The transverse thoracoepigastric cutaneous flap can also be used in this situation, and its donor site can be primarily closed with wide undermining. The safety and the rotation point of the thoracoepigastric flap can be improved by including the upper portion of the rectus abdominis muscle with the thoracoepigastric skin as a compound flap. This particular upper horizontal configuration is applicable only to low chest wall defects because this "high" placement of skin limits the arc of rotation of the flap. The large anterior fascial donor defect is similar for both the vertical and the upper horizontal rectus abdominis myocutaneous flaps. It may be possible to close the fascial defect primarily, but it is preferable to use Prolene® mesh if the closure is at all tight.

For purposes of breast reconstruction the vertical rectus abdominis myocutaneous flap is compared to the lower transverse rectus abdominis (TRAM) flap. The TRAM flap is more malleable and easier to shape. The TRAM flap reconstruction seldom requires an implant. Because of the deficient horizontal projection, it is usually necessary to use an implant with the vertical rectus myocutaneous flap. In a markedly obese patient the vertical flap can provide a satisfactory breast reconstruction without an implant because the flap should have suffi-

cient bulk to give the desired projection. It is still difficult to obtain a result which is comparable to the Hartrampf procedure using the vertical rectus abdominis flap because shaping of the vertical "sandwich" of skin and rectus abdominis muscle is difficult. When either type of rectus abdominis myocutaneous flap is used to reconstruct the breast without an implant, the long-term result can be expected to be superior to the latissimus dorsi breast reconstruction.

The inferiorly based rectus abdominis flap can be used to resurface the perineum completely and must be compared with the known results using the bilateral gracilis myocutaneous flaps and the posterior fasciocutaneous flaps of the thigh. The much larger inferior rectus abdominis flap should not be viewed as only a "back up" flap to these other reliable flaps. It now should be primarily considered as a single flap of choice for certain massive perineal and groin defects because of its size, reliability, and accessibility. For smaller problems in the groin or lower abdomen either the rectus femoris or TFL flaps are routinely chosen.

In the lateral abdomen very few flaps are available for resurfacing large defects. The proximally based latissimus flap will not reach this area at all. The groin flap and the thoracoepigastric flaps will not reach the most lateral aspects of the abdomen. The primary flap for comparison to the inferiorly based rectus abdominis flap is the distally based latissimus dorsi flap which is much less reliable and provides a much smaller area of coverage.

The inferior rectus abdominis myocutaneous flap is also a convenient and reliable source of tissue for total vaginal reconstructions. It is logical to use this anatomically convenient flap for "high" pelvic defects, but a laparotomy is required for the inset of the flap. If a laparotomy is already planned, this disadvantage is not relevant. The reliability and bulk of an inferior rectus abdominis flap cannot be matched by the smaller and more fragile gracilis myocutaneous flaps.

DISADVANTAGES

The primary disadvantage of any rectus abdominis myocutaneous flap is related to the abdominal wall donor site because the inclusion of fascia with this composite flap is obligatory. The anterior fascia should not be closed primarily unless it is a relatively tension-free closure. Even then it is a reasonable consideration to reinforce the fascial closure with an "onlay" patch of Prolene® mesh. If the actual fascial defect is more than seven to eight centimeters in width it should probably be repaired with an end-to-end patch of Prolene® mesh.

The superiorly based vertical rectus flap is more easily elevated than the TRAM flap, but it is harder to shape and usually requires a Silastic® implant for breast reconstruction. It is a reasonable method of breast reconstruction in the markedly obese patient, but the result will not be comparable to the TRAM flap reconstruction.

The inferiorly based rectus abdominis flap is quite reliable and will carry all of the skin overlying the muscle. One cannot depend on carrying the cutaneous portion of the superiorly based flap to the level of the pubis without a prior "delay." When the common femoral vessels are injured it can be presumed that the deep inferior epigastric vessels will also be injured. In this situation a contralateral rather than an ipsilateral flap should be chosen.

ADVANTAGES

The very reliable inferiorly based rectus abdominis flap provides massive amounts of coverage for the difficult areas of the lower quadrants of the abdomen, the groin, and the perineum. The superiorly based flap provides excellent lower chest wall and lower sternal coverage. Its generous size allows it to be used to resurface the entire sternum. The midline abdominal skin incision can usually be closed without any undermining whether the vertically oriented flap is superiorly or inferiorly based. For some reason there seems to be less abdominal morbidity with the vertical rectus abdominis flap than there is with the lower horizontal rectus flap. This difference in morbidity is probably related to the extensive undermining of the skin over the rib cage which is necessary for the closure of the horizontal skin defect.

COMPLICATIONS, PITFALLS, AND DONOR SITE

Flap loss has been rare and the vertical rectus abdominis flap does not seem to be particularly "cold sensitive." The mechanics of elevating either the superior or the inferior vertical rectus abdominis flap are straightforward until one enters the region of the dominant vasculature. The superior vessels can be injured as they pass beneath the muscle at the margin of the costal cartilage because they are sometimes difficult to identify. It is possible to injure the inferior vessels, but they are easily visualized on the undersurface of the rectus abdominis muscle. If there is a question of vascular patency because of previous trauma or irradiation to the flap vessels, a selective angiogram is in order. Although massive irradiation of the dominant flap vessels can lead to the total loss of the flap this has not been observed. It is still prudent to choose the opposite, nonirradiated flap electively in order to avoid this eventuality.

The functional loss of one rectus abdominis muscle is usually not significant in the nonathletic person because the external and internal oblique muscles are so much stronger than the rectus abdominis muscles. This difference in muscular strength is also suggested as the reason why incisional hernias are more common with vertical incisions than with horizontal incisions. The remaining lateral abdominal wall muscles exert a stronger muscular "pull" on the incision than the rectus abdominis muscles. The development of a postoperative hernia should be a rare complication following the use of this flap if the anterior fascia is carefully repaired.

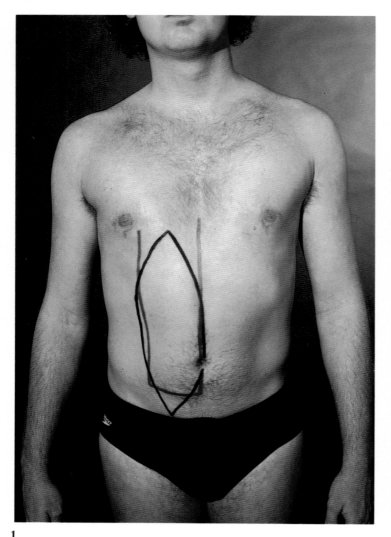

1

The primary territory of the vertical rectus abdominis myocutaneous flap is outlined. The superior vessels will reliably supply the upper two-thirds of the muscle.

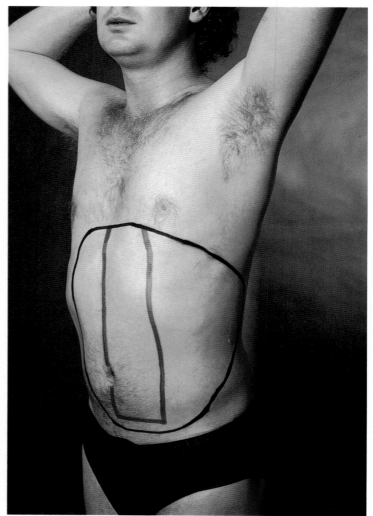

2

The rectus abdominis vascular territory provides the largest single myocutaneous flap in the body.

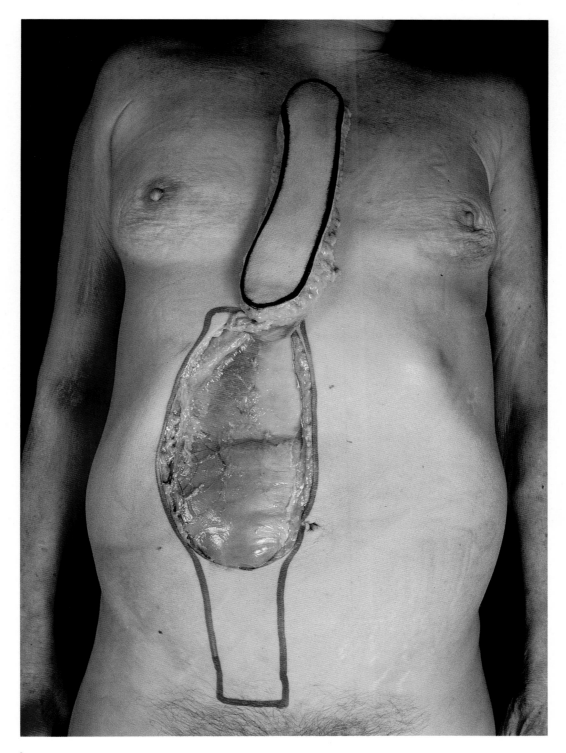

3

The primary territory of the vertical "island" rectus abdominis flap will easily cover the sternum. An anterior rectus fascial defect of this size will require reinforcement.

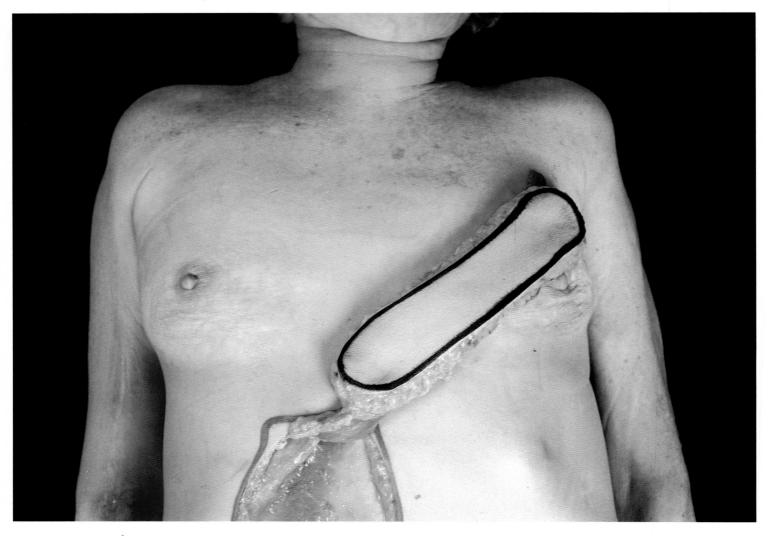

4

The vertical rectus flap will provide comparable coverage to either an ipsilateral or a contralateral lower chest wall defect.

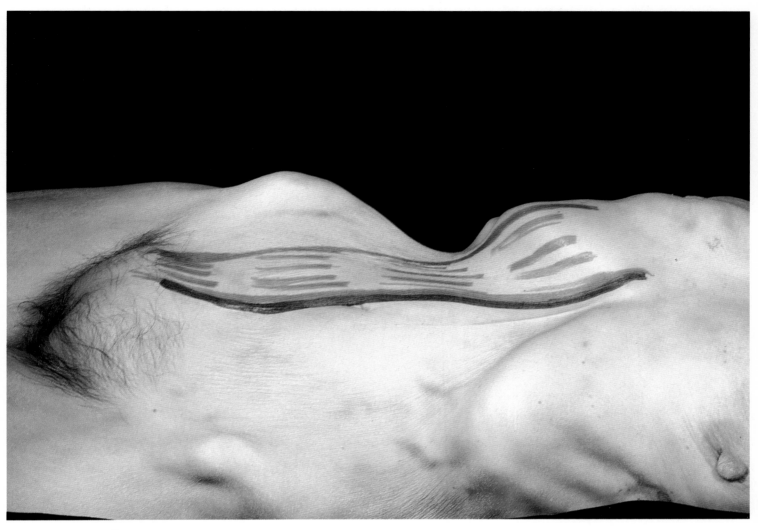

5

The right rectus abdominis muscle is outlined in red. A midline abdominal incision will be used to retrieve an inferiorly based muscle flap.

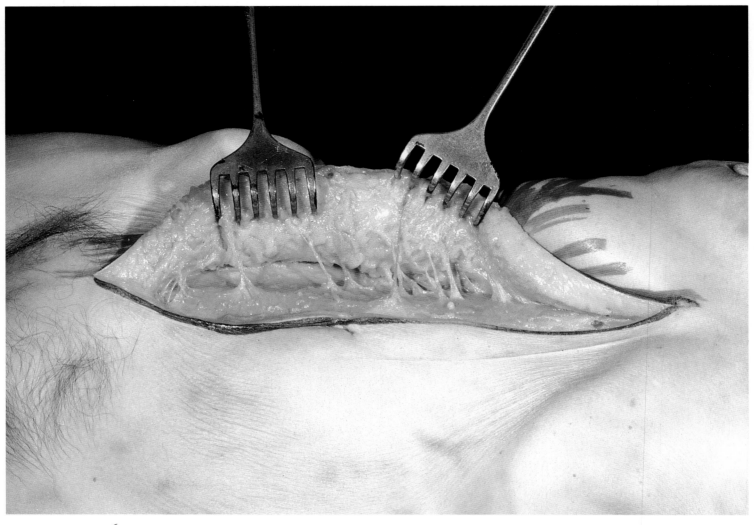

6

Exposure of the anterior rectus fascia.
Note that the rectus abdominis cutaneous
perforators are concentrated in the area
just above the umbilicus.

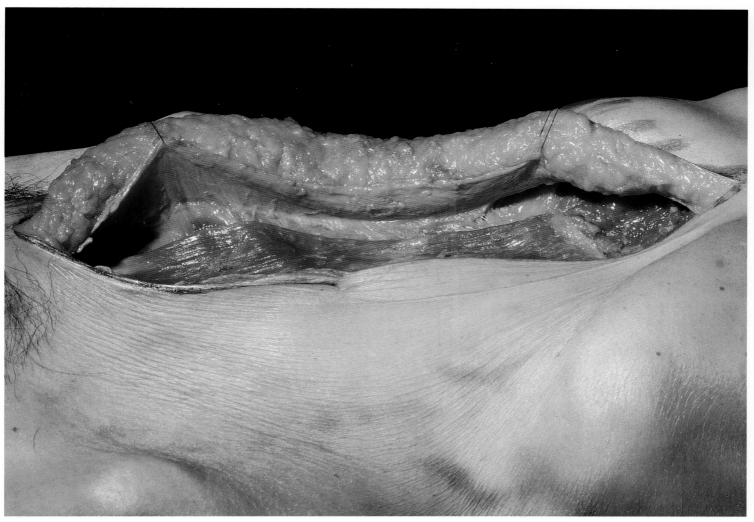

7

The anterior rectus fascia is retracted with sutures. The lateral border of the rectus abdominis muscle has been separated from the linea semilunaris ligaments.

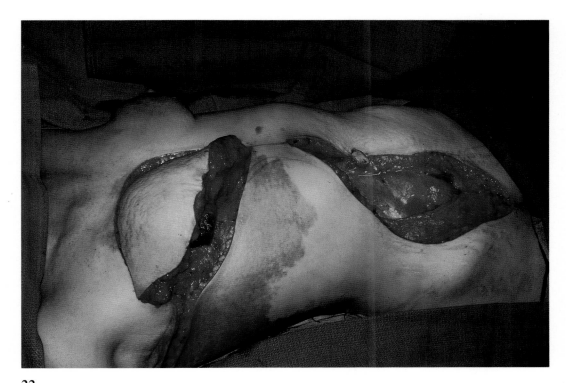

22

A triangular skin flap was designed to replace the lost breast tissue. Both the skin and fascial defects of the abdomen were primarily closed.

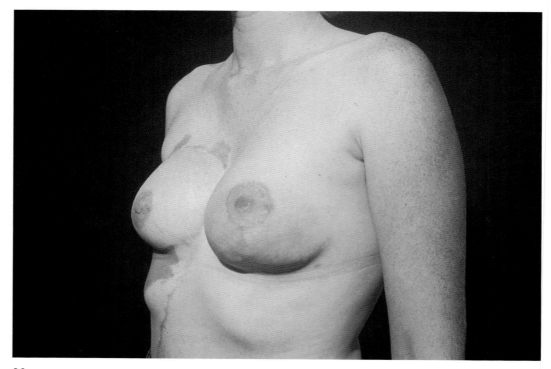

23

One year following the immediate reconstruction of the right breast and an opposite breast augmentation and mastopexy.

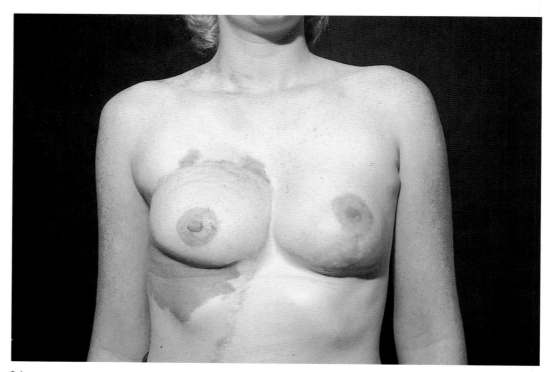

24

Because of the extensive skin removal, a
small implant was also used in the right
breast reconstruction. The overall breast
contour and symmetry are better than the
preoperative condition.

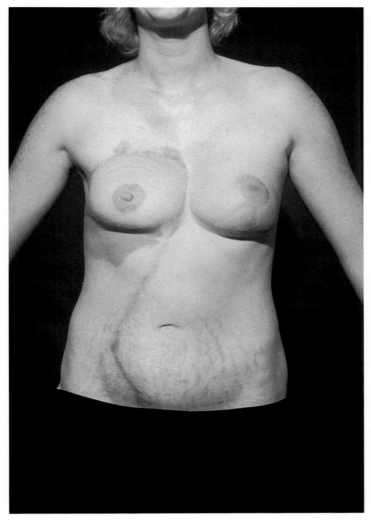

25

The abdominal skin was closed by advancement with relocation of the umbilicus. The abdominal wall has remained stable without mesh reinforcement.

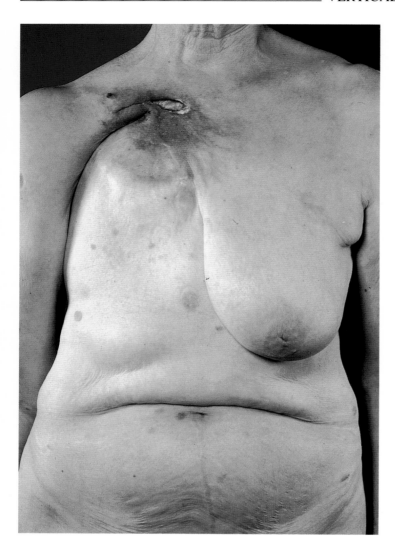

26

Seventy-year-old female who had undergone a right radical mastectomy and irradiation therapy twenty-five years earlier. An irradiation ulcer of the infraclavicular area was unresponsive to conservative therapy. A breakdown of the irradiated subclavian vessels was anticipated. (Case of P.G. Arnold)

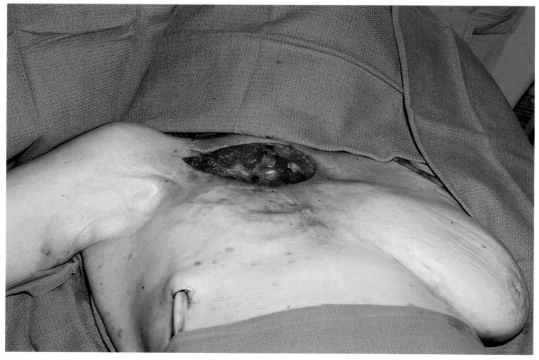

27

Full-thickness excision of the upper chest wall and clavicle with preservation of the subclavian vessels.

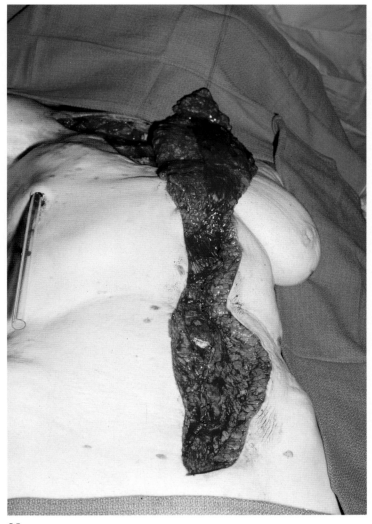

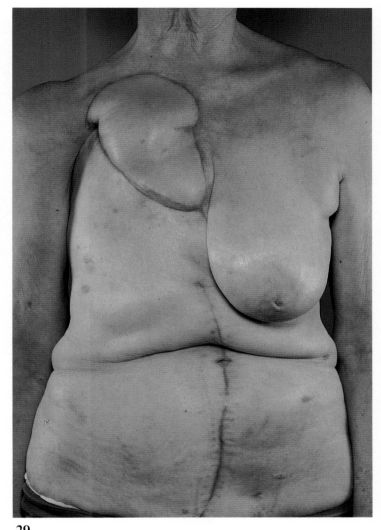

28

A contralateral rectus abdominis myocutaneous flap is elevated. The patency of the
left internal mammary vessel was determined by a preoperative angiogram.

29

Appearance at four months. Note the extent of the supraclavicular coverage. The
wound has remained healed for three
years.

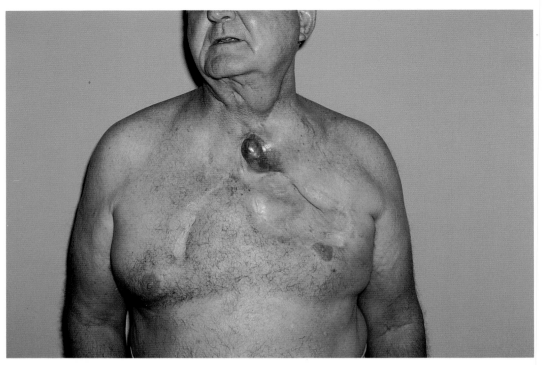

30

Fourth recurrence of a malignant histiocytoma which invaded the manubrium. Note the skin graft on the left pectoralis major muscle. (Case of P.G. Arnold)

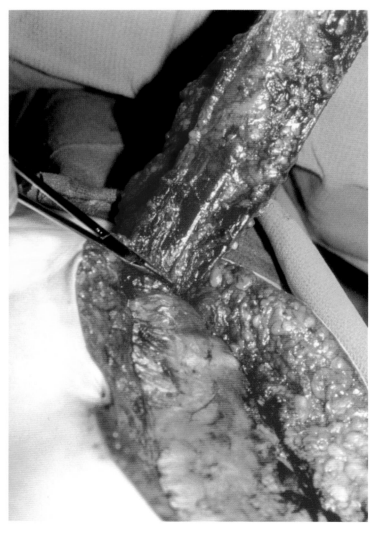

31

The left rectus abdominis muscle was elevated with the skin and subcutaneous fat, but it was far too bulky. The skin was removed from the flap and replaced as a graft.

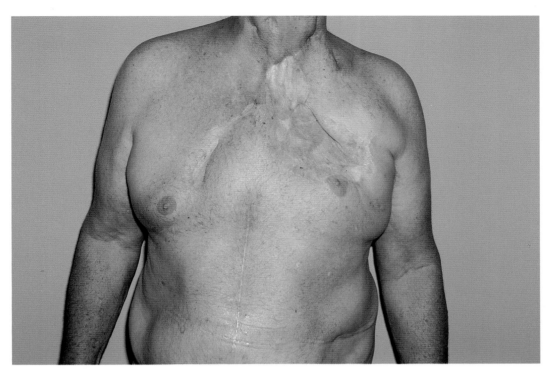

32

Skin-grafted rectus abdominis muscle flap
covering the upper sternum. Removal of
the manubrium did not cause any chest
wall instability.

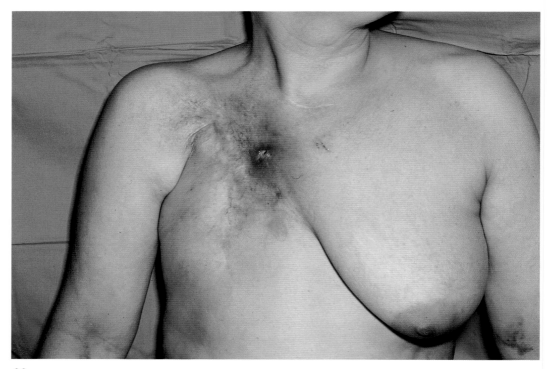

33

Forty-nine-year-old female with an extensive irradiation ulcer of the upper chest wall and sternum. (Case of P.G. Arnold)

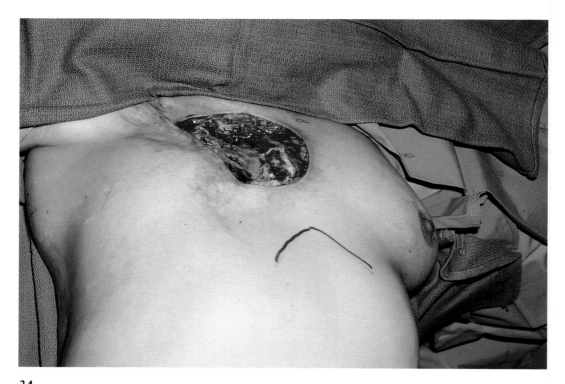

34

The chest wall resection included a portion of the sternum and three ribs.

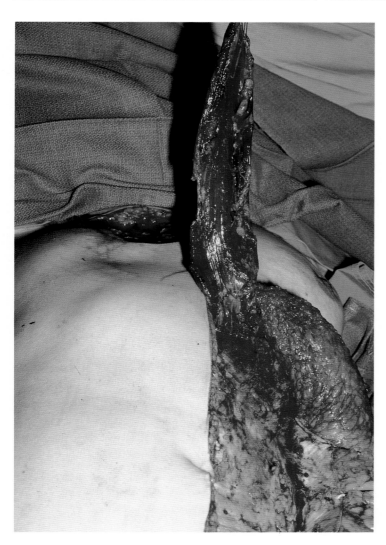

35

The left rectus abdominis muscle was raised as an "island" muscle flap.

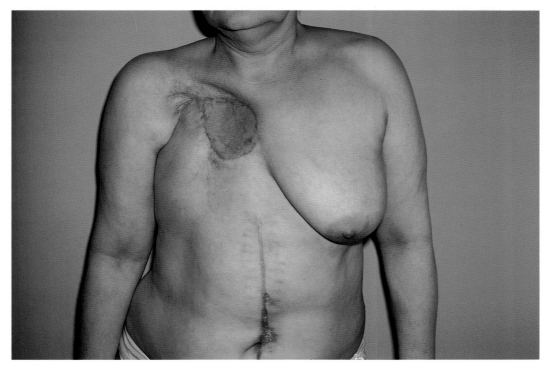

36

Appearance of the skin-grafted muscle flap closure of the chest wall at four months. The wound has remained healed for seven years.

291

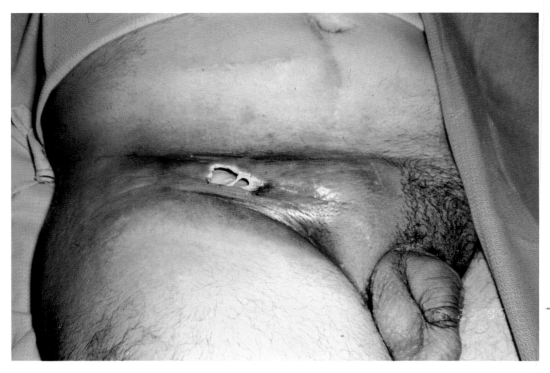

37

Fifty-one-year-old man with an extensive irradiation ulcer of the lower abdomen following a groin dissection. (Case of P.G. Arnold)

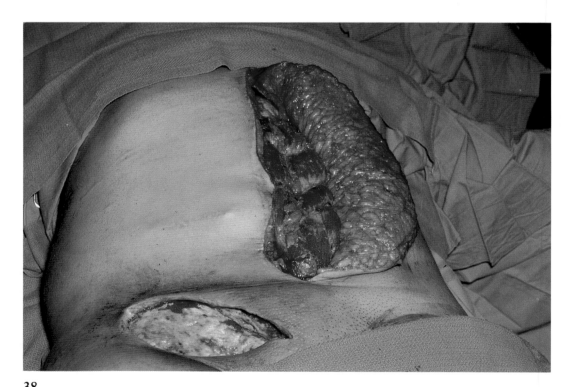

38

The contralateral rectus abdominis muscle was elevated on its inferior blood supply at the time of the debridement of the groin wound.

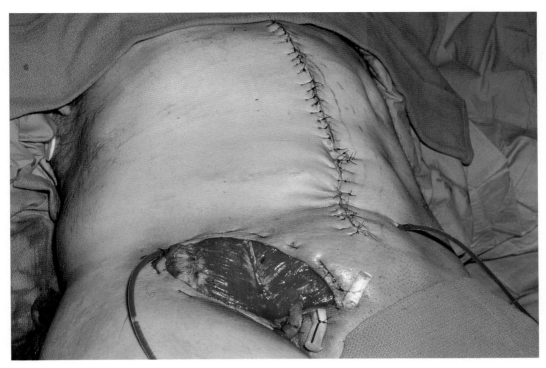

39
Inset of the left rectus abdominis muscle flap. Skin grafting was performed two days later.

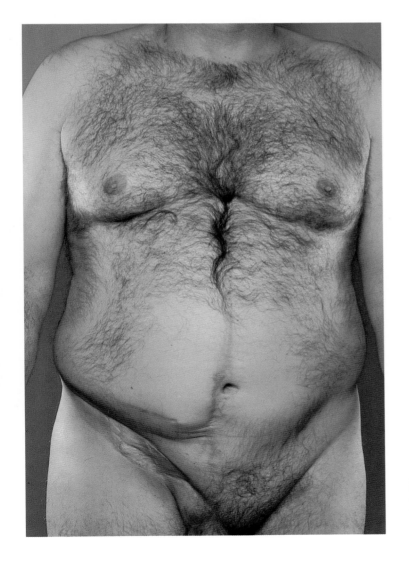

40
Appearance at one year. The anterior rectus fascial defect was closed without reinforcement.

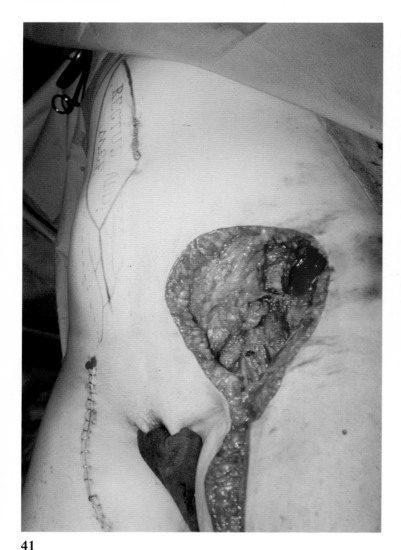

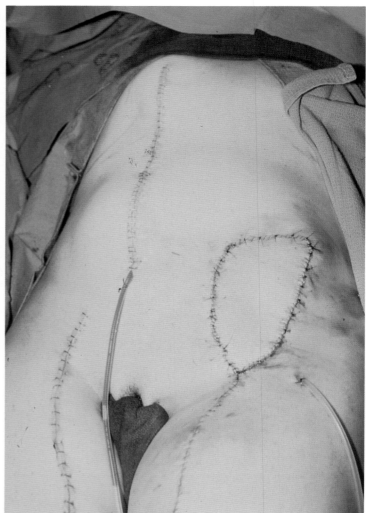

41

Shotgun wound of the left lower abdomen which destroyed the lower abdominal wall and the common femoral vessels. The right saphenous vein was used to reconstruct the left common femoral artery. Since the deep inferior epigastric vessels arise from the common femoral vessels, an ipsilateral rectus abdominis flap could not be used. (Case of J.B. McCraw and R. Russell)

42

A right inferiorly based rectus abdominis myocutaneous flap was used to provide muscle coverage for the femoral vessels and a fascial repair for the abdominal wall.

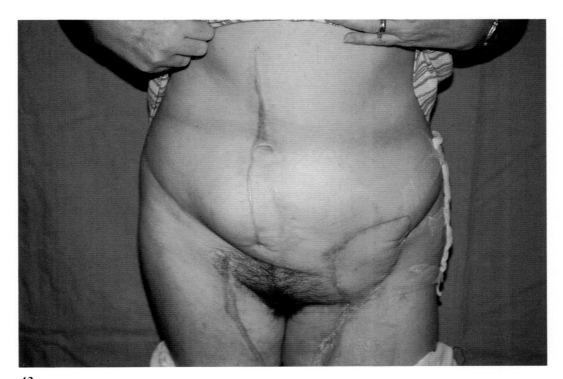

43

Healed flap at six weeks. The femoral
vessels have remained patent for four
years.

HORIZONTAL RECTUS

ANATOMICAL CONSIDERATIONS

See VERTICAL RECTUS

Vascular pattern

Hartrampf and his associates have clearly defined the physiological limits of the lower horizontal rectus myocutaneous flap in humans. The recent experimental work of Ian Taylor has demonstrated the distribution of the cutaneous perforating vessels in a definitive cadaver study which depicts the vast majority of perforating vessels as residing in the area of the umbilicus and decreasing in numbers as one moves away from the umbilicus. This anatomical study helps explain why the upper horizontal rectus abdominis myocutaneous flap is less viable than a flap which is placed closer to the umbilicus. Similarly, the lower horizontal flap can be designed so low on the abdomen that it exceeds the viable limits of the rectus abdominis muscular perforators. It is surprising that the transverse rectus abdominis (TRAM) flap survives as well as it does when one considers the multiplicity of systems which are directly capable of supplying the same area of skin. These vascular systems include the inferior deep epigastric vessels, the eighth through the twelfth lateral intercostal vessels, and the superficial inferior epigastric (vertical groin flap) vessels. Since the deep inferior epigastric vessels are relatively dominant over the superior deep epigastric vessels, it is likely that the superior system partially supplies this lower abdominal skin in a retrograde fashion by way of a reversal of flow through the inferior system. The deep epigastric system is quite capable of carrying any portion of the skin which is "primarily" supplied by the superior epigastric system. The rectus abdominis muscle will also survive on the eighth through twelfth lateral intercostal system even after the superior and inferior deep systems have both been divided. Finally, the small superficial inferior epigastric vessels, which supply the vertical groin flap described by Shaw and Paine can also nourish a major segment of lower abdominal skin extending from the iliac crest to the rib cage and past the midline.

The superior deep epigastric artery is a continuation of the internal mammary artery. After passing beneath the costal cartilages, this vessel perforates the central portion of the rectus abdominis muscle, but it can enter the muscle in its lateral third. This anatomical variation necessitates a careful search for the superior vessel instead of a "blind" acceptance of its expected position. The vessel usually splits in the upper portion of the muscle into a costomarginal branch which supplies the lateral margin of the rectus abdominis muscle. The deep superior epigastric vessels are usually visible on the undersurface of the rectus abdominis muscle for a distance of five to eight centimeters from the costal margin. Occasionally, it is difficult to identify this vessel until the level of the costal margin is reached. The "watershed" between the superior and inferior systems lies near the level of the umbilicus at the visible termination of the inferior vessels. The inferior deep epigastric vessels are easily visualized on the undersurface of the rectus abdominis muscle from the level of the "watershed" inferiorly. These vessels arise from the common femoral vessels, pass above the inguinal ligament, and enter the posterior rectus sheath just below the arcuate line. The eighth through the twelfth lateral intercostal vessels enter the posterior rectus sheath before penetrating the undersurface of the rectus abdominis muscle. Although these vessels vary in size and number, they anastomose with the superior and inferior deep systems within the muscle and act as a hemodynamic "buffer" to abrupt changes in the other two major systems. The most important cutaneous perforating vessels pass from the rectus abdominis muscle to the skin in the periumbilical region. The individual location of these vessels is quite variable, but the highest density of large vessels is found in an area which extends from approximately three centimeters above the umbilicus to eight centimeters below the umbilicus. These cutaneous perforators are organized into vertical rows which are predictable in their location. The medial row of cutaneous perforators is located approximately 2.5 centimeters lateral to the medial border of the rectus abdominis muscle. The lateral row is located approximately six to seven centimeters lateral to the medial border of the muscle. The medial group of cutaneous perforators consists of larger vessels than the lateral group of cutaneous perforators. Occasionally, there may be a significant number of large perforators in the lateral group. Terminally, the cutaneous perforators reach the subdermal plexus level where they interconnect hemodynamically with the other surrounding vascular systems.

Motor Nerves

Intercostal nerves five to twelve.

Sensory Nerves

Intercostal nerves five to twelve.

USES

The horizontal rectus abdominis myocutaneous (TRAM) flap is used primarily for reconstruction of the breast.

The standard Hartrampf flap, which carries the abdominal pannus, is usually chosen over the other varieties of rectus abdominis myocutaneous flaps because of its size and malleability. As one moves away from the major concentration of deep perforating vessels around the umbilicus, the reliability of the horizontal rectus abdominis flap diminishes. This is particularly true of the very high upper horizontal rectus abdominis flap. The survivability of the horizontal flap can be improved either by using a double rectus abdominis muscle pedicle or by reanastomosing the deep inferior epigastric vessels in their new location.

REGIONAL FLAP COMPARISONS

Although the reliable pectoralis major and latissimus dorsi flaps are usually chosen for chest wall defects, the horizontal rectus abdominis flap also has certain applications. The upper horizontal rectus flap donor site can be primarily closed, and it is in close proximity to the lower chest. Unfortunately, there is approximately a 20% incidence of flap necrosis in most hands. The reasons for this are unknown, but this is probably related to the variability of the deep muscular perforators in the upper abdomen. The superiorly based vertical rectus abdominis flap is usually a better choice in these situations since it is almost totally reliable. This is particularly true in the case of chest wall resections where any partial flap loss could contribute to a life-threatening event. The standard Hartrampf flap can provide a massive amount of tissue for the anterior chest wall, but its dissection is more time-consuming and tedious. It is a safe flap to use for major anterior chest wall defects if the superior vessels are intact and if a double rectus abdominis muscle pedicle is used.

The lower horizontal rectus abdominis (Hartrampf) flap is used almost exclusively for reconstruction of the breast. It is best compared to the latissimus dorsi myocutaneous flap breast reconstruction. The latissimus dorsi flap is obviously more reliable, but it usually requires an implant with the attendant problems of a known foreign body. In fact, 70% of our post-mastectomy (modified and radical) latissimus reconstructions have developed Baker Class III encapsulations with time. Sadly enough, most of these patients experienced a good early result only to be disappointed by the capsular problems after three to five years. There are several situations in which the TRAM flap breast reconstruction is superior to the latissimus dorsi reconstruction. These include a very *large defect* which would require a massive skin replacement, *combinations* of infraclavicular, axillary, and lower chest wall deformities which cannot be adequately repaired by the latissimus dorsi flap, and such *marked obesity* that an implant placed beneath either the pectoralis or latissimus muscles would not be expected to produce symmetry with the opposite breast. The flap is also useful in the pectoralis or latissimus breast reconstruction *"cripple"* with unacceptable contour, shape, or repeated scar capsule formations. Whenever there is adequate abdominal fat and skin available to reconstruct the breast without an implant, the results with the TRAM flap are clearly superior to the best results with the latissimus dorsi method of breast reconstruction.

Since symmetry is such a major consideration, both breasts should probably be treated similarly in regard to silicone implants. For instance, if an opposite total mastectomy is done and reconstructed with a silicone implant, it may be inconsistent to use autogenous abdominal tissue for the other breast. Whenever possible it seems more reasonable to reconstruct both breasts with either silicone implants or with bilateral horizontal rectus abdominis flaps since the eventual results of shape and softness are quite different with each of these types of procedures.

DISADVANTAGES

The upper horizontal rectus abdominis flap has an unexpectedly high incidence of flap necrosis of approximately 20%. The donor site skin can be closed primarily, but this limits the width of the flap to approximately ten centimeters in thin patients and fourteen centimeters in moderately obese patients. Since all of the anterior rectus fascia overlying the rectus abdominis muscle must remain in continuity with the skin, a Prolene® or Marlex® mesh end-to-end replacement is usually necessary for the structural repair of the abdominal wall.

The lower horizontal rectus abdominis flap may be associated with a significant amount of discomfort from the tight abdominal closure and the extensive subcostal dissection. Implants are seldom necessary, but when they are, capsule formation occurs in some thirty percent of these cases. This is surprising because one would think that this fatty flap would be "protective." Flap necrosis is very infrequent if the appropriate limits of flap dimensions are observed. Although an excellent contour is usually achieved, the flap is technically difficult to shape. Some secondary flap revision has been necessary in approximately half of our cases. The reasons for this are distributed fairly equally between problems of the inframammary fold and problems of either excessive or deficient upper fullness. At the first stage it is sometimes difficult to create a proper inframammary fold in the medial breast because the muscular pedicle crosses this area and cannot be constricted. Fat stiffness is related to fat necrosis of the "opposite" abdominal skin of the flap, and it will usually require a secondary excision when it occurs.

The donor site complications are clearly the dominating negative aspect of the TRAM flap. Hernias should be rare if the anterior fascial defect is properly repaired and bolstered with Prolene® or Marlex® mesh. The abdominal contour is seldom as satisfactory as in the esthetic abdominal lipectomy, and it should not always be considered a "bonus." The donor site scar can also be poor if it is necessary to close the skin wound under significant tension. Prolonged abdominal drainage — over seven days — is common, but seroma formation is rare. These patients deserve the same diligent care which one would offer any patient undergoing a major intra-abdominal procedure.

ADVANTAGES

The upper horizontal flap can give an adequate breast reconstruction, but an implant is almost always required. It is still a good secondary choice for an opposite breast reconstruction. However, it is more difficult to shape, and the inset of the flap into a transverse mastectomy scar is awkward. The lower transverse rectus abdominis flap provides an excellent breast reconstruction in patients with very large defects or in obese patients. When one attempts to gain symmetry with a large opposite breast, this is more easily done with the lower transverse rectus abdominis flap than with the latissimus flap. In the latissimus reconstruction the mandated large implant produces a round and wide breast rather than the desired cone shape offered by the rectus abdominis flap. The latissimus flap cannot be expected to correct a combination of defects, including the loss of the anterior axillary fold and the entire pectoralis muscle, because the latissimus muscle is not sufficiently large enough to correct all of these defects. Even in the most favorable postmastectomy situations, the results with the latissimus reconstruction are surpassed by the results with the TRAM flap procedure.

COMPLICATIONS, PITFALLS, AND DONOR SITE

Most complications have been related to the inexperience of the surgeon and are avoidable. The question of how to "delay" the flap or whether "delay" is effective is unsettled. We have occasionally attempted this maneuver when a large amount of tissue has been required. We have not experienced any flap loss with a "delay," but flap loss is not very common in any case. The method of "delay," which we have used is to complete the lower incision, to elevate the ipsilateral skin flap, and to partially ligate the deep inferior epigastric vessels. In a combined (J.B. McCraw and P.G. Arnold) personal series of more than two hundred cases, total flap loss has occurred in one case and partial flap losses have occurred in six cases. All of these cases were *early* cases. There have been no flap losses in the later cases. The differences may be ascribed to luck, but they are more likely related to operative experience. Any portion of the flap with questionable viability should be discarded. If a large amount of tissue is required, it is safer to use a double muscle pedicle.

Certain technical points should be reemphasized. Since the flap is "cold sensitive," the dissection of the entire upper abdomen and the recipient site should be completed prior to the final flap elevation. Warm packs are used throughout the procedure to maintain the flap temperature. A heating blanket, leg and arm wraps, heated inspired air, and heated intravenous fluids are used to maintain the "core" temperature of the body. The large surface exposed during the operation easily allows the "core" temperature to drop to 95 degrees. This temperature is the level at which flap problems will be encountered.

A safe abdominal closure constitutes the most critical area of concern. Hartrampf's method of preserving the linea semilunaris ligaments and repairing the anterior rectus abdominis fascia should be followed religiously. Further, the pyramidalis muscle and the anterior rectus fascia below the arcuate line should be left undisturbed. If there is any question about a safe closure of the abdominal donor site, the use of the TRAM flap must be carefully weighed. This is certainly the case in some obese patients or patients who have had previous intra-abdominal operations.

Flap elevation can be carried out in a number of ways. Although it is important to preserve the semilunaris ligaments in the course of flap elevation, it does not seem critical either to leave or to take a lateral strip of the rectus abdominis muscle. Approximately 1.5 centimeters of anterior rectus fascia should be left adjacent to the midline, and it is seldom necessary to remove more than four centimeters of the fascia lateral to this point. The anterior rectus fascia is usually elevated with the upper part of the rectus abdominis muscle in order to speed the dissection and to provide a strengthening layer for the fragile muscle. Completion of the skin elevation and division of the lower muscle is done only when the flap is ready to be inset. Upward retraction of the flap facilitates the final dissection of the superior epigastric vessels. It is not necessary to elevate the rectus abdominis muscle away from the chest wall because the division of the anterior rectus fascia on either side of the muscle (on the chest wall) provides for adequate upward flap mobility. The rectus abdominis muscle should be transposed in a gentle "S" fashion, and there should be no reason for torsion or tension on the transposed muscle pedicle. The value of fluorescein examination of the flap is debatable because many times a viable flap does not fluoresce well. This response is probably related to the cold sensitivity of the flap, but the non-fluorescence can be unnecessarily traumatic for the compulsive surgeon. Brisk red bleeding at the cut dermal edge is an equally good test of flap viability.

Postoperative care is similar to any other major abdominal wall reconstruction even though the abdominal cavity is not entered from a technical standpoint. Intense pulmonary care is necessary, and smoking is always interdicted. A Foley catheter is used for the first one to two days, and walking is encouraged the day following surgery.

Most of our concerns have been related to the donor site. If only four centimeters of anterior fascia are removed, it can routinely be directly reapproximated. Even in this favorable situation it is reasonable to use an overlay of artificial mesh to bolster the primary fascial repair. Very large anterior fascial defects usually do require an end-to-end or an overlapping mesh repair. Seromas can be troublesome, but their resolution is usually spontaneous. The contour of the abdomen can be a problem because of excessive fat in the epigastrium or flanks when compared to the lower abdominal contour. These have been treated by suction-assisted lipectomy or by direct fat excision. Although the horizontal scar may not be good and a vertical scar may be necessary, neither of these deficiencies has been a source of significant patient complaints.

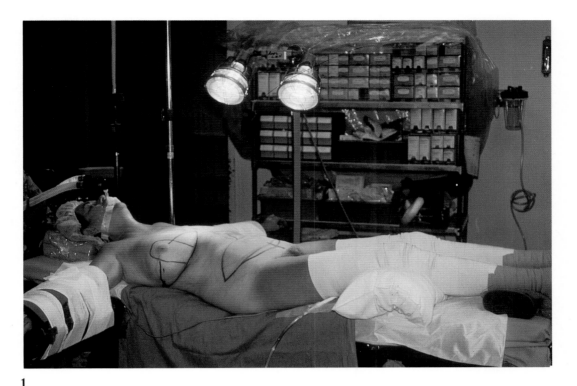

1

Intraoperative preparation. The legs, arms, and head are carefully padded and slightly flexed. The exposure to cold is limited by preoperative markings and skin preparation. The "core" temperature is maintained by a heating blanket, heated inspired air, and "french fry" lights. The legs are wrapped with ace bandages to promote vascular stability in the upright position.

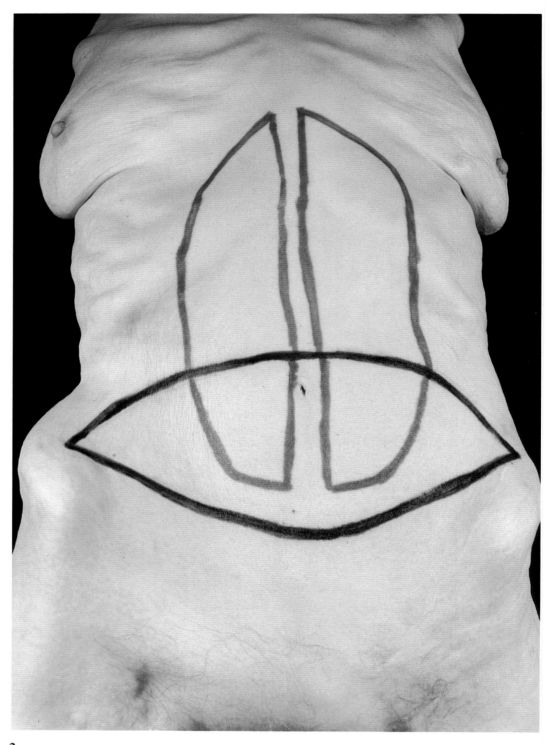

2

The TRAM flap is centered over the peri-umbilical perforators. A double muscle pedicle will be used to carry the entire skin ellipse.

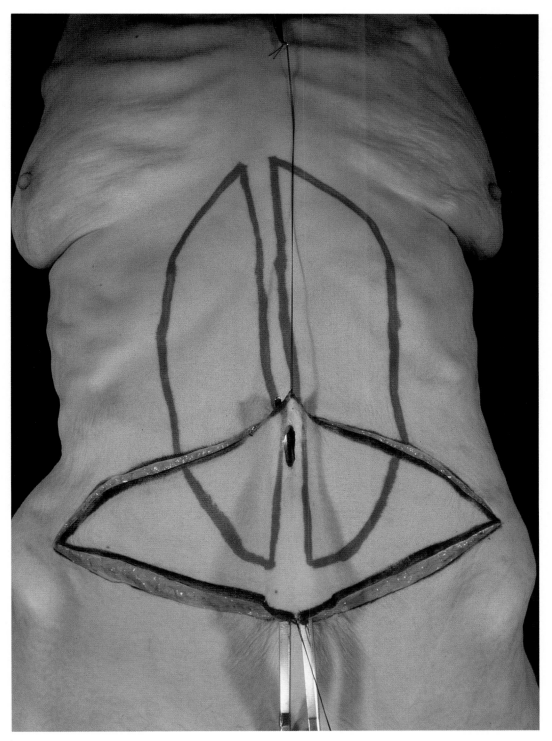

3

Scissors are used to elevate the skin from the avascular midline fascia blindly. This dissection is carried 1.5 centimeters lateral to the medial border of each rectus muscle.

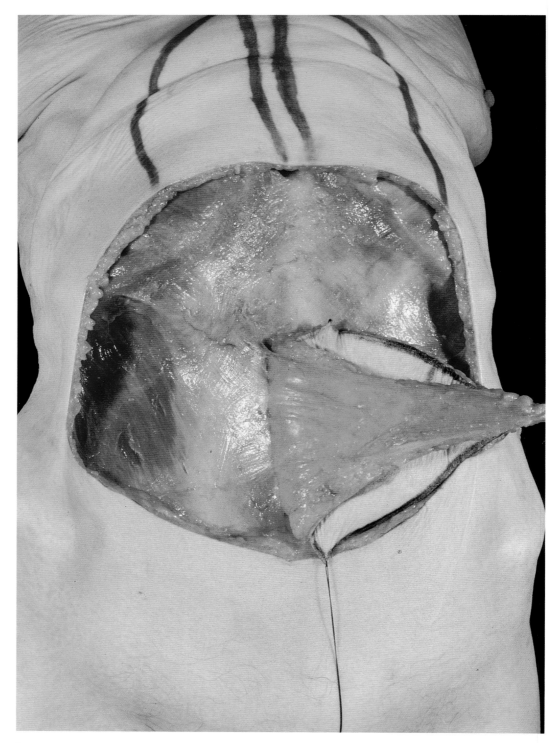

4

The lateral row of perforators is identified
and ligated. The dissection is then carried
medially until the more prominent medial
row of perforators is encountered.

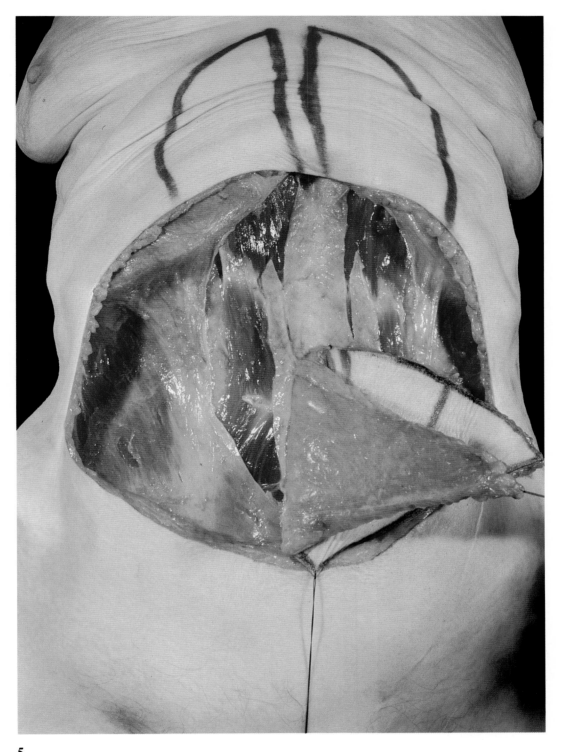

5

The upper abdominal skin and the two rectus muscles are completely dissected prior to the final elevation of the flap. A small strip of anterior rectus fascia is left on the surface of the rectus muscle to protect the muscle and to speed the dissection.

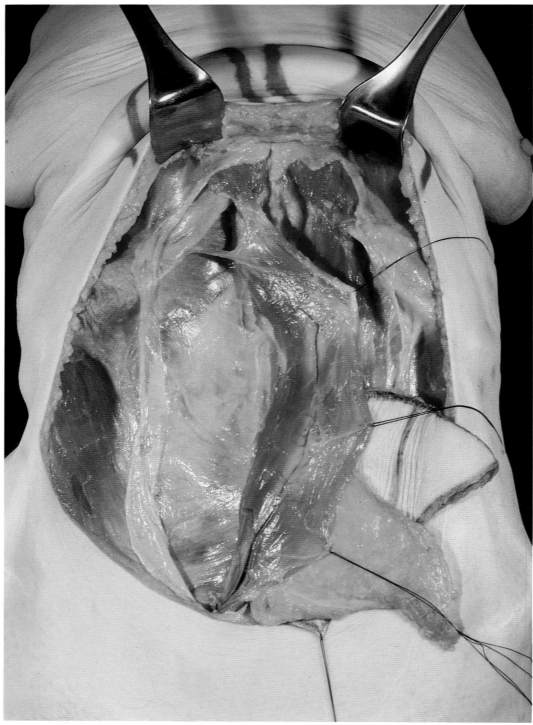

6

The right rectus abdominis muscle is rotated medially to expose the deep inferior epigastric vessels. This exposure is used to divide the anterior rectus fascia (from behind), approximately 1.5 centimeters lateral to the midline. This leaves a total anterior fascial defect of no more than four to five centimeters in width.

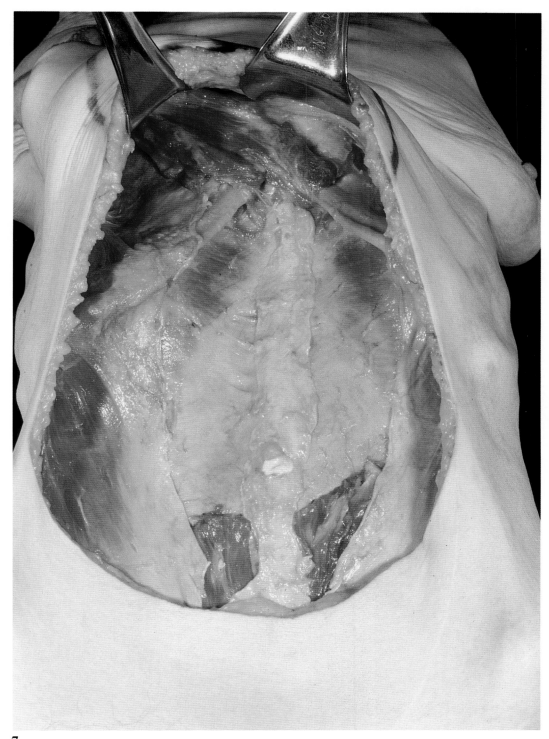

7

The flap is tunneled onto the chest without any torsion or tension on the vascular pedicles. The two muscular pedicles are visible in their course to the right breast area.

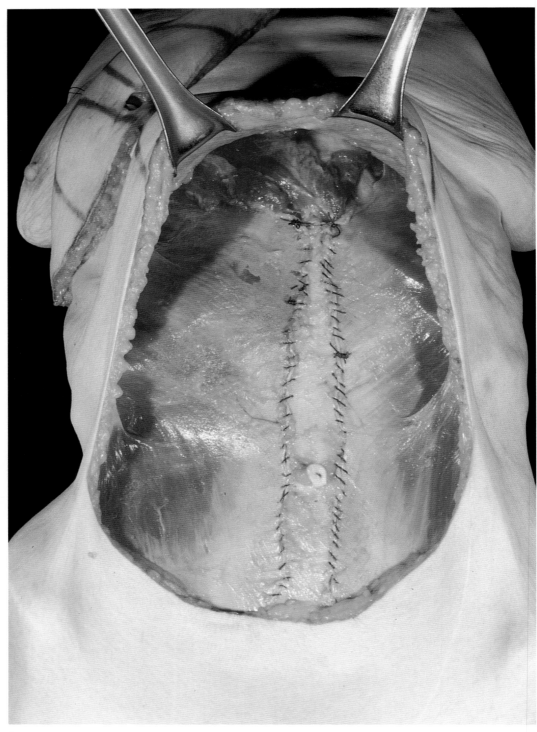

8

The bilateral anterior fascial defects are individually repaired and usually reinforced with an overlay of Prolene® mesh. The abdominal closure is equally as important as the shaping of the reconstructed breast.

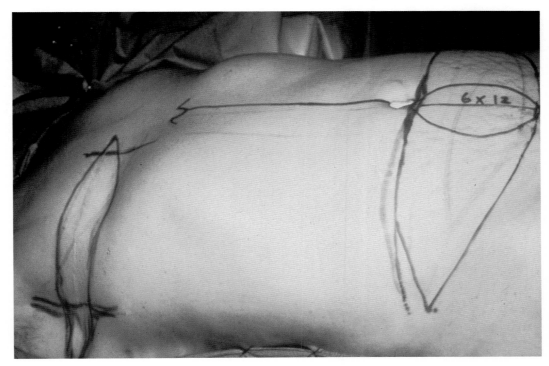

9

Forty-five-year-old female two years following a modified radical mastectomy and irradiation. The mastectomy scar will be widely excised to remove the atrophic skin and the lateral "dog ear." A low TRAM flap is outlined. (Case of J.B. McCraw)

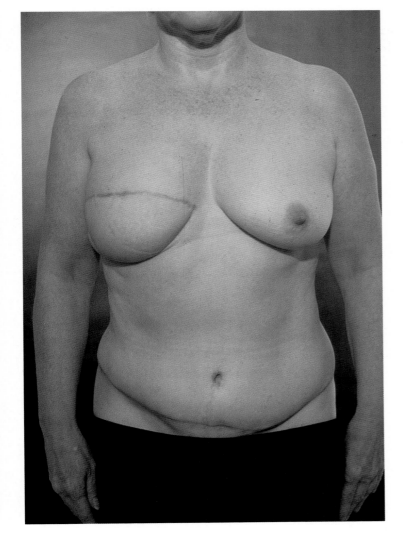

10

The flap was inset at the inframammary fold and contoured to match the opposite breast. The transverse mastectomy scar must be accepted as the upper line of closure.

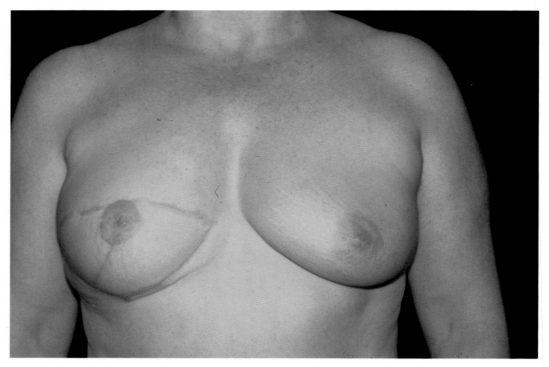

11

A nipple-areola reconstruction was done at a second stage. A vertical wedge "mastopexy" was also performed on the reconstructed breast to improve the symmetry with the normal breast.

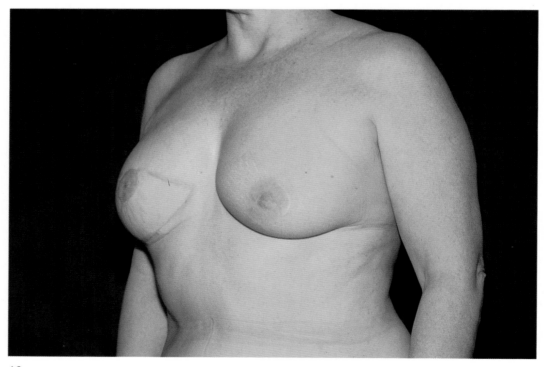

12

The "upper fill" provided by the buried TRAM flap is demonstrated.

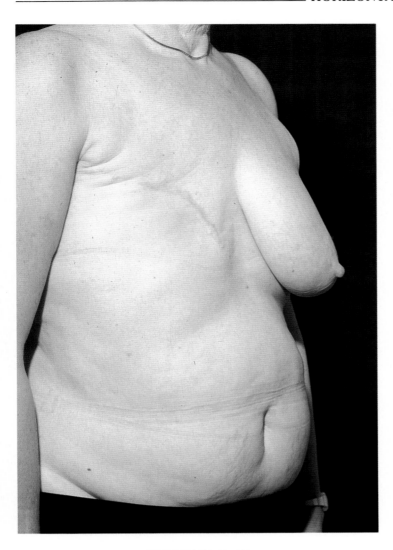

13

Obese fifty-year-old female with a large and ptotic opposite breast. A TRAM flap was chosen as the best method to gain symmetry with the opposite breast. (Case of J.B. McCraw)

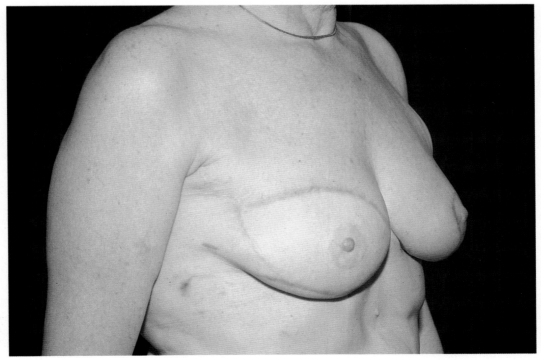

14

Even though a small reduction mammoplasty was performed on the opposite breast, it was necessary to emphasize the ptosis in the reconstructed breast.

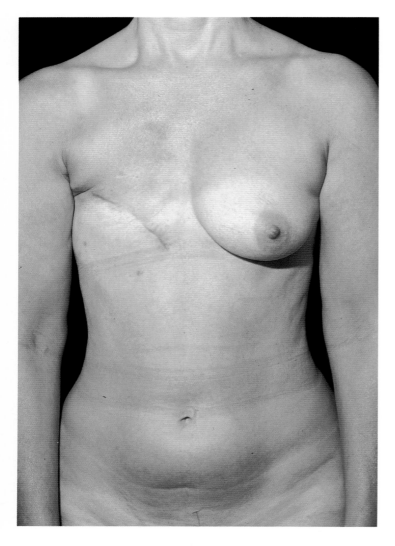

15, 16

Youthful patient with a favorable mastectomy scar and a denervated pectoralis major muscle. The normal breast is only slightly ptotic. A double muscle pedicle will be used to carry the entire abdominal pannus in this thin patient. (Case of J.B. McCraw)

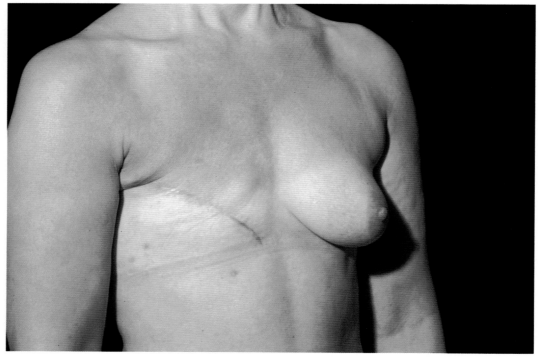

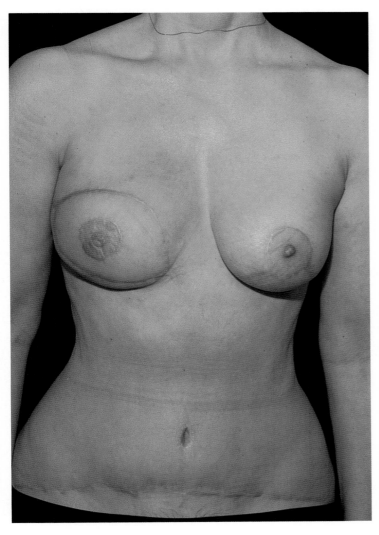

17, 18

The upper mastectomy scar was converted from a straight line into a "C" shape to broaden the central portion of the reconstructed breast. A mastopexy was performed on the opposite breast at the time of the nipple reconstruction. The postoperative abdominal contour was improved by the use of the double muscle TRAM procedure.

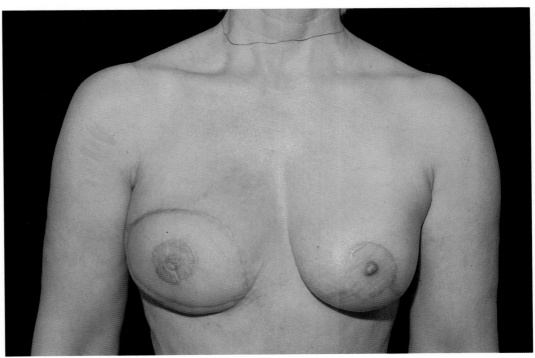

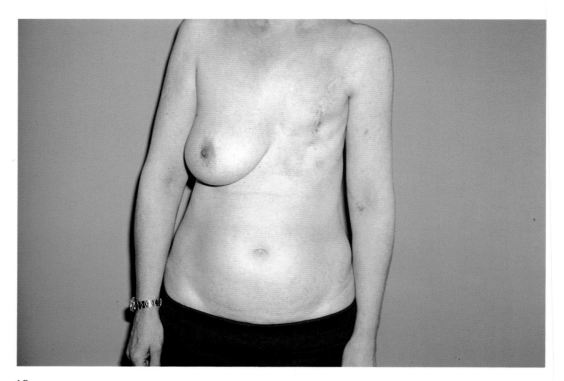

19

Fifty-one-year-old female who had undergone a radical mastectomy and irradiation. The left breast reconstruction was made complicated by the vertical mastectomy closure and the thin mastectomy flaps. (Case of P.G. Arnold)

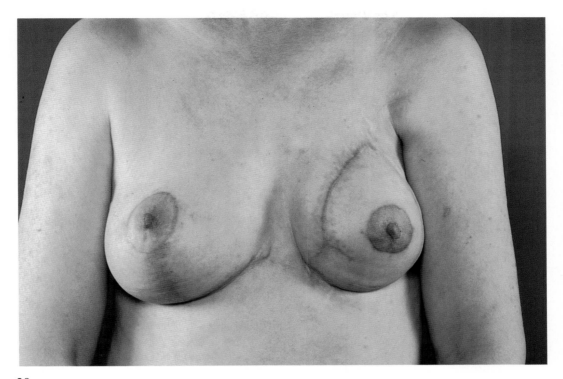

20

The volume of the single pedicled TRAM flap was not adequate to reconstruct the anterior axillary fold, to recreate the upper ''fill,'' and to replace the lost skin.

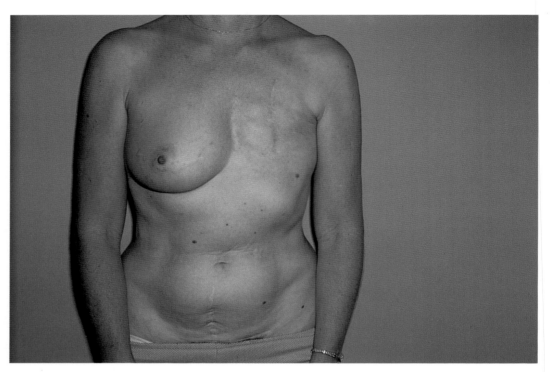

21

Fifty-one-year-old female who had undergone a modified mastectomy with a very medial vertical closure. A right lower paramedian scar limits the amount of abdominal tissue which can be transposed. (Case of P.G. Arnold)

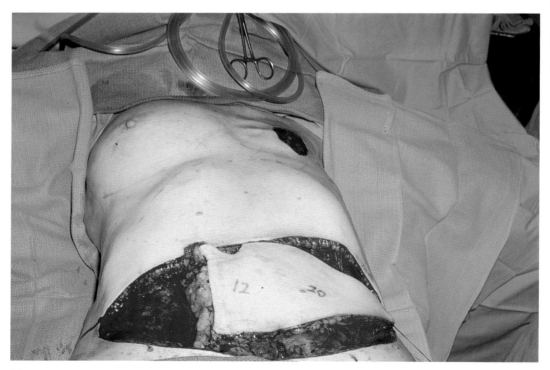

22

An ipsilateral TRAM flap was used because of the previous lower abdominal scar. Note the thinness of the mastectomy flaps.

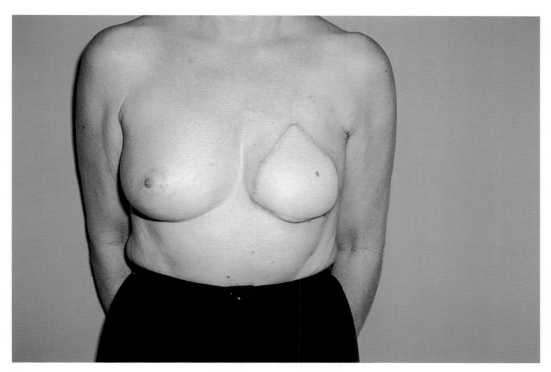

23

The TRAM flap was vertically oriented to accommodate the mastectomy closure. The midline margin of the abdominal flap was inset at the inframammary fold.

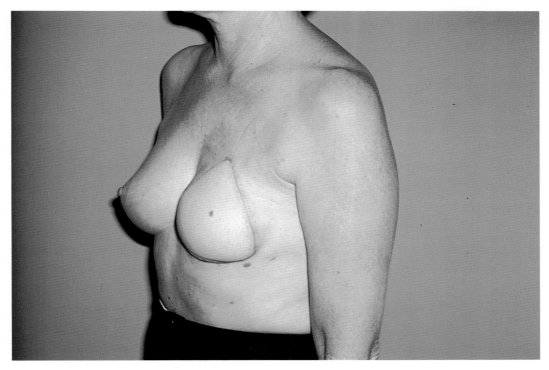

24

The TRAM flap produced good symmetry with the opposite breast and satisfactorily reconstructed the inframammary fold.

317

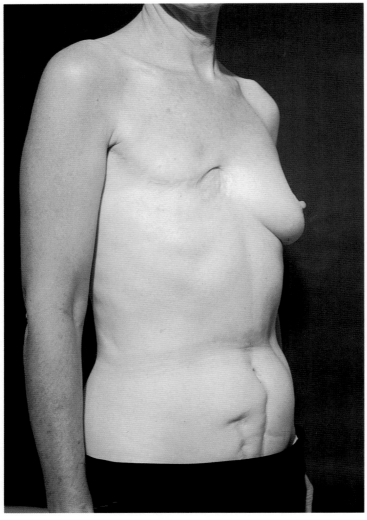

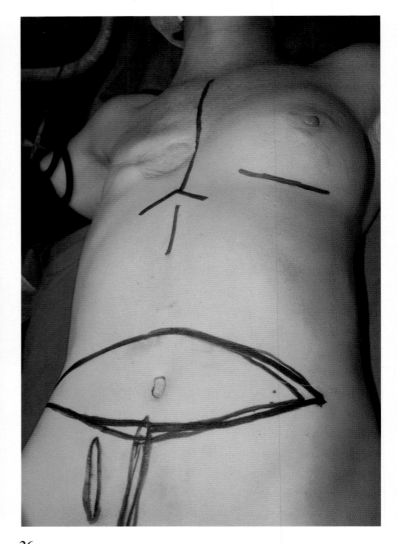

25

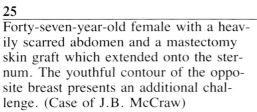

Forty-seven-year-old female with a heavily scarred abdomen and a mastectomy skin graft which extended onto the sternum. The youthful contour of the opposite breast presents an additional challenge. (Case of J.B. McCraw)

26

A high TRAM flap is outlined because this case predates the double muscle pedicle. Under no circumstances will the vasculature of the TRAM flap traverse a vertical abdominal scar.

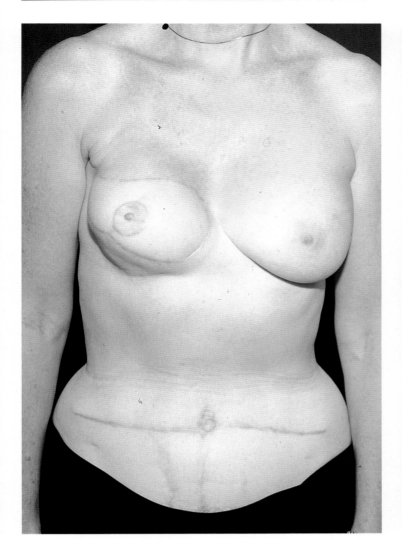

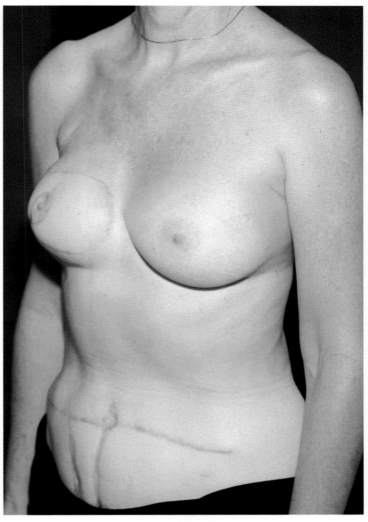

27, 28

The high abdominal closure through the umbilicus gives a predictably poor scar. The volume of the TRAM flap was insufficient to obtain symmetry with the normal breast. A double muscle pedicle would have provided the desired volume and allowed a lower abdominal closure.

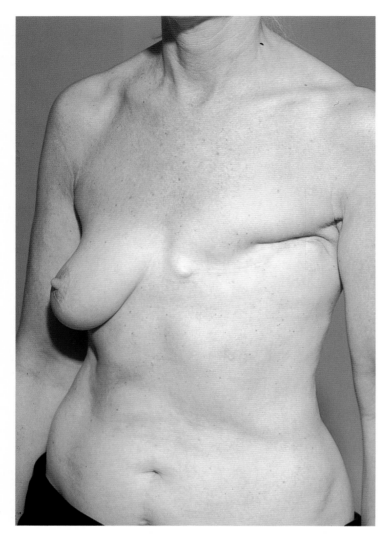

29, 30

Forty-six-year-old female with an extensive mastectomy and a lower midline abdominal scar. The small abdominal pannus was not adequate both to replace the deficient breast skin and to produce an acceptable volume. A tissue expander was used to stretch the existing chest wall skin. (Case of J.B. McCraw)

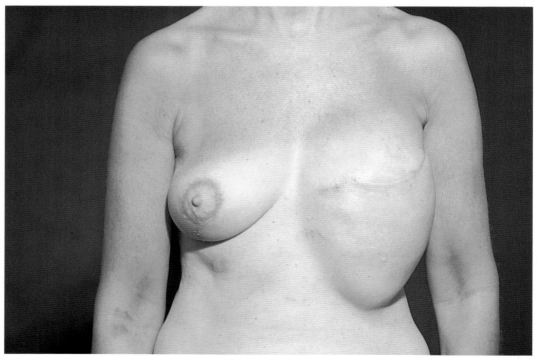

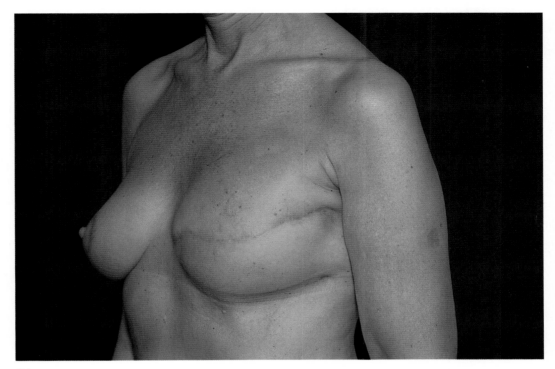

31

The 1000 cc tissue expander corrected the skin deficiency and helped to recreate the inframammary fold.

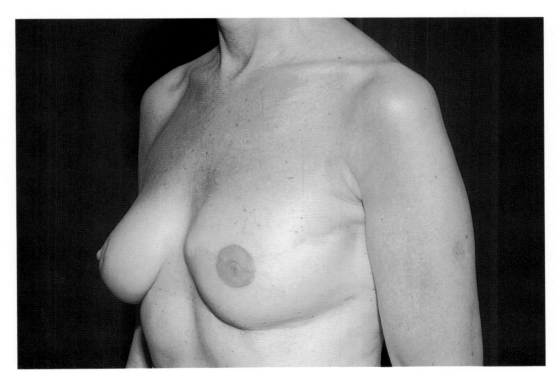

32

The TRAM flap was completely deepithelialized and buried for volume replacement. The symmetry with the ptotic breast is acceptable.

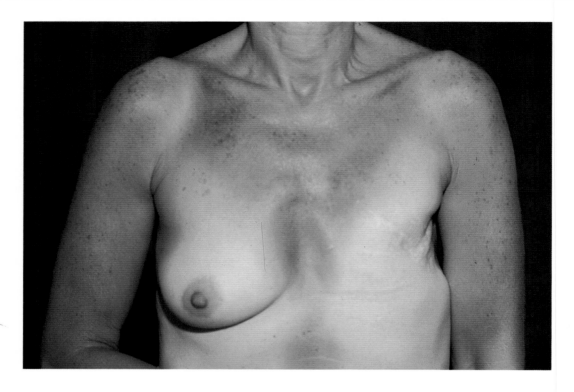

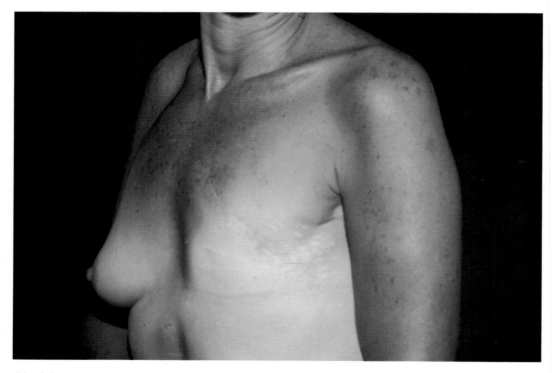

33, 34

Fifty-four-year-old female following an extensive modified radical mastectomy with a "T" closure and "pie crusting" of the mastectomy flaps. (Case of J.B. McCraw)

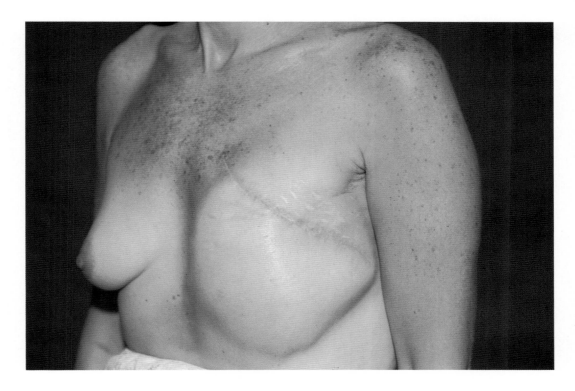

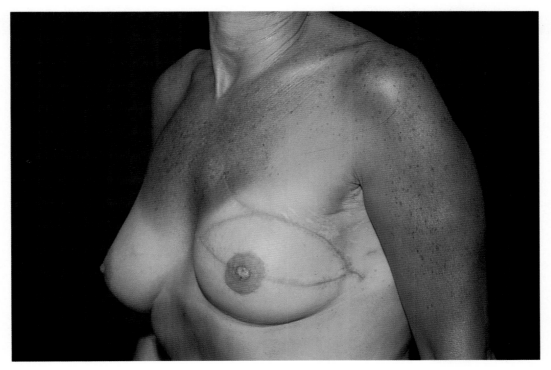

35, 36

A 1000 cc tissue expander partially replaced the deficient skin. It was still necessary to use a portion of the TRAM flap
for skin replacement.

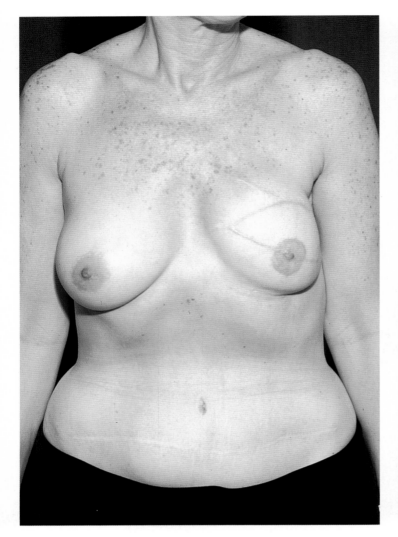

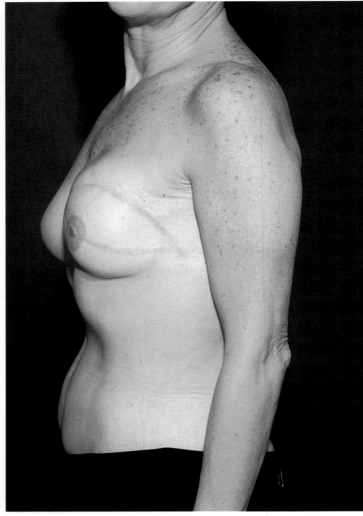

37, 38

Two years postoperative. The abdominal contour and closure are good. A double muscle pedicle would have eliminated the need for the tissue expander.

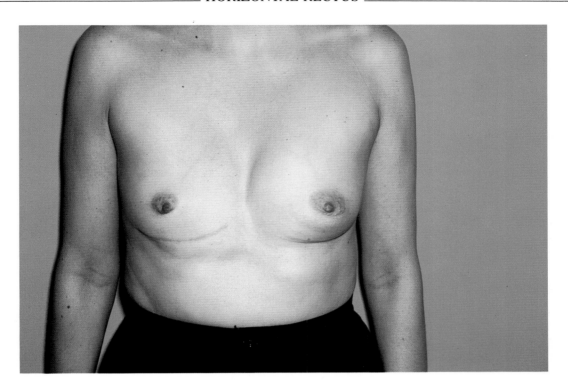

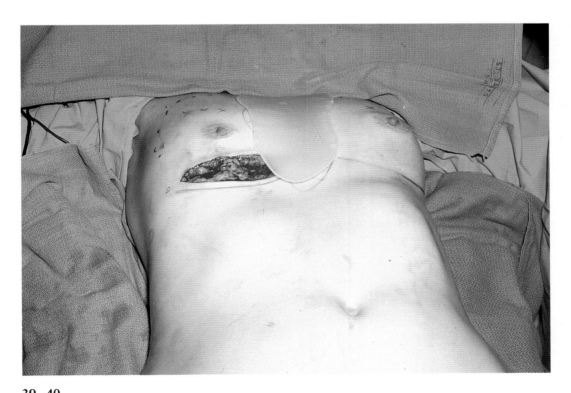

39, 40

Thirty-five-year-old female with pectus excavatum and a congenitally small right breast. This was previously treated with a disproportionate augmentation mammoplasty and a custom Silastic® sternal implant. Unfortunately, all three pockets communicated. (Case of P.G. Arnold)

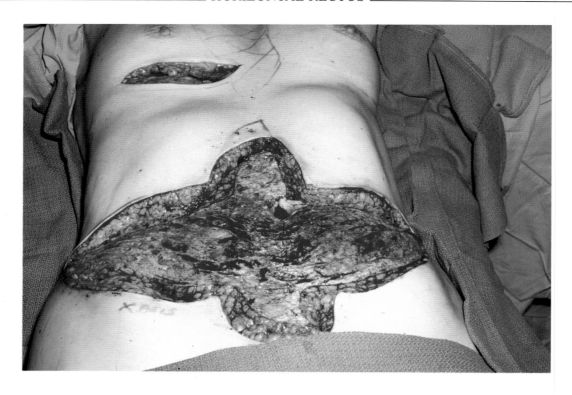

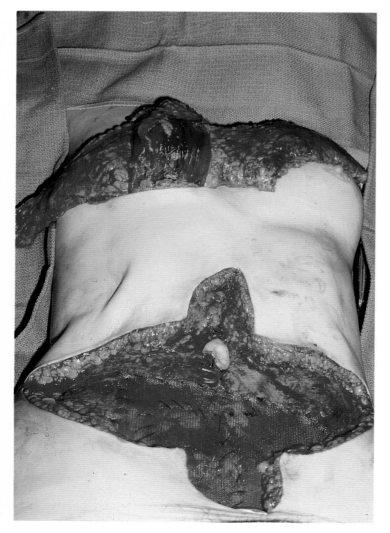

41, 42

The entire TRAM flap was deepithelialized. The vertical component of the flap was used to correct the pectus deformity, and the remaining flap was used to augment the right breast. The left breast implant was removed.

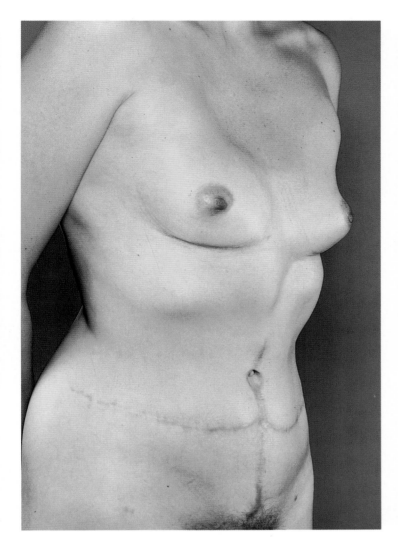
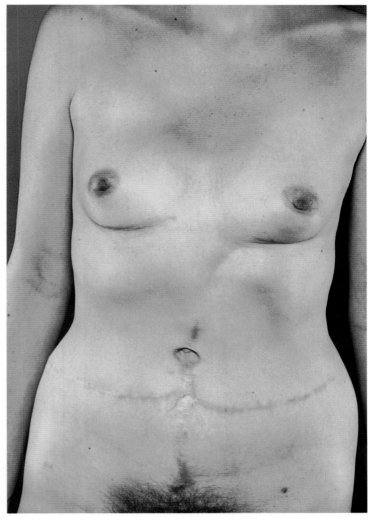

43, 44

Reasonable breast symmetry was obtained, and the pectus deformity was corrected. The abdominal contour is acceptable, but the vertical closure is less than ideal.

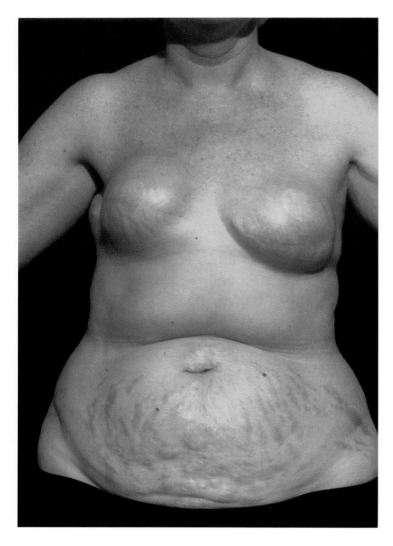

45, 46

Forty-six-year-old female ten years following bilateral mastectomies and prepectoral implants. The very large abdominal pannus was adequate for a bilateral breast reconstruction without implants. (Case of J.B. McCraw)

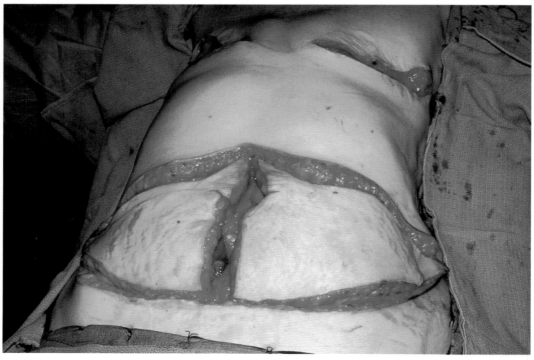

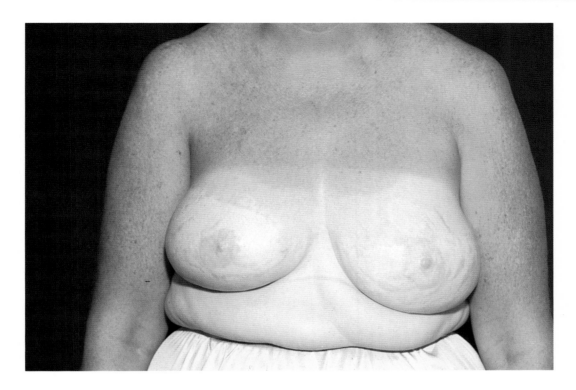

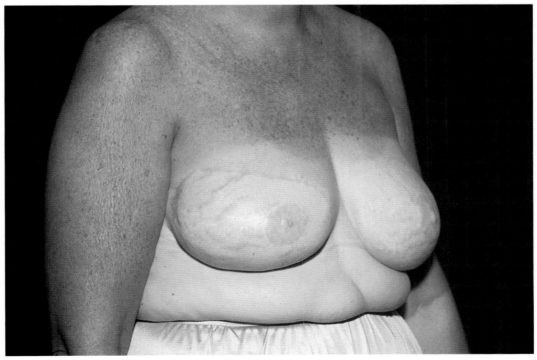

47, 48

Only the bilateral TRAM procedure can be expected to provide such a large reconstructed breast with normal ptosis. The patient was happy to reach a definitive solution to her implant problems.

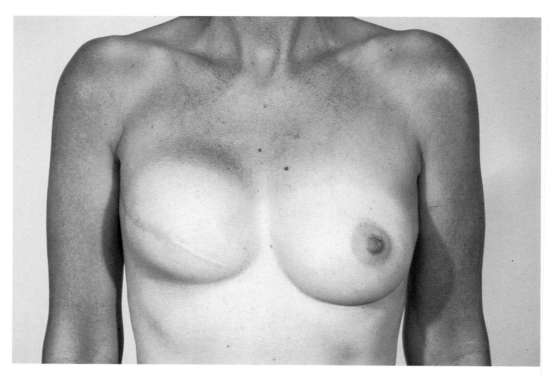

49

Forty-two-year-old female following a modified mastectomy and a subpectoral breast reconstruction. A capsular contracture persisted despite several open capsulotomies. (Case of J.B. McCraw)

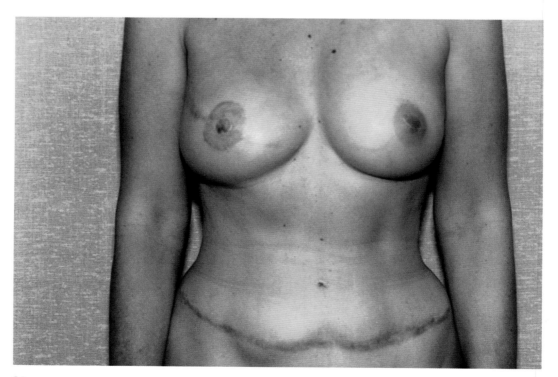

50

The right breast implant was replaced with a deepithelialized TRAM flap. The nipple was reconstructed in a second stage.

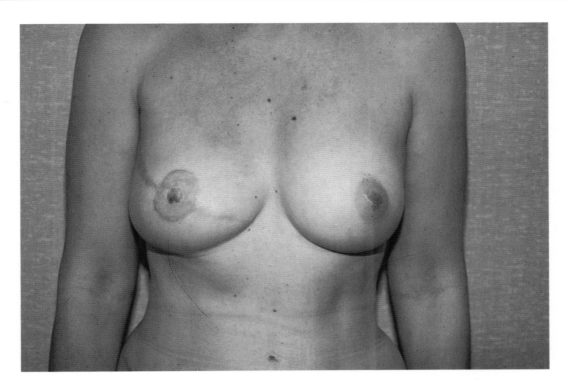

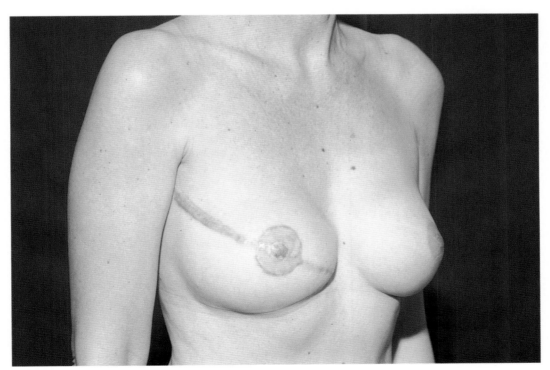

51, 52

Nearly ideal symmetry is achieved with the normal breast. The previous right subpectoral implant obviated the need for external skin replacement.

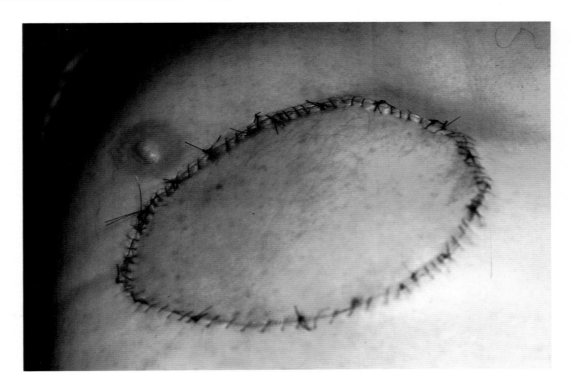

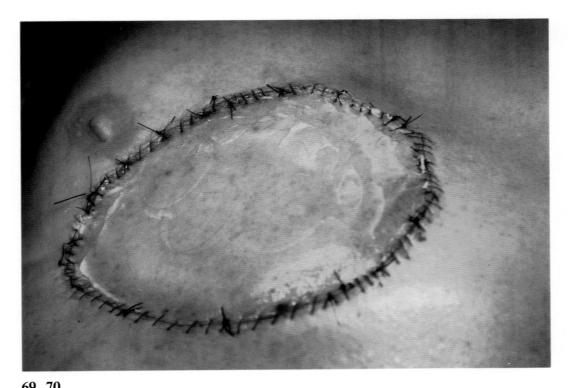

69, 70

The inset flap did not fluoresce well. Since this was not thought to be a mechanical problem, nitroglycerin paste was applied to the flap. Note the improved flap color and fluorescence within a two minute period.

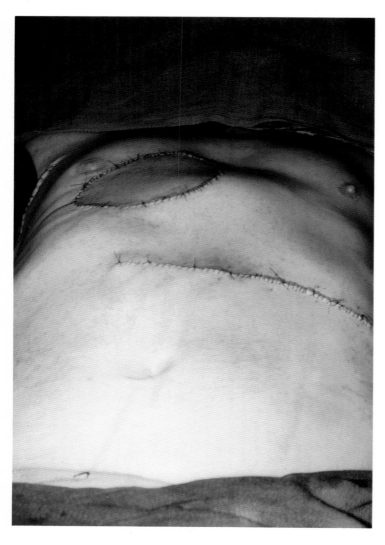

71, 72
Primarily closed donor site and inset flap. The color match and contour restoration are excellent in this patient. The quality of the reconstruction and the faster healing time cannot be matched by a skin graft.

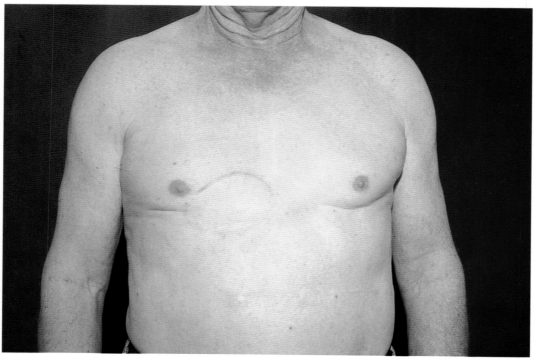

EXTERNAL OBLIQUE

ANATOMICAL CONSIDERATIONS

Surface Markings

The external oblique muscle encompasses the entire abdominal wall, extending from the midback to the lateral margin of the rectus abdominis muscle. It is easily palpated throughout its course.

Origin and Insertion

The muscle originates from the posterior aspects of the sixth to the twelfth ribs and runs obliquely downward to its broad attachment at the linea semilunaris and the inguinal ligament. The strength of the lateral abdominal wall musculature far exceeds that of the rectus abdominis muscles. This is probably the reason a ventral hernia is more common with a vertical incision than with a horizontal incision. Even though the external oblique muscle is functionally expendable, every attempt should be made to reestablish its muscular insertion.

Adjacent Muscles

The external oblique is the largest and the strongest of the flat abdominal wall muscles. It overlies the internal oblique muscle throughout its course and is partially covered by the latissimus dorsi and serratus anterior muscles posteriorly.

Vascular Pattern

The blood supply to the external oblique muscle arises from the multiple deep perforators from the sixth through the twelfth posterior intercostal vessels. These intercostal vessels enter the undersurface of the muscle near the posterior axillary line and diffusely arborize throughout the muscle. Because of this diffuse arborization it is possible to divide one or more of these major supplying vessels without harming the viability of the external oblique muscle flap. It is important to note that only a few inconsequential intercostal perforating vessels are seen anterior to the midaxillary line.

Motor Nerve

Sixth through twelfth intercostal nerves.

Sensory Nerve

Sixth through twelfth intercostal nerves.

USES

Since the external oblique muscle will "carry" all of its overlying skin, it is usually transposed to the lower anterior chest wall as a composite myocutaneous flap.

This composite flap will easily reach the level of the inframammary fold and the ipsilateral fourth rib, which is the primary application of the myocutaneous flap. This not only provides an esthetic reconstruction of the lower chest wall but also provides innervated skin and muscle. The external oblique muscle flap can also be rotated inferiorly to close a hemipelvectomy defect in the absence of the ipsilateral thigh musculature.

REGIONAL FLAP COMPARISONS

When it is available, the latissimus dorsi muscle flap is the first choice for high and lateral chest wall defects. The opposite upper horizontal rectus abdominis myocutaneous (Psillakis) flap can also be used for lower anterior chest wall defects, but the rate of flap necrosis may exceed 20%, which is unacceptable for coverage of a full thickness chest wall defect. The lower horizontal rectus abdominis myocutaneous flap will predictably supply a large amount of skin to the chest wall and sternum, but it provides very little muscle bulk for the coverage of prosthetic material or exposed bone. The vertical rectus abdominis myocutaneous flap offers an excellent alternative for defects of the lower chest wall or sternum when the internal mammary vessels are intact. It can be rapidly elevated and carries a ten centimeter width of anterior rectus fascia for structural reconstitution. Although the extensive anterior rectus fascial donor site usually requires a prosthetic repair, the midline skin closure can be accomplished without undermining.

The external oblique muscle can also be directly transposed into the hemipelvectomy defect. This inferior rotation is accomplished by simply separating the external oblique muscle from its lower chest wall attachments and relocating its muscular insertion. Only the opposite inferiorly based rectus abdominis myocutaneous flap will provide comparable coverage in the absence of the ipsilateral leg musculature. When a colostomy is required, the inferiorly based rectus abdominis flap is not as desirable for the closure of a hemipelvectomy defect because prosthetic mesh is needed to repair the rectus abdominis donor defect.

DISADVANTAGES

The primary disadvantage of the external oblique flap is its limited arc of rotation, which restricts its usefulness. The multiplicity of the intercostal blood supply is more an apparent than a real disadvantage. It would be

343

difficult to harm these vessels unless the dissection is carried beyond the posterior axillary line. The donor site closure offers a potential site for hernia formation, but this has not been observed.

ADVANTAGES

The primary advantage of this flap is that it will close a significant lower anterior chest wall defect with skin of similar color and texture without distorting the level of the breast. This is a positive esthetic consideration in women. It is a thin musculocutaneous flap which maintains its sensation and motor capabilities.

COMPLICATIONS, PITFALLS, AND DONOR SITE

The complications associated with the external oblique flap include those which can be expected from any extensive dissection: hemorrhage, infection, and seroma formation. If the external oblique muscle is separated from the overlying skin, it is important to leave the superficial fascia with the skin layer. This separates the musculocutaneous flap into a muscle flap and a fasciocutaneous flap. Inclusion of the fascia with the skin ensures the best possible blood supply to the skin. It is also helpful to include a small strip of anterior rectus fascia with the external oblique muscle flap. This provides a dense fascial layer for suturing this friable muscle.

The donor site can be closed in a V-Y fashion, but a small skin graft is also quite acceptable in the lower abdomen. Hernias have not occured with the simple transposition of the external oblique muscle flap, but great care must be exercised to avoid denervating the rectus abdominis muscle because this can result in a central abdominal weakness.

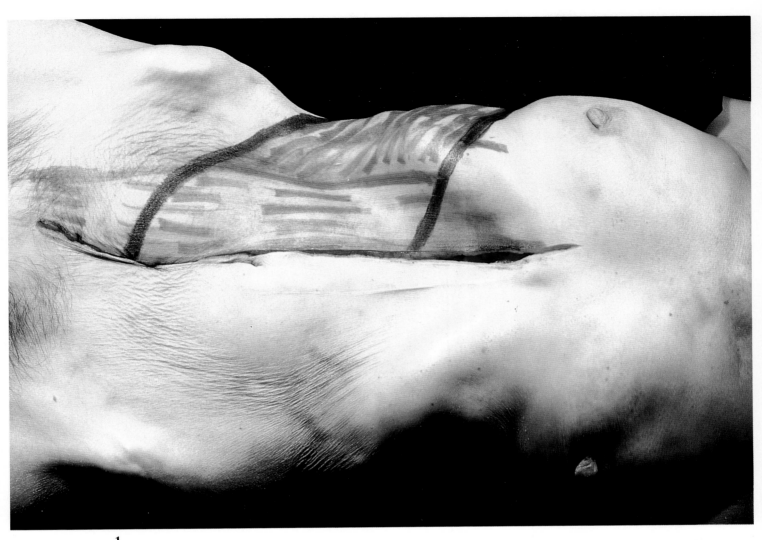

1

The fibers of the right external oblique muscle are marked in red and outlined in black. The vertical fibers of the right rectus abdominis muscle are also marked in red.

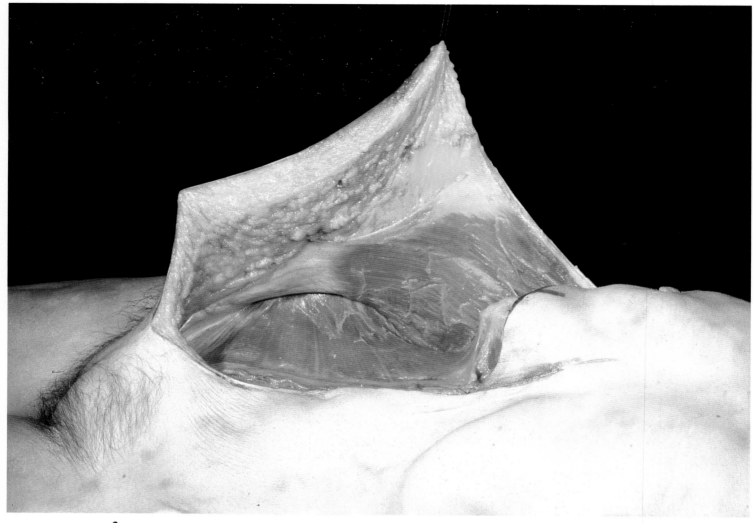

2

Elevation of the musculocutaneous flap is begun at the midline. The external oblique muscle has been elevated away from the internal oblique muscle after the semilunaris ligament has been detached. Note the easy plane of dissection between the external and internal oblique muscles.

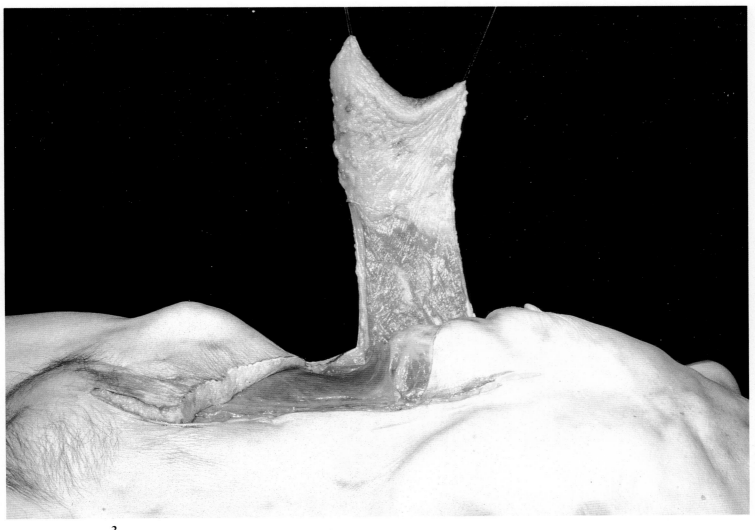

3

The external oblique musculocutaneous
flap is elevated to the level of the anterior
axillary line.

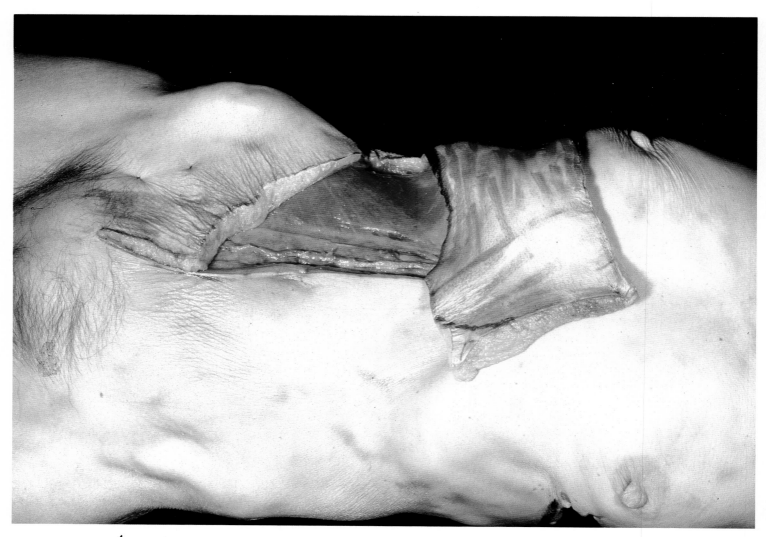

4

Musculocutaneous flap rotated superiorly
to the level of the inframammary fold.
Note the coverage of the lower sternum.

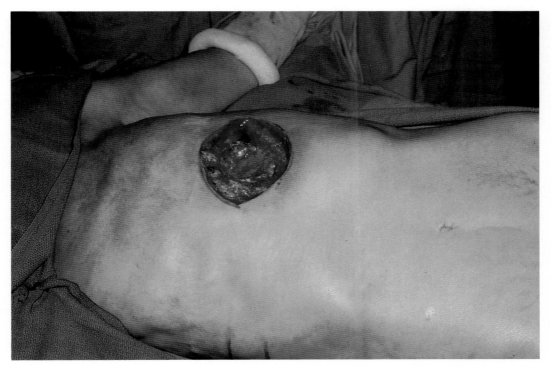

5

Sixty-two-year-old female following a wide excision of a radiation ulcer of the lower chest wall. The patient had previously undergone a bilateral mastectomy and irradiation therapy. (Case of P.G. Arnold)

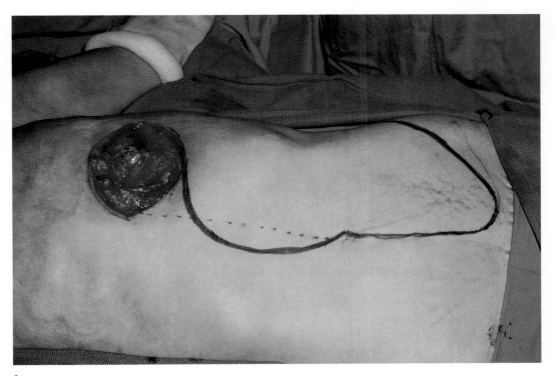

6

Outline of an external oblique myocutaneous flap which extends past the midline.

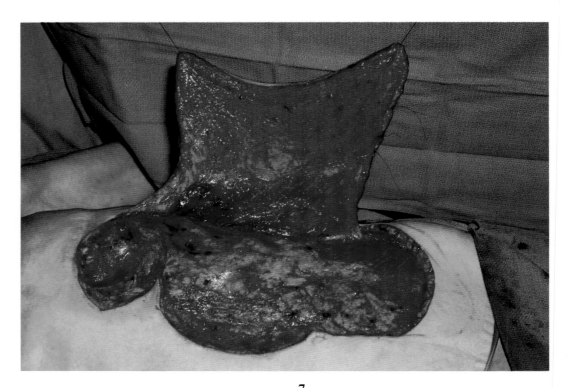

7

External oblique flap elevated to the level of the midaxillary line.

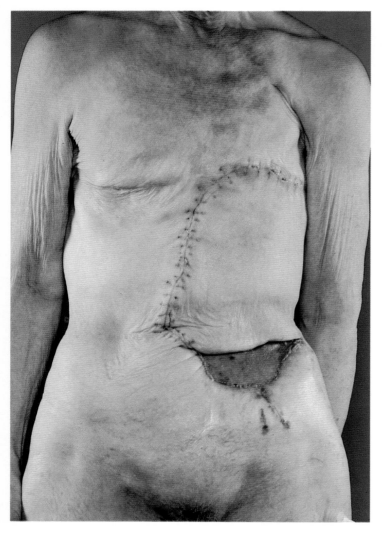

8

Postoperative view at three weeks. Healing skin graft on the internal oblique muscle.

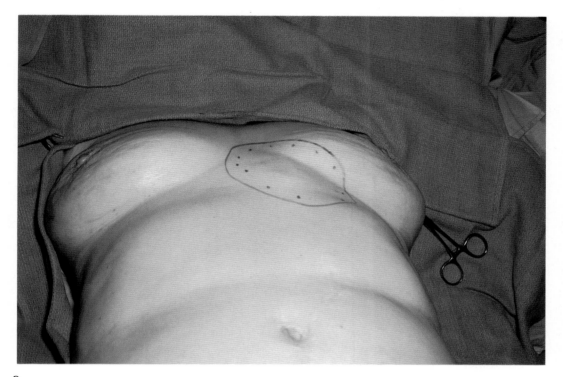

9

Forty-year-old female with a biopsy proven desmoid tumor of the lower chest wall. The extent of the lesion is marked in blue. (Case of P.G. Arnold)

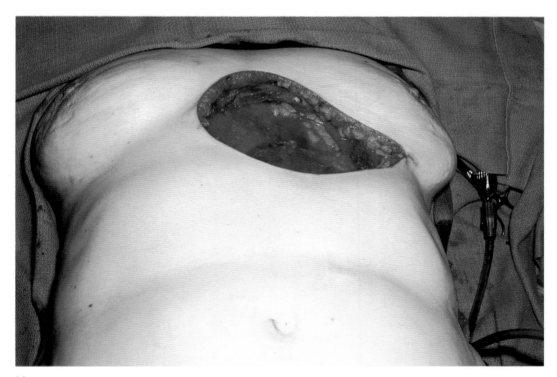

10

Defect following the wide excision of the lesion including the chest wall.

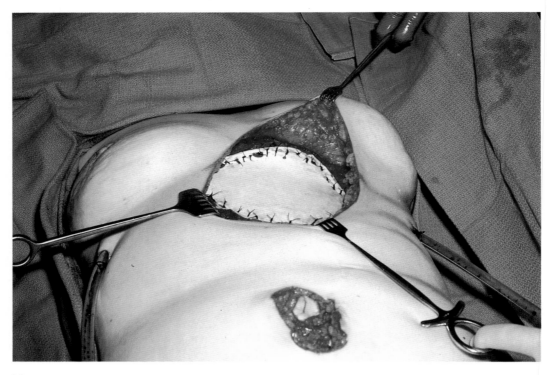

11

The chest wall defect was reconstructed with a Gortex® patch.

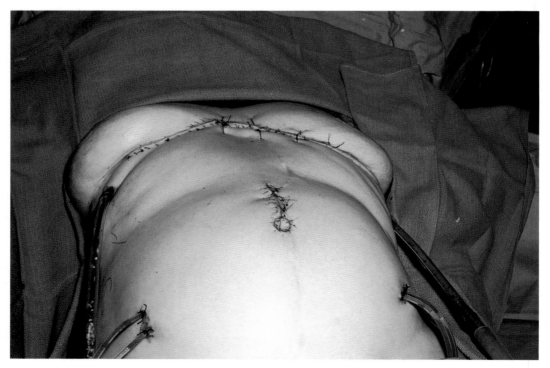

12

Bilateral external oblique musculocutaneous flaps were advanced superiorly for a distance of seventeen centimeters and closed as a "reversed" abdominoplasty.

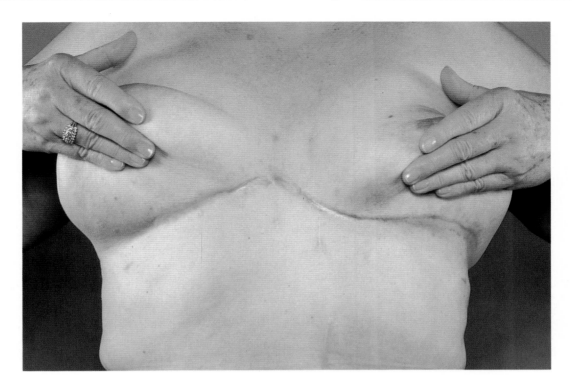

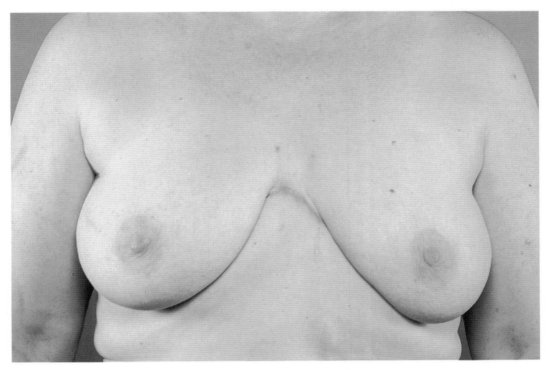

13, 14

Appearance of the patient one year later demonstrating the inframammary closure and the undisturbed breast contour.

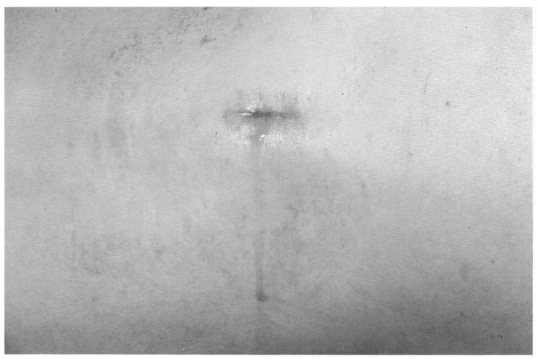

15

Infected axillo-femoral bypass graft. A thrombectomy incision site is draining in the midportion of the graft. (Case of J.B. McCraw and R.T. Gregory, Jr.)

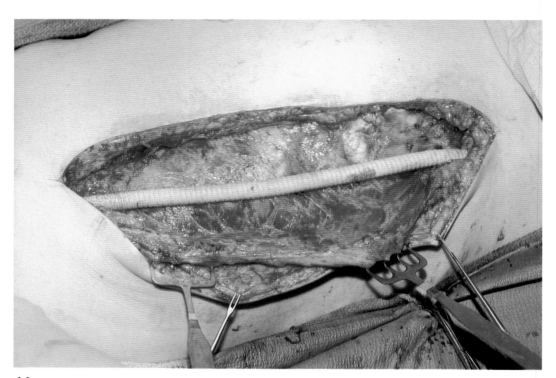

16

The pseudosheath was completely excised and the wall of the Dacron® graft was found to be uninfected. The vascular graft was then transposed from a subcutaneous location to a submuscular location beneath the external oblique muscle, which is retracted.

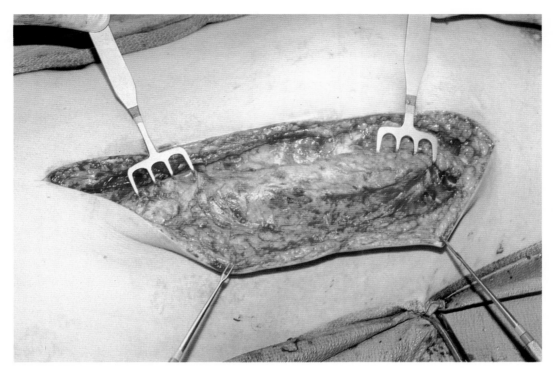

17

Demonstration of the external oblique muscular coverage of the midportion of the graft.

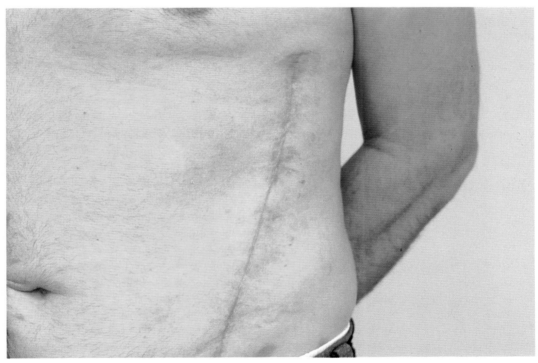

18

Healed incision at three months. The axillo-femoral graft was salvaged for a period of three years.

GLUTEUS MAXIMUS

ANATOMICAL CONSIDERATIONS

Surface Markings

The belly of the gluteus maximus muscle forms the bulk of the buttock. The medial margin is densely attached to the sacrum, and the inferior margin loosely creates the gluteal fold. The superior edge is palpable at the posterior border of the iliac crest.

Origin and Insertion

The majority of the muscle originates from the lateral margin of the sacrum and from the posterior superior iliac crest. To a lesser extent, it arises from the coccyx and the sacrotuberous ligament. The width of this quadrilateral shaped muscle is maintained throughout its course as it passes anterior to the greater trochanter and into the iliotibial tract. The muscle inserts more extensively into the iliotibial tract than it does into the greater trochanter. Unlike the vertically oriented gluteus medius and tensor muscles, which act as abductors and internal rotators of the hip, the gluteus maximus muscle is the strongest external rotator and extensor of the hip. These two motions are effected through the bidirectional insertion of the gluteus maximus muscle. The upper half of the muscle ''wraps'' horizontally around the greater trochanter and contributes to stair climbing and jogging. The lower half of the muscle inserts vertically into the iliotibial tract. Although both of these insertions contribute to abduction of the thigh at the hip joint, the upper half of the gluteus maximus muscle is more important to this function.

Adjacent Muscles

In its superior half the gluteus maximus overlies the gluteus medius muscle. Below this it covers the piriformis, obturator, and quadratus femoris muscles. The sciatic nerve is the most important structure in this area as it passes beneath the piriformis muscle and over the obturator internus and obturator externus muscles. The inferior gluteal nerve arises from the sciatic nerve to supply the gluteus maximus muscle while the superior gluteal nerve supplies the gluteus medius and gluteus minimus muscles. In the upper half of the buttock there is a distinct plane between the gluteus maximus and gluteus medius muscles, but in the lower half of the buttock the plane between the gluteus maximus muscle and the deeper muscles is less distinct. For this reason, the gluteus maximus muscle is initially identified at either the posterior iliac crest or the lateral sacral margin. The vertically oriented muscle fibers of the gluteus medius muscle and the transversely oriented fibers of the gluteus maximus muscle facilitate the identification of each muscle.

Vascular Pattern

The gluteus maximus muscle has a dual blood supply from the superior and inferior gluteal vessels which arise from the internal iliac vessels. The piriformis muscle serves as the landmark which separates these two sets of vessels. The superior vessels pass above the piriformis muscle, and the inferior vessels pass below it. The superior vessels can be predictably located at a point three centimeters lateral to the sacrum and five centimeters below the posterior superior iliac spine. The larger inferior gluteal vessels pass beneath the piriformis muscle just medial to the sciatic nerve at a point five centimeters from the sacral edge. There is usually a duplicate branch of the inferior gluteal vessels which passes to the lower half of the muscle. Even though the inferior gluteal vessels are dominant, the excellent intramuscular vascular connections allow the gluteus maximus muscle to be supplied by either set of vessels.

Motor Nerve

Inferior gluteal nerve (L-5, S-1, S-2).

Sensory Nerves

Superior, medial, and inferior clunial nerves.

USES

The gluteus maximus myocutaneous flap serves as the primary choice for coverage of the sacrum and as a secondary flap source for the ischium. In either case it can be used as a rotational flap, but it is more often moved in a V to Y fashion. For sacral coverage problems the flap is usually rotated on the superior gluteal vessels. However, the inferior gluteal vessels are more often used to supply the flap for ischial coverage. When bilateral V to Y flaps are employed for sacral defects, it is seldom necessary to divide either set of vessels or to release the muscular insertions.

The gluteus maximus muscle can also be split in the line of its fibers into caudal and cranial ''island'' myocutaneous flaps. An isolated ''island'' of skin can be placed on the lateral aspect of the gluteus maximus muscle and the donor site can be primarily closed. The cranial split ''island'' flap will reach the lumbar area and it has also been employed as a ''free'' flap donor site for breast reconstruction. The caudal split island flap can be used to transfer skin to the ischium and the central perineum because of the proximate rotation point of the inferior gluteal vessels. The gluteus maximus is rarely used as an isolated muscle flap because the amount of coverage provided by the pure muscle flap is disappointing and because a skin grafted muscle flap seems to be less durable than a standard myocutaneous flap.

REGIONAL FLAP COMPARISONS

The gluteus maximus musculocutaneous flap is the predominant flap chosen for coverage of the sacral area. As a bilateral V-Y flap it can cover essentially any sacral defect and later be readvanced to solve a subsequent sacral problem. Both the "reversed" latissimus dorsi myocutaneous flap and the intercostal "island" flap will reach the lower lumbar and upper sacral areas. However, both offer significant disadvantages in their complicated dissections, and neither will cover a large central sacral defect. The intercostal flap requires a preliminary "delay" and a complex intrathoracic dissection, but it does provide sensibility to its site of inset. Although the "reversed" latissimus flap is reasonably reliable, the dissection of the deep perforating vasculature is tedious and the arc of rotation is variable. It certainly is not applicable to most sacral defects. A transverse back flap is seldom considered because it is much less reliable than the gluteus maximus myocutaneous flap and because it leaves a skin-grafted donor site. Because of its better survivability, the cranial split "island" gluteus maximus myocutaneous flap would always be preferentially considered over both the "reversed" latissimus and the transverse back flaps.

Although the gluteus maximus myocutaneous flap can be used for ischial coverage problems, it must be compared to the equally reliable and less complicated V to Y biceps femoris myocutaneous flap. The V-Y biceps femoris flap is electively chosen for an isolated ischial ulcer, leaving the unique gluteus maximus flap in "reserve" for a subsequent sacral ulcer. When the biceps femoris flap is unavailable for coverage of an isolated ischial ulcer, the gluteus maximus flap can also be "saved" by using either the vastus lateralis muscle flap or the tensor fascia lata flap. The caudal split gluteus maximus "island" myocutaneous flap is another alternative for isolated ischial and perineal defects. Fortunately, it does not preclude the use of a V-Y gluteus maximus myocutaneous flap for a subsequent sacral defect.

One recent addition to our sacral coverage armamentarium is the combined gluteus maximus myocutaneous and posterior thigh fasciocutaneous flap, which is supplied by the inferior gluteal vessels. The inferior gluteal vessels will reliably supply the majority of the skin of the posterior thigh, and this combined unit can be rotated as an "island" flap to resurface the sacrum and the ischium at the same time.

DISADVANTAGES

The gluteus maximus muscle is an important muscle in the ambulatory person because it is the primary extender and abductor of the hip. Strong hip "stabilization" is necessary for climbing, rising from a "stooped" position, and standing on one leg. The total loss of this muscle leaves a significant functional deformity which is described as a "gluteus limp." This can be prevented by "splitting" the gluteus maximus muscle and leaving a portion of the muscle undisturbed. If the gluteus maximus myocutaneous flap is used as a rotation flap rather than as a V-Y flap, it may be necessary to skin graft the exposed gluteus medius muscle. This adds some morbidity to the procedure because skin grafts in this area usually increase the healing time. Bilateral V-Y gluteus advancement flaps are preferred for large sacral defects since the donor defects can be primarily closed. The gluteus maximus muscle is seldom used without its overlying skin, because of the disappointing amount of coverage provided by the muscle alone.

ADVANTAGES

Because of its dual blood supply, the gluteus maximus is an extremely dependable musculocutaneous flap. It can be raised as an "island" flap on either artery or the muscle can be split into two halves as separate "island" flaps. "Splitting" the muscle is useful in the ambulatory individual as this usually circumvents any functional loss. Most large sacral ulcers can be closed with bilateral V-Y myocutaneous flaps without dividing the trochanteric and iliotibial tract insertions since the majority of flap movement is obtained by elevating the muscle away from the sacrum. One added advantage of the V-Y flap is that it can be "re-advanced" to cover a recurrent sacral ulcer.

COMPLICATIONS, PITFALLS, AND DONOR SITE

Definition of this muscle in the quadriplegic may be difficult because of muscle atrophy. The plane between the gluteus maximus and gluteus medius muscles is best identified either at the posterior iliac crest or at the sacral margin. Alternatively, the plane between these two muscles can be identified by tracing the sciatic nerve up to the piriformis muscle. Once the plane between the gluteus medius and maximus muscles is established, the gluteal vessels should be located. The larger inferior vessels are identified below the piriformis muscle, and the smaller superior gluteal vessels are identified approximately three centimeters above the piriformis muscle. The advancement of the V-Y flap is facilitated by separating the gluteus maximus away from the gluteus medius muscle. The most significant medial release comes from the division of the fascial attachments of the gluteus maximus muscle to the sacrum. Further advancement is obtained by dividing the gluteus maximus muscular insertions. It should be unusual to injure the sciatic nerve since it is easily identified and well removed from the usual plane of dissection. This is a real consideration in spastic paraplegics because sciatic motor innervation may be important in ''transferring'' activities.

The donor site of the primarily closed V-Y flap rarely causes any problem if it is properly closed. The flap must be sufficiently mobilized to provide a tension-free closure, and large sutures must be used. Horizontal mattress #2 nylon retention sutures tied over 4 x 4 bolsters are effective in obliterating the deadspace and preventing wound disruptions. These large sutures are unsightly, but they obviate the need for buried sutures which may potentiate wound infections.

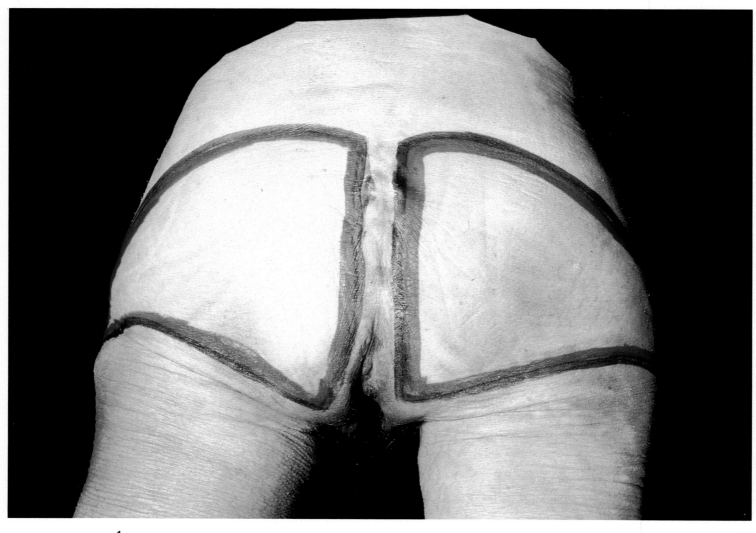

1

Outline of the margins of the gluteus
maximus muscles.

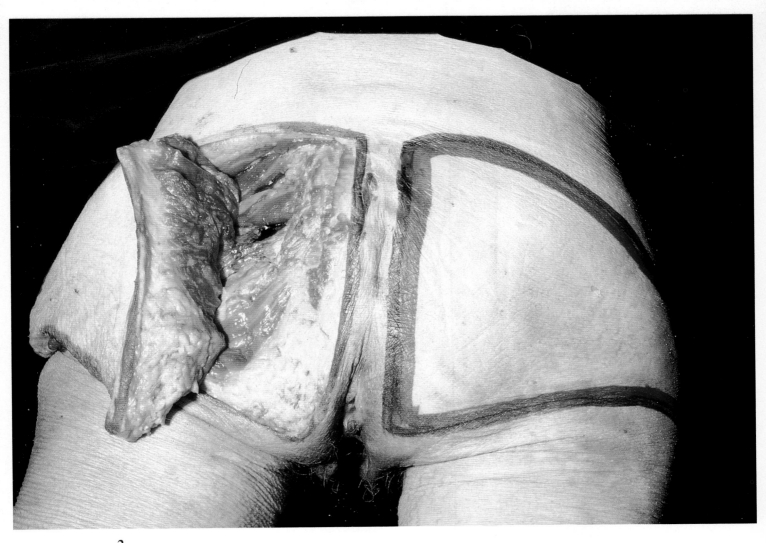

2

The skin incision is completed, and the gluteus maximus muscle is partially elevated away from the gluteus medius muscle. The gluteus maximus muscle has been detached from the sacrum and iliac crest attachments but not from the greater trochanter.

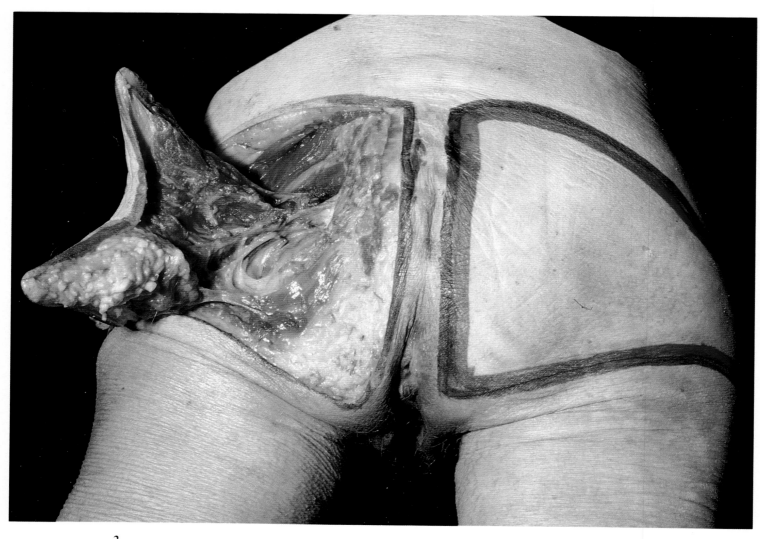

3

Completion of the "island" flap elevation, demonstrating the superior and inferior gluteal vessels.

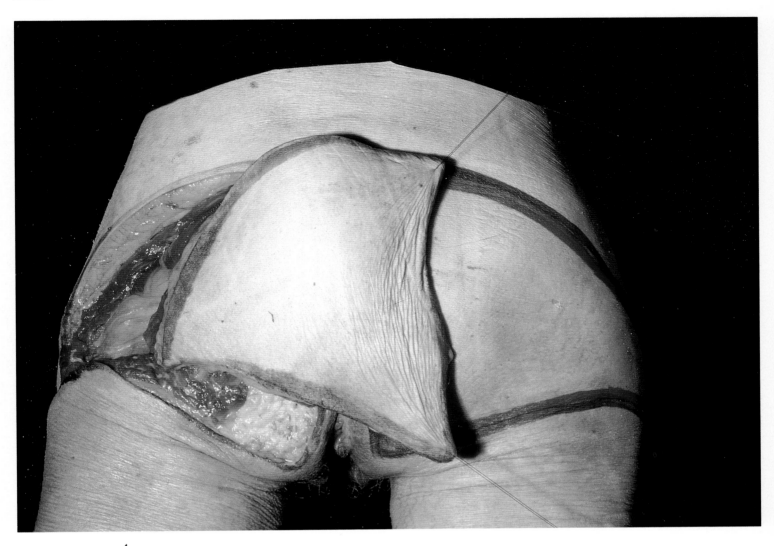

4

Central advancement of the "island" gluteus musculocutaneous flap after the division of the muscular insertion. It is usually not necessary to divide the muscular insertion when bilateral myocutaneous flaps are centrally advanced.

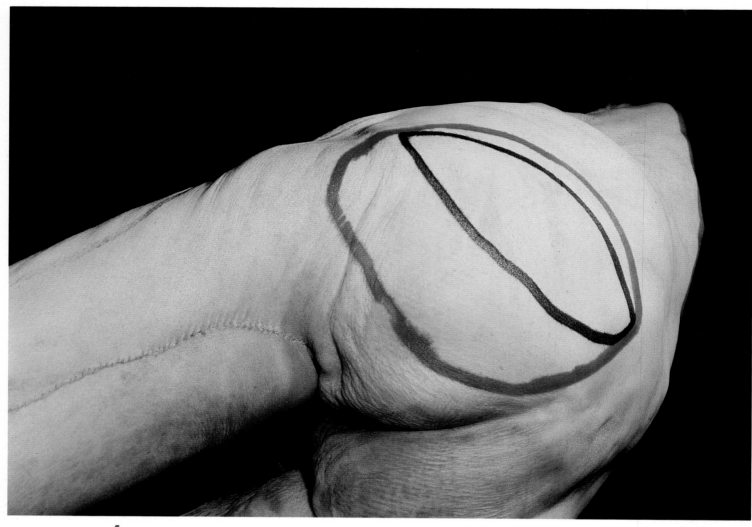

5

Outline of a gluteus maximus "island"
flap. The muscle is outlined in red.

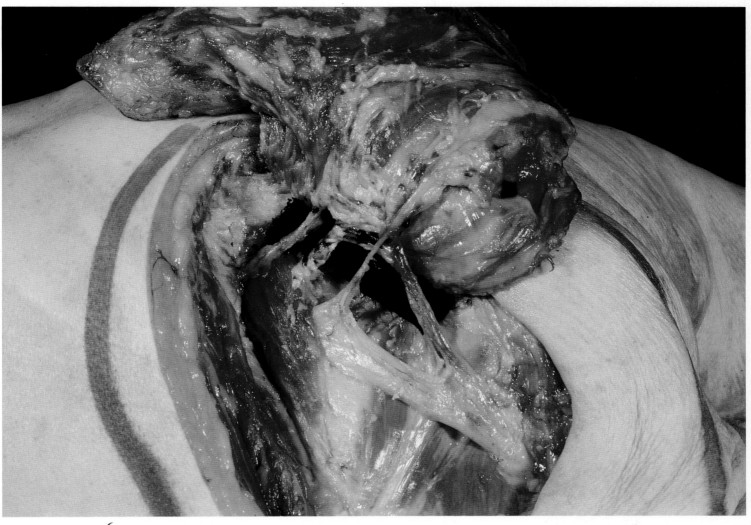

6

The sciatic nerve is seen passing beneath
the piriformis muscle. The superior and
inferior gluteal vessels are seen on either
side of the piriformis muscle.

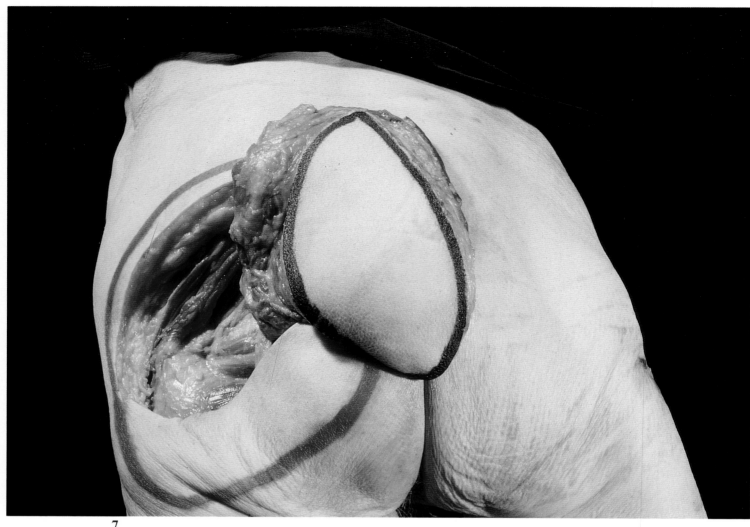

7

A single "island" flap can be rotated
onto the sacrum. This results in a significant donor site deformity unless the skin
can be primarily closed. Bilateral V-Y
advancements are generally preferred for
major sacral defects.

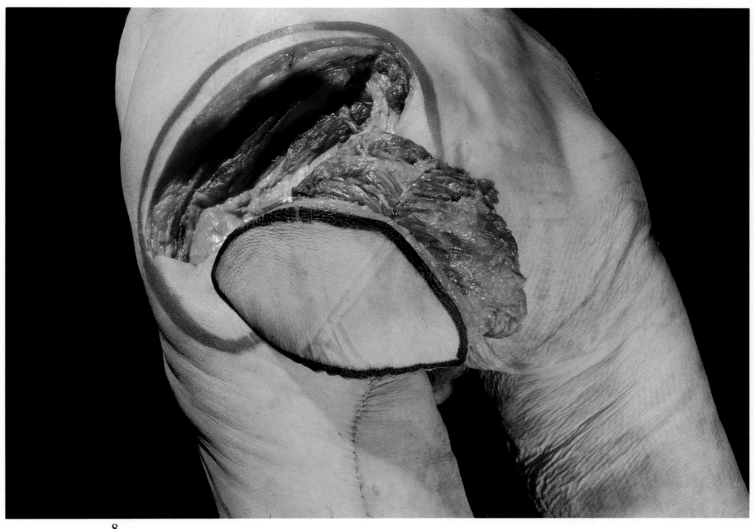

8

The "island" flap can also be rotated inferiorly to cover the ischium. It is rarely used for this purpose.

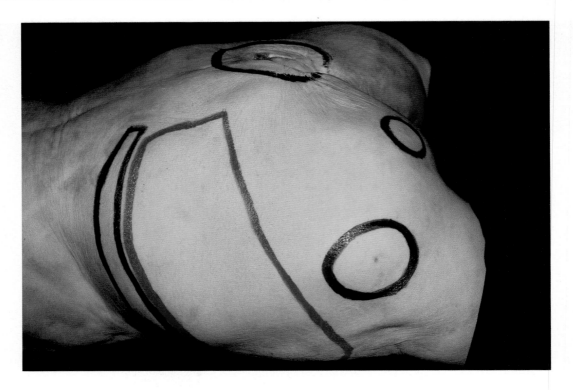

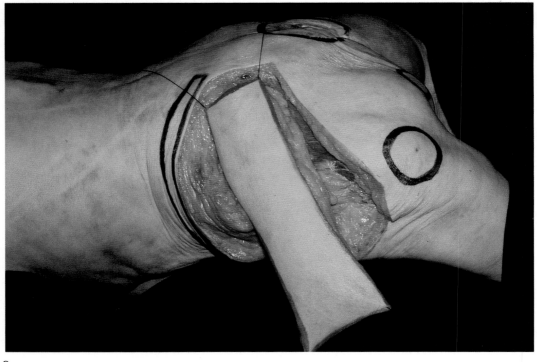

9

Outline of the upper gluteus maximus myocutaneous flap. The cutaneous segment (red) overlies the cranial or superior half of the gluteus maximus muscle and extends well beyond the anterior crest. An ulcer of the lower sacrum is outlined in black along with the locations of the ischial tuberosity and the greater trochanter. Flap elevation is begun by dividing the deep fascia. Note the anterior extent of the flap.

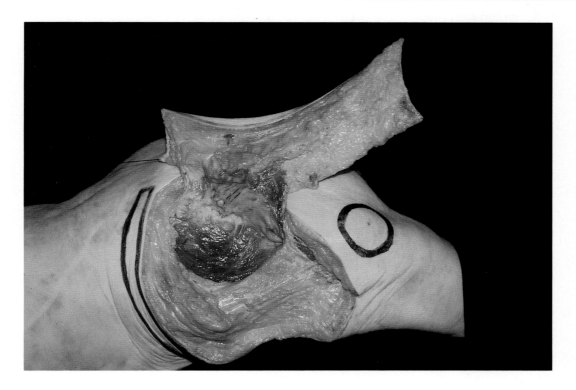

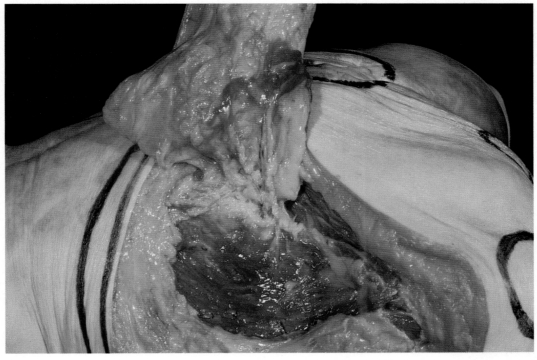

10

The gluteus maximus muscle is first separated from its origin at the iliotibial tract and elevated away from the vertically oriented gluteus medius muscle. The superior gluteal vessels are seen on the under- surface of the cranial half of the gluteus maximus muscle, which has been ''split'' from the caudal half of the muscle. The ''island'' flap is completed by dividing the fascial attachments to the sacrum.

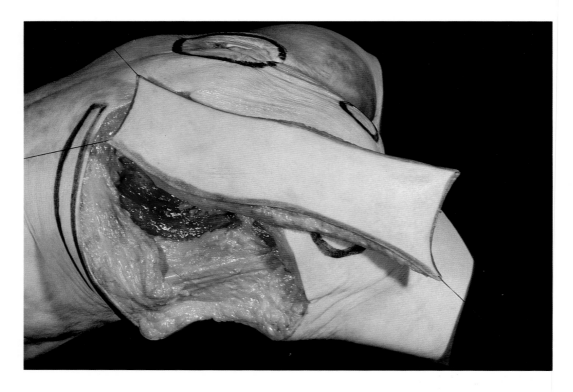

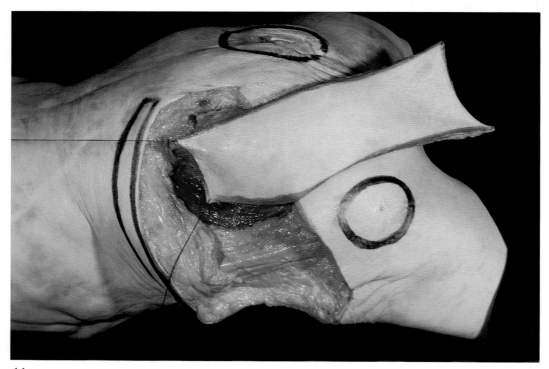

11

The flap is transposed inferiorly to cover the greater trochanter and the ischial tuberosity.

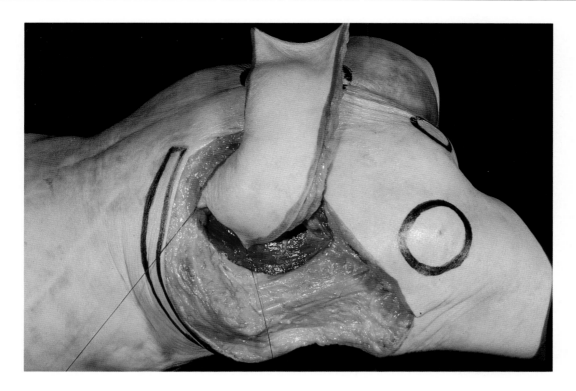

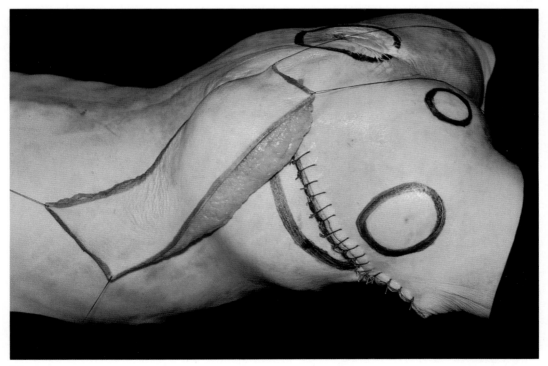

12

Rotation of the upper gluteus maximus myocutaneous flap onto the sacrum and the lower chest wall. The vertically oriented flap will also cover the lumbar area. The donor site is closed primarily.

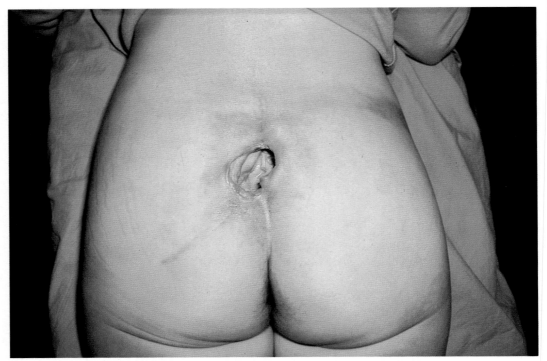

13

Fifty-four-year-old female with a recurrent chondrosarcoma following three major excisions and extensive irradiation to the sacral area. Note the scar on the left buttock which will be included in the gluteus maximus myocutaneous flap. (Case of P.G. Arnold)

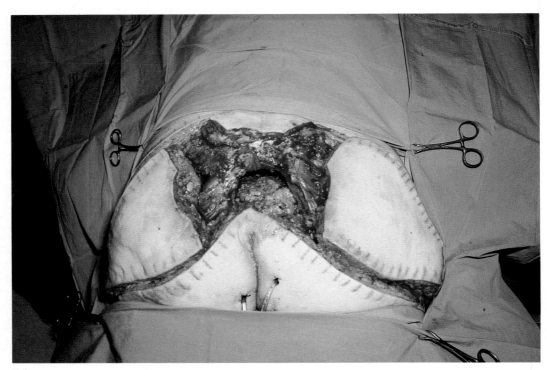

14

Bilateral gluteus maximus flaps were incised at the time of an abdominoperineal resection three days earlier. In this second operation the recurrent sarcoma of the sacrum was widely excised and repaired with V-Y gluteus maximus advancement myocutaneous flaps. The cutaneous "delay" was unnecessary, but it was still a reasonable "test" of the flaps in this precarious situation.

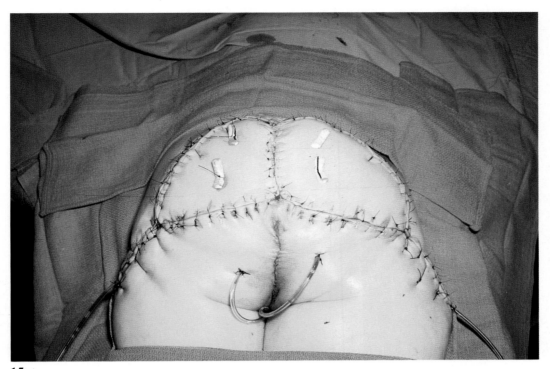

15

The gluteus maximus flaps were advanced to the midline. Fluorescein examination predicted complete flap viability. Large surface sutures were used to avoid using deep absorbable sutures.

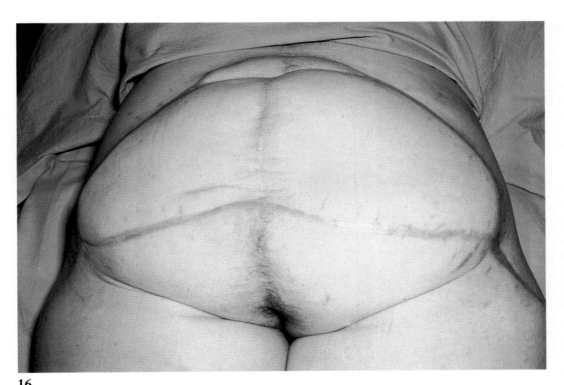

16

Healed V-Y flaps at six months.

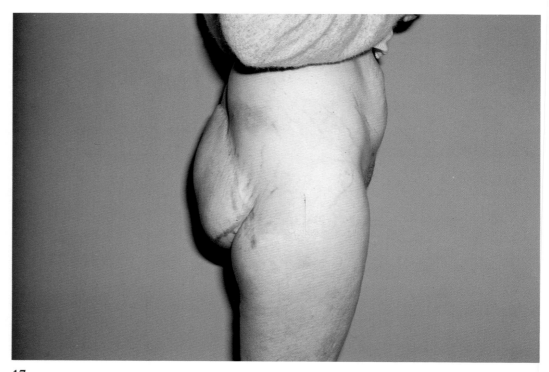

17

Lateral view at eight months. The patient is still able to ambulate, swim, and play golf without difficulty. The closure remains stable at six years.

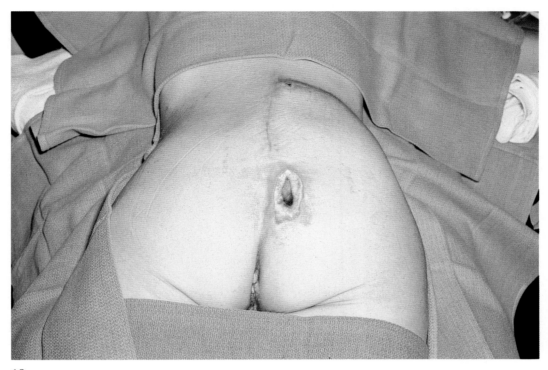

18

Thirty-eight-year-old female with a pressure sore following an extensive resection of an osteogenic sarcoma of the lumbosacral area. (Case of P.G. Arnold)

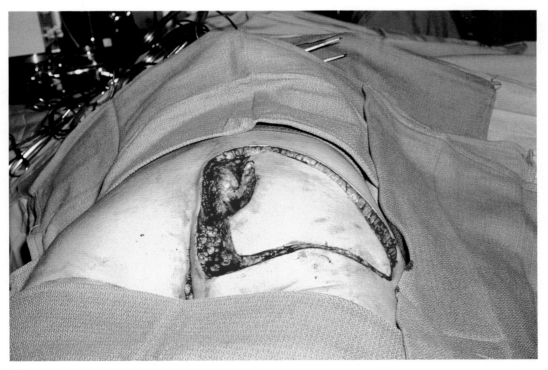

19

The pressure sore was excised, and a single gluteus maximus myocutaneous flap was prepared for V-Y transposition and primary closure. Note that the V-Y flap is significantly wider than the area of excision to incorporate both vessels and to ensure the flap's viability.

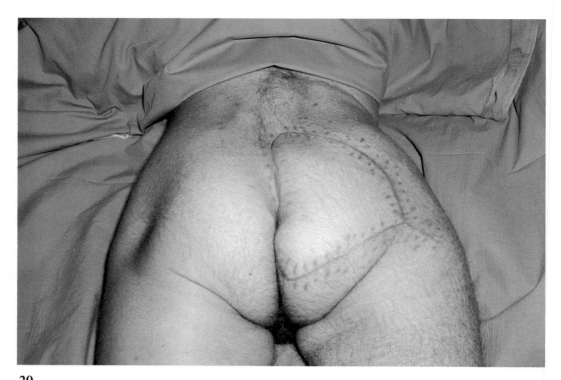

20

Healed V-Y gluteus maximus transposition at four months. The wound has remained healed for five years.

BICEPS FEMORIS

ANATOMICAL CONSIDERATIONS

Surface Markings

The biceps femoris is the most lateral of the "hamstring" muscles as it courses from the ischial tuberosity to the lateral aspect of the knee. The lateral border of the muscle can be palpated at the margin of the vastus lateralis muscle and the lateral intermuscular septum. The medial border of the muscle forms a visible boundary of the popliteal fossa.

Origin and Insertion

The long head of the biceps femoris muscle originates from the ischial tuberosity along with the semitendinosus and semimembranosus muscles. The short head has a deeper origin from the linea aspera of the femur and the lateral supracondylar line of the femur. Distally the muscle passes over the lateral head of the gastrocnemius muscle and inserts into the head of the fibula and the lateral condyle of the tibia. The biceps femoris tendon directly overlies the fibular collateral ligament of the knee joint.

Adjacent Muscles

The biceps femoris muscle is fused with the more medial semitendinosus and semimembranosus muscles through their combined origin from the ischial tuberosity. In the midthigh these two hamstring muscle groups are separated by the sciatic nerve. In the lower thigh the semitendinosus muscle diverges away from the biceps femoris muscle as the two muscles separate to form the upper borders of the popliteal fossa. Laterally, the biceps femoris muscle is densely fused to the lateral intermuscular septum and the vastus lateralis muscle. The intimate relationship of the biceps femoris muscle to the sciatic and the common peroneal nerves should be recognized. The sciatic nerve passes beneath the biceps femoris muscular origin and then bisects the two hamstring muscle groups in the midline of the thigh. The common peroneal nerve passes beneath the biceps femoris tendon in its course to the fibular head.

The functional importance of the biceps femoris muscle is still debated. The biceps femoris tendon does tighten the flexed iliotibial tract, which is an important lateral knee stabilizer. The contributions of the lateral collateral ligaments and the iliotibial tract are probably more important than the biceps femoris tendon in lateral knee stability, but the biceps femoris is a major external rotator of the knee. As an isolated muscle, it is expendable as a knee flexor except in certain athletic situations. In an anecdotal number of cases, we have encountered lateral knee instability with the use of the tensor fascia lata flap but not with the biceps femoris flap.

Vascular Pattern

The biceps femoris is a classic example of a muscle which is supplied almost totally by multiple segmental vessels. These deep perforating vessels arise from the profunda femoris vessels in the upper two-thirds of the muscle while the lower one-third of the muscle is supplied by the popliteal vessels. Because of the lack of intramuscular vascular connections, each deep muscular perforator supplies only an isolated segment of the biceps femoris muscle. For this reason the muscle is usually employed as an advancement flap so the majority of the perforating vessels can be left intact. Since the distal perforating vessels are relatively dominant, only a distally based "island" flap of any size is feasible. A proximal muscle flap can be used to obliterate an ischial cavity, but the vascularity of the proximal muscle flap is variable.

Motor Nerve

Sciatic nerve.

Sensory Nerve

Posterior cutaneous nerve of the thigh.

USES

The biceps femoris V-Y myocutaneous flap is used primarily for ischial pressure sores. It is the flap of choice for the isolated ischial ulcer so that the gluteus maximus myocutaneous flap can be preserved for later sacral coverage problems. Bilateral myocutaneous advancement flaps can also provide a remarkable amount of soft tissue for central perineal defects. The segmental vasculature of the biceps femoris muscle limits the applicability of "island" muscle flaps. Although a turnover muscle flap in combination with a laterally based skin flap is a reasonable option for ischial ulcers, it is less reliable than the V-Y myocutaneous advancement flap. The distally based biceps femoris muscle flap is occasionally considered for popliteal and suprapatellar defects when the gastrocnemius muscle is unavailable.

REGIONAL FLAP COMPARISONS

The biceps femoris V-Y advancement flap has several advantages over other local flaps in the paraplegic patient. Although the vastus lateralis muscle flap and the gluteus maximus musculocutaneous flap are just as useful for ischial defects, their dissection is more tedious, and they are preferably reserved for later hip and sacral problems. For poorly understood reasons, the biceps femoris V-Y flap is more reliable in the paraplegic patient than either the TFL or the gracilis myocutaneous flap. Neither of the latter flaps is useful to obliterate the usual ten by ten centimeters ischiectomy cavity.

DISADVANTAGES

The V-Y advancement myocutaneous flap has a limited (ten centimeters) upward mobility, which can present a problem in a very large ischial or buttock defect. This mobility can be improved by elevating the entire posterior calf musculature and also by dividing the sciatic nerve in the paraplegic patient. It is necessary to use bilateral V-Y flaps for large central perineal defects; however, both of the donor sites can be primarily closed. Although distally based and proximally based biceps femoris muscle flaps can be designed, their reliability is always in question and their vascular axis and arc of rotation cannot be determined until the time of exploration.

ADVANTAGES

The advantages of the biceps femoris V-Y myocutaneous advancement flap derive from its demonstrated simplicity and reliability. The distally based muscle flap offers a distinctly secondary muscle flap source for suprapatellar or popliteal defects because the gastrocnemius muscle flap is more easily dissected and is obviously more reliable. The functional loss of the biceps femoris muscle as a lateral knee stabilizer and knee flexor is not noticeable if the adjacent muscles are undisturbed.

COMPLICATIONS, PITFALLS, AND DONOR SITE

The complications associated with the V-Y advancement flap are seldom related to flap necrosis unless there is an excessive sacrifice of the segmental vessels. This should rarely be encountered since it is not usually necessary to divide any of these deep perforators in the V-Y flap advancement. Wound disruptions have occurred following ischiectomy and a biceps femoris myocutaneous flap closure because the functional ischial skin deficit is always much larger than the surface ischial ulcer. It is tempting to obliterate an ischial cavity with a biceps femoris muscle flap and to close the skin directly. However, a deficiency of expansile skin over the ischium contributes to an exceedingly high incidence of wound disruption with a direct closure. It is better to prevent an ischial wound disruption by replacing the lost ischial skin completely and avoiding any hip flexion for a period of two weeks. The flotation bed is routinely used to dissipate the harmful effects of direct pressure on the flap in the supine position. Although the flotation bed will dissipate this direct pressure paraplegic patients, and quadriplegic patients in particular, are frustrated by their inability to turn in this bed. This has resulted in a sensation of claustrophobia which is manifested by extreme agitation. The V-Y biceps femoris myocutaneous flap donor site has not yielded any significant complications in our experience.

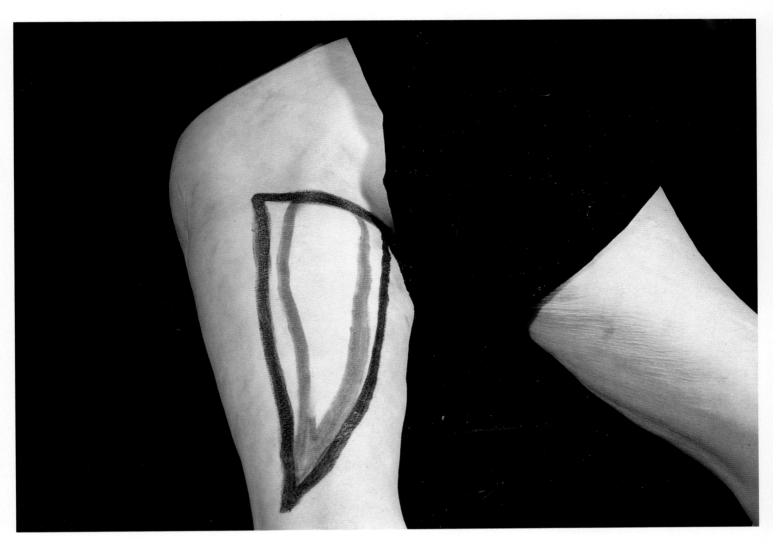

1

Outline of the biceps femoris V-Y advancement flap on the posterior thigh in the cadaver. The long head of the biceps femoris muscle is outlined in its course between the ischium and the knee. The upper margin of the flap lies at the level of the ischial tuberosity.

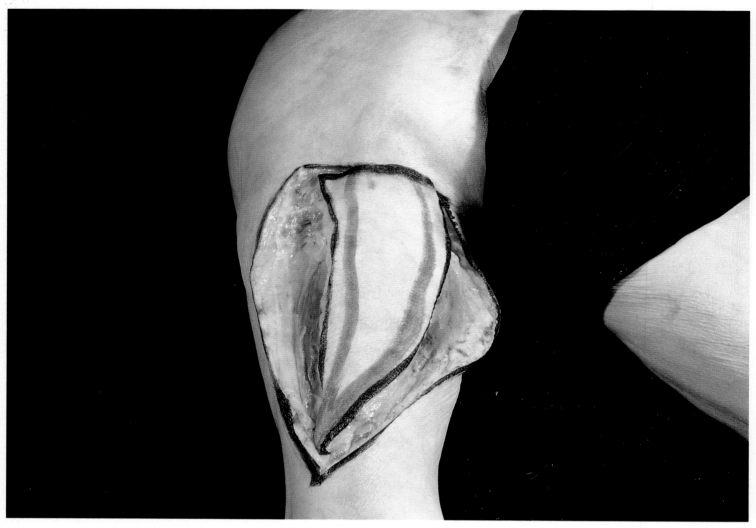

2

Elevation of the biceps femoris long and short heads with the overlying skin. The muscle has been separated from its fascial attachments to the vastus lateralis and the semitendinosus muscles on either side.

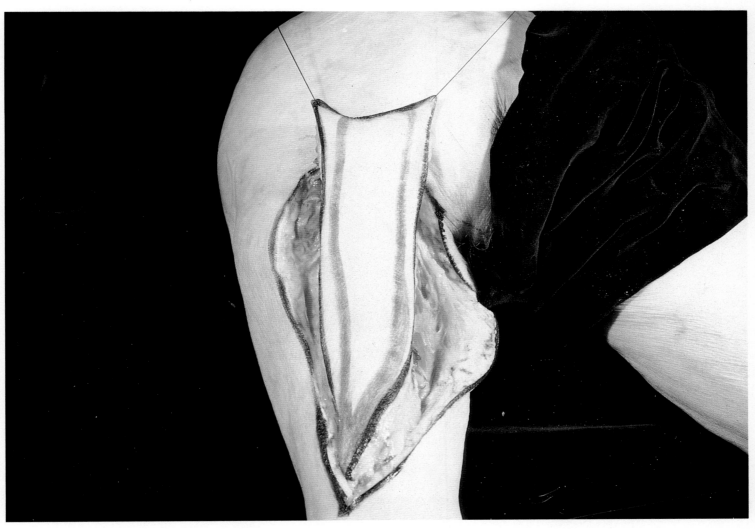

3

Once the biceps femoris tendon is divided, the myocutaneous flap unit can be advanced to cover the ischium. The donor site is closed in a V-Y fashion.

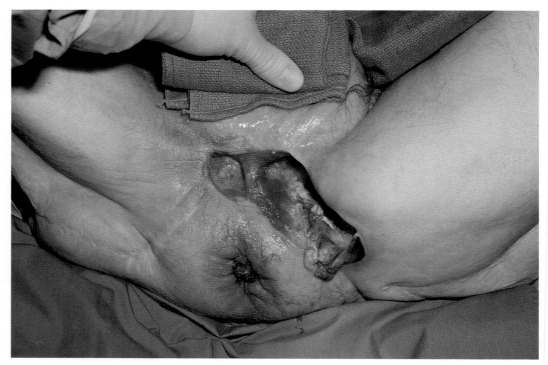

4

Massive perineal pressure sore in a sixty-year-old paraplegic with multiple sclerosis. The problem was complicated by erosion of the perineal urethra, which necessitated ligation of the bladder neck and permanent suprapubic drainage. (Case of P.G. Arnold)

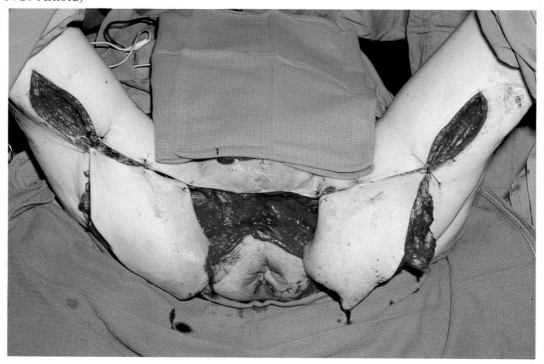

5

The perineal wound has been widely debrided. Bilateral biceps femoris myocutaneous flaps are ready to be advanced into the central perineum in a V-Y fashion.

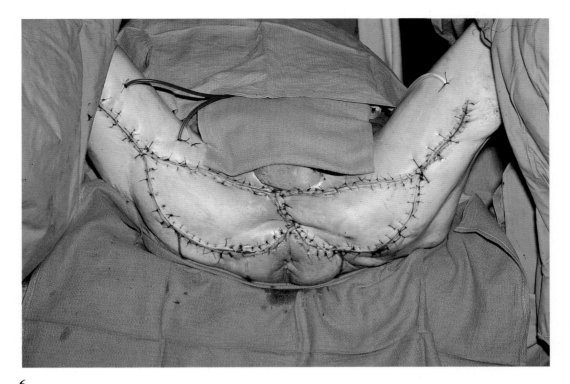

6

Note the amount of V-Y advancement
into the central perineum.

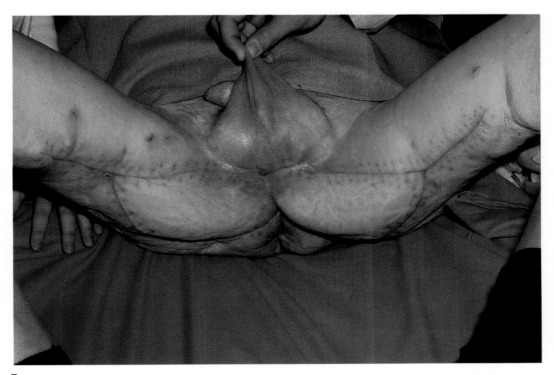

7

Completed healing six weeks following
perineal reconstruction. The patient returned to full time desk work following
this procedure.

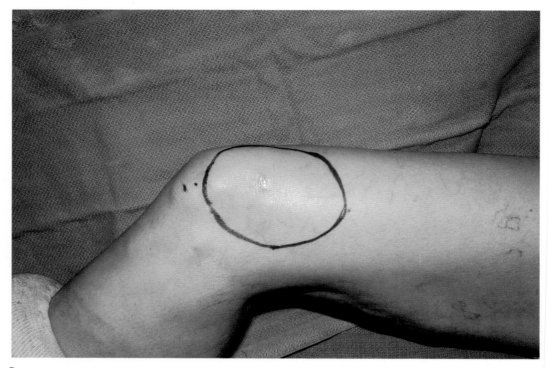

8

Forty-eight-year-old female with a biopsied level II melanoma of the suprapatellar area. The proposed tumor excision is outlined. (Case of J.B. McCraw)

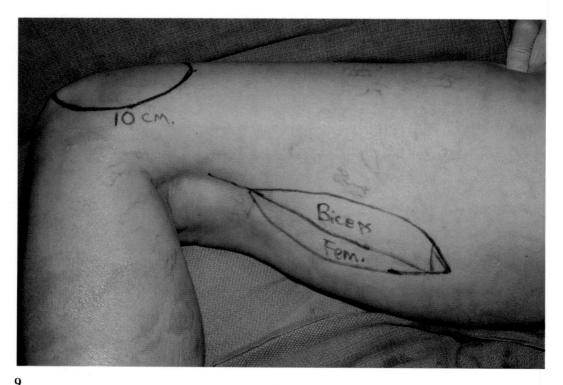

9

The long head of the biceps femoris is outlined as a "reversed" muscle flap.

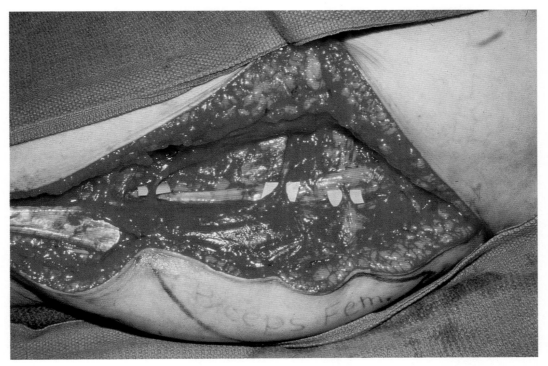

10

The segmental perforators of the biceps
femoris muscle are demonstrated with
blue backing just lateral to the sciatic
nerve. The two proximal perforators
shown here will be divided.

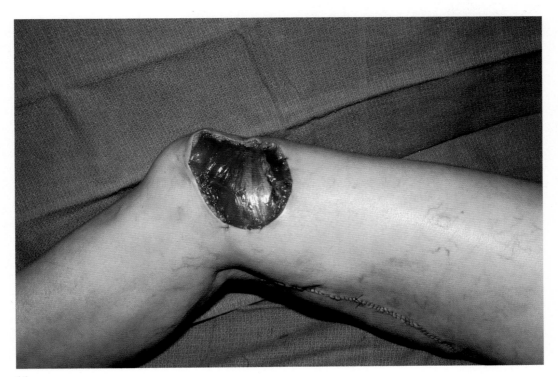

11

The ''reversed'' biceps femoris muscle
was rotated into the suprapatellar defect
to provide a pliable cover for the patellar
tendon.

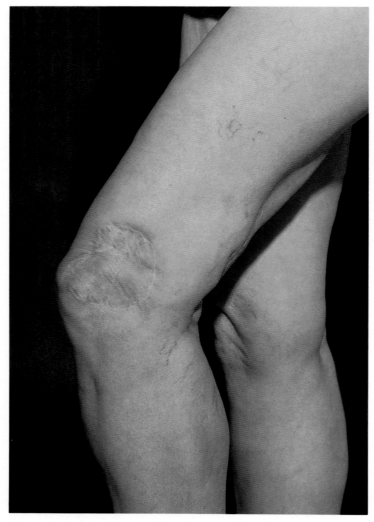

12

Skin-grafted muscle flap four years following surgery. The patient returned to full activity. There was no functional disability from the use of the biceps femoris muscle.

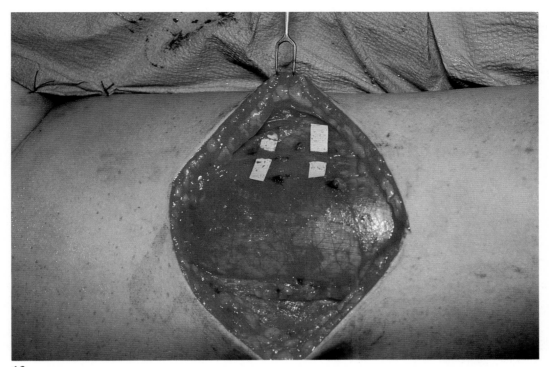

13

Twelve centimeter excision of a level II melanoma of the posterior thigh in an eighteen-year-old female. The posterior cutaneous nerve of the thigh has been preserved. (Case of J.B. McCraw)

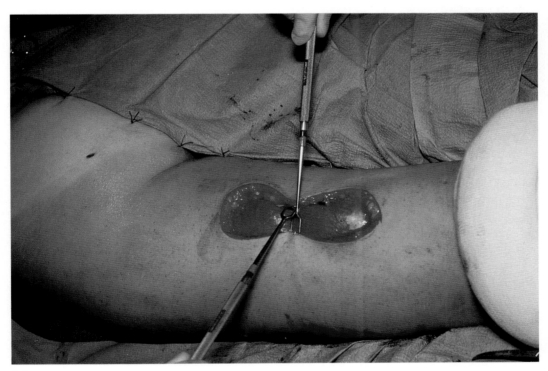

14

A primary closure was desirable for esthetic reasons. Note the transverse tension of the approximated posterior thigh skin.

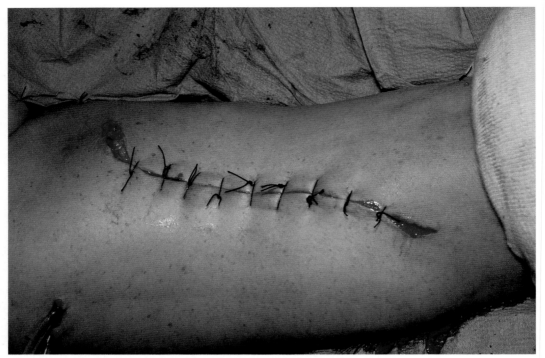

15

The temporary 2-0 silk sutures demonstrate the tension of the closure. The silk sutures were removed, and fasciocutaneous advancement flaps were used to give a nearly tension-free closure. To accomplish this, the fascia lata was incised medially, laterally, and distally. This allowed the skin and the fascia to advance into the defect.

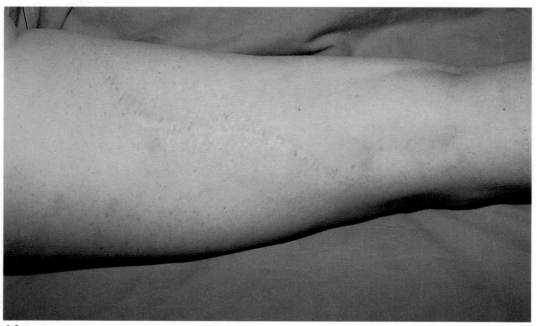

16

View of the scar at two years. The closure was dramatically facilitated by incising the fascia lata medially and laterally. This type of closure is simpler and faster than a ''simple'' skin graft.

GRACILIS

ANATOMICAL CONSIDERATIONS

Surface Markings

The cutaneous segment of the gracilis myocutaneous flap measures approximately six by twenty-four centimeters. It is centered on an imaginary line which passes between the pubic tubercle proximally and the semitendinosus tendon distally. The proximal gracilis muscle is difficult to palpate, but it can be identified adjacent to the fascial cleft which lies directly behind the prominent tendon of the adductor longus muscle. The distal tendon of the semitendinosus muscle, which lies between the gracilis and semimembranosus tendons, is easily palpated above the knee.

Origin and Insertion

The gracilis muscle originates from the pubic tubercle and the inferior ramus of the pubis and inserts into the pes anserinus at the medial knee. It functions as an accessory thigh adductor and knee flexor and is a totally expendable muscle.

Adjacent Muscles

The sartorius muscle lies anterior to the gracilis muscle, and the semimembranosus and semitendinosus muscles lie posterior to it in the distal thigh. In the upper thigh the adductor magnus muscle lies deep to the gracilis muscle and the adductor longus lies directly anterior to the gracilis throughout its course. The adductor longus muscle is the most important palpable landmark because its prominent proximal tendon forms a notable "cleft" with the gracilis muscle when the hip is forcibly adducted with the patient in the "frog leg" (externally rotated) position.

Vascular Pattern

The gracilis muscle has a proximal, dominant pedicle from the produnda femoris artery which enters the muscle approximately nine to ten centimeters below the inguinal ligament. The proximal vessels may enter the muscle as low as fifteen centimeters below the inguinal ligament. This can make the flap unusable. When a low proximal vessel is encountered in raising a gracilis flap, the opposite muscle should be explored since the vascular arrangement is not always symmetrical. There is usually a small vessel in the midpoint of the muscle which is inconsequential. A branch from the saphenous artery is the dominant blood supply to the distal one-third of the muscle and its overlying skin. As is the case in most long, thin muscles, the intramuscular collateralization and crossover between the proximal and distal vasculature is minimal. Nevertheless, the entire gracilis muscle can be safely transposed on the proximal vessels as an "island" muscle flap.

Motor Nerve

Femoral nerve.

Sensory Nerve

Medial cutaneous nerve of the thigh.

USES

The gracilis myocutaneous flap is used primarily for perineal defects including vaginal, scrotal, and penile reconstructions. It is still the myocutaneous flap of choice for a total vaginal reconstruction or for the abdomino-perineal defect. The flap also has some application in coverage of the medial two-thirds of the groin and in problems of the suprapubic area. It has occasionally been used for ischial pressure sores in paraplegics when the paralysis is "spastic" in nature and a reasonable amount of muscle bulk is preserved. If the paralysis is flaccid, the results with the denervated gracilis myocutaneous flap have been quite disappointing.

The gracilis muscle alone is an excellent "free" muscle flap for distal tibial osteomyelitis because of its long and narrow configuration. It is also quite useful for the vascularization of a neourethral full-thickness skin graft or as an interposition muscle flap for the correction of vesicovaginal or rectovaginal fistulae. Bilateral, crossed gracilis muscle flaps have been used for anal incontinence even though this provides an unphysiologic replacement for the sophisticated anal sphincter mechanism.

The primary criticism of the gracilis myocutaneous flap is that its viability in the distal third of the flap is variable. One must accept the fact that the cutaneous segment which can predictably be carried will not extend into the distal third of the thigh without a "delay." This same criticism does not apply to the muscle flap, which will survive entirely on the proximal vessels. If the gracilis myocutaneous flap is properly designed and carefully handled, it is a very reliable flap.

REGIONAL FLAP COMPARISONS

For surface defects of the central perineum the gracilis myocutaneous flap is compared primarily to the inferior gluteal fasciocutaneous flap, which is quite reliable, sensate, and technically undemanding to elevate. Although the fasciocutaneous flap provides excellent surface cover, bilateral gracilis myocutaneous flaps are more useful for major internal pelvic defects because of their size and bulk. Very large central perineal surface defects can also be corrected by the very reliable inferiorly based rectus abdominis myocutaneous flap, but it has the disadvantage of significant donor site morbidity. Neither the TFL flap nor the rectus femoris myocutaneous flap reaches the central perineum or the pelvis because of the limited arcs of rotation in this direction.

Even though bilateral gracilis myocutaneous flaps are usually employed for pelvic exenteration defects, the inferiorly based lower horizontal rectus abdominis myocutaneous flap can be used for these same defects. The rectus abdominis flap is more applicable to high pelvic defects because of its proximity, and it is by far the largest myocutaneous flap which will reach into the pelvis. If a laparotomy is anticipated, the inferiorly based rectus abdominis myocutaneous flap immediately becomes a reasonable alternative for major pelvic defects.

The gracilis myocutaneous flap is seldom considered for the usual ischial pressure sore because of the unpredictable survivability of the denervated gracilis myocutaneous flap. This is true even in the spastic paraplegic. The V-Y biceps femoris myocutaneous flap is considered to be a more reliable method of reconstruction in these individuals.

DISADVANTAGES

Vascular "spasm" poses the biggest threat to the gracilis myocutaneous flap because once it exists it is practically impossible to relieve. Significant vascular "spasm" will usually cause some loss of the cutaneous segment, but not of the muscle. Gentle dissection and avoidance of any stretch of the vessels are the most important measures for the prevention of "spasm."

Occasionally the dominant pedicle of the gracilis muscle may not lie as proximal as we would like. If the proximal pedicle falls fifteen centimeters or more below the inguinal ligament, the constricted arc of rotation can make the flap unusable. Some upward mobility can be gained by skeletonizing the dominant pedicle and dividing the intermuscular septum. The vasculature of the opposite gracilis muscle should be explored as the next option since it may have a completely normal vascular arrangement. The inferior gluteal fasciocutaneous flap can still be used even though a gracilis myocutaneous flap has been elevated in the same leg. Prior elevation and return of a gracilis myocutaneous flap does not harm the viability of the adjacent fasciocutaneous flap, and the donor site in the thigh can still be primarily closed.

ADVANTAGES

The gracilis myocutaneous flap is very useful for most perineal reconstructions even in the context of the reliable inferior gluteal fasciocutaneous flap. The gracilis myocutaneous flap has the advantage of providing muscle, skin, and bulk. It will reach a higher point in the pelvic cavity than any adjacent flap, except the inferiorly based rectus abdominis myocutaneous flap, which can be passed directly into the pelvis through the lower posterior rectus sheath. The gracilis myocutaneous flap can be used without harm to the other adjacent flaps of the thigh, and the donor site is inconsequential.

COMPLICATIONS, PITFALLS, AND DONOR SITE

The "island" gracilis myocutaneous flap must be respected for its intolerance to vascular "spasm." This is usually caused by undue torsion or tension on the flap vessels, and the lethality of this event is difficult to reverse. The improper placement of the cutaneous segment is another preventable surgical error. The gracilis muscle will only "carry" skin which directly overlies the muscle so the course of the muscle should be identified proximally and distally before a commitment is made determining the eventual location of the skin "island." The usual skin "island" measures six by twenty-four centimeters and does not include the skin overlying the distal one-third of the muscle. This distal skin is independently supplied by branches of the saphenous artery. It must be "delayed" in order to ensure its viability.

The donor site should be trouble free if it is carefully closed and adequately drained. Retention sutures of #2 nylon tied over 4 × 4 bolsters offer a secure closure of the deep layers and allow us to avoid buried sutures. The large nylon sutures should be removed by the fourth or fifth day to prevent permanent epithelialization of these sizable suture tracts. There is no functional loss from the sacrifice of the gracilis muscle, and its use does not compromise the later use of the other adjacent myocutaneous and fasciocutaneous flaps in the thigh.

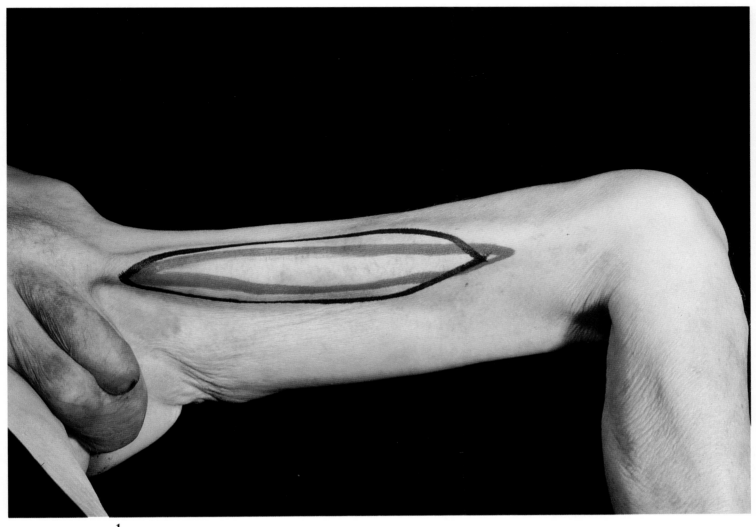

1

The leg is abducted to outline the gracilis
muscle in red and the overlying cutaneous
segment in black.

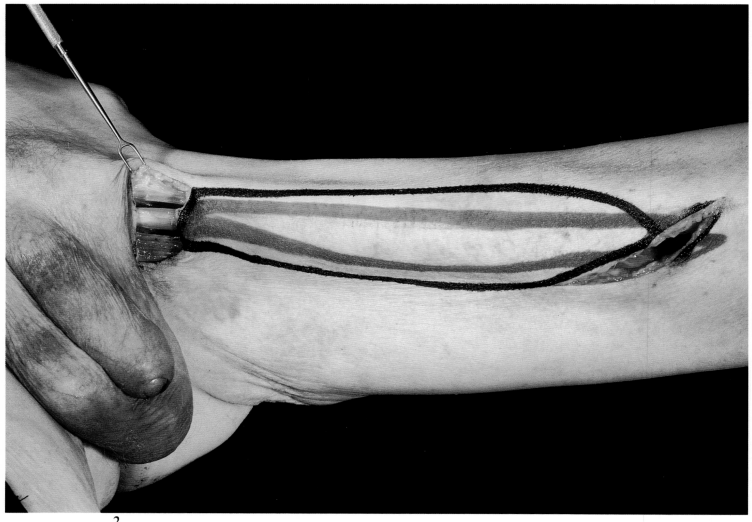

2

The proximal gracilis tendon is isolated. The hook retracts the adductor longus tendon. The distal incision is used to confirm the course of the gracilis muscle.

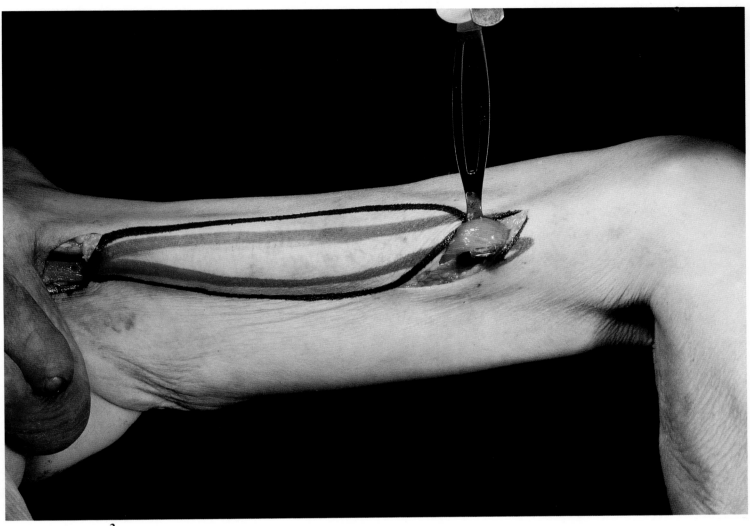

3

The distal gracilis muscle is identified between the semitendinosus tendon posteriorly and the sartorius muscle anteriorly. By "bow stringing" the gracilis muscle with a retractor, the proper location of the overlying skin can be demonstrated.

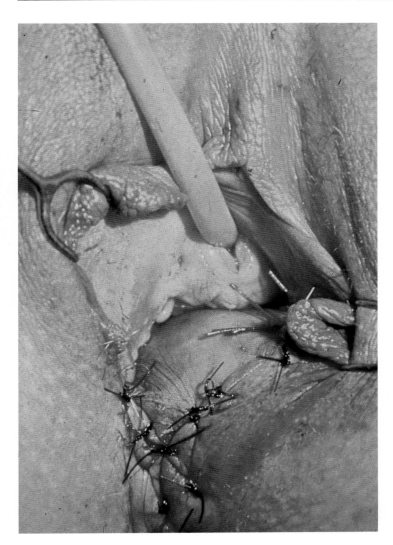

12
Inset of the gracilis flap to replace the posterior two-thirds of the vagina. It was possible to bury the flap and to close the perineal skin primarily.

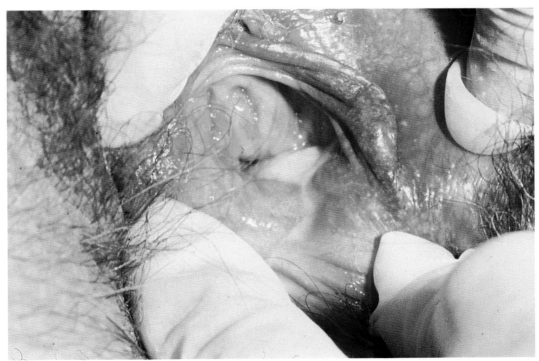

13
Close-up view of the healed gracilis myocutaneous flap (white) replacing the posterior wall of the vagina. Although the flap was in contact with secreting vaginal mucosa, it did not become macerated.

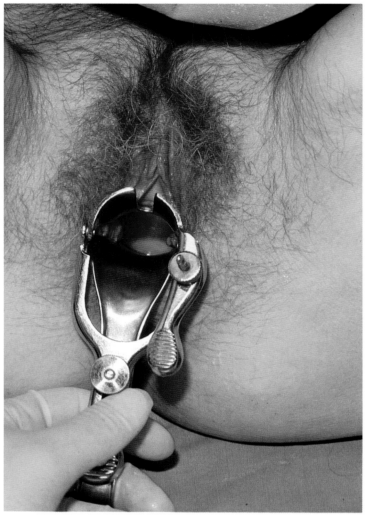

14

The size of the introitus was acceptable,
and the patient returned to normal
intercourse.

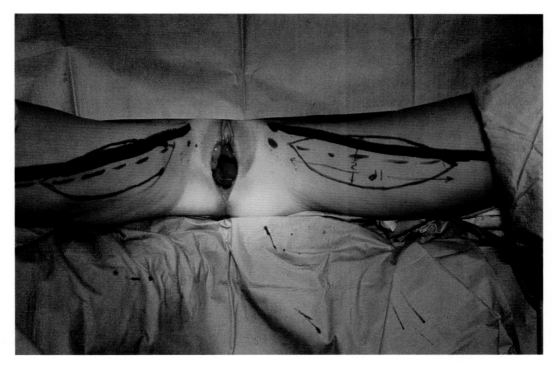

15

Thirty-nine-year-old patient with a recurrent carcinoma of the cervix following irradiation therapy which required a Wertheim hysterectomy. The reconstructive team was able to perform the vaginal reconstruction while the ileal loop was being constructed. This prevented any prolongation of the operative time, and it did not interfere with the completion of the abdominal closure. This case is of historical interest because it was the first immediate vaginal reconstruction performed at the Wilford Hall USAF Hospital in 1974. (Case of J.B. McCraw and F. Massey)

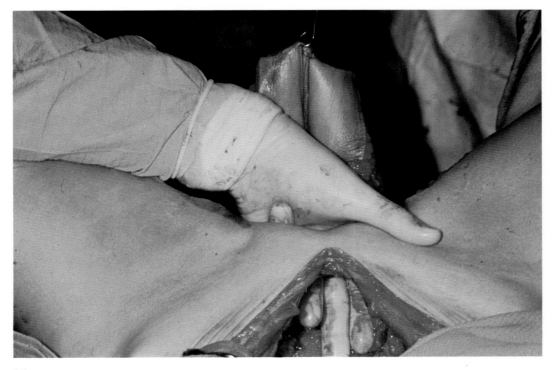

16

The extent of the pelvic defect is demonstrated at the time of the radical exenteration. The bilateral gracilis myocutaneous flaps effectively obliterate the massive pelvic dead space and prevent herniation of the small bowel.

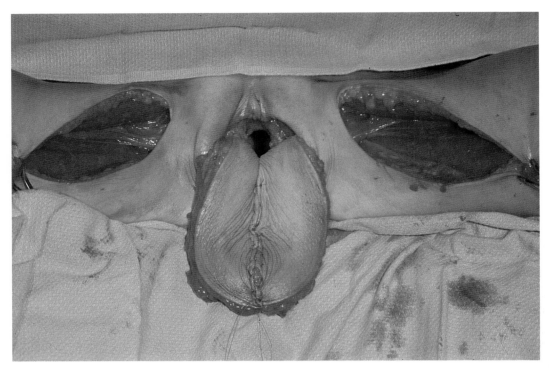

17

The bilateral gracilis myocutaneous flaps are approximated in the midline. Once the flaps are introduced into the pelvis, this suture line will become the anterior vaginal wall.

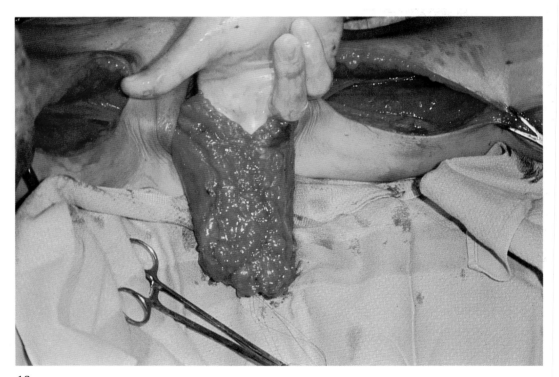

18

Completion of the posterior suture line closure recreates the neovaginal pouch. The gracilis muscles are seen on either side of the cutaneous closure.

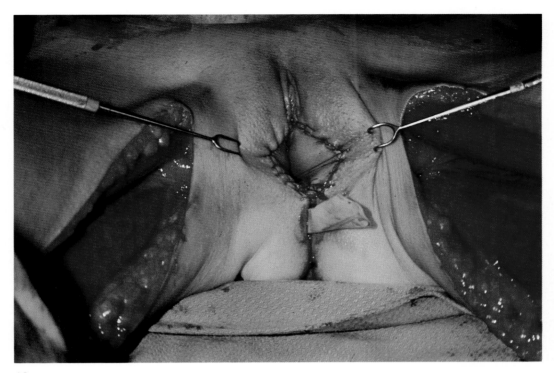

19

Immediate inset of the flaps into the pelvis. Internal suture fixation of the flaps is not necessary to prevent prolapse.

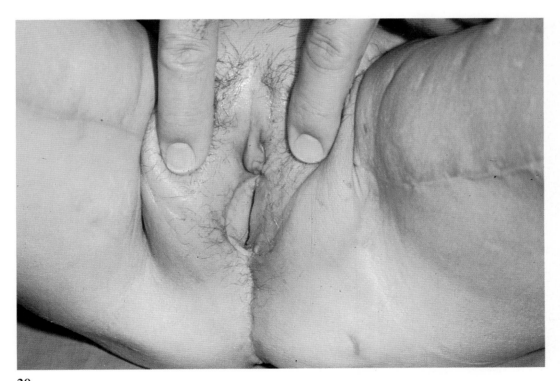

20

Late postoperative view of the introitus and the donor site. It is preferable to introduce some triangulation into the surface closure to prevent a circular scar contracture.

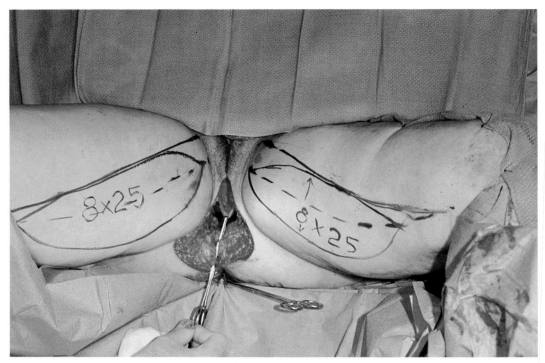

21

Forty-six-year-old patient with an extensive carcinoma of the anus. The resection included the rectum and anus as well as the posterior two-thirds of the vagina and the surrounding skin. The remaining cuff of anterior vagina is retracted with a clamp. Large gracilis flaps are outlined to provide adequate soft tissue for both vaginal reconstruction and perineal coverage. In the obese patient one must be careful to place the skin segment accurately on the muscle surface because the skin falls posteriorly in the supine position. (Case of J.B. McCraw and P.K. Carlton)

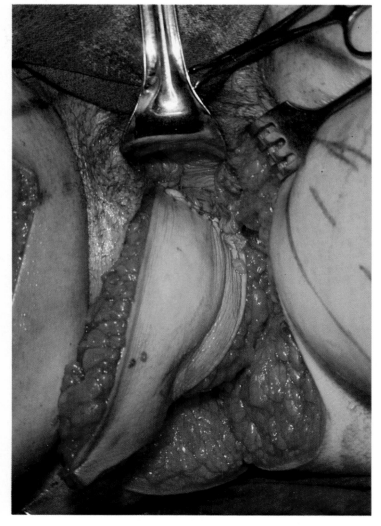

22

The right gracilis flap was used for the hemivaginal reconstruction. The left gracilis flap will be used to correct the remaining surface defect.

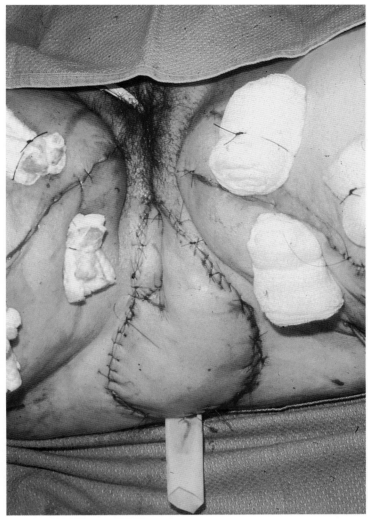

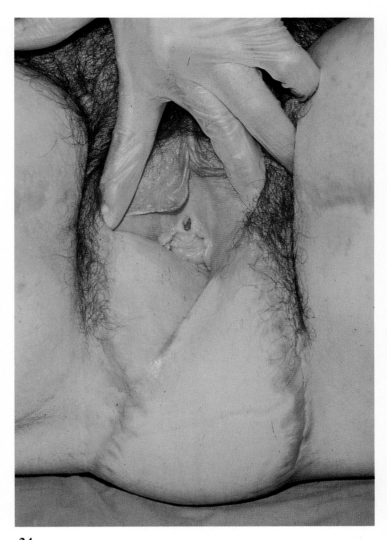

23

The majority of the perineal surface was replaced by the left gracilis myocutaneous flap. Only a small portion of the right gracilis myocutaneous flap is visible at the introitus. The donor sites were primarily closed with #2 nylon sutures with bolsters.

24

At six months the flaps were still bulky. They did provide a primarily healed wound and an adequate introitus.

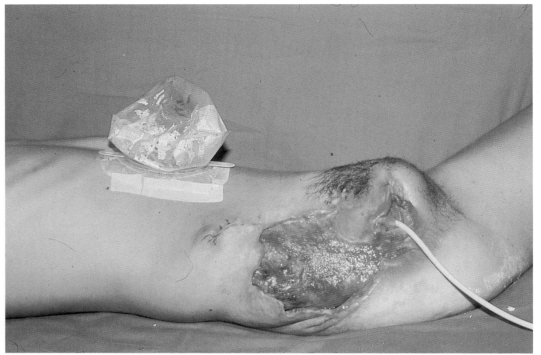

25

Nineteen-year-old patient who sustained a traumatic hemipelvectomy in a motorcycle accident. The ileum was totally avulsed from the sacrum and carried the iliac artery with the leg. In the process of secondary healing, the vagina and anus were lateralized and fused. The majority of the posterior vagina was also lost. This patient was extremely lucky to have survived the injury since only thirteen survivors have previously been reported in the world literature. (Case of J.B. McCraw and S. Philippakis)

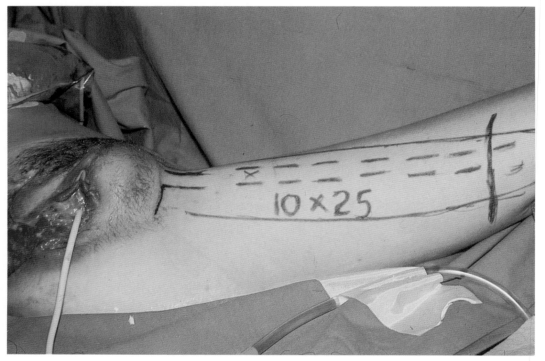

26

A very wide gracilis myocutaneous flap was outlined on the remaining leg to give an adequate amount of soft tissue to correct the perineal defect.

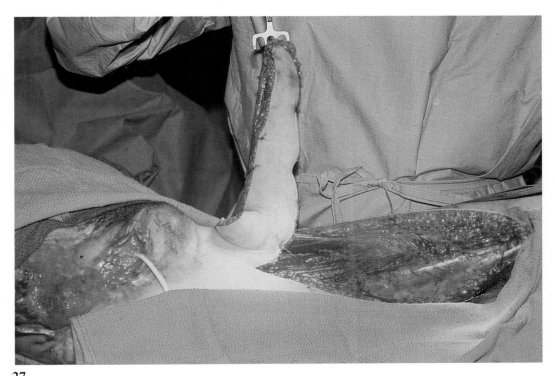

27

An "island" flap was not created in an effort to enhance the viability of the cutaneous segment. Every precaution was taken with this flap since it was thought to be the only flap available in the absence of the opposite inferior rectus abdominis flap.

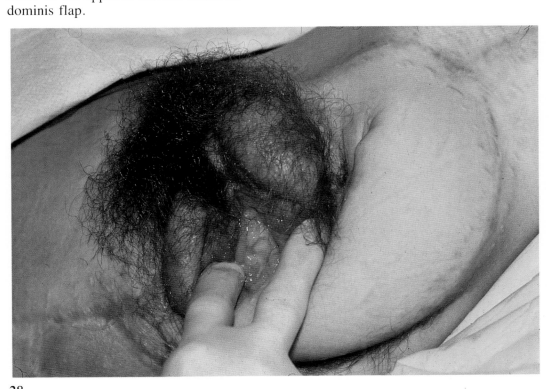

28

Close-up view of the introitus of the centrally relocated vagina. It was not necessary to replace the lost posterior vaginal wall after repositioning the vagina.

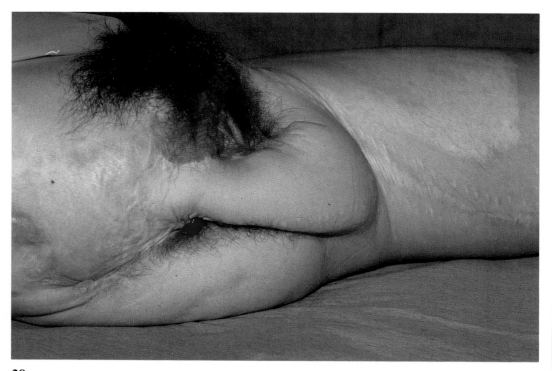

29

Lateral view of the healed gracilis flap
which separates the vagina and anus. The
adjacent pelvic wall defect was skin
grafted.

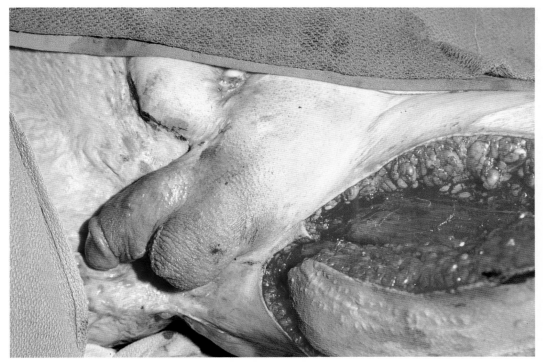

30

Nineteen-year-old male who sustained a high voltage electrical injury when he parachuted onto a high tension wire. This resulted in the loss of the medial right thigh musculature, the adjacent perineum, half of the scrotum, and the proximal urethra. A gracilis myocutaneous flap was elevated in the left thigh and examined with fluorescein prior to the recreation of the deformity. The scar in the left gracilis cutaneous segment is from the removal of the saphenous vein, which was used to repair the right femoral artery. It was not then known if this scar would harm the vascular connections between the muscle and the skin. (Case of J.B. McCraw, C.E. Horton, P.C. Devine and C.J. Devine, Jr.)

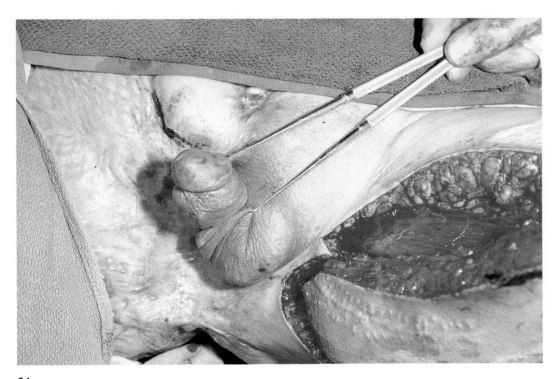

31

The penis and remaining scrotum are retracted to demonstrate the perineal contracture.

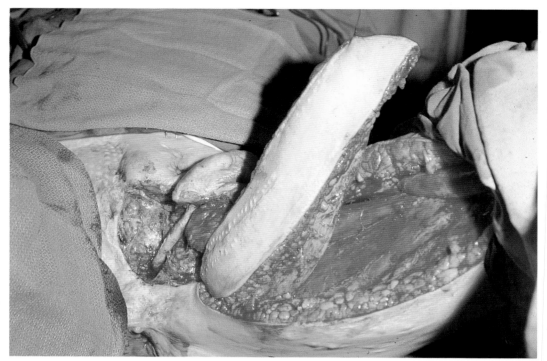

32

Elevated gracilis myocutaneous flap and the perineal deformity. The ten centimeter gap of urethra between the bladder neck and the penile urethra was replaced with a full-thickness tube graft. This case is memorable to the author because it was the first myocutaneous flap done in Norfolk in 1975.

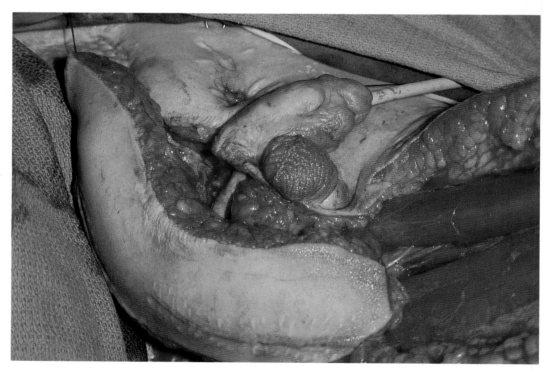

33

Rotation of the gracilis flap into the perineum. The distal one-third of the gracilis muscle was wrapped around the neo-urethral graft to facilitate its revascularization. The adductor longus, brevis, and magnus muscles are outlined in the donor thigh. The sartorius muscle crosses the distal wound.

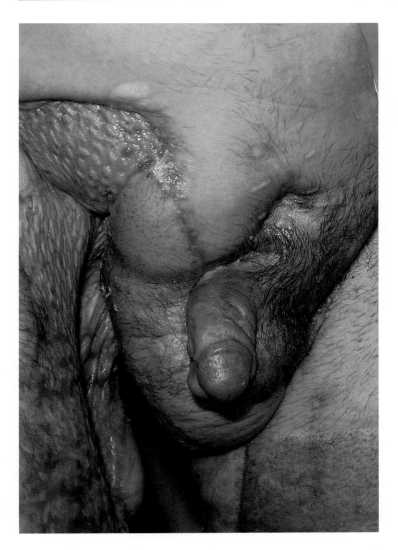

34

Healed gracilis myocutaneous flap which resurfaces the perineum and a portion of the suprapubic area. The patient developed urinary continence and a normal stream. A penile stiffener allowed the patient to have intercourse.

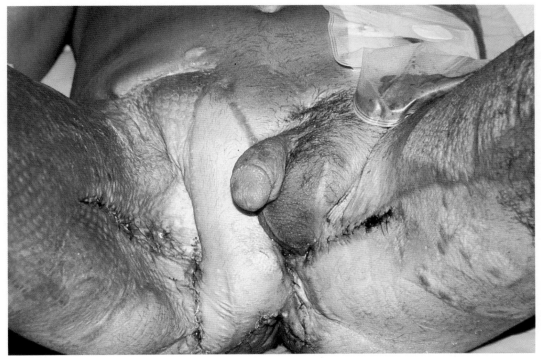

35

In a later stage the flap was turned into the perineum to release the anal contracture. The proximal muscle and the dominant blood supply of the flap were divided at this stage without harm to the flap.

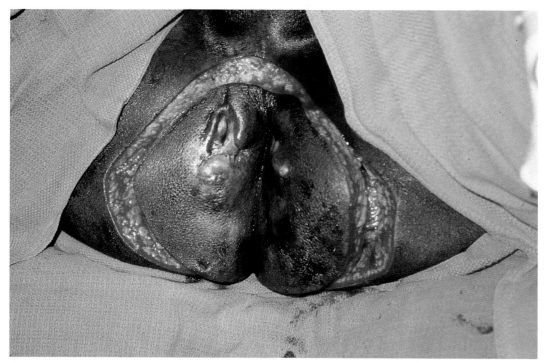

36
Fifty-eight-year-old man with Crohn's disease of the perineum. This was complicated by an anal carcinoma which invaded numerous sinus tracts. The carcinoma appeared to be unresectable. (Case of J.B. McCraw and G. Hoffman)

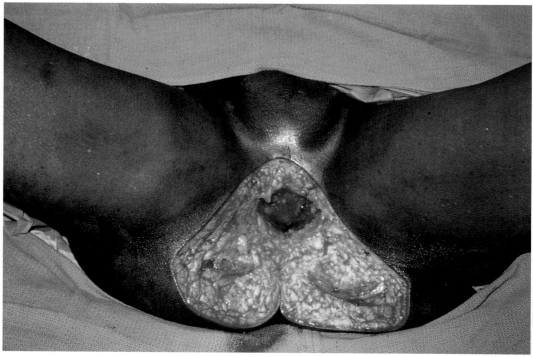

37
Perineal defect following resection. It was necessary to remove a large amount of buttock skin in order to excise the tumor infiltrated sinus tracts.

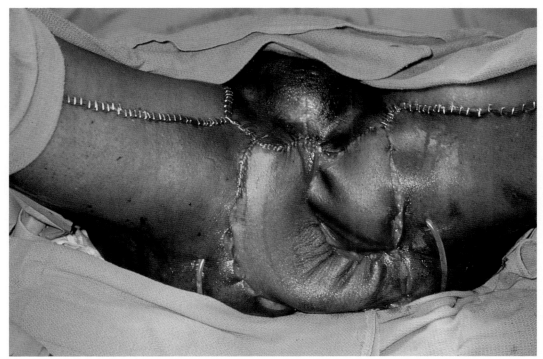

38

The right gracilis myocutaneous flap was used for perineal and posterior buttock coverage. The left gracilis myocutaneous flap was deepthelialized in its distal half to obliterate the pelvic dead space. The proximal portion of the left gracilis flap was used for perineal coverage.

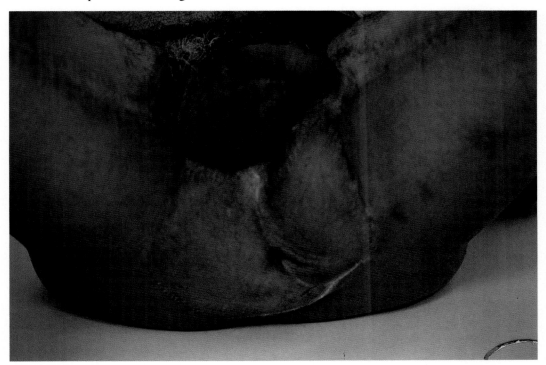

39

Healed gracilis flaps two years following resection of the anal carcinoma. The patient is alive and well six years following surgery.

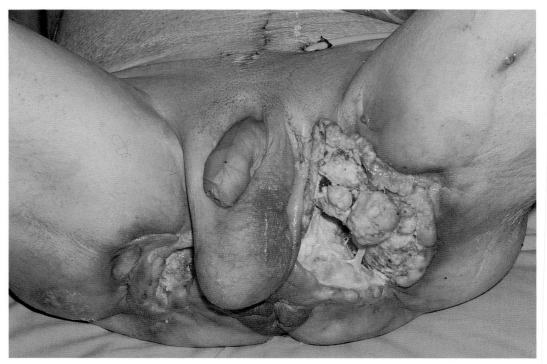

40

Fifty-five-year-old paraplegic male with a thirty-five-year history of bilateral ischial ulcers. Unfortunately all of the biopsies proved to be low-grade squamous cell carcinoma. A diverting colostomy was performed prior to the resection. (Case of P.G. Arnold)

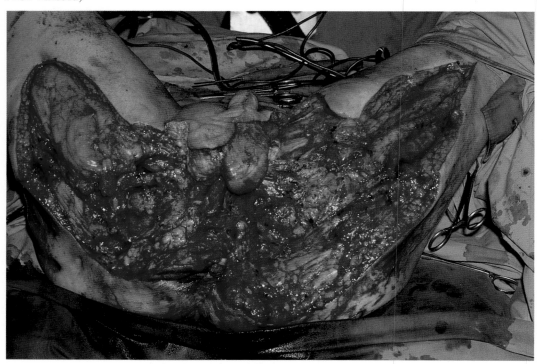

41

A wide excision of all of the tumor was carried out with histologic control of the margins. Because of the dimensions of the operative defect a total thigh flap was necessary to correct the massive deformity.

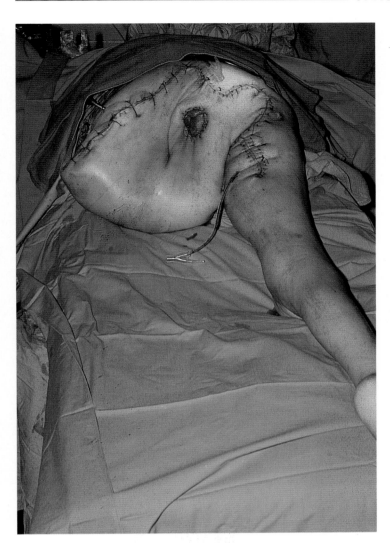

The anus was brought through the flap at the level of the patella. The defect on the right posterior thigh was closed directly.

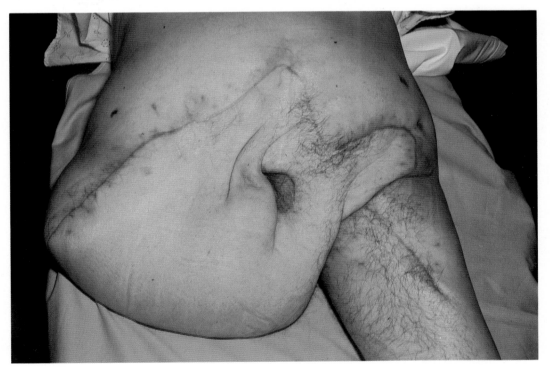

43

The wound healed primarily. The patient has survived for nine years.

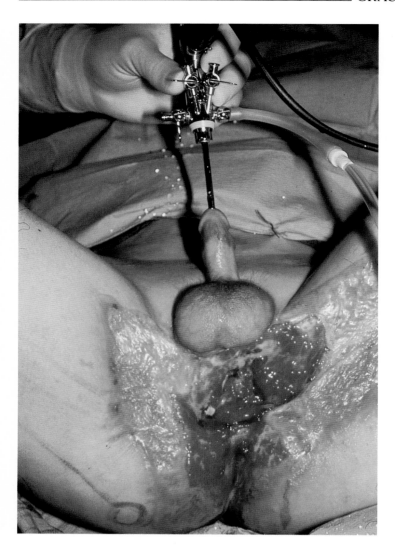

44

Eleven-year-old boy who sustained a fourth degree burn of the perineum while pinned beneath a hot muffler. The urethra between the bladder neck and the penis was totally lost. The anus was also destroyed. A colostomy had been done previously to protect the perineal burn and later skin grafts. (Case of J.B. McCraw, C.J. Devine, Jr., and G. Harkins)

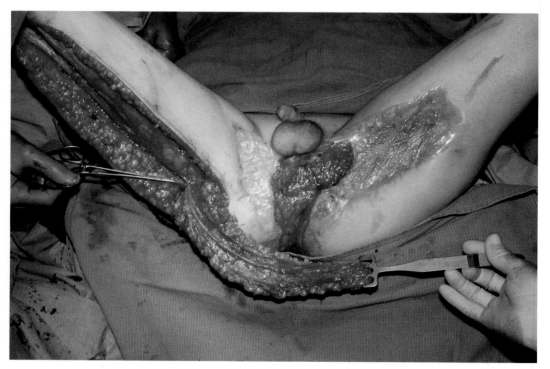

45

Elevated gluteal fasciocutaneous flap with the posterior cutaneous nerve of the thigh visible on the deep fascial surface. The neurovascular bundle is pointed out.

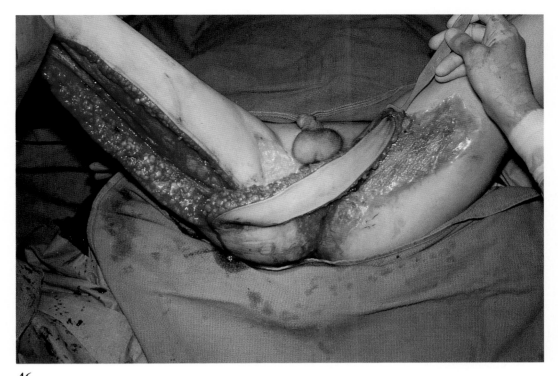

46

The posterior thigh flap was chosen for perineal coverage so the gracilis muscles could be preserved for a later reconstruction of the anal sphincter.

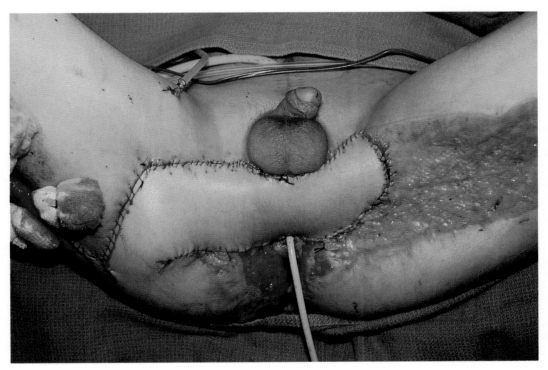

47

Transposed flap with the perineal urethrostomy in place. At the second stage, a ten centimeter tube graft urethroplasty was performed beneath the flap.

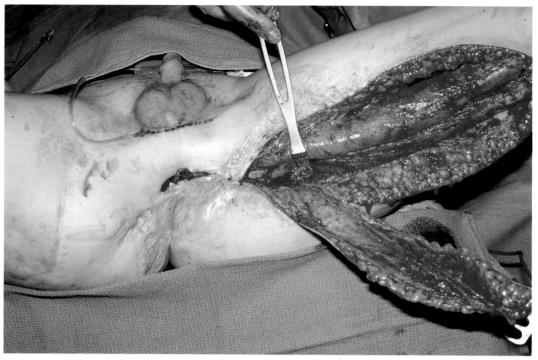

48

Identification of the inferior gluteal vessels at the ''base'' of the opposite posterior thigh flap which was covered with a skin graft. Since the posterior cutaneous nerve of the thigh was intact it was presumed that the deeply placed inferior gluteal vessels had survived the burn injury.

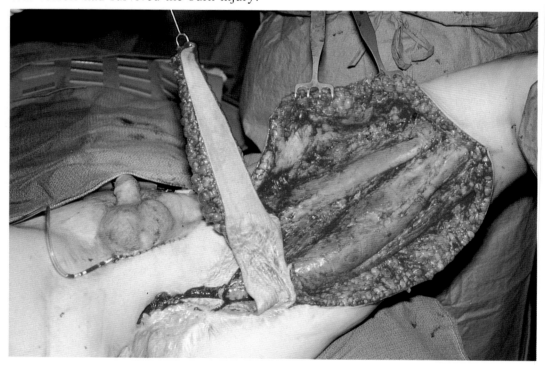

49

Elevated flap. Note the skin graft in the ''base'' of the fasciocutaneous flap. The skin graft had created a defacto ''island'' neurovascular flap.

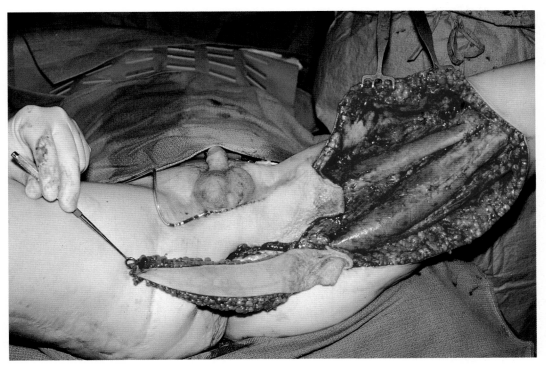

50

Flap transposed to the posterior perineum. The perineal urethrostomy was closed at this stage and urinary continence was reestablished.

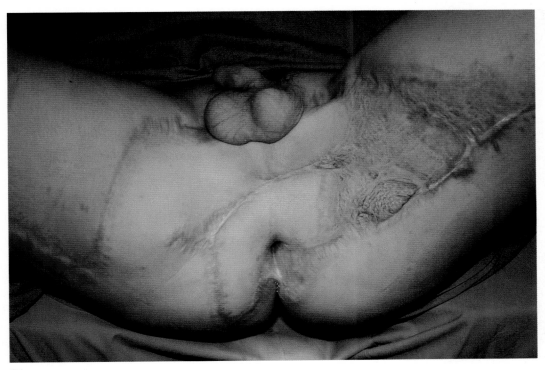

51

Healed flaps which resurfaced the entire perineum. The anal incontinence was corrected by a local plastic procedure, and the colostomy was removed. Bowel and bladder function was returned to normal.

TENSOR FASCIA LATA

ANATOMICAL CONSIDERATIONS

Surface Markings

If one draws a line passing from the greater trochanter to the midlateral aspect of the knee, this line should bisect the center of the tensor fascia lata (TFL) flap. The anterior border of the TFL flap extends to the margin of the rectus femoris muscle, and the posterior border extends to the margin of the biceps femoris muscle. The tensor muscle, itself, is usually palpable just distal to the greater trochanter.

Origin and Insertion

The tensor muscle originates partially from the anterior superior iliac spine but more extensively from the greater trochanter of the femur. The fascia lata extension of the small tensor muscle inserts into the lateral aspect of the knee and acts as a lateral knee stabilizer. This limits the usefulness of the TFL flap in an athletic individual because its sacrifice can contribute to lateral knee instability.

Adjacent Muscle

The tensor muscle lies between the biceps femoris and rectus femoris muscles. The vastus lateralis muscle is attached to the deep surface of the tensor fascia lata flap throughout its course.

Vascular Pattern

The tensor muscle is supplied by the lateral circumflex femoral vessels which also supply the rectus femoris and vastus lateralis muscles. All of these terminal vessels are end-arteries of the profunda femoris vessels and enter the three muscles approximately eight to ten centimeters below the inguinal ligament. There is a significant cutaneous vessel in the proximal skin of the flap, but the dominant blood supply to the TFL cutaneous segment is contributed by the extensive vascular network on both sides of the fascia lata. The skin in the distal and lateral one-third of the thigh is predominately supplied by direct cutaneous perforators from the vastus lateralis muscle. The relative dominance of these distal perforators limits the effective dimensions of the TFL flap, unless it is "delayed."

Motor Nerve

Inferior branch of the gluteal nerve L4-5.

Sensory Nerve

Lateral femoral cutaneous nerve, L1-3.

USES

Although the arc of rotation of the TFL flap extends from the ischium to the groin and, finally, to the abdomen, its applications are generally limited to the structural reconstruction of the abdominal wall and the replacement of groin skin. The tensor fascia will reach the chest wall margin if the tensor muscle is completely detached from its origin and raised as a pure "island" myofascial flap, as was first done by Waagensteen in 1933. Lower abdominal defects are more easily closed with the adjacent rectus femoris muscle flap which carries an even tougher fascial layer. A simple TFL rotation flap offers the most expeditious method to resurface major groin skin defects. Both the vastus lateralis muscle flap and the inferiorly based rectus abdominis muscle flap can be used for similar groin defects, but their dissection is more complex and their donor sites are even less desirable than that of the TFL flap. The TFL flap is exceedingly useful in spina bifida patients because of its ability to introduce cutaneous sensibility into the sitting area. It is seldom considered for a deep ischial ulcer because of its inability to obliterate the resulting excisional cavity.

REGIONAL FLAP COMPARISONS

The TFL flap is usually compared to the vastus lateralis muscle flap and the rectus femoris muscle or musculocutaneous flaps. The vastus lateralis muscle flap can be used to resurface exactly the same areas as the TFL flap, and it also has the advantage of adding muscular capabilities. The fascia of the vastus lateralis muscle is not as strong as the tensor fascia, but it is still adequate for a full-thickness abdominal defect. Unfortunately, the dissection of the vastus lateralis muscle flap is tedious and bloody. This limits its usefulness for abdominal wall and groin defects. The rectus femoris flap can also carry a similar amount of skin as the TFL flap if the anterior fascia lata is left attached to the rectus femoris muscle. It can be more useful for lower abdominal wall reconstructions because the fascia incorporated on the undersurface of the rectus femoris muscle is even stronger than the fascia lata of the TFL flap. For this reason the rectus femoris muscle alone is usually preferred over the TFL flap for lower abdominal defects or in situations where muscle is needed to obliterate a deep cavity. Even when the transposed rectus femoris muscle flap must be skin grafted, it is the simplest flap to use for osteomyelitis of the iliac crest and the hip joint. The V-Y biceps femoris myocutaneous flap is the traditional choice for standard ischial ulcers, unless one is attempting to introduce sensation into the sitting area with the TFL flap. The standard TFL flap will barely cover the ischial tuberosity, and it will not obliterate the usual ten by ten centimeter cavity which results from an ischiectomy.

DISADVANTAGES

The distal one-third of the lateral thigh skin receives its blood supply from the underlying vastus lateralis muscle perforators. This effectively limits the distal extent of the TFL flap unless it is "delayed." The TFL donor site usually can be primarily closed if the flap is no more than ten centimeters in width. When a skin graft is necessary, the "take" of the skin graft on the donor site (vastus lateralis muscle) is quite acceptable, but the esthetic deformity can be significant. Prolonged drainage from the donor site is a common problem; it can easily persist for several weeks when it occurs. A more significant disadvantage is the occasional knee instability which results from the loss of the lateral tensor band. In one case it was necessary to transfer the rectus femoris tendon into the distal tensor band to correct the lateral knee instability which resulted from the use of the TFL flap. It may be possible to circumvent knee instability by attaching the distal cut margin of the tensor band into the proximal fascia of the vastus lateralis muscle. It was initially thought that the use of rectus femoris flap would cause a greater functional loss than the TFL flap, but this has not been the case. Because it is primarily a fasciocutaneous flap, the TFL flap is not effective in correcting contaminated wounds or in obliterating cavities.

ADVANTAGES

The TFL unit is versatile because it can be used either as a fasciocutaneous or myofascial flap. It is innervated by a predictable sensory branch (lateral femoral cutaneous nerve), which is easily visualized between the iliac crest and the lateral border of the rectus femoris muscle. The lateral femoral cutaneous nerve has made the flap particularly useful for ischial coverage in meningomyelocele patients, since this L1-3 sensory area is spared in the majority of these patients and can be used to transfer sensate skin to the ischium. As a myofascial flap it is certainly the most useful tissue for middle and upper abdominal wall reconstructions, as well as for the difficult problem of the recurrent inguinal hernia.

COMPLICATIONS, PITFALLS, AND DONOR SITE

Excessive flap length and improper inset of the flap under tension should be recognized as the most common causes of flap necrosis in this normally robust flap. The flap can sustain a generous amount of either tension or torsion, but the combination of these two stressful events should be avoided. Flap elevation is straightforward, but one must carefully protect the dominant vessels and the lateral femoral cutaneous nerve. Since this sensory nerve enters the anterior border of the TFL flap, the TFL flap must be extended onto the lateral margin of the rectus femoris muscle if the nerve is to be included with the flap. Injury to the lateral femoral cutaneous nerve may result in the well known meralgia paresthetica complex of symptoms. Fortunately, the size and location of the dominant vessels to the flap are predictable.

Prolonged drainage has developed in a small number of patients. In a few cases serous drainage lasted for six or more weeks and was probably caused by a lymphatic fistula or a draining lymphocele. Lateral knee instability is an unusual complication, but it is correctable by the transfer of the rectus femoris tendon into the distal tensor band. It can probably be prevented by attaching the cut distal tensor band into the tendon of the vastus lateralis muscle.

There are very few pitfalls in the mechanics of flap elevation because the plane between the vastus lateralis muscle and the tensor fascia is easily defined. It is possible to injure the dominant vessels when raising the flap as an "island" flap, but their location is consistent. Vascular "spasm" can be caused by traumatic handling of the dominant vessels, and it may lead to partial flap necrosis. Rather than stretching the TFL vessels over the rectus femoris muscle, the origin of the rectus femoris muscle should be divided to increase the upward mobility of the TFL flap. Fortunately, this transection of the rectus femoris muscular origin does not affect the subsequent use of an "island" rectus femoris flap in the same muscle. The donor site is quite acceptable if it can be primarily closed. A skin-grafted donor site is remarkably unesthetic in appearance. Primary closure is facilitated by complete elevation and incision of the fascia lata on the medial aspects of the thigh anteriorly and posteriorly. This fascial "release" advances the skin margins of the remaining thigh skin by an additional five to six centimeters, which can make a critical difference in the donor site closure.

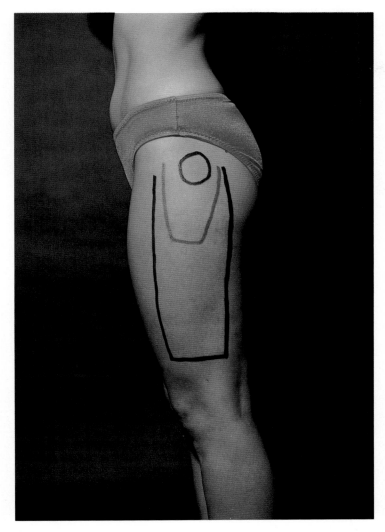

1

The disparity between the small size of
the tensor muscle and the surrounding
TFL flap dimensions is demonstrated in a
model. This donor defect will require a
skin graft for closure.

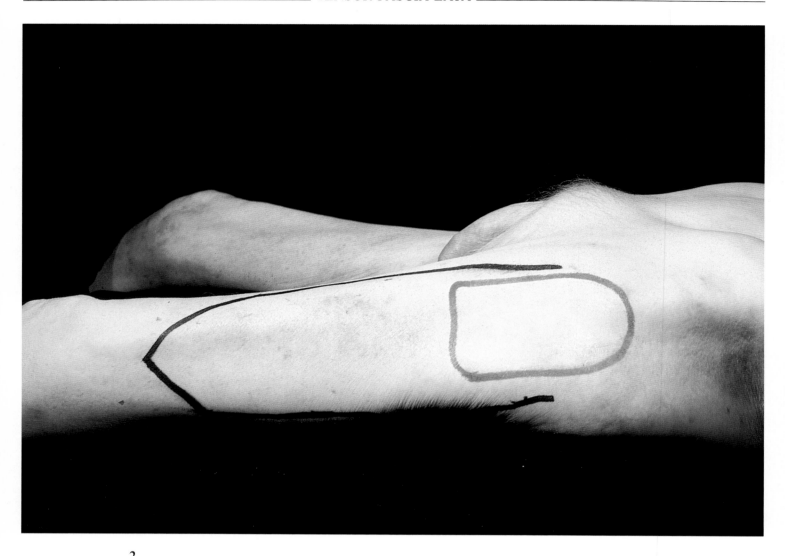

2

A very large TFL flap is outlined in the cadaver. This will create a defect which must be skin grafted. There is a cutaneous vessel which enters the proximal cutaneous ''base'' of the flap and provides a separate blood supply to the skin. It is unlikely that a longer flap would be reliable because of the relative dominance of the vastus lateralis perforators in the distal one-third of the thigh.

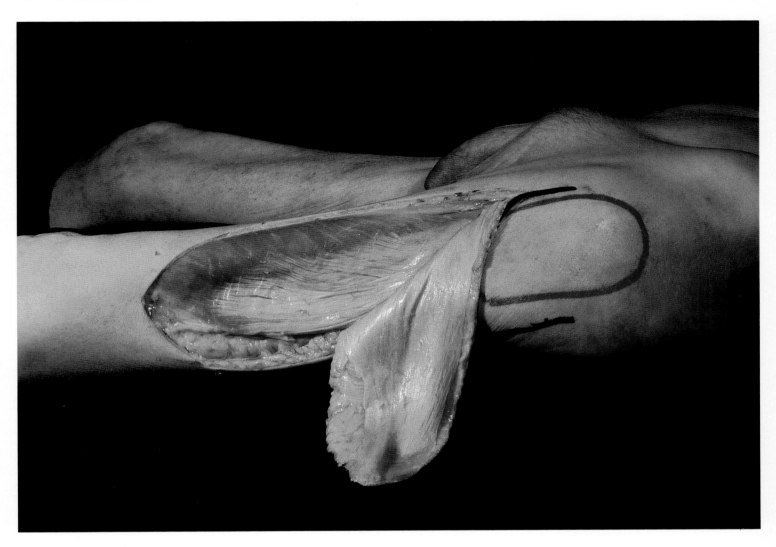

3

The outlined TFL flap extends from the margin of the biceps femoris muscle posteriorly to the midline of the thigh anteriorly. Note that the tensor fascia is deficient distally in the area of the biceps femoris tendon.

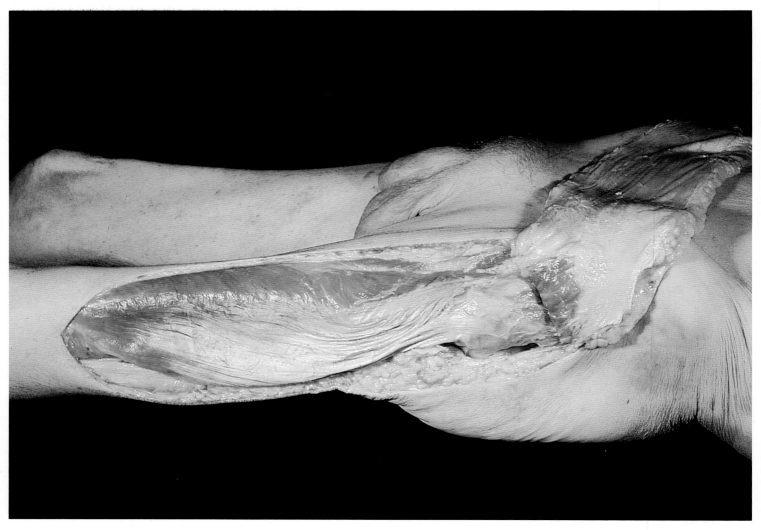

4

The tensor fascia is readily dissected away from the underlying vastus lateralis muscle. In this example the deep fascia was included from the margin of the rectus femoris muscle to the margin of the biceps femoris muscle. The small tensor muscle is partially elevated from its trochanteric origin.

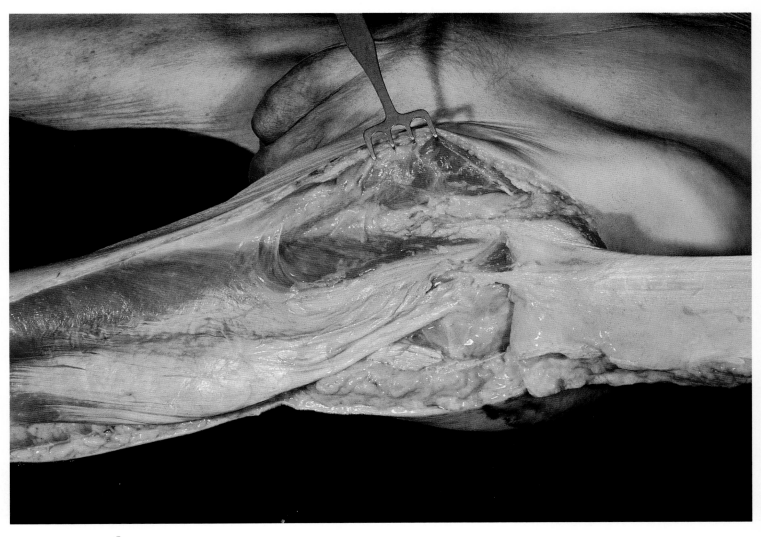

5

The TFL flap has been completely elevated away from the vastus lateralis muscle. The dominant vascular pedicle is seen piercing the proximal tendon of the vastus lateralis muscle and then entering the medial edge of the tensor fascia. The tensor muscle has been partially elevated away from its origin on the greater trochanter. It is safe to remove the tensor muscle from its origin completely since the dominant vasculature is not harmed by this maneuver.

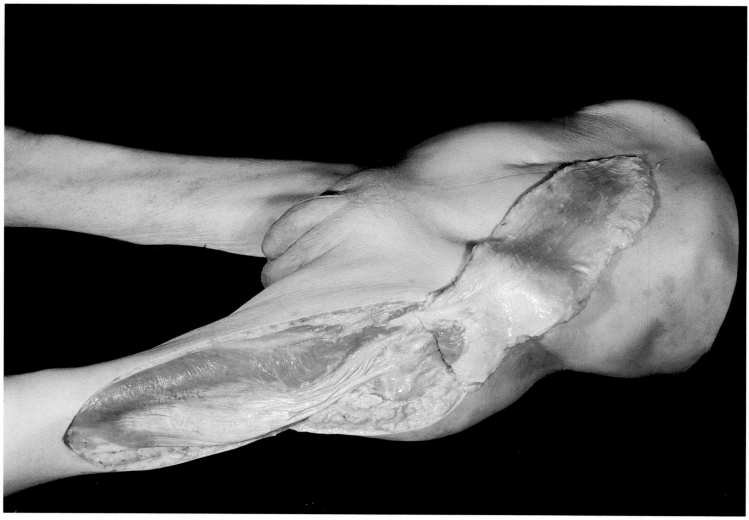

6

The fascial undersurface of the TFL flap is demonstrated. The lateral circumflex femoral vessels are seen entering the tensor muscle just medial to the greater trochanter. These vessels arise from the profunda femoris vessels and then pass beneath the rectus femoris muscle approximately ten centimeters below the inguinal ligament.

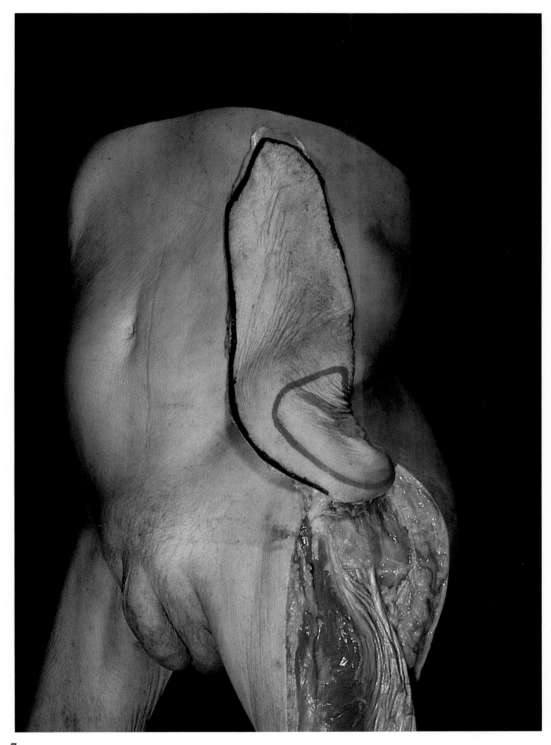

7

The tip of this flap reaches the lower
chest wall. Complete elevation of the tensor muscle from the greater trochanter
and the creation of a true "island" flap
will allow the most distal portion of the
tensor fascia to reach the xiphoid.

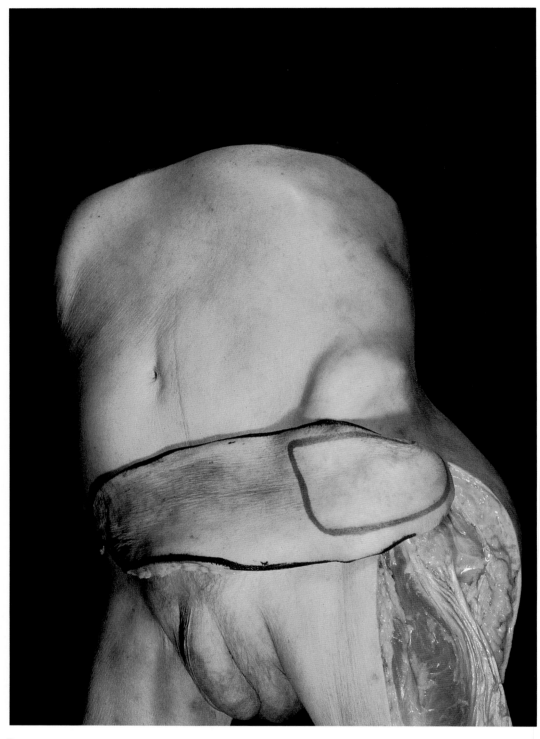

8

The entire suprapubic area can be resurfaced by the TFL flap.

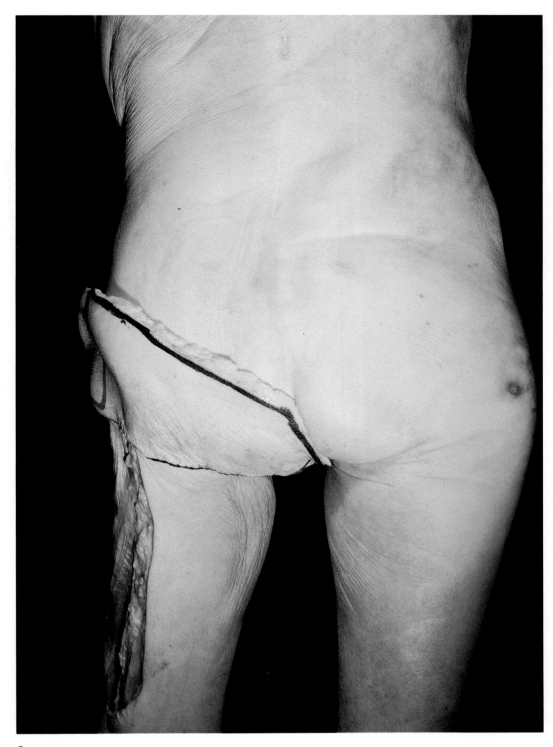

9

Generally the TFL flap will barely cover an ischial defect. This flap has an exceptional posterior excursion.

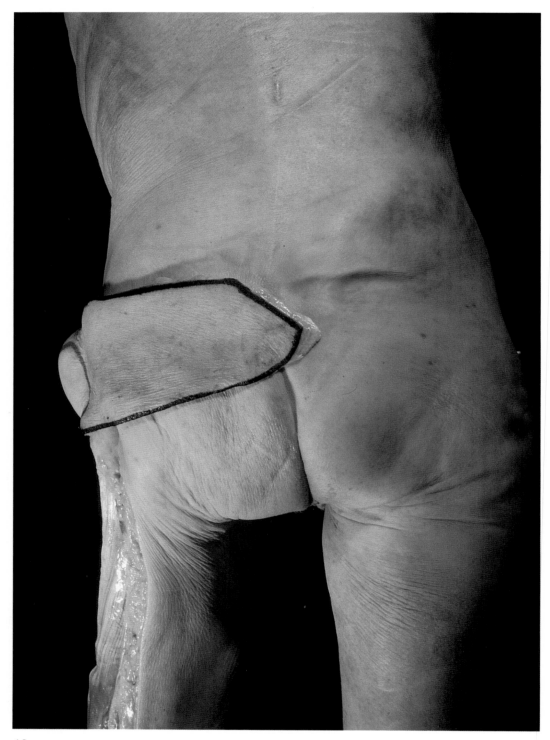

10

The posterior rotation shows the TFL flap
reaching the midsacrum. The long legs of
this cadaver provided an unusually
lengthy flap.

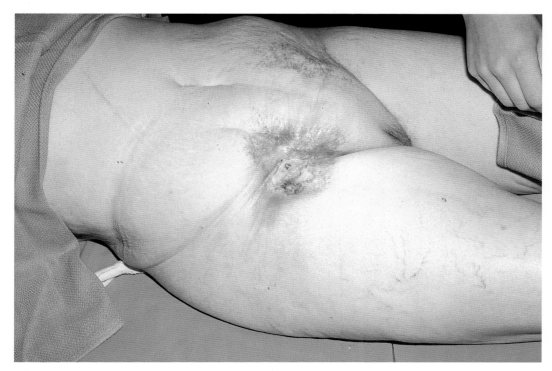

11

Seventy-eight-year-old woman with a carcinoma of the cervix treated with a radical hysterectomy and bilateral groin irradiation. The extensive irradiation ulcer of the right groin has been present for two years. (Case of P.G. Arnold and G. Irons)

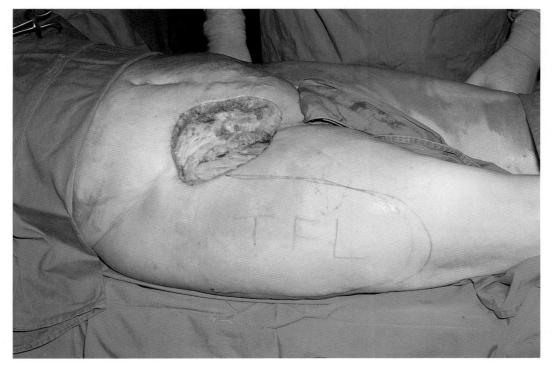

12

The irradiation ulcer of the groin and lower abdomen was excised. No tumor was found. A very wide TFL flap is outlined to accommodate the large excisional defect.

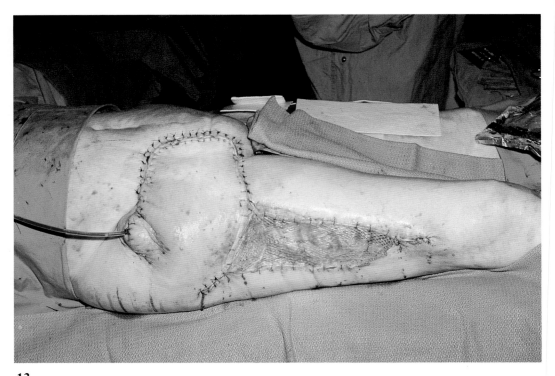

13

TFL flap rotated into the defect. The donor site was immediately grafted.

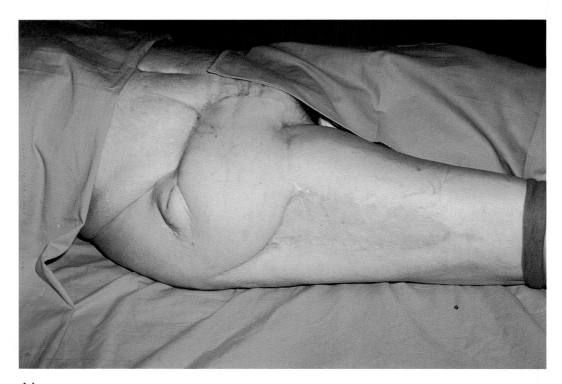

14

Appearance of the flap and donor site at three years. The wound has remained healed.

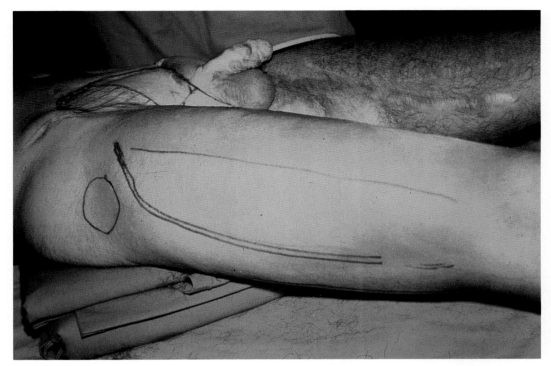

15

This twenty-six-year-old patient sustained a high voltage electrical injury to the perineum, abdomen, and right thigh. The full thickness of the left lower quadrant of the abdominal wall had been lost. A skin graft covered a herniated Marlex® mesh graft in this area. The anterior margin of the TFL flap is outlined. The posterior margin (double line) of the flap will be defined after the ability to close the donor site has been determined. (Case of J.B. McCraw, C.E. Horton, and G. Hoffman)

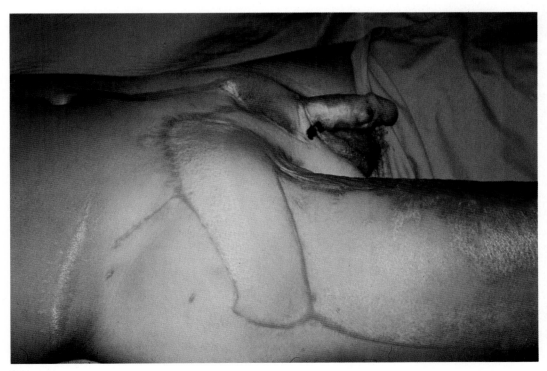

16

The "island" TFL flap is rotated into position. Primary closure of the donor defect was facilitated by anterior and posterior incisions of the deep fascia. The fascia on the undersurface of the TFL flap was used to repair the abdominal wall defect. The cutaneous portion of the flap was used to replace the skin graft of the lower quadrant. The closure of the donor defect was somewhat difficult because the entire medial thigh had previously been skin grafted.

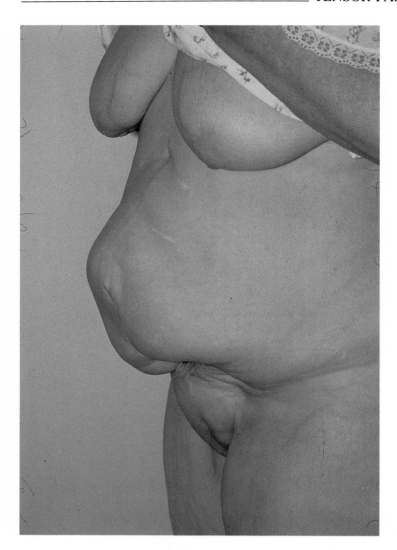

17

This sixty-nine-year-old patient was left with a recurrent abdominal hernia after six abdominal repairs with artificial mesh. The patient had also undergone cobalt irradiation for carcinoma of the cervix, which resulted in an irradiation ulcer in the suprapubic area. (Case of J.B. Mc-Craw and M. Greenspan)

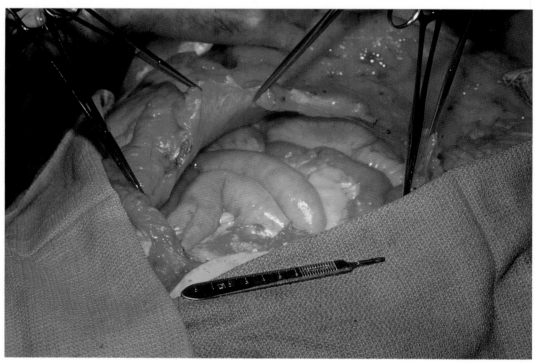

18

The huge abdominal wall defect could not have been closed primarily.

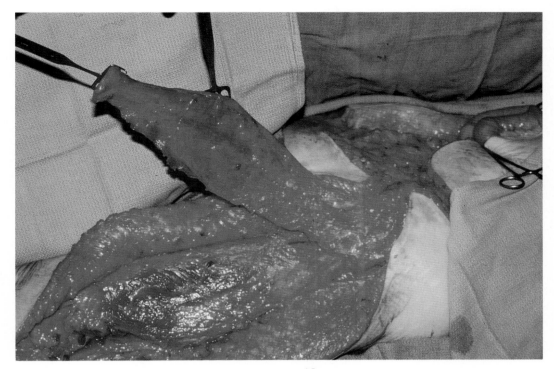

19

A tensor myofascial flap is elevated as a pure "island" flap.

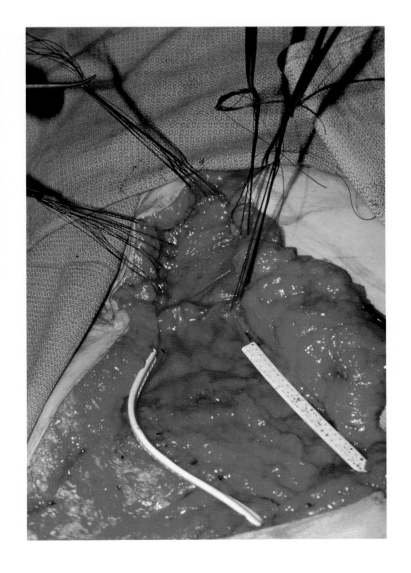

20

The tensor fascia was used as an end-to-end patch, interposed between the two rectus abdominis muscles.

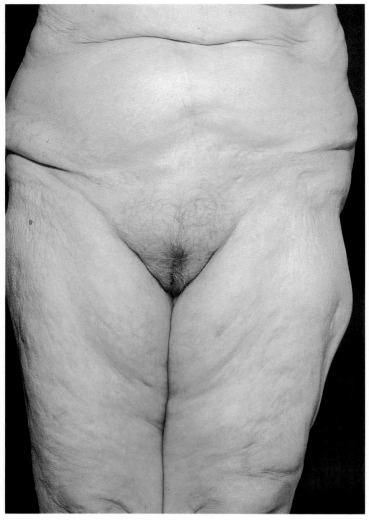

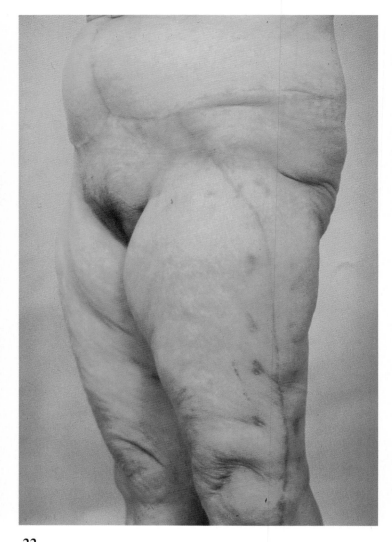

21

Postoperative view demonstrating good abdominal wall stability. This is the same procedure described by Dr. Owen Waagensteen in 1933.

22

Healed donor site.

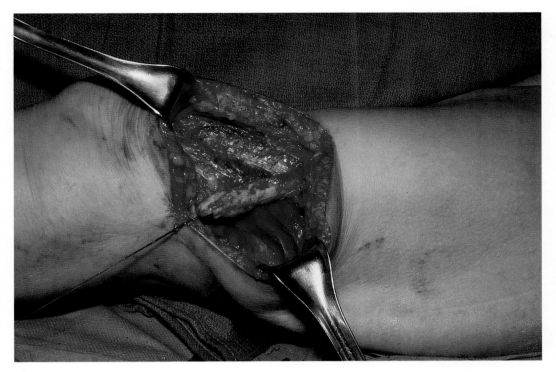

23

Two years later the patient developed left lateral knee instability. The rectus femoris tendon is elevated for transfer into the distal tensor band.

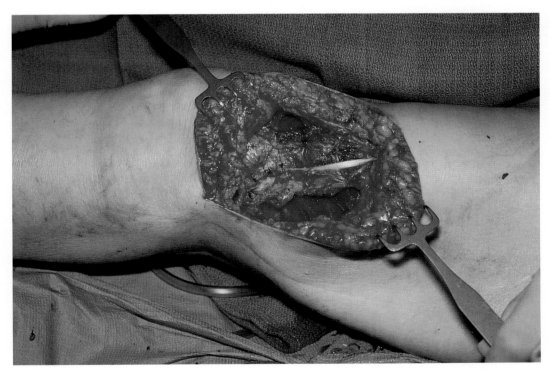

24

The rectus femoris tendon transfer adequately corrected the deficient lateral knee stability that had resulted from the use of the TFL flap.

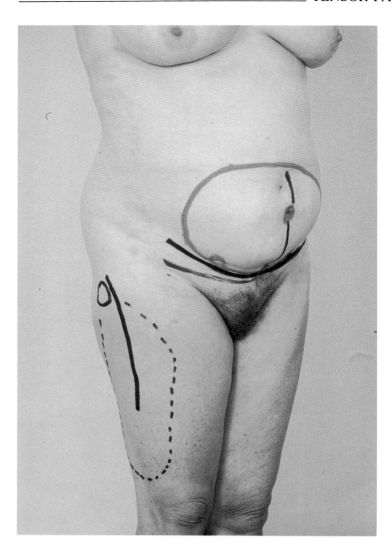

25

Infected Marlex® mesh repair of an abdominal hernia in a severe asthmatic. A tensor myofascial flap is outlined. (Case of J.B. McCraw and G. Hoffman)

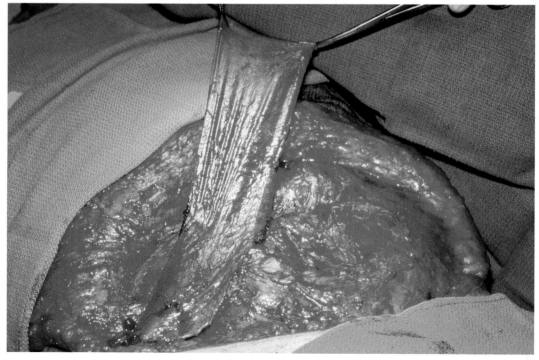

26

''Island'' tensor myofascial flap transposed into the abdominal defect.

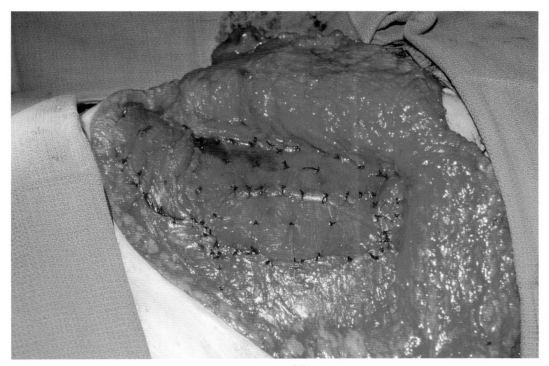

27
Lateral view of the end-to-end repair of
the abdominal fascial defect.

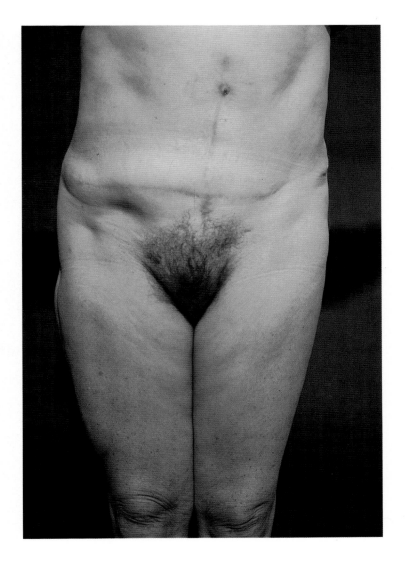

28
Solid abdominal repair at one year. Note
the unsightly bulge of the tensor muscle
in the right groin. This fullness decreased
very little with time and could have been
avoided by trimming the tensor muscle
initially.

RECTUS FEMORIS

ANATOMICAL CONSIDERATIONS

Surface Markings

The course of the rectus femoris muscle follows a line which passes directly between the anterior superior iliac spine and the patella. It is easily palpated during forcible extension of the knee.

Origin and Insertion

The rectus femoris muscle originates from the anterior inferior iliac spine and the upper border of the acetabulum and inserts into the patellar tendon. It is densely fused with the vastus lateralis and vastus medialis muscles through musculotendinous connections in the distal one-third of the thigh. The primary function of the rectus femoris muscle is in the terminal 15-20 degrees of knee extension.

Adjacent Muscles

The vastus lateralis and vastus medialis muscles parallel the rectus femoris muscle, and the vastus intermedius muscle is directly subjacent throughout its course. In the upper-third of the thigh the tensor muscle abuts on the lateral surface of the rectus femoris muscle, and the sartorius muscle crosses the proximal one-third of the rectus femoris muscle from lateral to medial.

Vascular Pattern

The rectus femoris muscle has a purely proximal vascular pattern with no minor pedicle distally. The profunda femoris vessels supply all of the anterior thigh musculature. These profunda femoris branches enter the anterior thigh muscles approximately eight to ten centimeters below the inguinal ligament. Branches of the lateral circumflex femoral vessels supply the tensor, vastus lateralis, and rectus femoris muscles after exiting the profunda femoris vessels. Just before entering the deep surface of the rectus femoris muscle, the lateral circumflex femoral artery divides into two major branches which are each two to three millimeters in diameter. The proximal branch primarily supplies the proximal one-third of the muscle while the distal branch supplies the distal two-thirds of the muscle. The "end-artery" nature of this vascular pattern suggests that the integrity of both of these branches should be preserved, but the viability of the rectus femoris muscle flap is apparently not harmed by the sacrifice of the distal set of vessels. An independent fasciocutaneous vessel enters the proximal cutaneous segment near the inguinal ligament so the preservation of the proximal skin bridge may enhance the viability of the rectus femoris myocutaneous flap.

Motor Nerve

Femoral nerve.

Sensory Nerve

Intermediate cutaneous nerve of the thigh.

USES

The rectus femoris myocutaneous flap is used primarily for lower quadrant and suprapubic abdominal coverage problems, particularly when it is desirable to transpose muscle and dense fascia. A musculofascial flap is the usual choice in reconstruction of the lower abdominal wall since skin replacement is seldom necessary. The lateral rotation of the "island" rectus femoris muscle flap easily extends to the greater trochanter and to the hip joint. It should be noted that the rectus femoris myocutaneous flap does not reach the central perineum, bladder, or vagina.

REGIONAL FLAP COMPARISONS

For suprapubic and lower abdominal coverage, the rectus femoris myocutaneous flap is preferred over the TFL flap because of its proximity, reliability, and ease of elevation. The TFL donor site is also associated with greater morbidity, and frequently requires skin grafting. Compared to the standard TFL flap, the rectus femoris myocutaneous flap does not serve as well for groin coverage. In addition, it will not reach the upper abdomen for purposes of abdominal wall reconstruction. The vastus lateralis muscle provides a larger muscle and a broader area of coverage than the rectus femoris flap. However, the vastus lateralis flap is much more difficult to elevate, and the fascia of the vastus lateralis muscle is less dense than the fascia of the rectus femoris muscle. The rectus femoris muscle flap alone is usually sufficient to correct recalcitrant hip wounds following the loss of a hip prosthesis.

DISADVANTAGES

The potential loss of terminal knee extension should not be realized if the vastus medialis and lateralis muscles are carefully centralized and repaired above the patellar tendon. The functional "reserve" of the strong quadriceps mechanism compensates for the loss of this single anterior thigh muscle in all but the athletic individual.

ADVANTAGES

If the dominant vessels are not stretched or otherwise injured, the rectus femoris myocutaneous flap is one of our most dependable flaps. The cutaneous segment can be expanded safely to approximately three times the width of the rectus femoris muscle by including the adjacent fascia lata. This fasciocutaneous "extension" of the myocutaneous flap encompasses the majority of the anterior thigh skin. Although the muscle is only six centimeters in width, the associated muscle fascia is strong enough to reconstruct a much larger (e.g. fifteen to twenty centimeters) full-thickness defect of the abdominal wall.

COMPLICATIONS, PITFALLS, AND DONOR SITE

One must be careful not to place too much tension or torsion on the dominant vessels because they are subject to vascular "spasm." This caused a significant loss of the cutaneous segment of the flap in one case, but flap necrosis has not been encountered in any other case. The dissection is straightforward, but entry into the su-prapatellar bursa should be carefully avoided. One should also take extreme care to protect the femoral nerve which lies on the surface of the vastus intermedius muscle and provides the motor supply to the entire quadriceps muscular mechanism. Since the dominant vessels are the limiting factor in upward flap rotation, division of the muscular origin does not facilitate upward mobility of the flap. To prevent any loss of active knee extension, the vastus medialis and vastus lateralis muscles should be approximated in the midline for a distance of approximately fifteen centimeters above the knee.

The donor site is quite favorable when it can be closed primarily. It holds the same disadvantages as the TFL donor site if it must be skin grafted, but this is rarely necessary. For some reason, seroma formation and prolonged drainage have not occurred with the rectus femoris donor site as frequently as they have with the TFL donor site. The permanent loss of muscular function has not been detectable by any measurable means in our cases, even in the aged patient. Despite this favorable experience, one might expect that the use of this "important" muscle would result in some disability in the athletic individual.

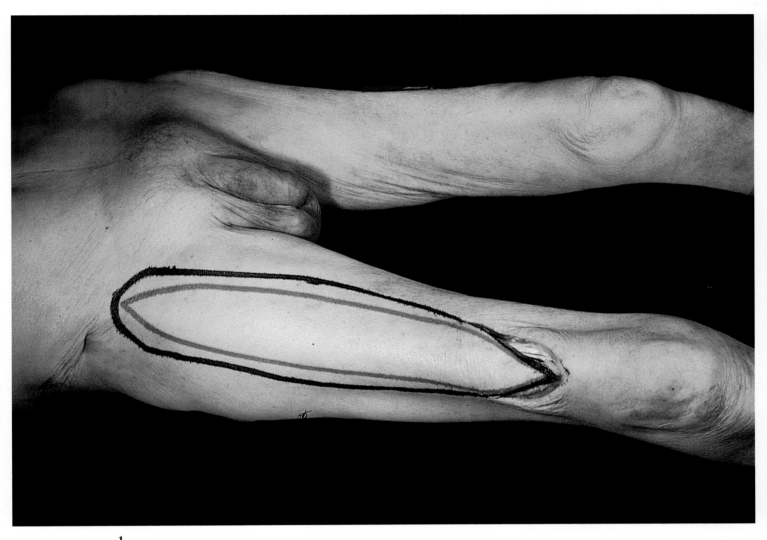

1

The course of the rectus femoris muscle is depicted on a line between the patellar tendon and the anterior iliac spine. The standard cutaneous segment is outlined in black. A much larger cutaneous segment can be carried if the adjacent fascia lata is included with the myocutaneous flap.

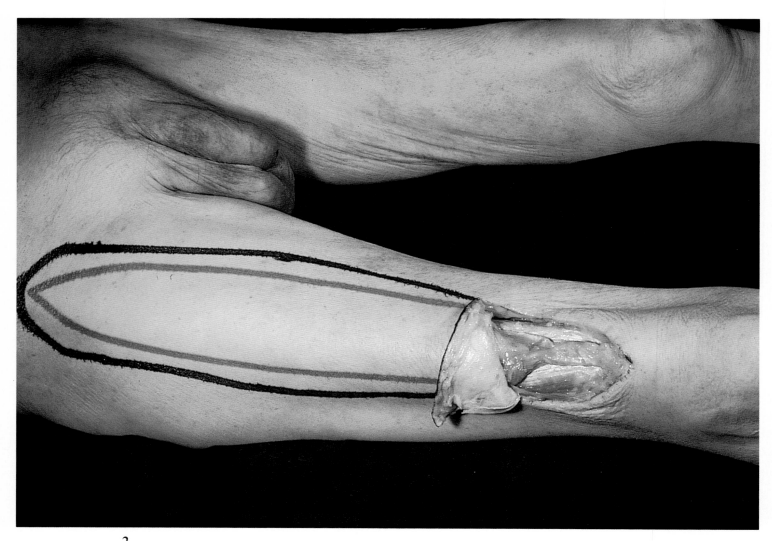

2

The rectus femoris tendon is isolated on the surface of the vastus intermedius muscle after it is separated from the tendinous attachments of the adjacent vastus medialis and vastus lateralis muscles. The integrity of the suprapatellar bursa is protected in this part of the dissection.

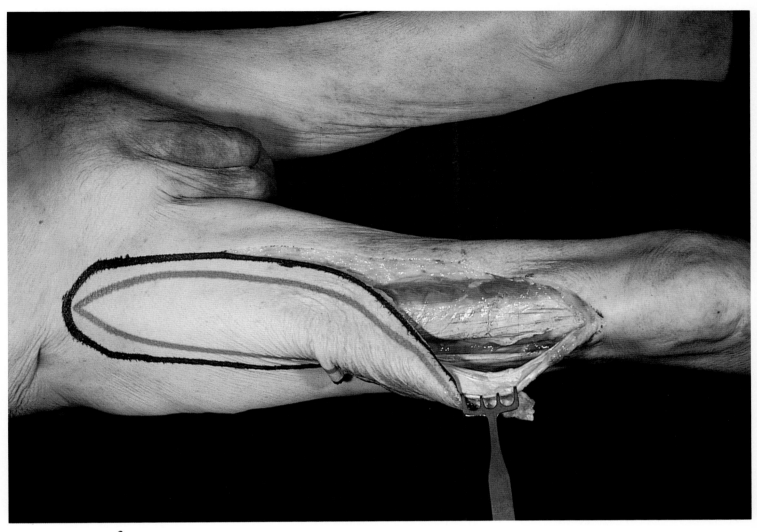

3

The rectus femoris muscle is elevated away from the underlying vastus intermedius muscle once the attachments of the vastus medialis and vastus lateralis muscles have been divided. The loose areolar plane between the rectus femoris and vastus intermedius muscles is easily developed.

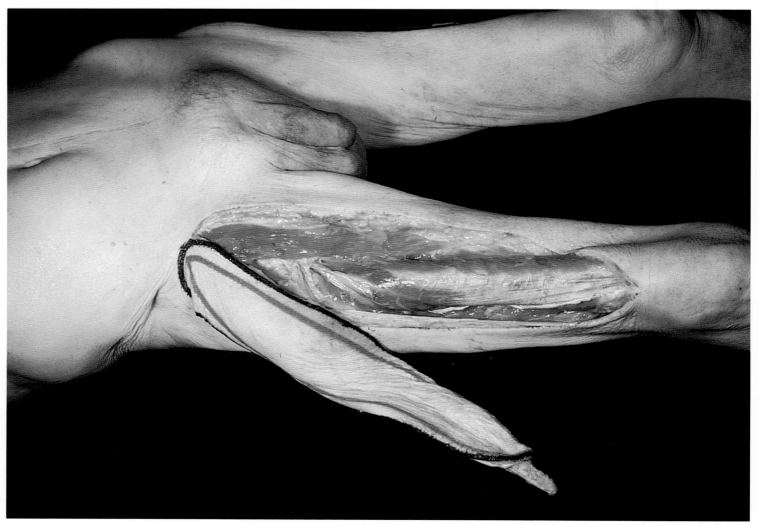

4

The lateral circumflex femoral vessels and the femoral nerve are seen on the surface of the vastus intermedius muscle. These dominant vessels pass beneath the sartorius muscle approximately ten centimeters below the inguinal ligament. Note the remaining fascial margin on the vastus lateralis and vastus medialis muscles. This dense fascia will be used to approximate the two muscles in the midline of the thigh.

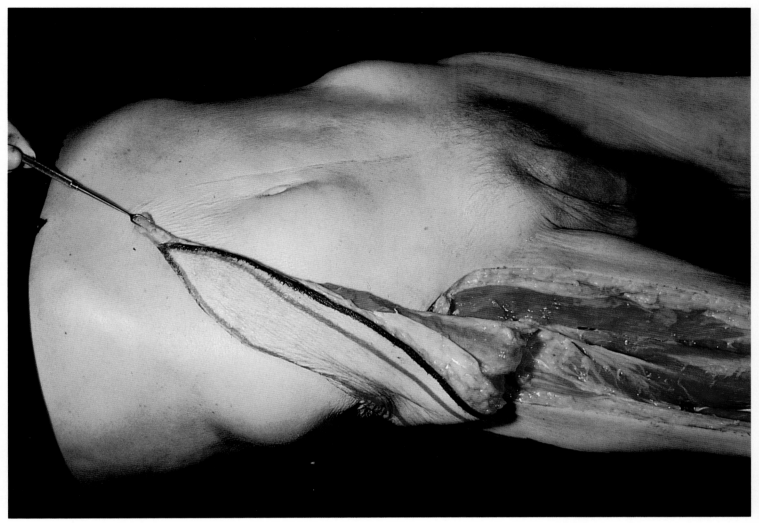

5

The upward mobility of the flap is limited
by the vascular pedicle, which is seen
passing beneath the lateral margin of the
sartorius muscle. The flap excursion is
not enhanced by the division of either the
muscular origin or the proximal skin
bridge. The tip of the myocutaneous flap
reaches a point between the umbilicus and
the xiphoid.

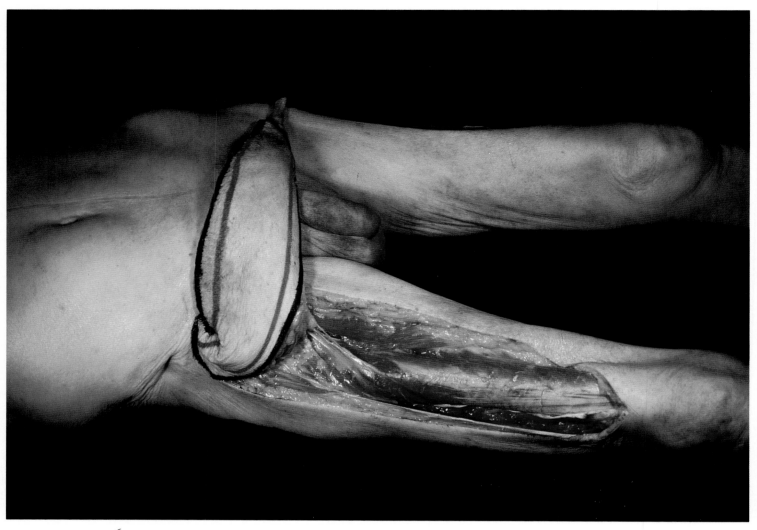

6

The rectus femoris flap is most useful for the repair of lower abdominal wall defects. The flap covers the suprapubic area and reaches the opposite anterior spine of the iliac crest.

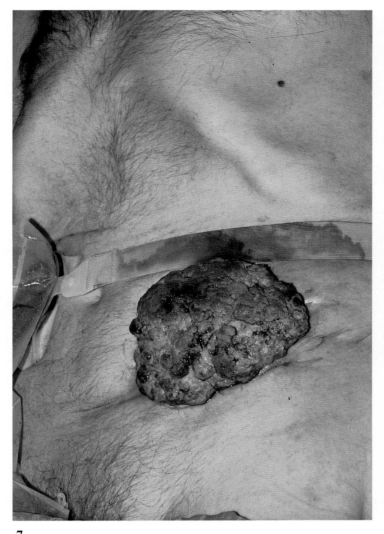

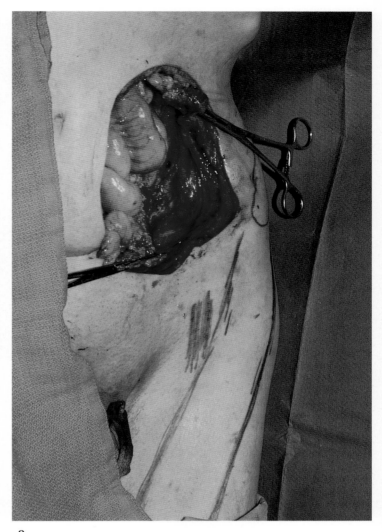

7

Sixty-year-old man with a fungating adenocarcinoma arising from the left colon and invading the abdominal wall. The patient previously had undergone a right colectomy for an adenocarcinoma of the colon. This new tumor represented a second metachronous adenocarcinoma of the left colon. The patient was considered to be a candidate for curative resection, but it was feared that the massive abdominal defect would be lethal to a man with severe chronic lung disease unless the structural component of the abdominal wall could be immediately reconstructed. (Case of J.B. McCraw and R. Ludwig)

8

An en bloc resection of the left colon and the abdominal wall was carried out. The fifteen by twenty centimeter abdominal defect extended from the inguinal ligament to the iliac crest inferiorly and to a point five centimeters above the umbilicus superiorly. The resection also included the left rectus abdominis muscle.

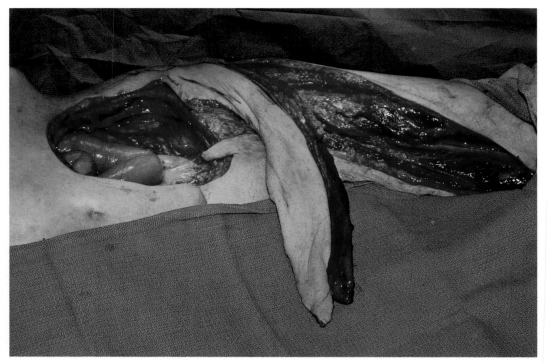

9

The rectus femoris flap was raised after the extirpation was completed. The flap dimensions of this early case (1975) helped to dispel the prevailing ''length-width'' theory of the day.

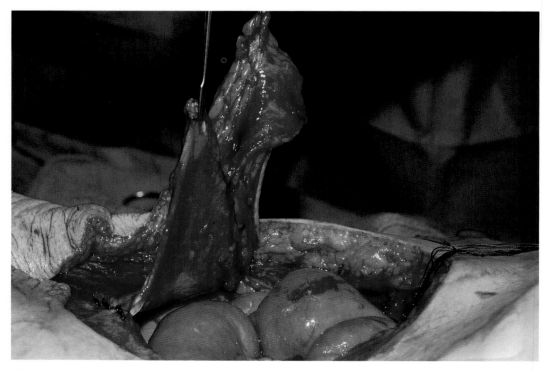

10

The dense fascia of the rectus femoris muscle was strong enough to accommodate a tense closure of the large abdominal wall defect.

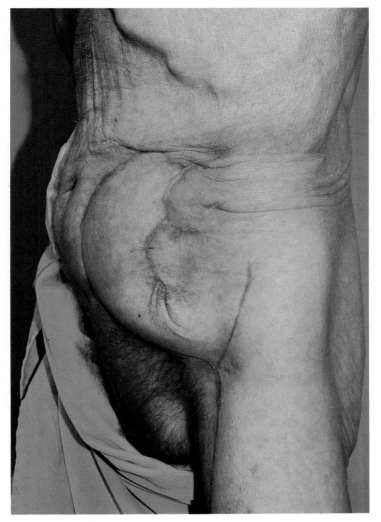

11

Healed flap and donor site at six months. The abdominal wall was stable. The patient was killed in a motor vehicle accident two years following the surgery.

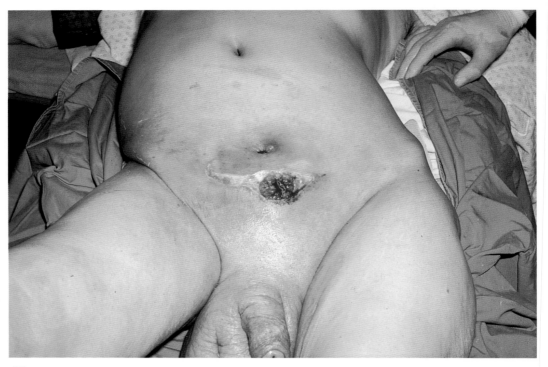

12

Fifty-four-year-old paraplegic man with a squamous cell carcinoma of the bladder involving the suprapubic tube tract. (Case of P.G. Arnold)

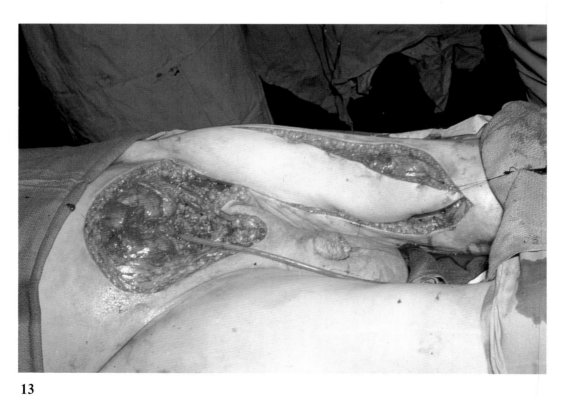

13

The anterior half of the urinary bladder and the overlying abdominal wall were resected en bloc. The remaining bladder wall was repaired around the suprapubic catheter.

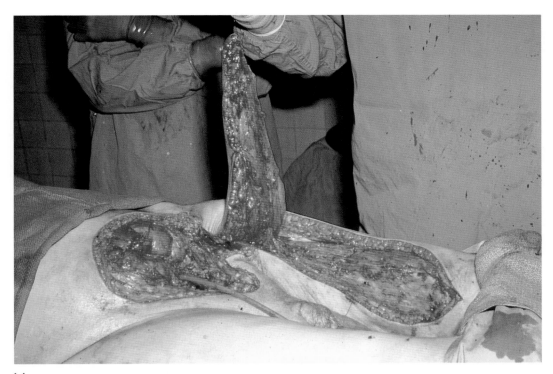

14
A left rectus femoris myocutaneous flap
is elevated for the abdominal wall
closure.

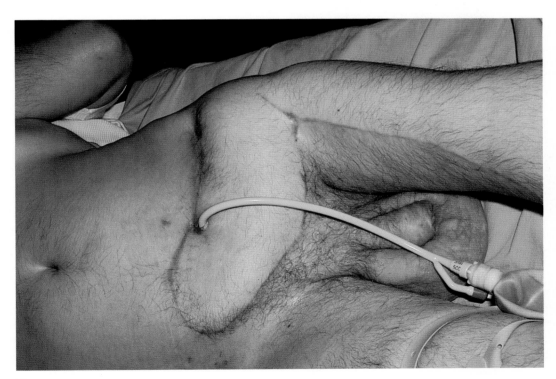

15
Healed wound at six months. The patient
has done well for seven years.

457

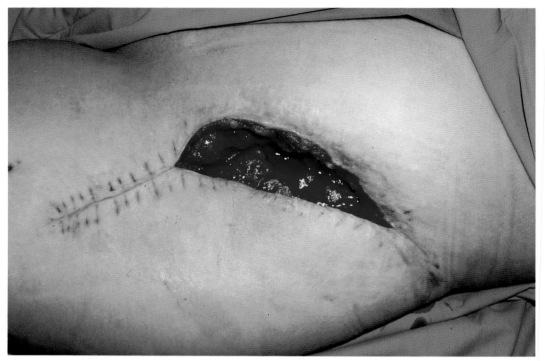

16

Fifty-three-year-old female with osteo-myelitis of the iliac crest following the harvesting of a bone graft for an ankle fusion. The osteomyelitis had been resistant to multiple attempts at direct closure and the patient was referred for definitive treatment. (Case of P.G. Arnold)

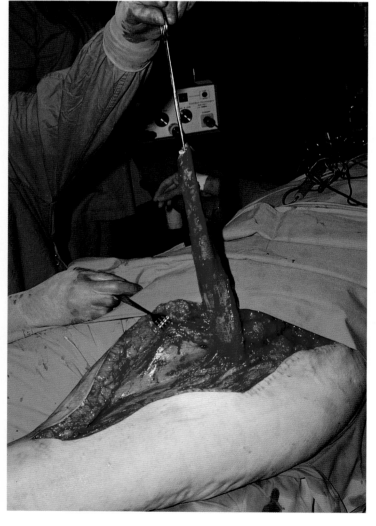

17

The adjacent rectus femoris muscle was elevated through an extension of the previous incision.

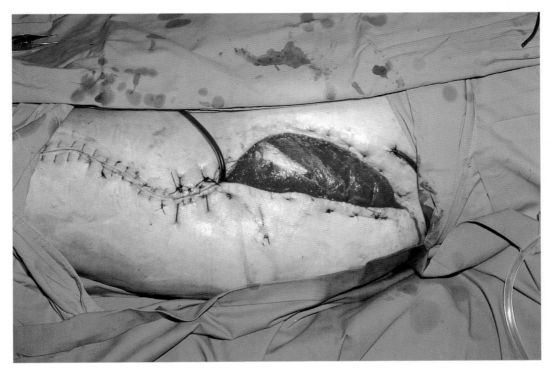

18

The transposed rectus femoris muscle completely obliterated the iliac crest defect. The muscle was skin grafted two days later.

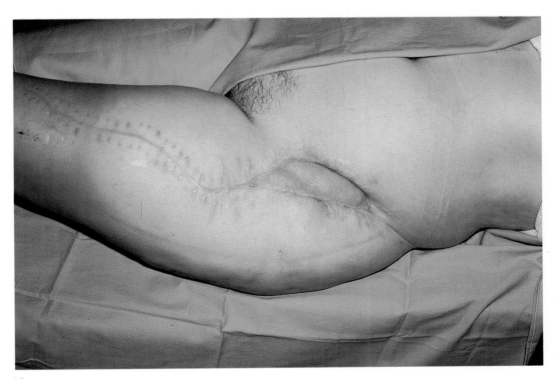

19

Healed wound at three years. The osteomyelitis has not recurred over a nine-year period.

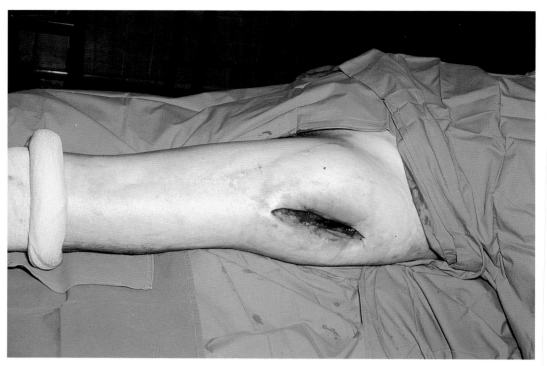

20

Sixty-year-old man with a failed total hip procedure. The osteomyelitis involved both the femur and the acetabulum. A previous TFL flap closure had been unsuccessful. (Case of P.G. Arnold)

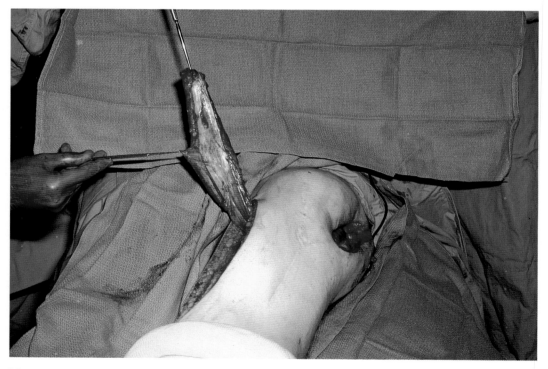

21

Elevated rectus femoris muscle flap. A generous tunnel was created for the muscle flap transposition.

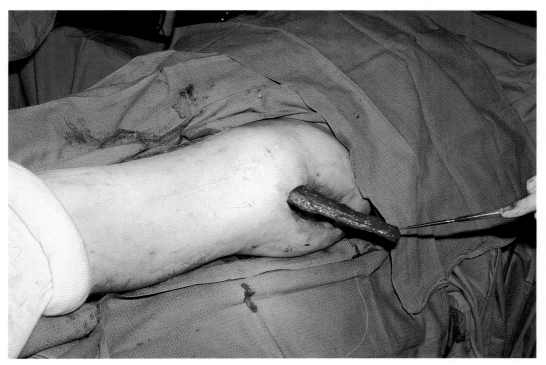

22

Rectus femoris muscle flap passed into the "total hip" defect. Approximately half of the rectus femoris muscle is visible beyond the hip defect.

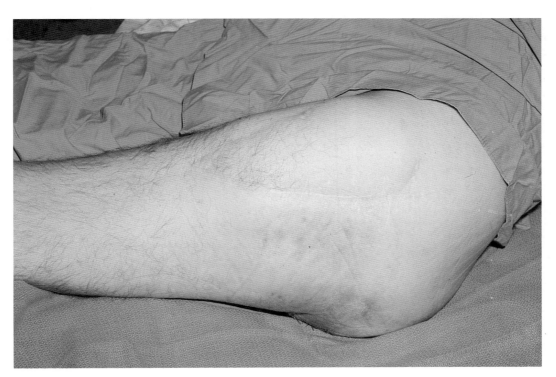

23

Healed skin closure over the buried muscle flap. The wound has remained stable for seven years.

VASTUS LATERALIS

ANATOMICAL CONSIDERATIONS

Surface Markings

The contracted vastus lateralis muscle can be palpated between the lateral margins of the rectus femoris and biceps femoris muscles. The cleft between the biceps femoris and vastus lateralis muscles is easily visualized in most legs. The anterior margin of the vastus lateralis muscle can best be palpated at the lateral border of the rectus femoris muscle in the lower thigh.

Origin and Insertion

Anteriorly the vastus lateralis originates from the lateral surface of the greater trochanter and the trochanteric line of the femur. Posteriorly it originates from the lateral lip of the linea aspera and the intermuscular septum. It inserts into the tendon of the rectus femoris, the upper border of the patella, and the lateral condyle of the tibia, thereby forming a part of the lateral patellar retinaculum. The vastus lateralis muscle functions as an accessory knee extensor and lateral knee stabilizer. It is functionally expendable if the rectus femoris and tensor muscles are intact.

Adjacent Muscles

The vastus lateralis muscle lies between the rectus femoris and biceps femoris muscles and encompasses the whole of the lateral thigh. The vastus intermedius muscle surrounds the femur and lies deep to the vastus lateralis muscle throughout its course. The overlying tensor fascia provides a "sausage casing" which is loosely adherent to the surface of the vastus lateralis muscle.

Vascular Pattern

The proximal vastus lateralis muscle is supplied by the lateral circumflex femoral artery, a branch of the profunda femoris artery. Branches of the same vessel also supply the tensor and rectus femoris muscles. The majority of the vastus lateralis muscle is nourished by this proximal vasculature, but the distal one-third of the muscle is independently supplied by deep perforating branches of the superficial femoral vessels. Although it may be possible to carry the entire muscle on the proximal vessels, only the proximal two-thirds of the muscle can be reliably carried by the lateral circumflex femoral system. Like other broad, flat muscles, the extensive intramuscular vascular network will support either a distally based or a proximally based muscle flap.

Motor Nerve

Femoral nerve

USES

The primary use of the vastus lateralis muscle is in situations which require muscle coverage, rather than skin or fascial replacement. The arc of rotation is almost identical to the TFL flap and includes the ischium, the greater trochanter, the hip, the groin, and the lower abdomen. The tensor fascia can also be "carried" on the surface of the vastus lateralis muscle in order to provide a supplemental "living" fascial replacement for the abdominal wall. As a practical matter, the vastus lateralis muscle flap is seldom used for abdominal wall replacement because it is more difficult to elevate than either the rectus femoris or TFL flaps. It does provide an unparelleled volume of muscular tissue for deep defects of the hip, femur, and groin.

REGIONAL FLAP COMPARISONS

The vastus lateralis muscle flap is primarily used to introduce a large amount of muscle into areas of low-grade infection or irradiation damage. Enthusiasm for the use of this large muscle flap has been tempered only by the bloody dissection which is necessary for its retrieval. When the biceps femoris V-Y flap is unavailable, the vastus lateralis muscle flap is useful for the obliteration of an ischiectomy defect. Like the smaller rectus femoris muscle flap, the "island" vastus lateralis muscle flap will reach the iliac crest and the hip joint. The more accessible rectus femoris muscle flap is usually chosen for these adjacent defects when it is thought to be large enough to correct the deformity. When combined with the vastus medialis muscle flap, the vastus lateralis muscle flap can simultaneously be used to restore knee function and resurface the distal anterior thigh. The vastus lateralis muscle and the TFL flap have nearly identical arcs of rotation, but the TFL flap is much more easily manipulated. Even though the vastus lateralis muscle can be used to reconstruct the abdominal wall, it is more reasonable to use the rectus femoris muscle flap for the lower abdomen and use the "island" tensor myofascial flap for the upper abdomen.

DISADVANTAGES

Only the proximal two-thirds of the muscle can be carried reliably by the proximal pedicle because the distal one-third of the muscle is supplied by segmental branches of the superficial femoral vessels. This is not so much a disadvantage as it is a recognized reality of the existing blood supply. Still, it can be a cause of distal muscle flap necrosis. The vastus lateralis muscle has a dense fascial layer on both its superficial and deep surfaces, but it is not as strong as the fascia included with the TFL or rectus femoris flaps. Like the TFL flap, the donor site is subject to prolonged drainage. The dissection of this muscle is much more tedious and bloody than the dissection of either the rectus femoris or TFL flaps because it is difficult to define the distal limits of the muscle. Although it is possible to injure the proximal vascular leash, it is easily visualized and reasonably predictable in its location. If these proximal vessels are accidentally divided there is no secondary blood supply to fall back on. In this event, the proximally based flap will be totally lost.

ADVANTAGES

The vastus lateralis muscle can be completely removed through a single incision with a primary closure of the donor site. There is no noticeable depression in the area of its removal, and we have not noticed any functional loss from its use. It is certainly expendable when the adjacent thigh muscles are intact. The vastus lateralis muscle is quite broad (fifteen centimeters wide) and provides an excellent new blood supply for its expected areas of coverage. A skin graft on the surface of the transposed muscle offers a very acceptable esthetic result, and neither muscle bulk nor lymphedema have marred the eventual results in our cases. The vastus lateralis muscle can also be raised as a myocutaneous flap since there are numerous cutaneous perforators in the distal half of the muscle which pass directly to the skin. This vastus lateralis myocutaneous flap offers a mechanism to transpose the distal thigh skin to a remote site, but the skin-grafted donor site is usually less desirable than a skin-grafted muscle flap. It can also be used as a distally based "salvage" flap for the anterior knee because of the independent superficial femoral vasculature.

COMPLICATIONS, PITFALLS, AND DONOR SITE

Some loss of part of the distal one-third of the muscle can be expected if an attempt is made to carry the entire muscle on the proximal vasculature. Torsion on the proximal vessels has been the apparent cause of partial flap necrosis. If our experience with other muscle flaps can be translated to this flap, external compression should also be expected to be a potential cause of flap necrosis.

Clearly, there are several recognized pitfalls in the elevation of this muscle flap. The proper sequential dissection of the muscle is crucial to the success of the

flap transfer. First, the vastus lateralis muscle should be identified at the lateral margin of the rectus femoris tendon and the distal tendons of these muscles should be carefully separated. Once this is done, the plane between the vastus intermedius and vastus lateralis muscles becomes readily apparent. The dominant vascular leash can then be isolated by retracting the proximal belly of the rectus femoris muscle. The remaining dissection of the distal thigh is bloody and imprecise because the distal vastus lateralis muscle is fused with both the vastus intermedius and the biceps femoris muscles. Rather than attempting to identify these three fused muscles in the distal thigh, it is preferable to divide the vastus lateralis muscle above this area of muscular fusion. If these surgical steps are not taken sequentially, one can injure the proximal vessels or incorrectly define the limits of the vastus lateralis muscle. Special attention should also be given to the femoral nerve since it is the sole motor nerve for the anterior thigh musculature. The femoral nerve is intimately related to the lateral circumflex femoral vessels but it is easily identified on the surface of the vastus intermedius muscle in the femoral triangle.

Unless a TFL flap is used in combination with the vastus lateralis muscle flap, the donor site can be primarily closed. Prolonged serous drainage from the donor site, as in the case of the TFL flap, occasionally occurs. Overall, the donor site is favorable and presents very few problems.

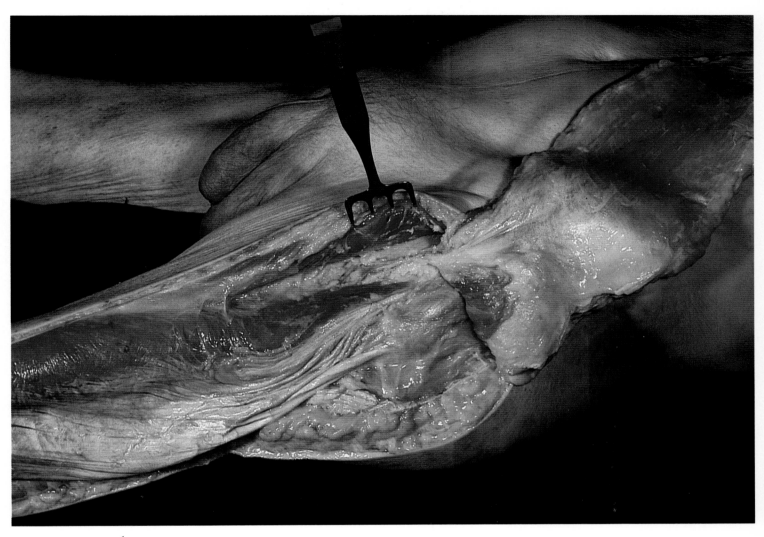

1

The overlying TFL flap is elevated for illustrative purposes. The proximal vasculature is first identified by separating the (retracted) rectus femoris muscle from the vastus lateralis muscle. Note the dense fascial attachments of the vastus lateralis muscle to the greater trochanter and the upper femur.

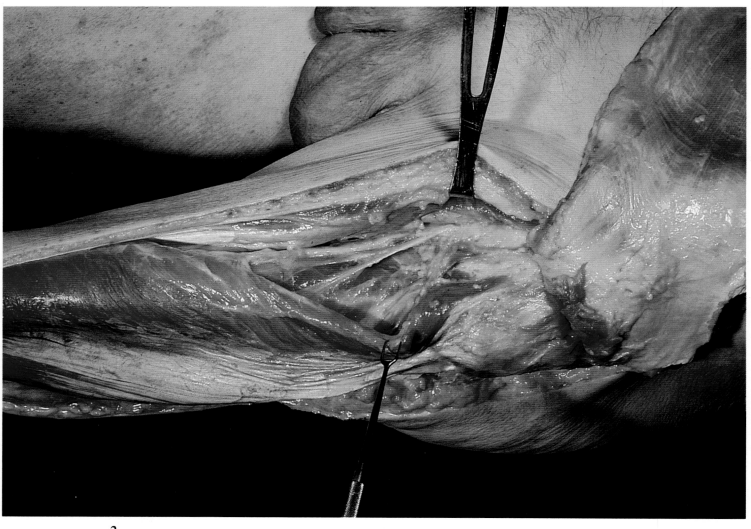

2

The dominant vessels enter the under surface of the vastus lateralis muscle after passing beneath the rectus femoris muscle. The neurovascular bundle is seen between the two retractors. Note the femoral nerve on the surface of the vastus intermedius muscle.

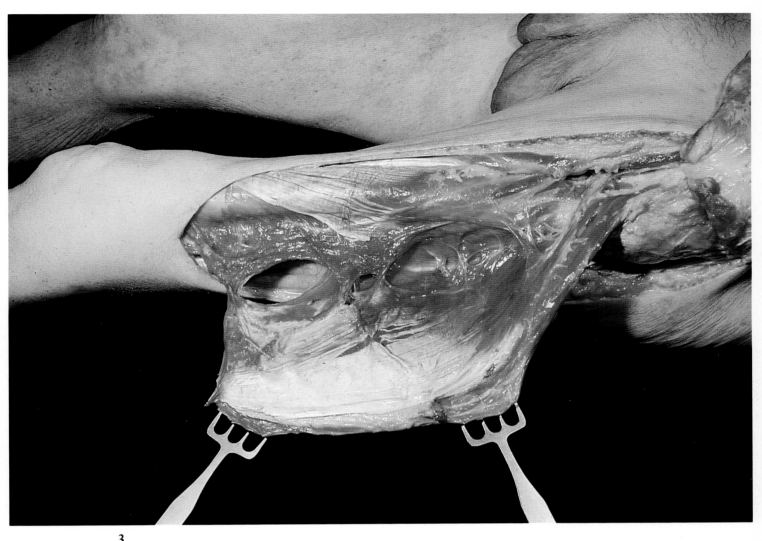

3

The vastus lateralis muscle is elevated away from the vastus intermedius muscle. The two muscles are still attached by numerous deep muscular perforators. Note the dense fascia on the undersurface of vastus lateralis muscle.

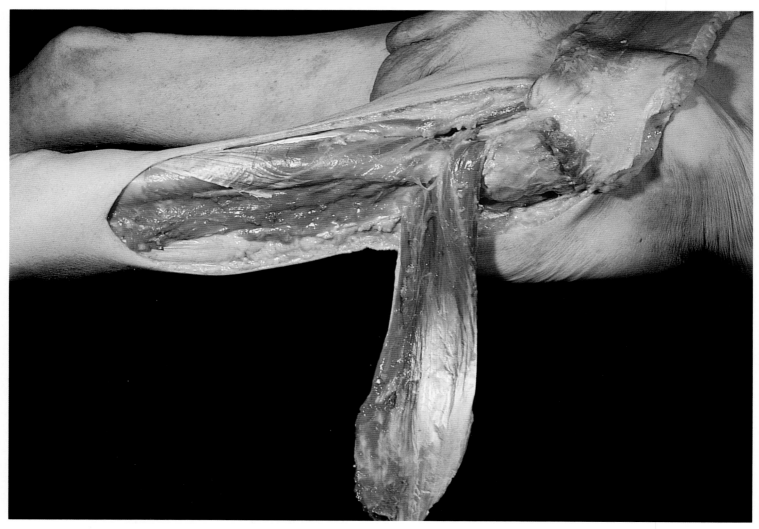

4

The vastus lateralis muscle is elevated away from the biceps femoris and vastus intermedius muscles. The extensive upper femoral origin is still intact. The dominant vessels are seen on the undersurface of the muscle after they circle the proximal femur.

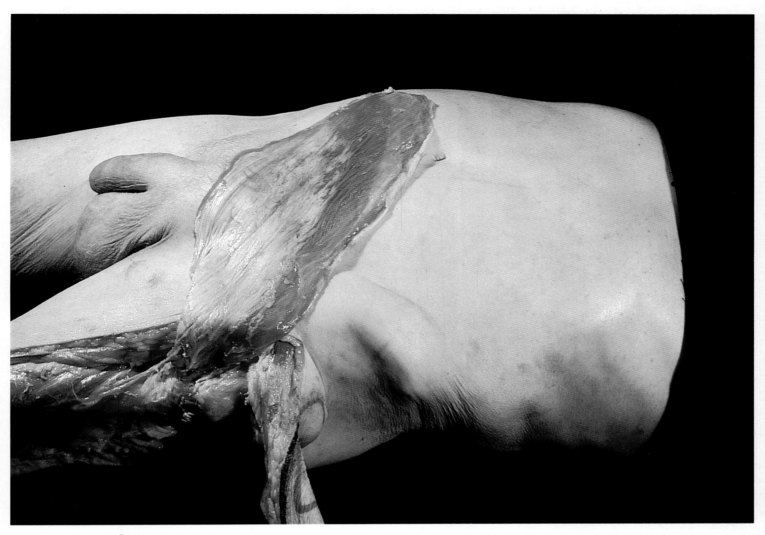

5

Upward mobility of the "island" vastus lateralis muscle flap after the muscular origin has been divided. The deep muscular fascia is visible on the surface of the vastus lateralis muscle. The anterior arc of the flap includes the groin, the middle abdomen, and the hip joint.

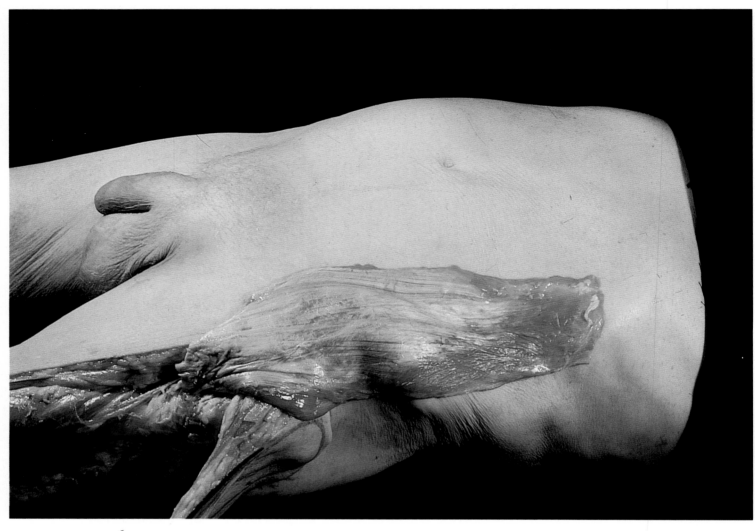

6

The muscle flap will barely reach the lower chest wall, but it easily covers the entire iliac crest. The fifteen centimeter width of the vastus lateralis muscle is remarkable.

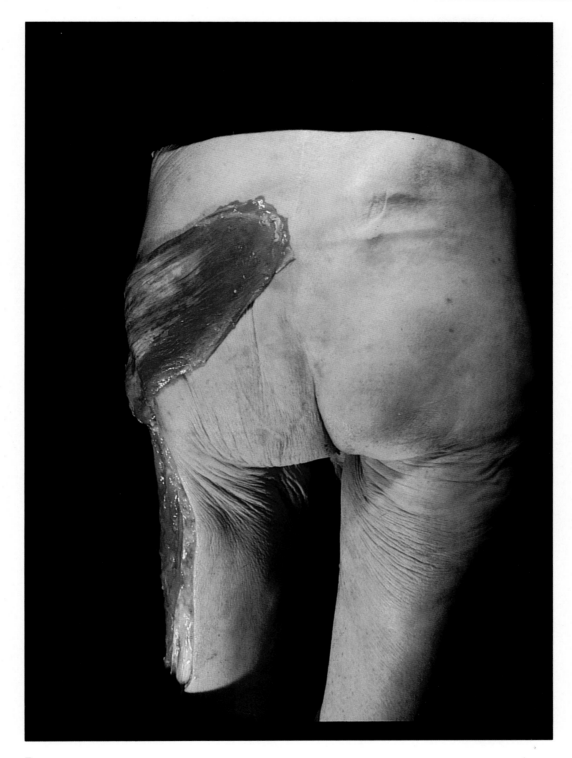

7

Rotation of the flap onto the posterior
iliac crest. The vastus lateralis muscle
flap cannot be extended onto the sacrum.

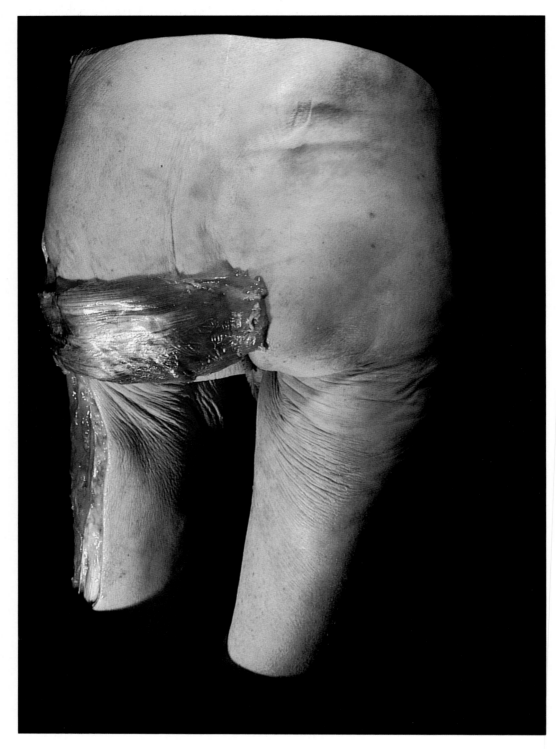

8

Posterior rotation of the flap into the area of the ischial tuberosity. Although the flap dissection is tedious, a significant volume of muscle can be transposed into a hip defect or an ischial cavity.

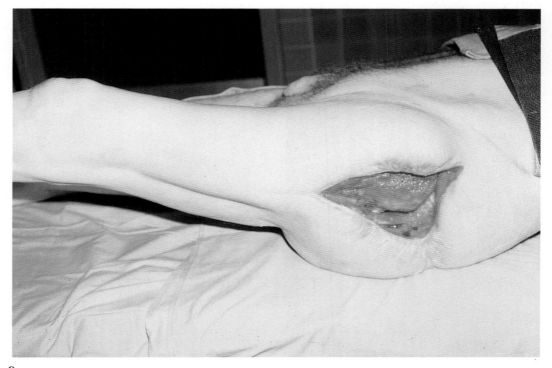

9

Massive hip defect following the removal of a total hip prosthesis. Both the proximal femur and the acetabulum were grossly infected. (Case of P.G. Arnold)

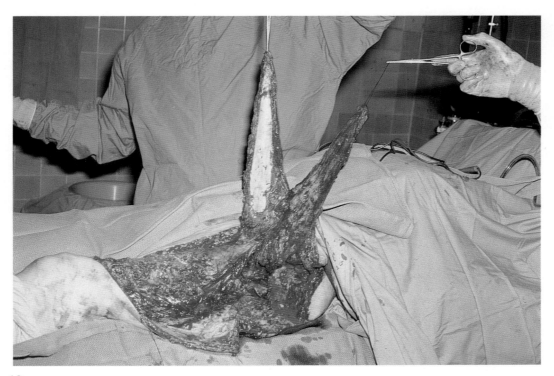

10

Lateral view of the thigh, which has been exposed through a midlateral incision. The vastus lateralis muscle is retracted with a suture. The rectus femoris muscle is retracted with forceps.

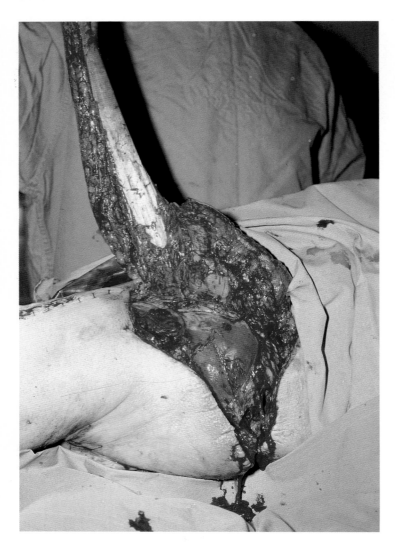

11

The vastus lateralis muscle has been transposed into the infected hip cavity. The retracted rectus femoris muscle will be used to obliterate the remaining surface defect.

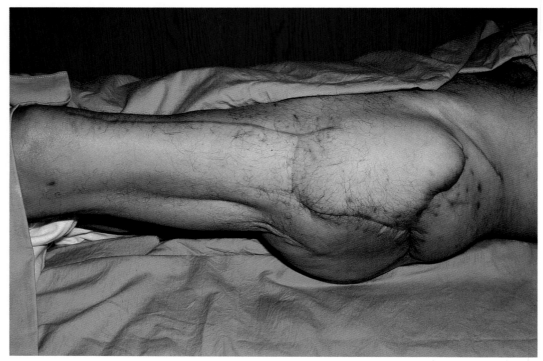

12

"Random" skin rotation flaps were used to provide surface coverage for the transposed muscle flaps. Note the healed donor site incision in the anterolateral thigh. The patient is ambulatory, and the recalcitrant osteomyelitis has not recurred over a period of six years.

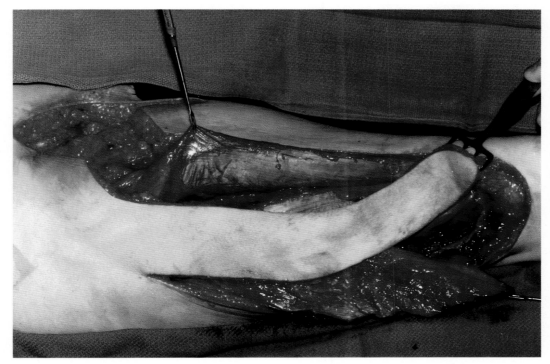

13

Fifty-eight-year-old patient with an infected Dacron® vascular graft in the groin. A vastus lateralis muscle flap and a TFL flap are elevated in combination. The rectus femoris muscle is retracted with the double hook. (Case of J.B. McCraw and R.T. Gregory, Jr.)

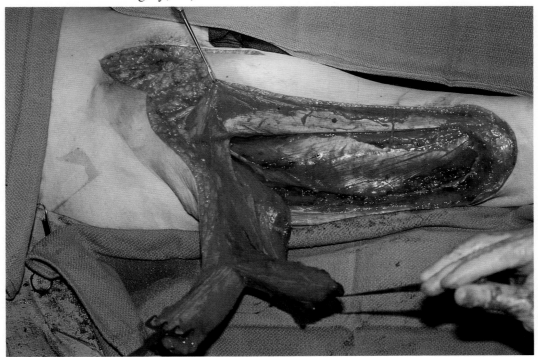

14

The combined flap has been elevated away from the rectus femoris, vastus intermedius, and biceps femoris muscles. Note the "hamburger" appearance of the remaining distal vastus intermedius muscle. The groin defect is seen above the retracted rectus femoris muscle.

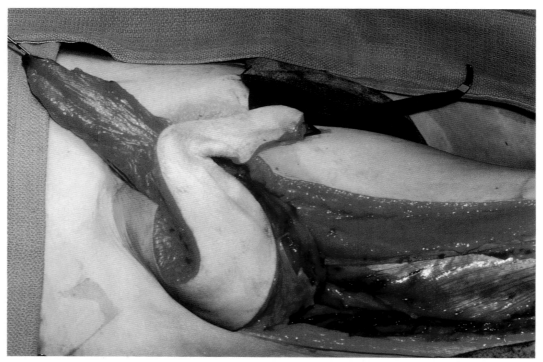

15

The vastus lateralis muscle is readied for passage beneath the inguinal ligament to cover both the superficial femoral and common femoral vessels. The associated TFL flap will be used for surface cover of the groin skin defect.

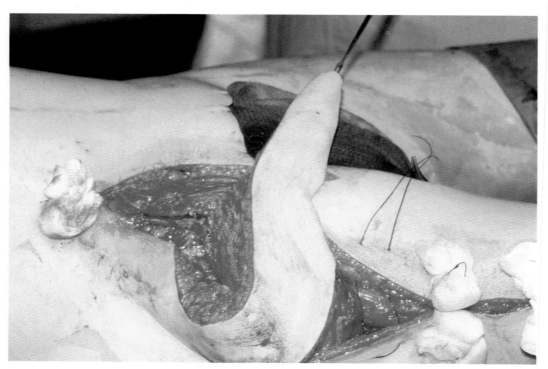

16

Inset of the vastus lateralis muscle into the groin defect in an "L" shape. The muscle was passed beneath the inguinal ligament to also cover the common femoral vessels.

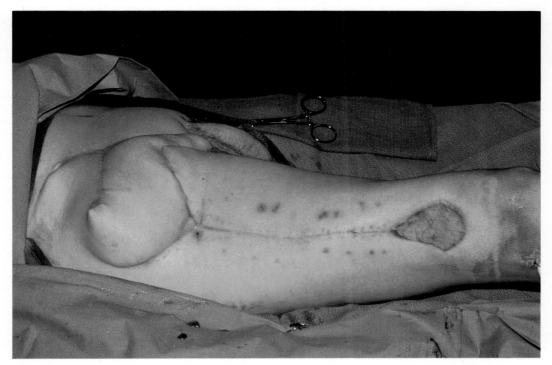

17

Healed TFL flap on the surface. The vastus lateralis muscle salvaged the infected Dacron® graft. A skin-grafted vastus lateralis muscle flap would have provided a simpler solution with a more esthetic result. The combined TFL flap seemed like a good idea at the time.

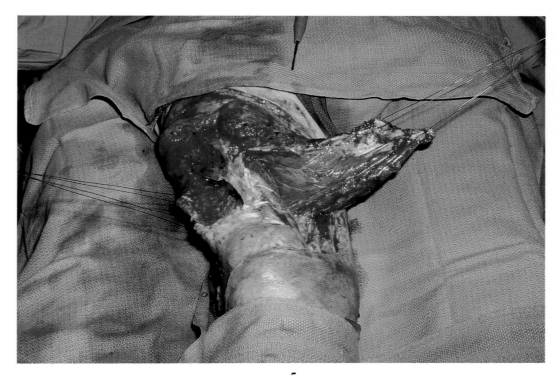

5

Elevated vastus medialis muscle flap. The remnant of the vastus lateralis muscle is retracted laterally.

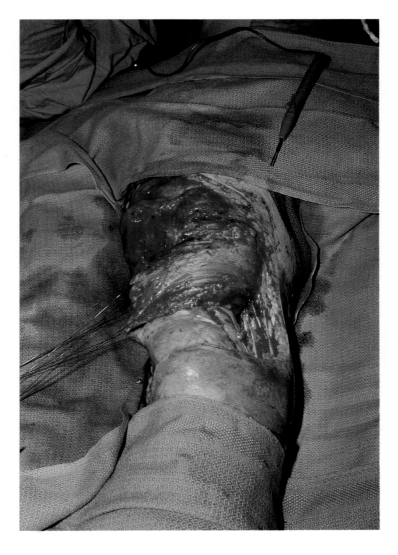

6

Vastus medialis muscle flap transposed into the suprapatellar area.

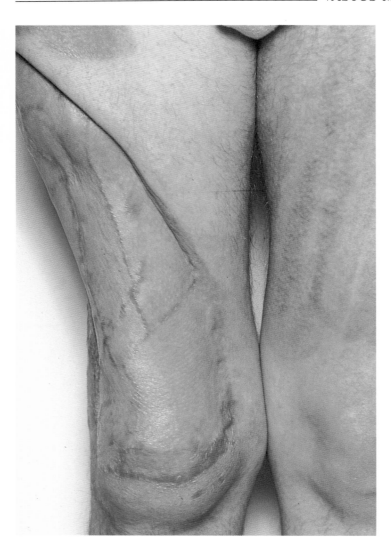

7

Appearance of the skin-grafted vastus medialis muscle flap at six months. Since the rectus femoris and vastus lateralis muscles were lost, the vastus medialis muscle was used both to cover the knee joint and to reestablish knee extension.

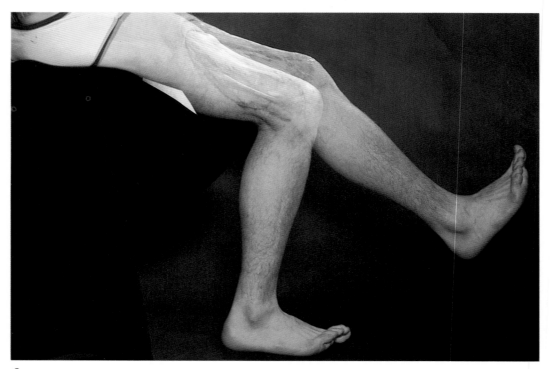

8

Double-exposed photographic demonstration of active knee extension following the functional vastus medialis muscle flap transfer. The patient is able to walk with a normal gait despite the devastating injury.

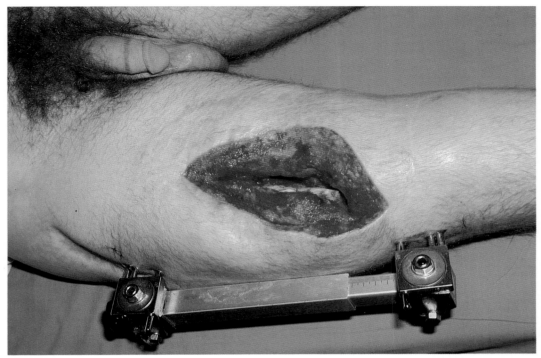

9

Twenty-five-year-old male with an open fracture of the femur complicated by clostridial myositis. The fracture of the femur was grossly infected, and the rectus femoris muscle had been totally excised. (Case of P.G. Arnold)

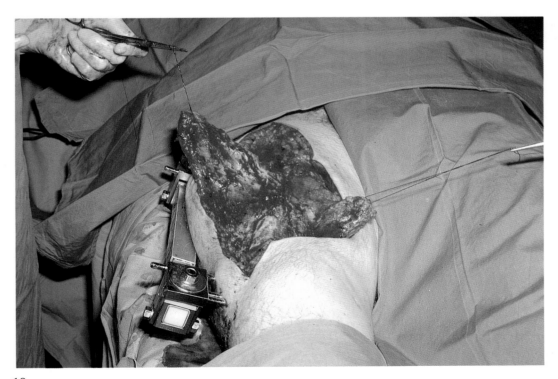

10

The vastus medialis and lateralis muscles were transposed over the infected femur and sutured together into a midline closure. The approximated muscles were then reattached to the patellar tendon to reestablish active knee extension.

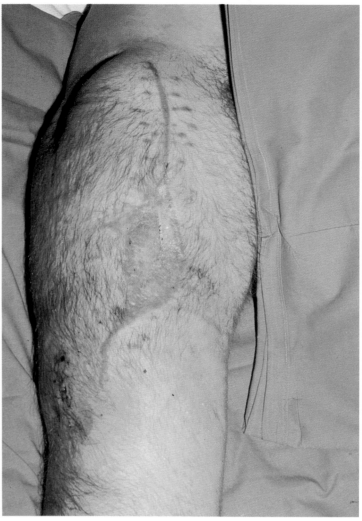

11

Appearance of the skin-grafted vastus medialis and lateralis muscle flaps at six months. The muscular reconstitution of the quadriceps mechanism allowed the complex femoral fracture to heal. Full active knee extension was maintained in the absence of the rectus femoris muscle.

GASTROCNEMIUS MUSCLE AND MUSCULOCUTANEOUS FLAPS

ANATOMICAL CONSIDERATIONS

Surface Markings

Each gastrocnemius muscular head can be vividly outlined by forcibly flexing and extending the foot. The two muscles are separated by an imaginary line in the posterior calf where a ''stocking-seam'' would normally be. The medial head is clearly the larger of the two muscles.

Origin and Insertion

The muscle originates from the femoral condyles and inserts into the Achilles tendon some five centimeters proximal to the soleus muscular insertion. The two heads of the muscle are partially fused in the midline of the calf where the course of the sural nerve represents the imaginary ''stocking-seam'' separation. At the level of the Achilles tendon, the gastrocnemius and soleus muscles are densely adherent to each other over a distance of about five centimeters. The isolated function of one head of the gastrocnemius muscle is totally expendable. Normal ambulation can also be expected after the sacrifice of the soleus muscle and one head of the gastrocnemius muscle.

Adjacent Muscles

The soleus muscle lies directly beneath the gastrocnemius muscle and the Achilles tendon. The plantaris tendon is identified on the surface of the soleus muscle in the plane between the soleus muscle and the medial head of the gastrocnemius muscle. The lateral compartment musculature is separated from the lateral head of the gastrocnemius muscle by the lateral intermuscular septum.

Vascular Pattern

The gastrocnemius muscle is the definitive example of a muscle with a single proximal, dominant vascular pedicle. The sural artery is a branch of the popliteal artery which passes directly into the proximal portion of both heads of the gastrocnemius muscle. The sural artery arborizes in the proximal one-third of each muscle, enabling one to either trim or ''split'' the distal and peripheral gastrocnemius muscle at the time of transposition. The posterior calf skin is supplied by direct musculocutaneous perforators proximally and by the deep fascia distally. The medial gastrocnemius myocutaneous flap can be carried to a point five centimeters above the flare of the medial malleolus. The lateral myocutaneous flap can be carried to a point ten centimeters above the flare of the lateral malleolus. Fasciocutaneous flaps of comparable size can be outlined in the calf, but their safe dimensions are presently ill-defined. Even though exceedingly lengthy fasciocutaneous flaps can be raised in the posterior calf, their viability is enhanced by preserving the direct musculocutaneous perforating vessels from the underlying gastrocnemius muscle.

Motor Nerve

Popliteal nerve.

Sensory Nerve

Sural and saphenous nerves.

USES

Although the gastrocnemius muscle can be used either as a muscle flap or a musculocutaneous flap with equal ease, it is almost always employed as a pure muscle flap because of the donor site considerations. Either the medial or lateral head of the gastrocnemius muscle (or both heads) can be used to cover the difficult areas of the upper tibia, the knee joint, and the popliteal fossa. The primary application of the medial head of the gastrocnemius muscle is for coverage problems in the proximal one-third of the tibia, but the soleus muscle is more commonly used for defects of the middle one-third of the tibia. The medial gastrocnemius myocutaneous flap can also be used for middle one-third defects, but the donor defect requires a skin graft for closure. Generally speaking, it is preferable to transpose the gastrocnemius muscle as a pure muscle flap since the skin-grafted muscle offers a durable surface. The muscle flap can also be tailored at the time of inset to provide an appropriate contour restoration.

The musculocutaneous flap is usually employed as a fasciocutaneous flap (without elevating the muscle) to repair defects of the middle and lower tibia. It is occasionally useful as a cross-leg flap, particularly in reconstruction of the contralateral Achilles tendon area. The deep fascia of the leg is always included with the distal cutaneous segment, and half of the Achilles tendon can be carried safely with the myocutaneous flap to reconstruct the opposite Achilles tendon. Bilateral myocutaneous anterior advancement flaps of both the medial and lateral gastrocnemius heads provide excellent mid-tibial coverage with a very acceptable posterior calf "stocking-seam" donor site. One other application of the musculocutaneous flap is the distal V-Y advancement into the Achilles area. The V-Y musculocutaneous flap is elevated as a pure "island" flap after the muscular origin has been divided from the femur. Release of the muscular origin advances the distal tip of the cutaneous segment for an additional three to four centimeters. This simple maneuver can obviate the need for a "free" flap or a cross-leg flap for the small Achilles tendon defect.

REGIONAL FLAP COMPARISONS

The medial and lateral heads of the gastrocnemius muscle cover similar areas, but the medial head is approximately twice the size of the lateral head. This anatomical difference should be recognized when dealing with a sizable defect. The only other muscle which can give similar upper-third tibial coverage is an "island" soleus muscle flap. The standard soleus muscle flap is more often used for defects of the middle-third of the tibia because of its accessibility and ease of transfer. Bilateral gastrocnemius myocutaneous flaps are ideally suited for lengthy pretibial defects which are less than four centimeters in width. Massive upper-half defects of the tibia usually dictate the use of a soleus muscle flap in combination with a medial gastrocnemius muscle flap.

DISADVANTAGES

Even though it might be expected, the use of one head of the gastrocnemius muscle does not cause any detectable functional loss. Neither should the combined use of the medial head of the gastrocnemius muscle and the soleus muscle cause a noticeable functional loss, except in the athletic person. The skin-grafted donor site of the gastrocnemius musculocutaneous flap offers a significant esthetic disadvantage, particularly in women.

ADVANTAGES

Of all the muscles in the lower extremity, the gastrocnemius is certainly the most comfortable and reliable muscle to transpose. Its proximal, dominant blood supply is protected in the popliteal fossa and is difficult to injure. In fact, it is seldom seen in the process of trans-

position because simple separation of the two heads of the gastrocnemius muscle is usually sufficient to effect an adequate muscle transposition. If more length is needed, the origin of the muscle can be separated from the femur, and the muscle can be converted into a true "island" flap. Because of the distinct arborization of the dominant vasculature in the proximal one-third of the muscle, the muscle can be trimmed at the time of transposition to accommodate the defect precisely. The muscle can also be split in half both to obliterate a cavity and to correct a surface defect. The fascia on either side of the muscle can be "scored," as is done with the galea, or it can be excised to "expand" the muscle and allow it to be spread over a wider area. When the muscle is used to correct a low-grade infection, it is always advisable to remove this fascia to expose the raw muscular surface. The muscular fascia is also routinely removed to facilitate the "take" of a skin graft on the muscle flap.

Bilateral, bipedicle musculocutaneous flaps can be advanced together into long and narrow anterior tibial defects. This dissection is usually done from the anterior approach, but the midline separation of the muscular heads can be done more precisely through a "stocking seam" incision. The posterior access incision is usually skin grafted, but it is possible to close it primarily if the anterior tibial defect is less than four centimeters in width.

COMPLICATIONS, PITFALLS, and DONOR SITE

Because the gastrocnemius muscle flap is such a hardy flap, the infrequent surgical disappointments are usually caused by the operator and not by the muscle. For instance, even minor errors of surgical technique will cause failures in dealing with osteomyelitis of the tibia, because a 95% successful correction of the infection often equates with a 100% failure. This is usually related to an inadequate debridement of the bone, an incomplete obliteration of the dead space, or an imperfect immobilization of the inset muscle. Like most muscle flaps the gastrocnemius muscle is extremely sensitive to external pressure. It should never be tunneled beneath a "tight" skin bridge. In fact, external pressure has been the only cause of muscle flap necrosis in our experience.

When dissecting in the popliteal fossa, one should always be cognizant of the adjacent nerves. The important common peroneal nerve is intimately involved with the lateral head of the gastrocnemius muscle and can easily be injured. The tibial nerve is readily identified in the midline of the popliteal fossa between the two heads of the gastrocnemius muscle. Distally, it is important to protect the posterior tibial nerve since it lies in close proximity to both the soleus muscle and medial head of the gastrocnemius muscle. Even the seemingly dispensable sural nerve should be preserved because the loss of sensation on the lateral aspect of the foot can be bothersome.

The gastrocnemius musculocutaneous cross-leg flap takes at least twice as long to gain a new blood supply, when compared to the standard cross-leg flap. This seems to be related to the robust blood supply which exists in the musculocutaneous unit and its lesser ''need'' to obtain a new blood supply from the recipient location. For this reason the flap should not be divided in a single stage, and its viability should be tested with fluorescein prior to the final separation of the legs. This is done by placing a tourniquet on the donor (flap) leg and then administering intravenous fluorescein. If the inset flap fluoresces, one can presume that this is the result of ''local'' blood supply, not the inherent flap blood supply.

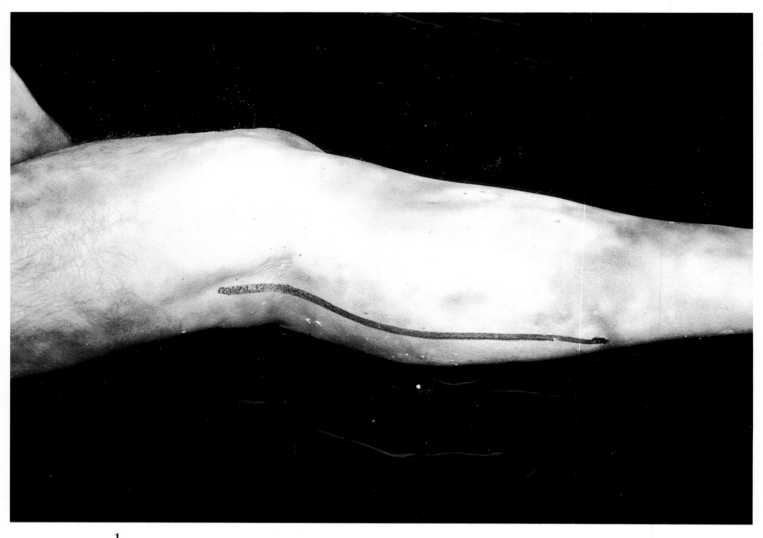

1

Cadaver dissection of the gastrocnemius
muscle using a ''stocking-seam'' incision.

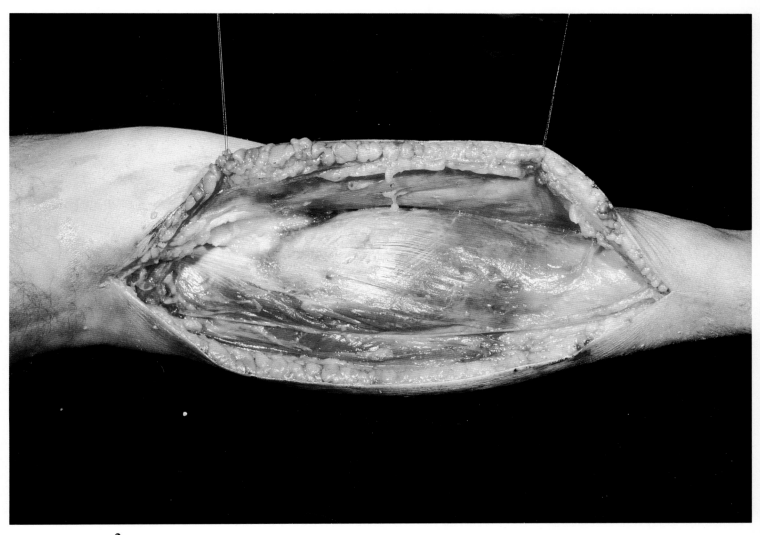

2

View of the medial head of the gastrocnemius muscle with the sural nerve at its
lateral border.

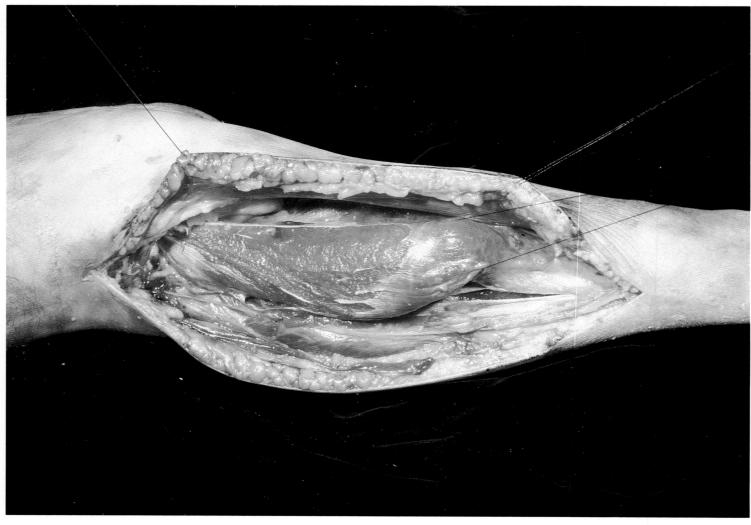

3

The medial head of the gastrocnemius is elevated with sutures after the muscle fascia has been removed from its external surface.

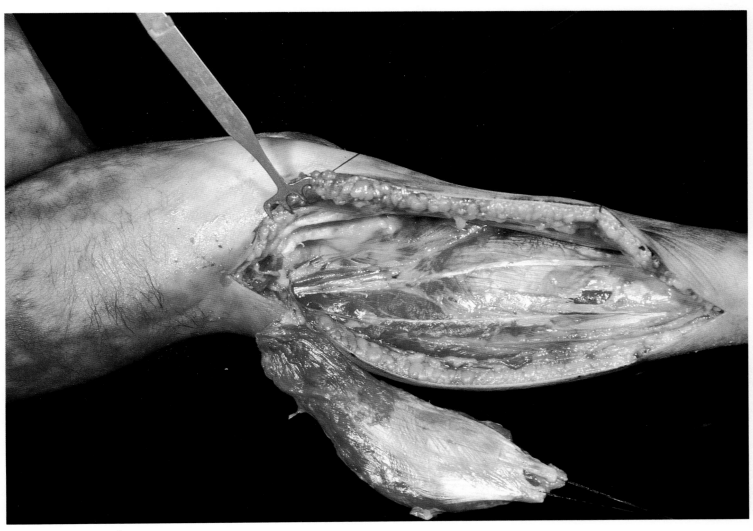

4

The medial head is converted into a true "island" flap by division of its origin from the femur. Note the dense fascia on the undersurface of the muscle. This fascia can be "scored" or completely excised to "expand" the area of muscle coverage.

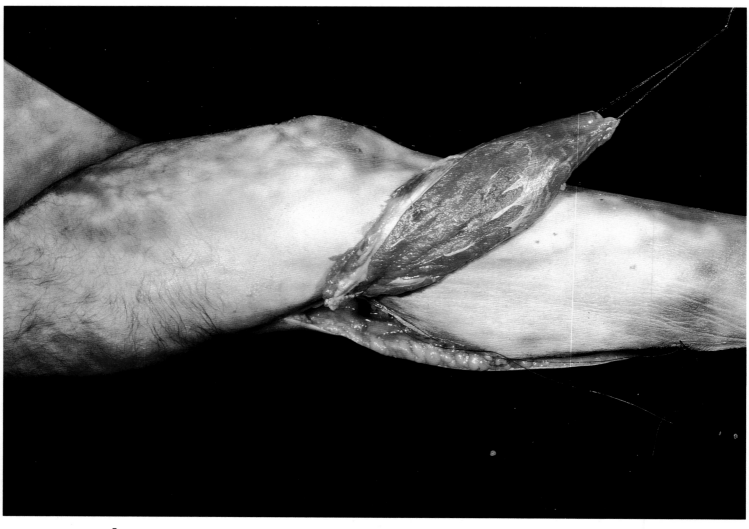

5

Muscle coverage of the upper one-third of
the tibia by the "island" gastrocnemius
muscle flap.

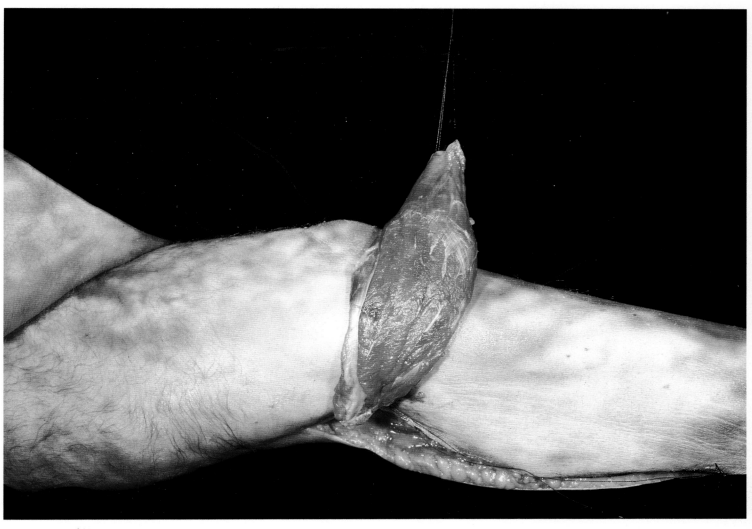

6

Both the tibial tubercle and the patella are easily covered by the medial head.

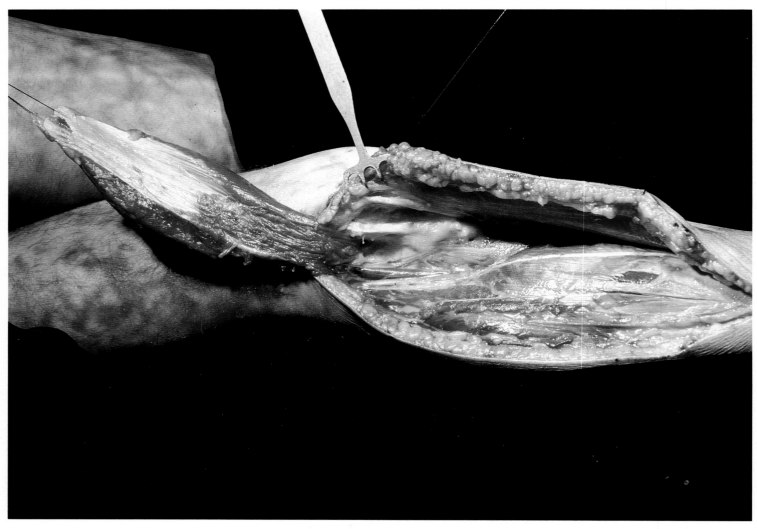

7

The transposed muscle flap reaches well above the patella, which lies at the level of the retractor.

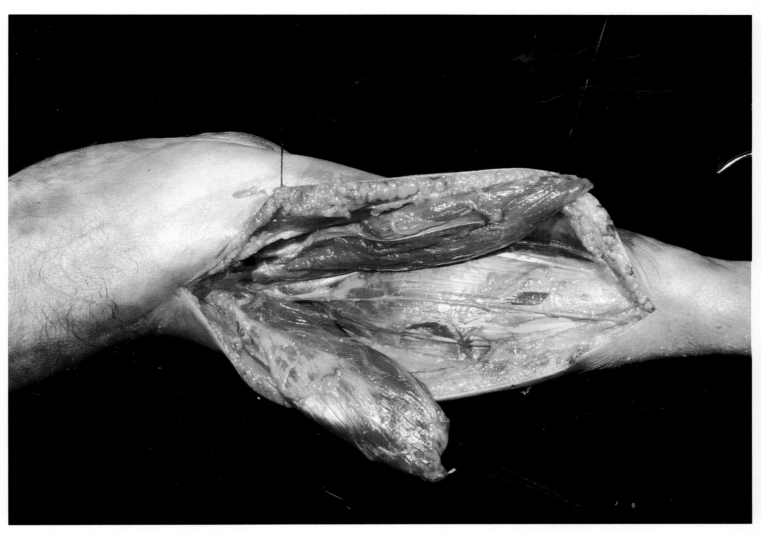

8

Elevation of both heads of the gastrocnemius muscle through a ''stocking-seam'' approach. Note the intact sural nerve on the surface of the soleus muscle (in the midline) and the plantaris tendon anterior to this.

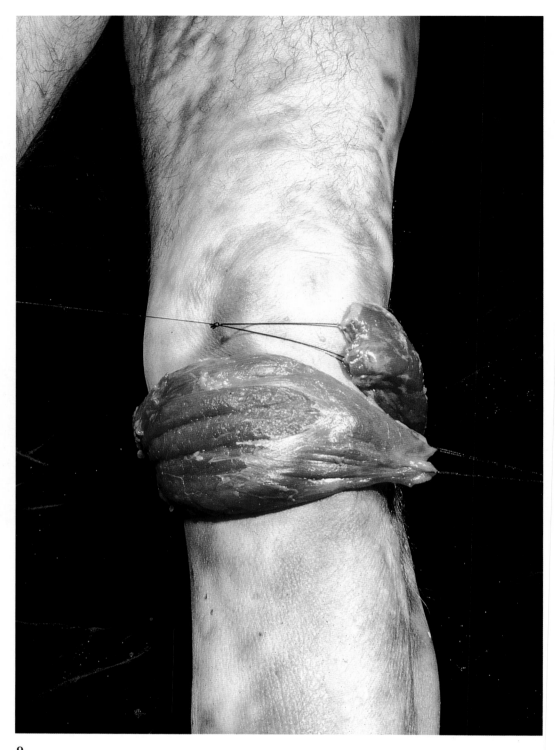

9

Anterior view of the medial and lateral
heads of the gastrocnemius muscle transposed into the patellar area. The medial
head is the larger of the two heads.

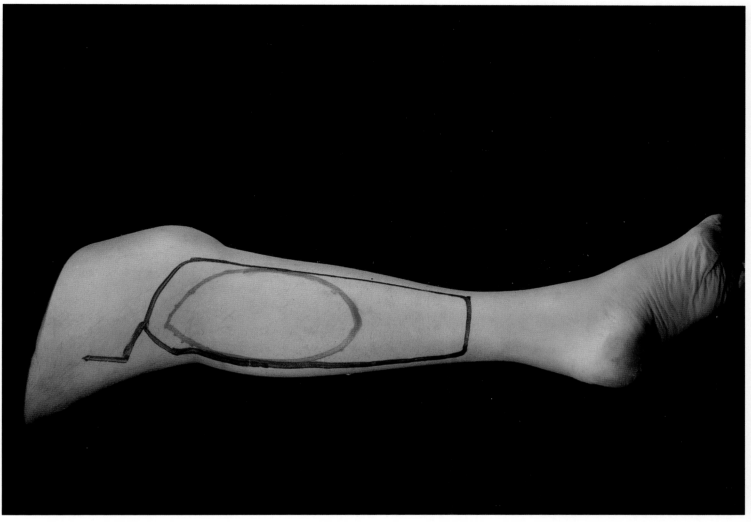

10

The medial gastrocnemius myocutaneous flap is outlined in black with an optional popliteal incision marked for division of the muscular origin. The anterior border of the flap parallels the medial margin of the tibia, and the posterior margin is near the midline of the calf. The distal flap margin extends to a point approximately five centimeters above the ''flare'' of the medial malleolus.

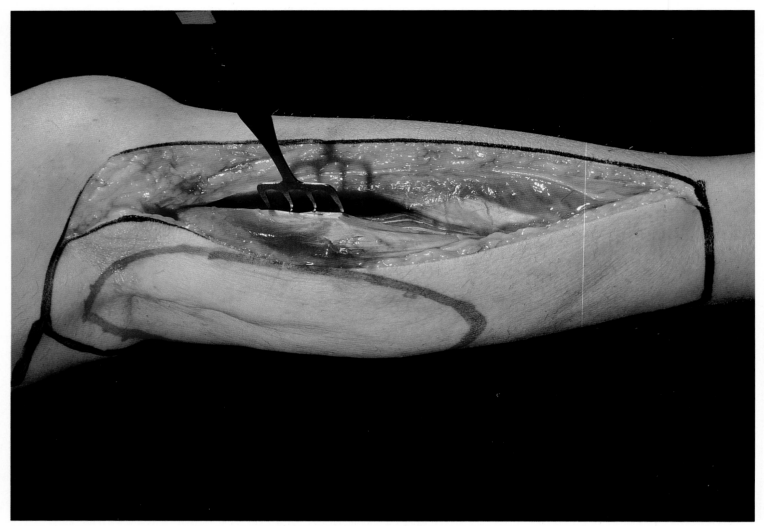

11

The separation between the gastrocnemius and soleus muscles is first identified proximally, and the dissection is then carried distally. The medial head of the gastrocnemius muscle is retracted away from the adjacent soleus muscle with the ''face lift'' retractor.

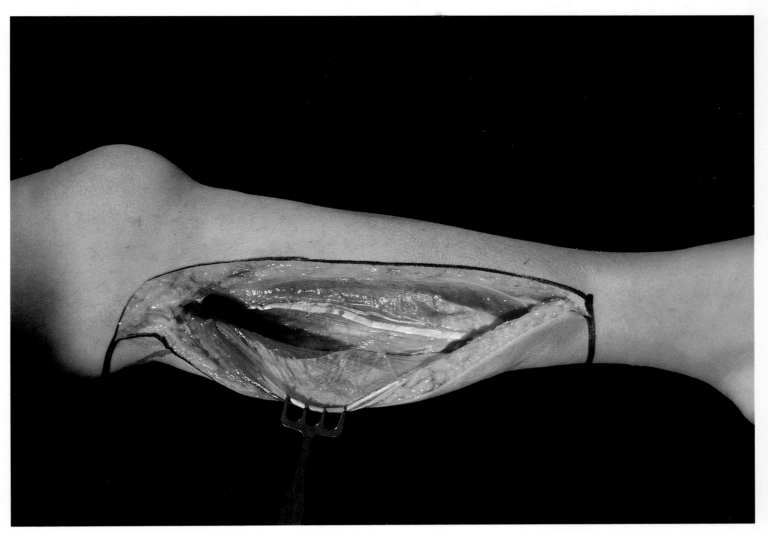

12

The medial head of the gastrocnemius muscle and the deep fascia of the calf are retracted. The separation between the medial and lateral heads of the muscle can be found from this anterior approach, but it is more accurately identified using a posterior approach.

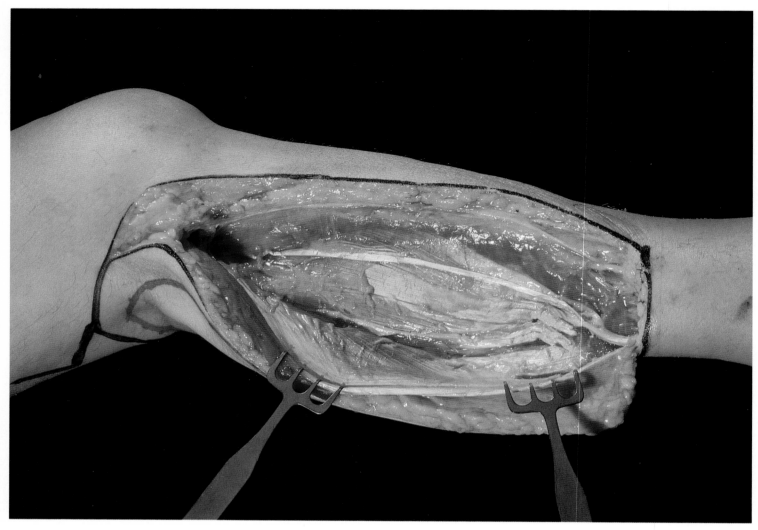

13

The areolar plane between the gastrocnemius and soleus muscles is bluntly dissected down to the level of the Achilles tendon. At this point the two muscles become fused and must be sharply separated. Note the plantaris tendon on the surface of the soleus muscle.

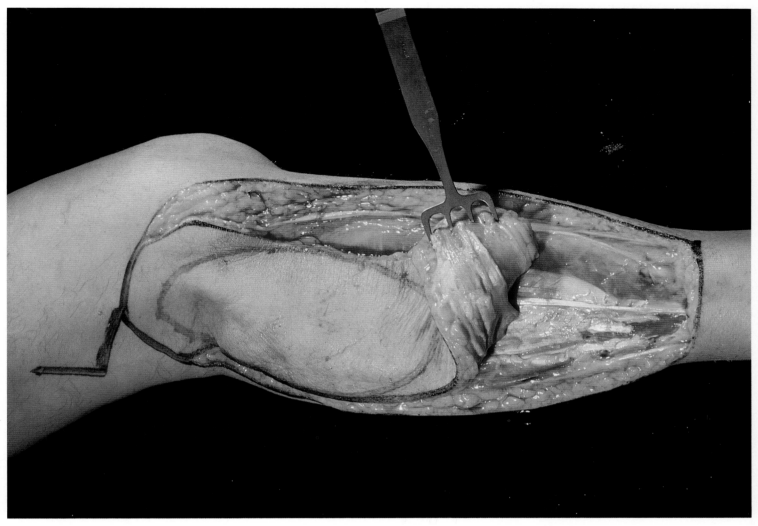

14

The deep fascia of the calf is always included with the cutaneous segment of the gastrocnemius myocutaneous flap. A portion of the Achilles tendon can also be included with the flap without harming its physical strength. The lesser saphenous vein and the sural nerve are identified posteriorly, but are not included with the flap.

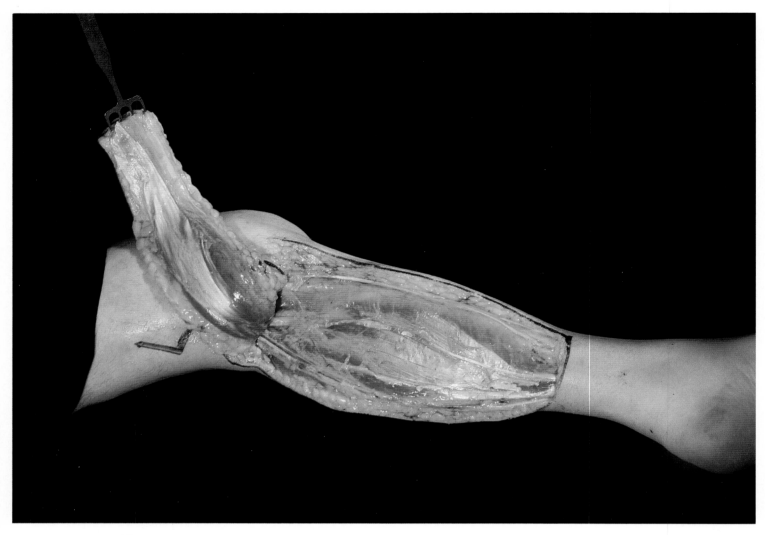

15

The medial gastrocnemius myocutaneous
flap is elevated up to the level of the
muscular origin. When only the distal
half of the cutaneous segment is needed
for coverage it can be safely raised as a
pure fasciocutaneous flap.

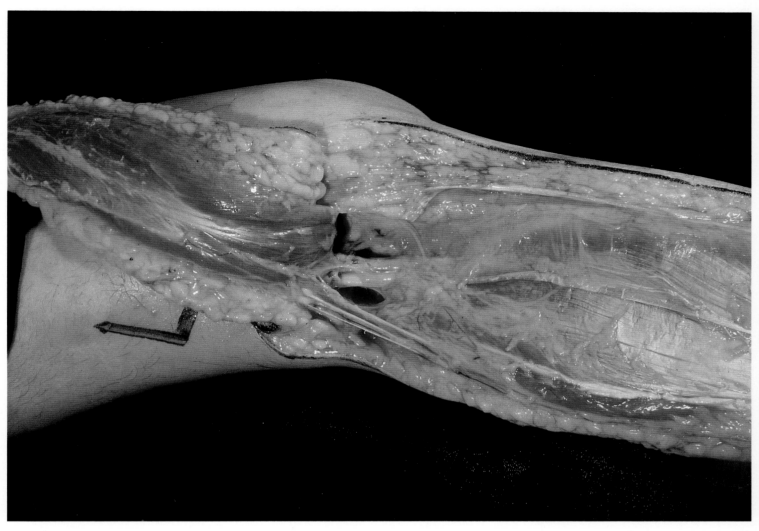

16

Close-up view of the popliteal neurovascular structures. The sural nerve and lesser saphenous vein are seen posteriorly.

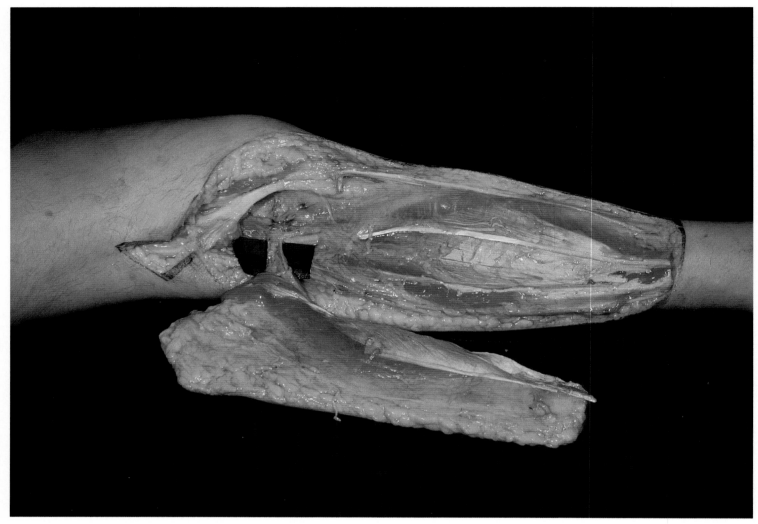

17

Demonstration of the ''island'' medial gastrocnemius myocutaneous flap. Black felt is used to outline the neurovascular bundle. Division of the muscular origin from the femur will increase the distal excursion of the flap by three to four centimeters without harming its viability.

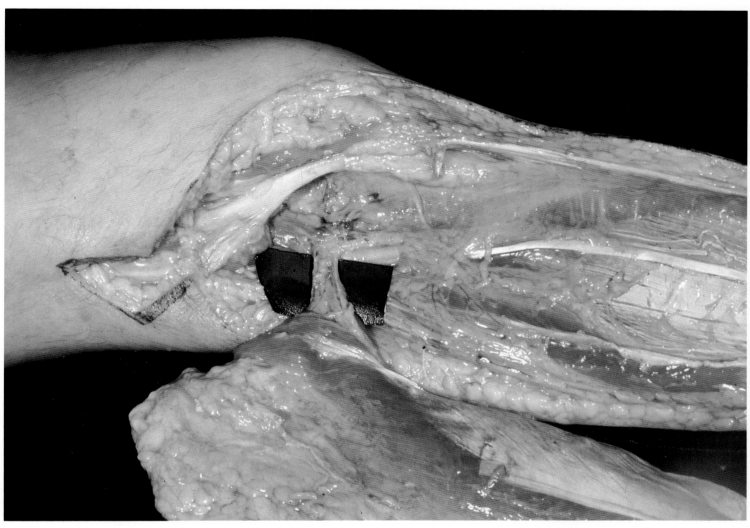

18

Close-up view of the popliteal neurovascular bundle after the muscular origin has been divided. Note the pes anserinus (''goose's foot'') tendinous expansion just anterior to the popliteal vessels.

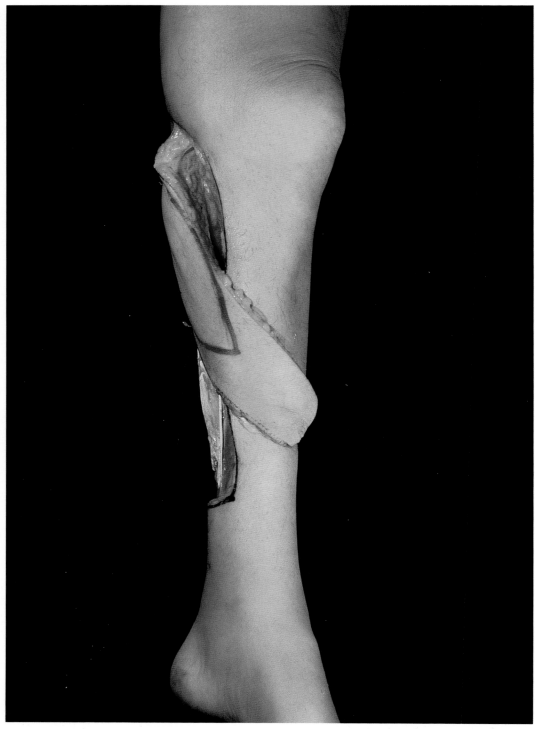

19

Pretibial coverage as a fasciocutaneous flap without elevation of the gastrocnemius muscle.

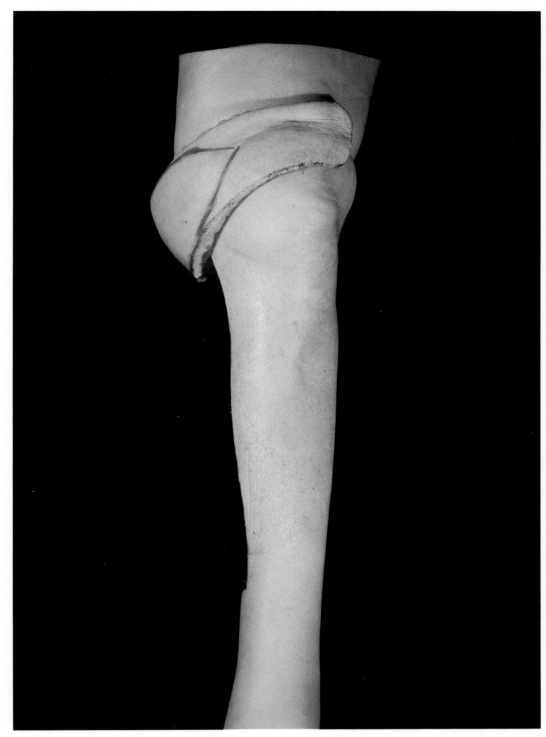

20

Suprapatellar extension of the medial gastrocnemius myocutaneous flap. The ''island'' medial gastrocnemius muscle flap will also cover this same area.

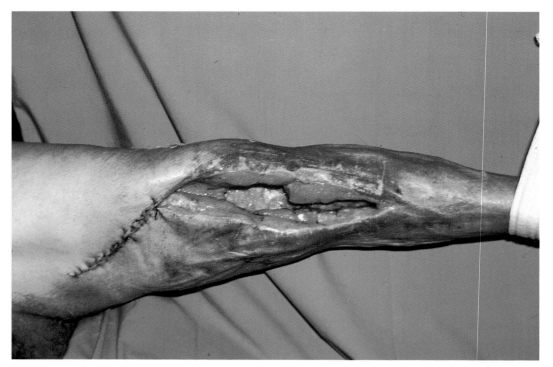

21

Sixty-eight-year-old retired professional football player who had undergone three total knee prosthetic replacements. Each attempt had failed because of osteomyelitis. A previous knee fusion was successful, but this large pretibial osteomyelitic defect remained. (Case of P.G. Arnold)

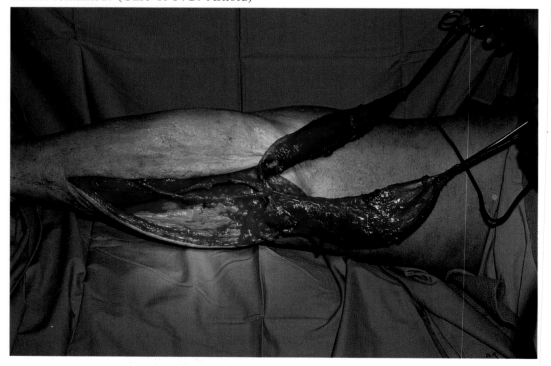

22

Both heads of the gastrocnemius muscle were mobilized as pure "island" flaps through a posterior "stocking-seam" incision. Note the larger size of the medial head.

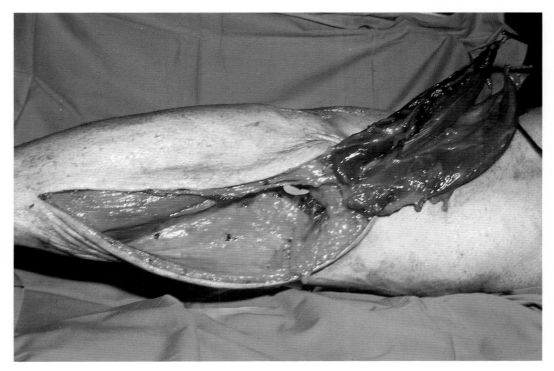

23

A "window" was made in the fused knee
joint so the two gastrocnemius muscles
could be directly transposed into the pretibial wound.

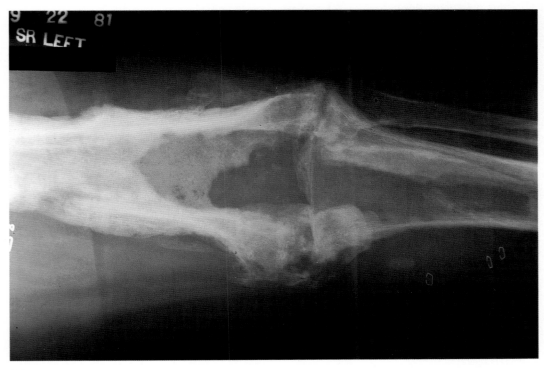

24

X-ray of the fused knee joint and the
"window" created for the muscle transposition. The unsightly knee fusion was
stable and allowed normal weight
bearing.

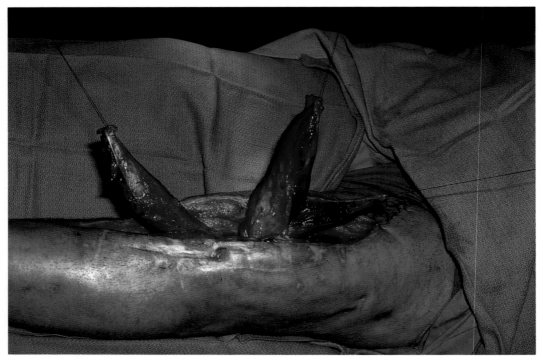

25

The medial and lateral heads were both "split" to fill the marrow cavity defect as well as cover the exposed tibial surface. The larger medial head is seen proximally in the pretibial wound.

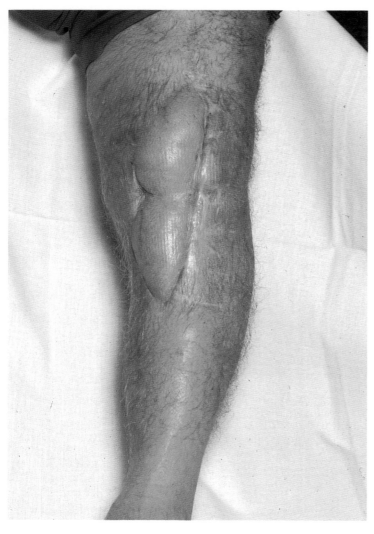

26

Healed muscle flaps at three years. The osteomyelitis has not recurred and the patient is active and ambulatory.

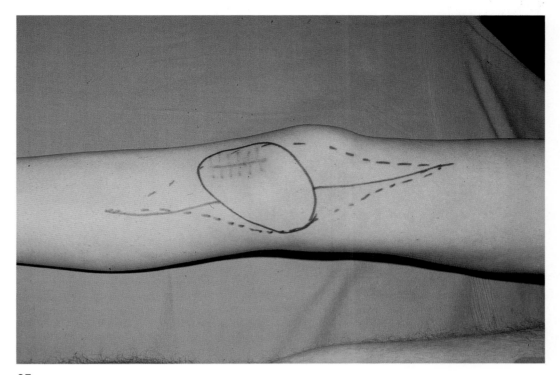

27

This young man had a biopsy-proven osteogenic sarcoma of the proximal tibia. (Case of P.G. Arnold)

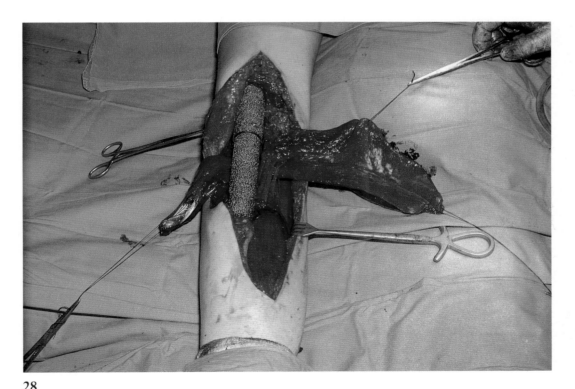

28

The distal femur and the proximal tibia were widely excised, and the knee joint was replaced with a fibrometallic prosthesis. Both heads of the gastrocnemius muscle are elevated. The two muscle flaps will be used to cover the prosthesis and to nourish the surrounding bone grafts.

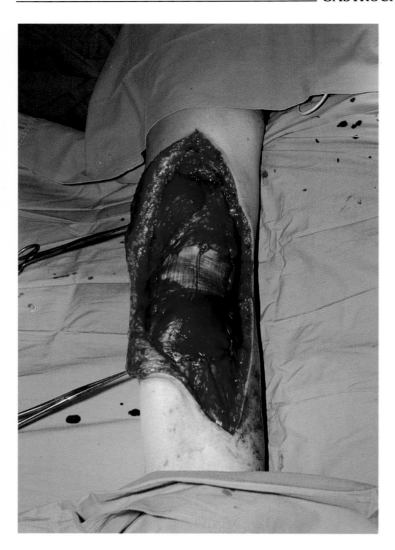

29

The two heads of the gastrocnemius muscle were wrapped around the fibrometallic prosthesis and the bone grafts in a ''barber pole'' fashion. The onlay bone grafts were used to prevent rotation of the prosthesis.

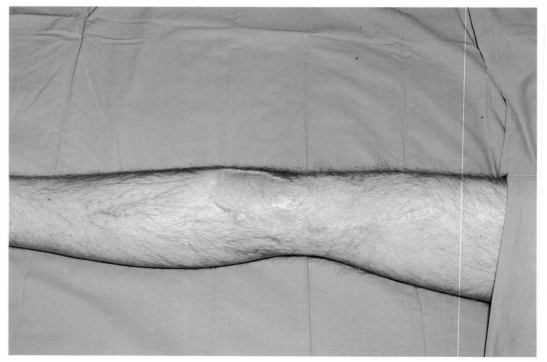

30

The skin-grafted medial and lateral gastrocnemius muscle flaps have provided excellent coverage of the bone-grafted metallic prosthesis for five years. The patient is fully ambulatory.

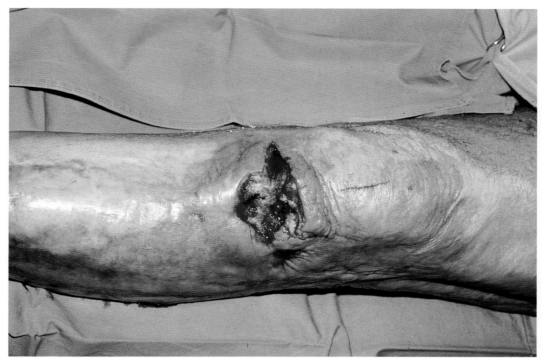

31

This fifty-three-year-old man sustained a major burn of the leg, which was allowed to heal secondarily during childhood. Trauma to the knee resulted in an infrapatellar abscess which destroyed the lower patellar tendon mechanism. (Case of P.G. Arnold)

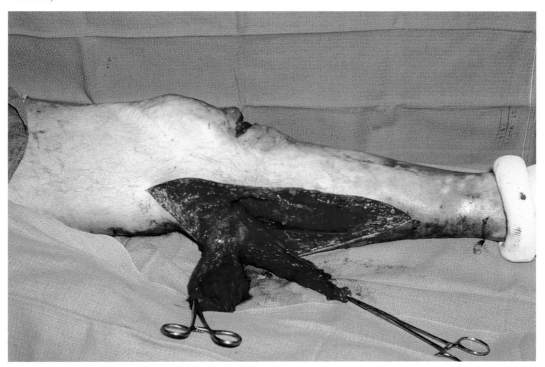

32

The medial head of the gastrocnemius muscle was "split." The larger segment of the medial head was used to obliterate the osteomyelitic cavity. The remaining muscle was used to bolster the secondary patellar tendon repair, which was accomplished with a plantaris tendon graft.

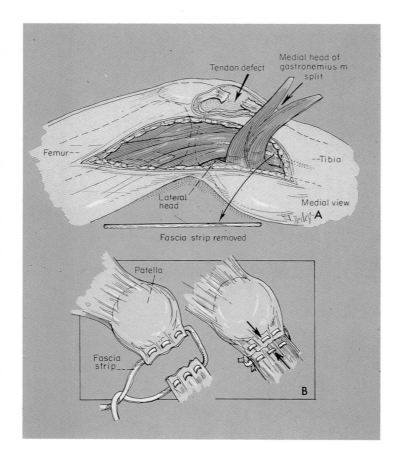

33

Illustration of the "split" gastrocnemius muscle and the patellar tendon repair.

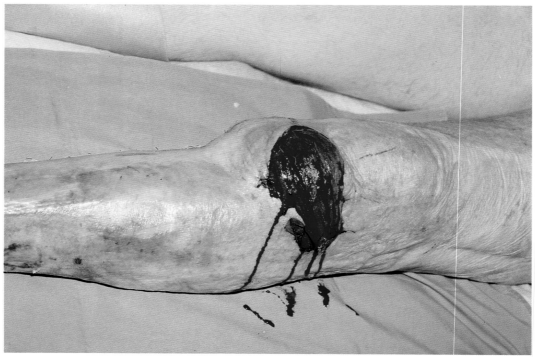

34

The reconstructed infrapatellar tendon became the "meat" in the sandwich of the "split" medial head of the gastrocnemius muscle.

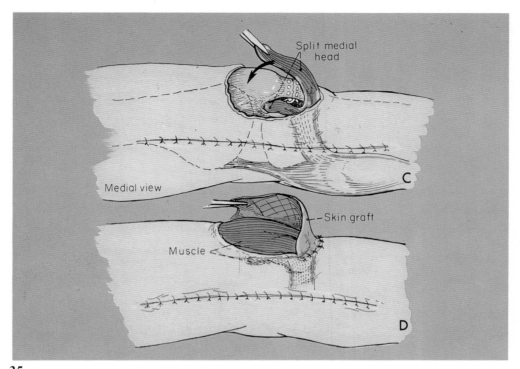

35

Illustration of the "split" medial gastrocnemius muscle, which surrounds the tendon repair.

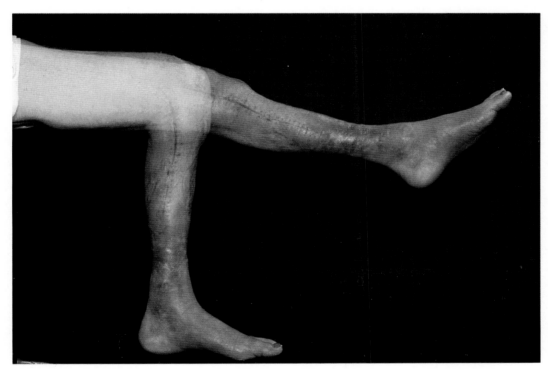

36

The wound healed without incident. The active range of motion is demonstrated by this double exposure.

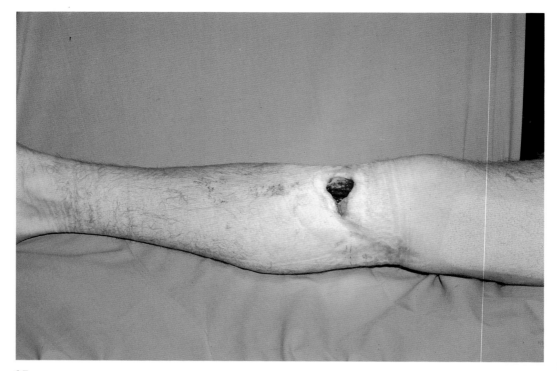

37

Osteomyelitis of the proximal tibia in a
forty-five-year-old man following a shotgun injury. There is a small but significant bony defect following the wound debridement. (Case of P.G. Arnold)

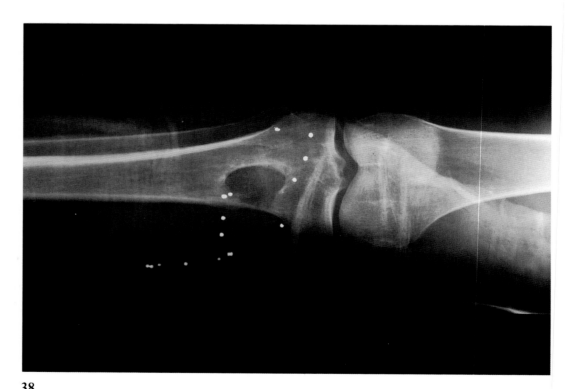

38

Tibial defect following the
sequestrectomy.

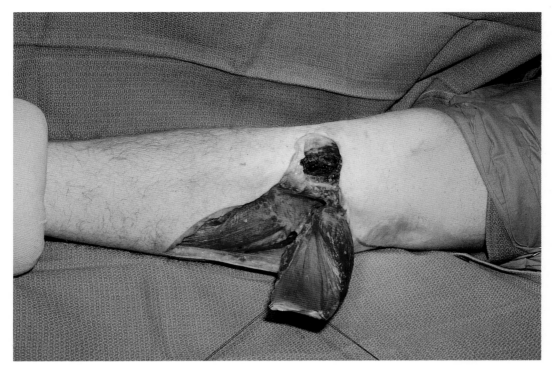

39

The mobilized medial head of the gastrocnemius muscle is clearly too large to fit the circumscribed pretibial bony defect.

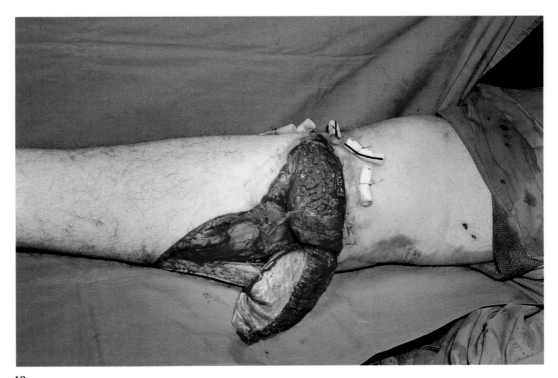

40

The medial head was "split" into two segments. Only part of the muscle was needed for the bony defect. The remaining gastrocnemius muscle was returned to the donor site.

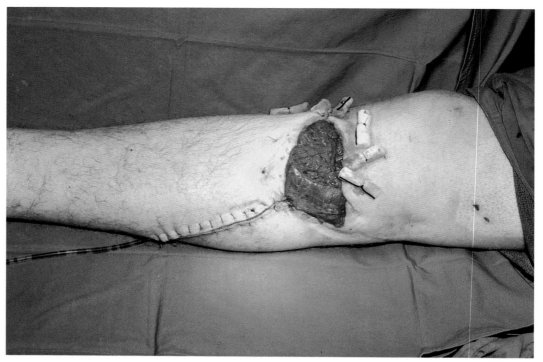

41

The gastrocnemius muscle flap was initially trimmed to improve the contour. Appearance of the transposed muscle flap at the time of skin grafting.

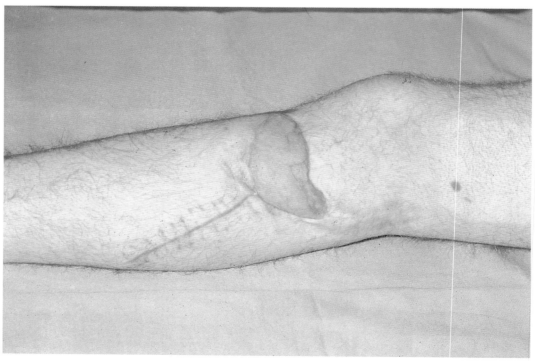

42

Appearance at six months. The patient is fully ambulatory, and the wound has remained healed for six years.

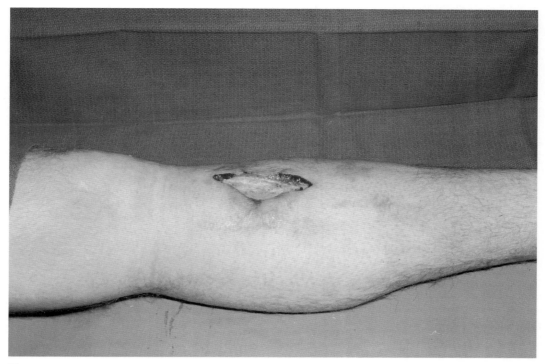

43

Twenty-four-year-old man with osteomyelitis of the upper tibia. Note the vertical
skin scar just medial to the tibial wound.
(Case of P.G. Arnold)

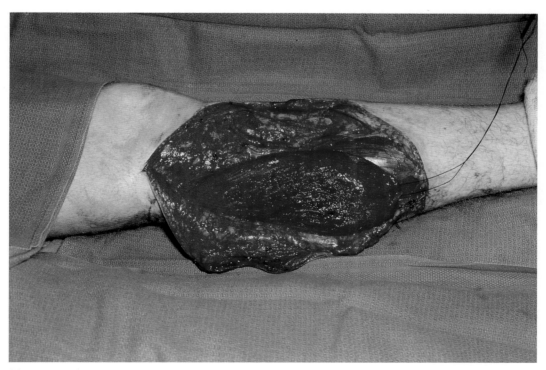

44

The medial head of the gastrocnemius
muscle is separated from the underlying
soleus muscle and denuded of its muscular fascia. A portion of the distal fascia,
which normally attaches to the Achilles
tendon mechanism, was retained to hold
sutures.

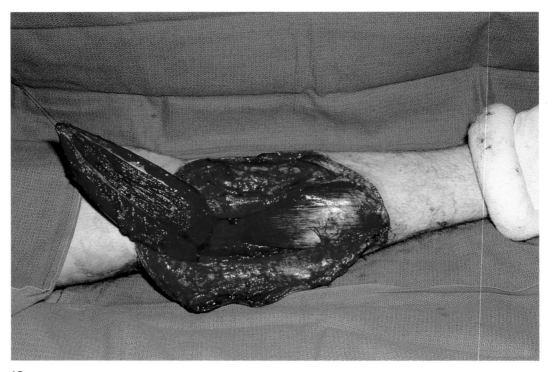

45

Elevated medial gastrocnemius muscle flap. The deep muscle fascia has also been removed.

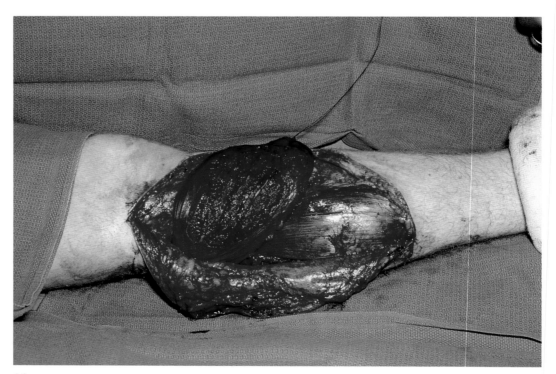

46

Gastrocnemius medial head transposed over the pretibial defect. The soleus muscle is seen beneath the gastrocnemius muscle.

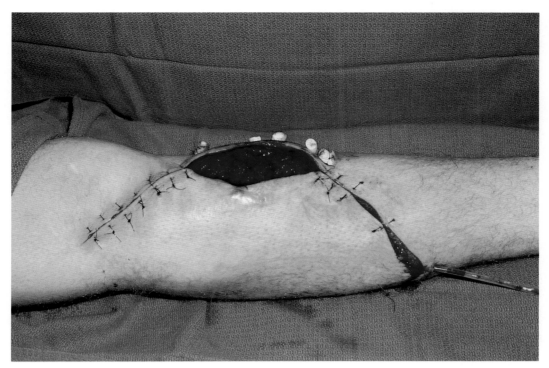

47

The muscle was sutured into place with through and through sutures tied over cotton rolls. The muscle flap was skin grafted two days later.

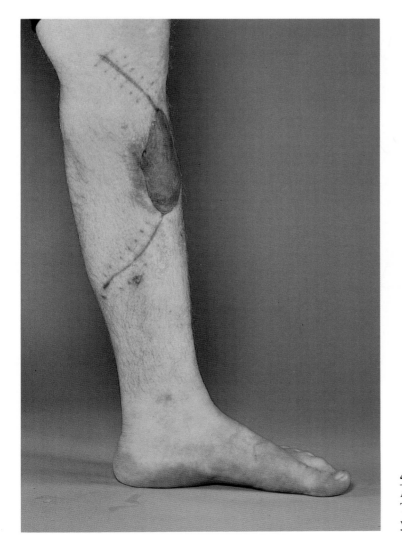

48

Appearance of the wound at six weeks. The wound has remained healed for four years.

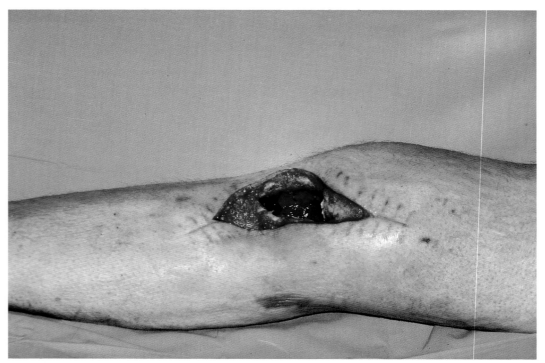

49

This giant cell tumor of the upper tibia was treated by curettage and immediate bone grafting. The wound became acutely infected and the bone grafts were lost. (Case of P.G. Arnold)

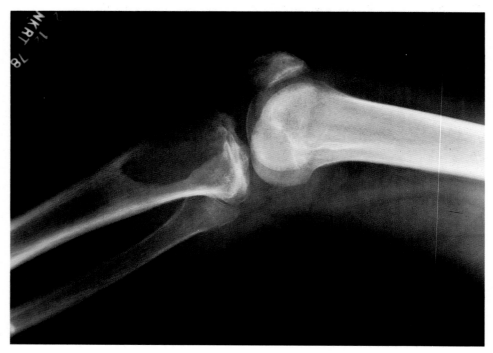

50

X-ray appearance of the bony defect of the tibia.

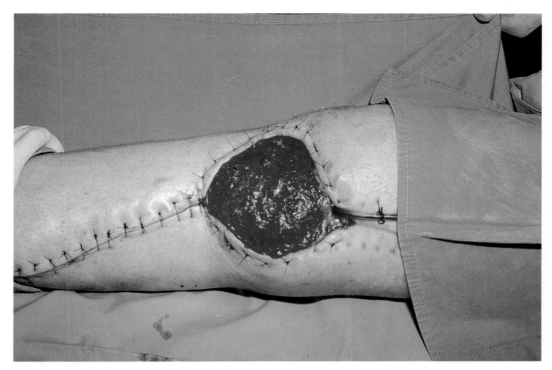

51

The medial head of the gastrocnemius muscle was rotated into the tibial defect. Healing muscle flap at the time of delayed skin grafting.

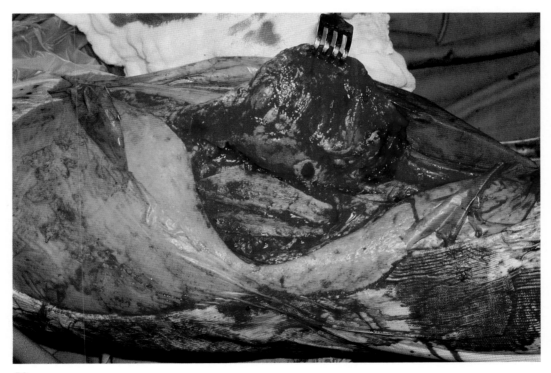

52

Eight weeks later, the medial gastrocnemius muscle flap was reelevated, and iliac bone grafts were used to fill the tibial cavity.

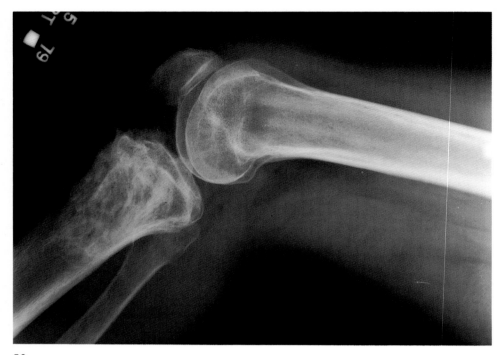

53

Three years following the secondary bone grafts. The upper tibia was completely reconstituted.

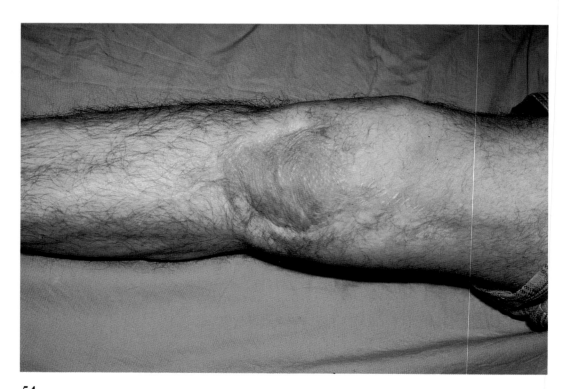

54

Appearance of the leg at five years. The patient has normal knee motion and is pain free. The reconstruction has remained stable for ten years.

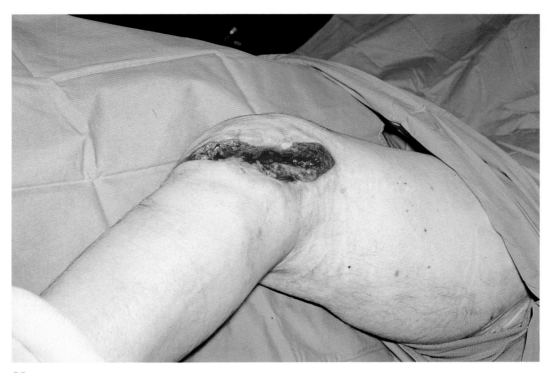

55

Avulsion injury to the anterolateral aspect of the knee. The debridement included the capsule of the knee joint and the lateral stabilizing ligaments. (Case of P.G. Arnold)

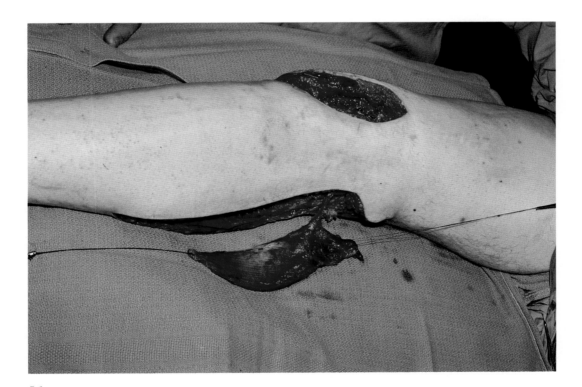

56

After the wound was clean, the lateral head of the gastrocnemius muscle was mobilized as a pure "island" muscle flap.

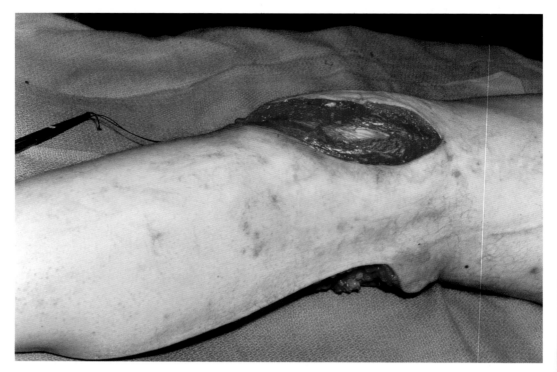

57

The lateral head of the gastrocnemius muscle was passed beneath a generous skin bridge and immediately inset. The deep muscular fascia was used to replace the joint capsule and the lateral ligamentous structures of the knee.

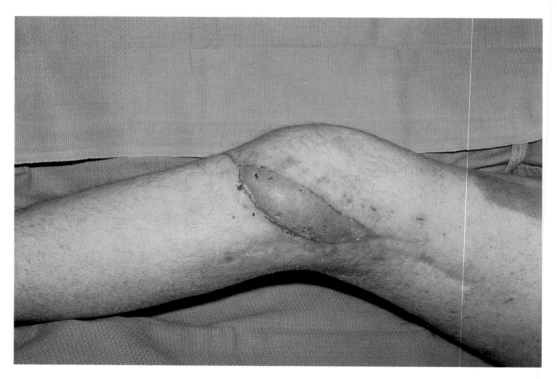

58

Stable knee joint at six months. The wound has remained healed for six years.

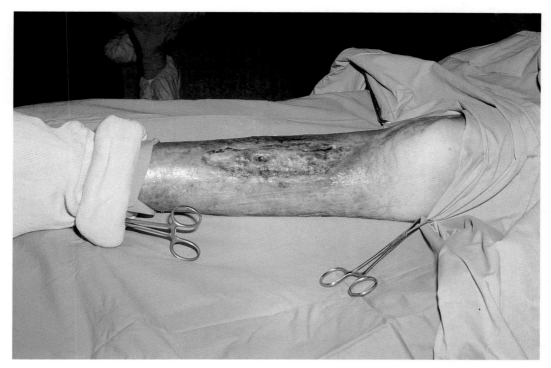

59

Sixty-two-year-old man with long-standing osteomyelitis involving the central two-thirds of the anterior tibia. The pretibial defect was ideally suited for bilateral gastrocnemius advancement flaps. (Case of P.G. Arnold and S. Eisengart)

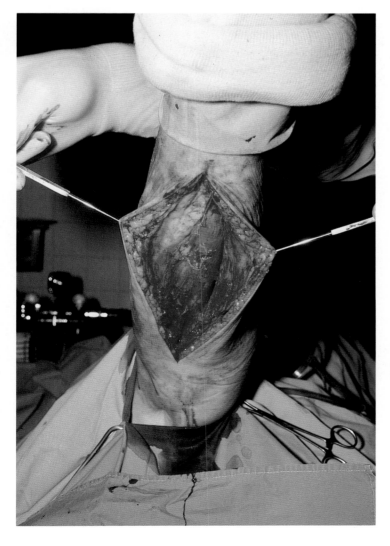

60

A "stocking-seam" incision was used to separate the two heads of the gastrocnemius muscle, which were left attached to their overlying skin. The deep dissection was carried beneath the gastrocnemius muscle and the deep calf fascia. The bipedicled myocutaneous flaps were finally advanced into the pretibial defect by dividing the gastrocnemius muscular insertion at the Achilles tendon.

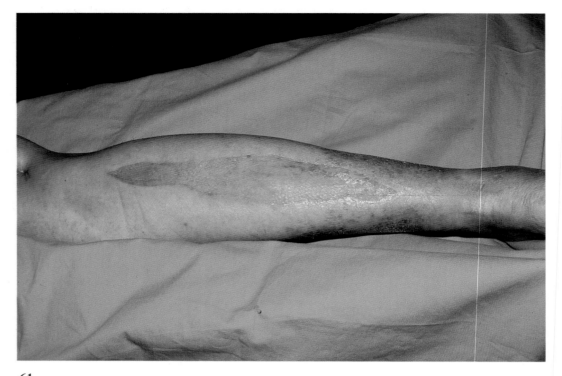

61

Skin-grafted ''stocking-seam'' donor site. Ambulation was not affected by the anterior transposition of the entire gastrocnemius muscle.

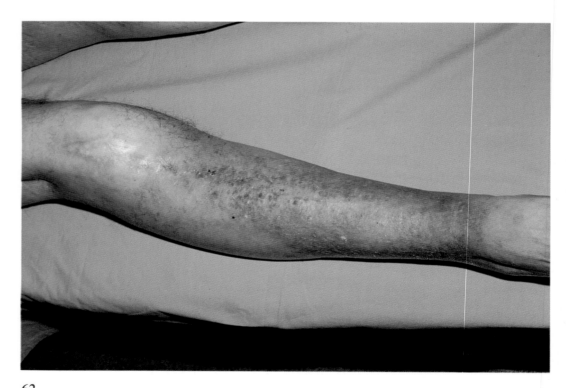

62

The bipedicled gastrocnemius myocutaneous advancement flaps were closed primarily over the pretibial defect. The wound has remained healed for eight years.

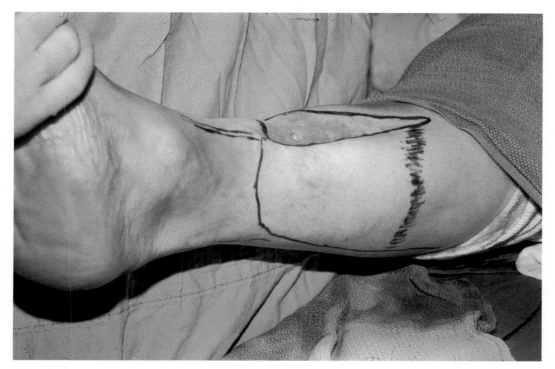

63

Minimal pretibial osteomyelitis surrounded by an area of atrophic epithelium in a forty-five-year-old female. A medial gastrocnemius fasciocutaneous flap is outlined. (Case of J.B. McCraw)

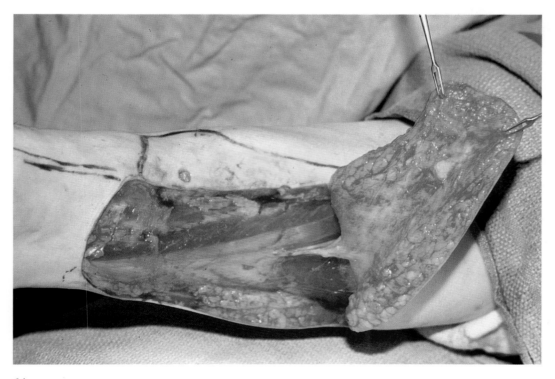

64

The fasciocutaneous flap is elevated away from the underlying soleus muscle but left completely attached to the medial head of the gastrocnemius muscle. Note the prominent vessel passing from the gastrocnemius muscle to the fasciocutaneous flap.

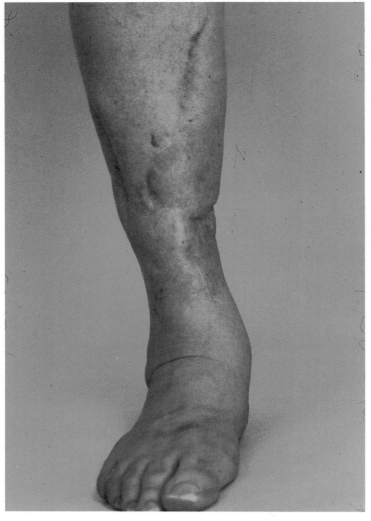

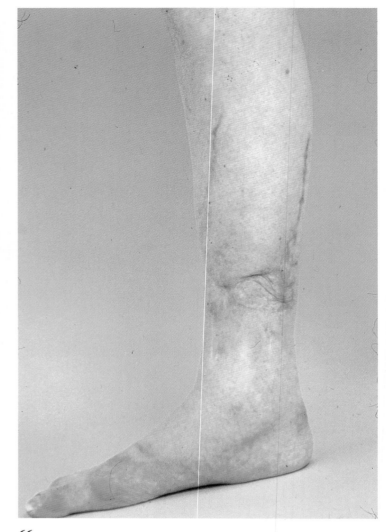

65
Anterior view of the low pretibial flap coverage.

66
Medial view of the transposed flap. Although the appearance of the skin-grafted donor site is not good, it is smaller than the pretibial defect which was repaired.

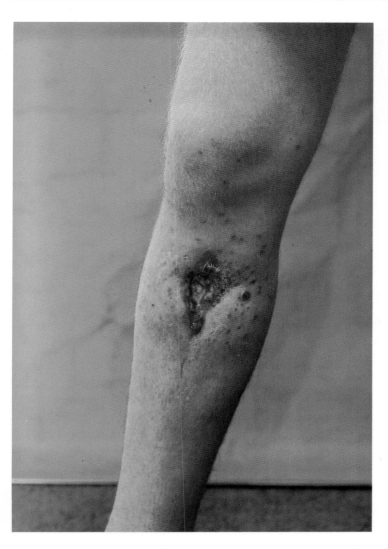

67
Nineteen-year-old man who sustained a shotgun wound at close range in a hunting accident. The tibial osteomyelitis went untreated for a period of six months. (Case of J.B. McCraw)

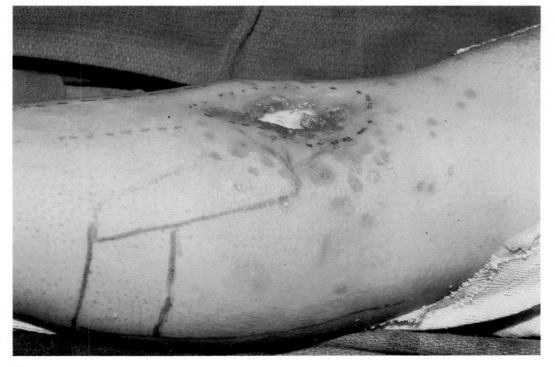

68
A small medial gastrocnemius myocutaneous flap is outlined. The cutaneous segment was included so the pellet-filled skin could be replaced at the time of the bony debridement.

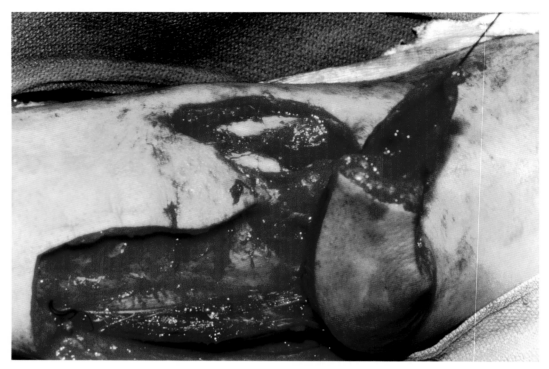

69

The medial head of the gastrocnemius muscle was ''split'' and tailored to fit the tibial defect. The muscle was used to eradicate the bony dead space, and the overlying skin of the flap was used for surface cover.

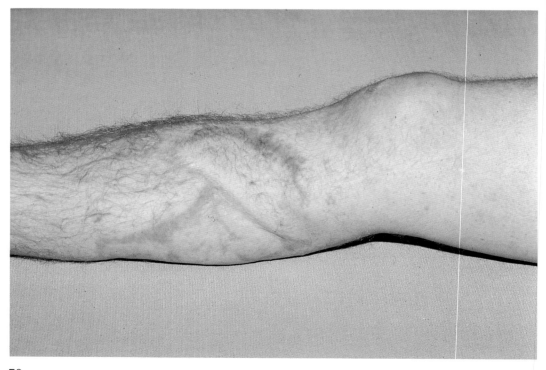

70

Eighteen months following surgery. The wound has remained healed for nine years. The donor site on the posterior calf is acceptable.

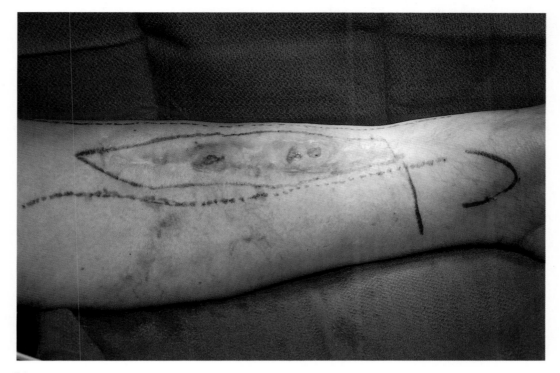

71

Seventy-one-year-old patient with a sixty-nine-year history of osteomyelitis of the central tibia from a systemic staphylococcal infection as a child. The patient was otherwise healthy and physiologically very young. Bipedicled gastrocnemius myocutaneous flaps are outlined. (Case of J.B. McCraw)

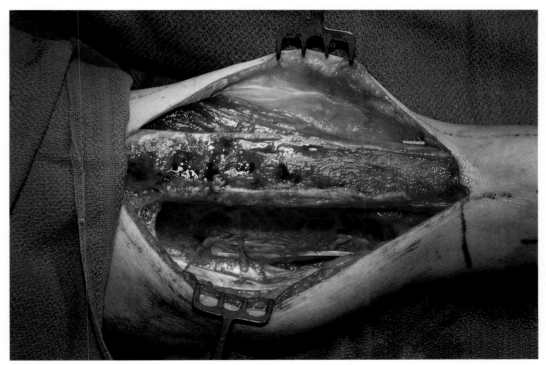

72

Debrided tibia and elevated gastrocnemius myocutaneous flaps. Excellent exposure of the deep surface of both heads of the gastrocnemius muscle was obtained without resorting to a posterior calf incision in this narrow (three centimeter) pretibial defect.

venous outflow. This muscular swelling then becomes self-perpetuating and eventuates in a fatally decreased arterial inflow. This same intolerance of constrictive pressure precludes the use of a "stent" to secure a skin graft on the surface of the soleus muscle flap.

If there is any question about the viability of the muscle, it should be placed on the recipient site and left ungrafted for a few days. An immediate skin graft may obscure the nonviability of the muscle flap for five to seven days because one may be erroneously led to believe that the skin graft is "taking." In this situation, it is better to observe the muscle directly for two to three days. Any nonviable muscle can be electively trimmed and the skin graft can be placed in a delayed fashion.

Hematoma and seroma formations have been unusual, but they will occur if the wound is not properly drained by suction catheters. The donor site is inconsequential both from functional and esthetic standpoints.

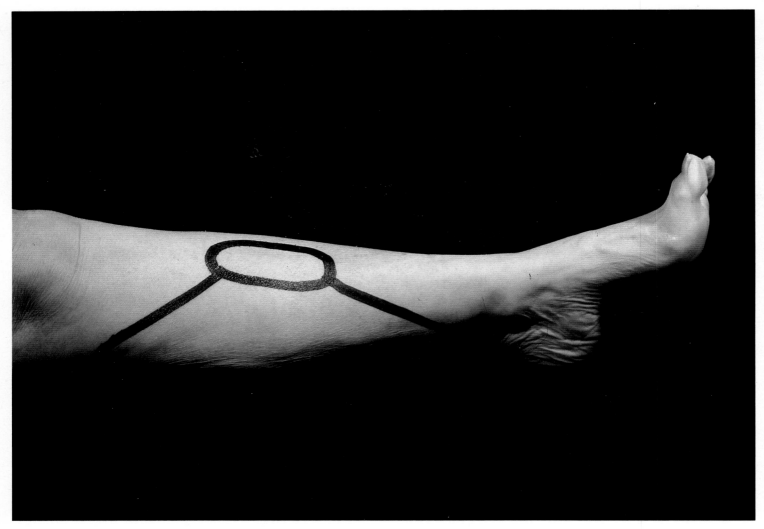

1

Medial approach to the soleus muscle with a ''typical'' area of coverage circled in the midtibial region. This direct approach to the muscle avoids a constricting skin bridge over the transposed muscle flap.

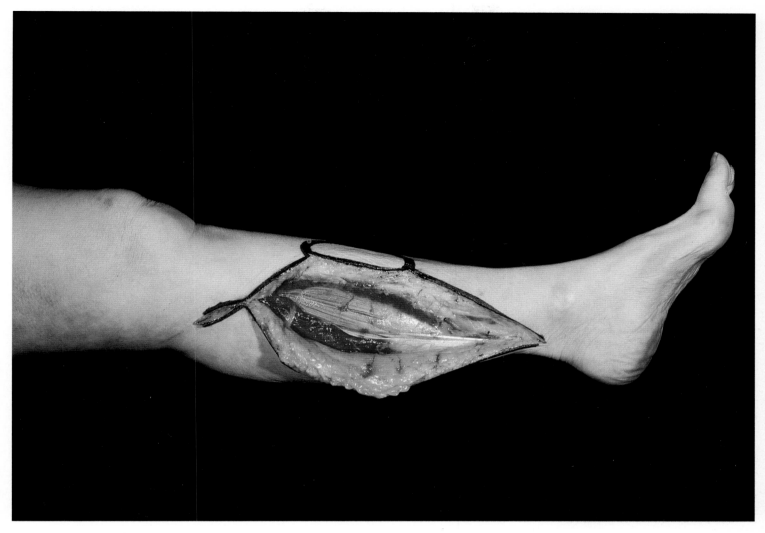

2

The separation between the soleus and gastrocnemius muscles is first identified in the midcalf. This separation can also be found near the Achilles tendon, but the plane of dissection is less clearly defined. Note the plantaris tendon on the surface of the soleus muscle indicating that the plane of dissection between the two muscles is correct.

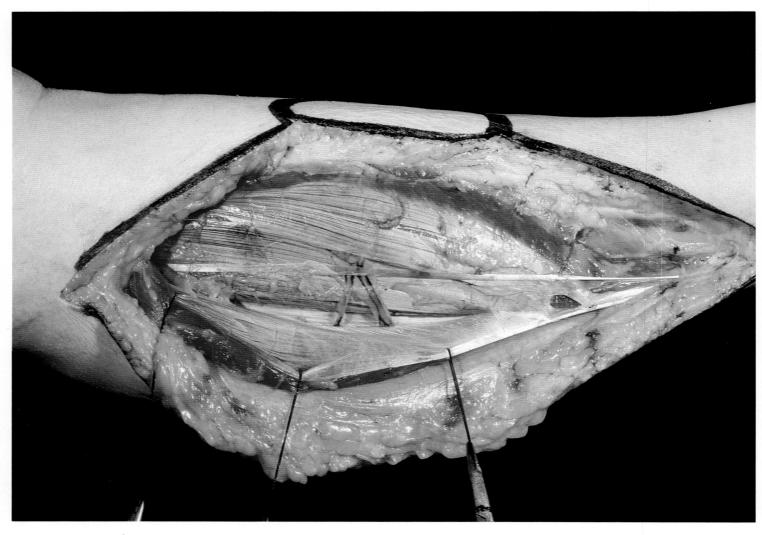

3

Close-up view of a deep muscular perforator passing from the soleus muscle to the undersurface of the gastrocnemius muscle, which is retracted with sutures. The soleus muscle is next separated from its medial attachment to the tibia starting at the point where the plantaris tendon crosses the distal muscle. In the area of the Achilles tendon, the soleus muscle must be sharply separated from the gastrocnemius muscle and the Achilles tendon.

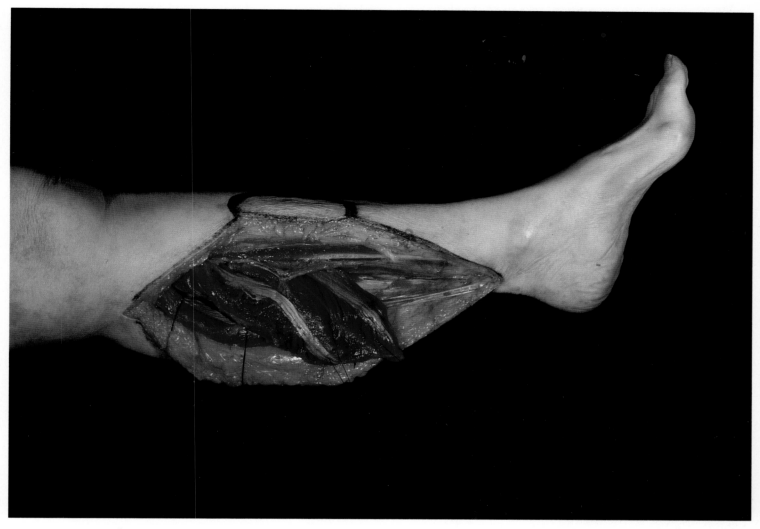

4

The soleus muscle has been separated from the Achilles tendon. It is still attached to most of the deep perforating branches from the posterior tibial artery. These deep perforators may be divided if it is necessary to increase the upward excursion of the muscle, but if they can be left intact, the blood supply to the muscle flap is obviously enhanced.

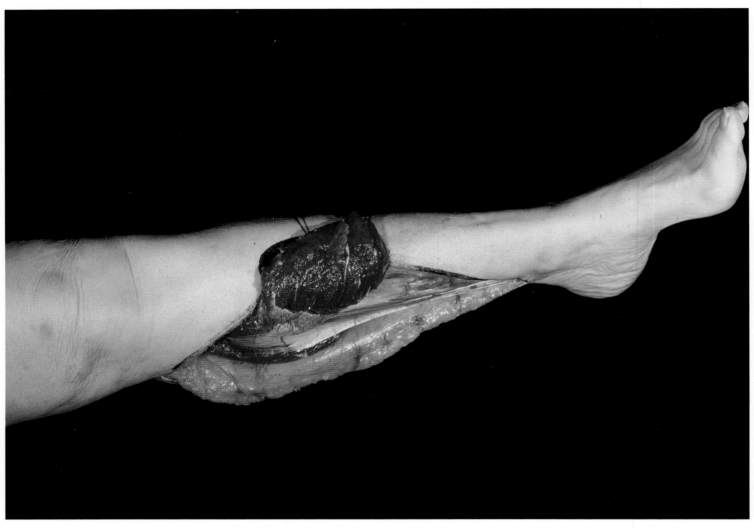

5

With this limited dissection the soleus muscle can be readily transposed into a midtibial defect. Coverage of a larger defect by the soleus muscle requires a more extensive dissection.

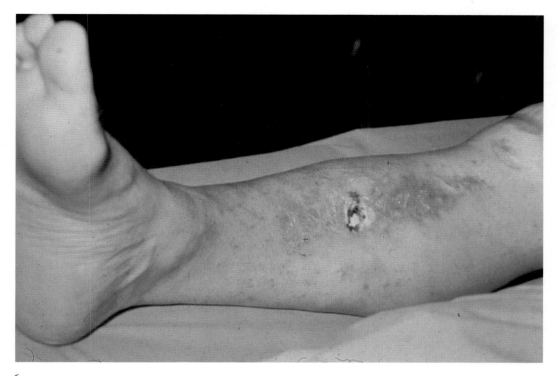

6

Twenty-two-year-old man with a superficial osteomyelitis of the tibia following an open fracture. This is a historical case for the authors since it was the first soleus muscle flap done at the Henry Grady Memorial Hospital in Atlanta. (Case of J.B. McCraw and L.O. Vasconez)

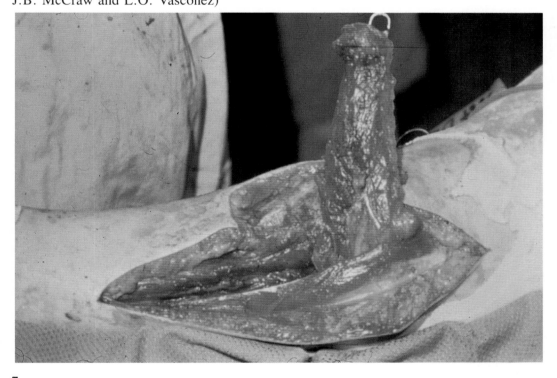

7

The soleus muscle is retrieved through a medial access incision following the debridement of the tibia.

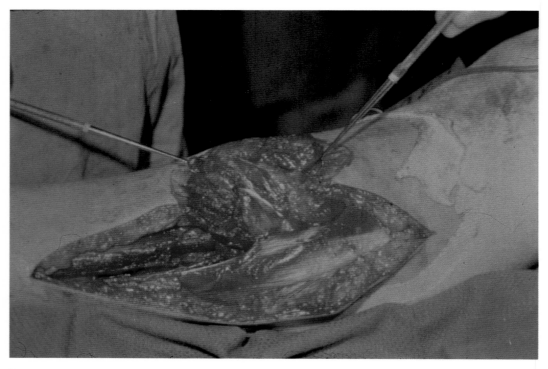

8

The soleus muscle is rotated into the pretibial defect. Skin grafting was delayed
for two days.

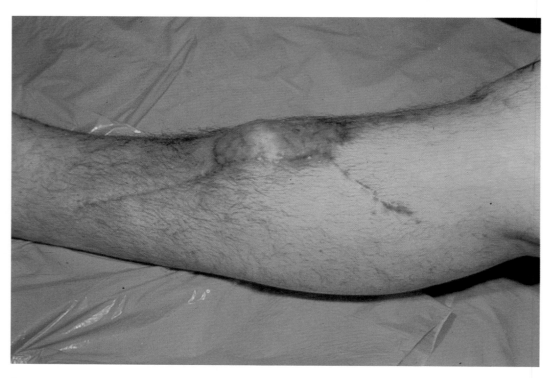

9

Skin-grafted muscle flap and primary closure of the donor site. The skin closure
must be effected without any muscular
constriction since the soleus muscle is
very sensitive to external pressure. It is
remarkable that our methods have not
changed since 1972. It is even more remarkable that this same method was used
by Professor Stotz in World War I.

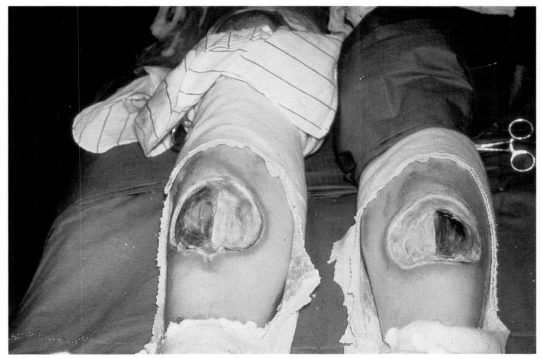

10

Twenty-four-year-old housepainter who sustained a high voltage injury to both midpretibial areas while standing in contact with a metal ladder. The anterior compartment musculature was necrotic, and the tibia was exposed in both legs. Bilateral cross-leg flaps would have been quite difficult, and this 1975 case predated reliable "free" tissue transfers to the lower leg. (Case of J.B. McCraw)

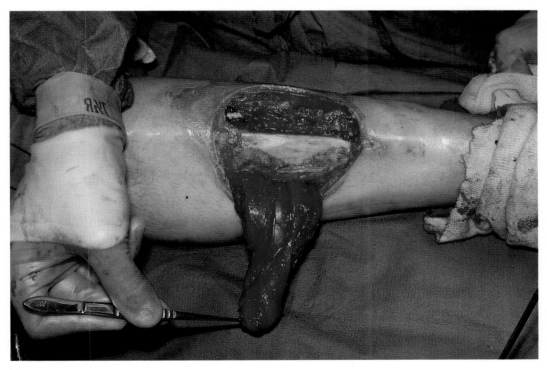

11

The tibial cortex was tangentially excised, and the necrotic anterior compartment musculature was debrided. It was possible to raise a soleus muscle flap at the time of the initial debridement because the viable margins of the injured tissues were adequately delineated.

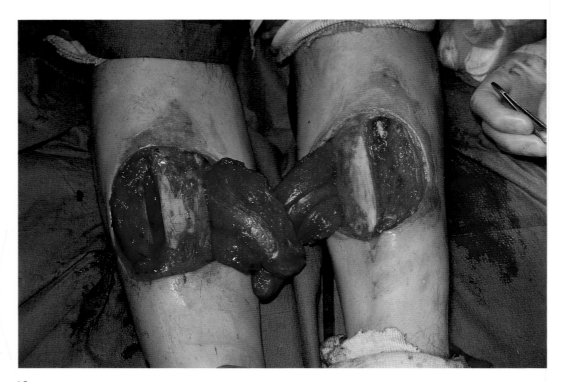

12

Bilateral soleus muscles elevated and
readied for transfer into the pretibial
defects.

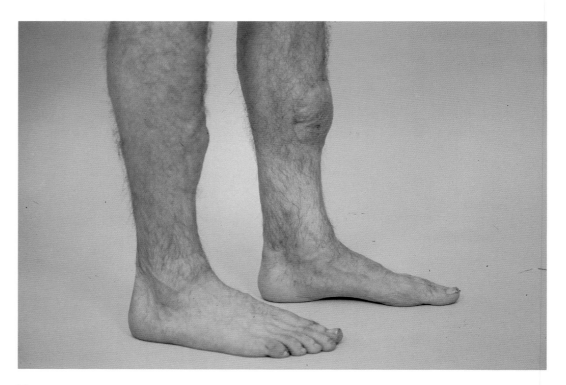

13

Early postoperative view of the skin-
grafted soleus muscle flaps. The patient
was very upset by the appearance of the
flaps and threatened a lawsuit. He never
recognized the potential gravity of his situation. Needless to say, the flaps were
never revised.

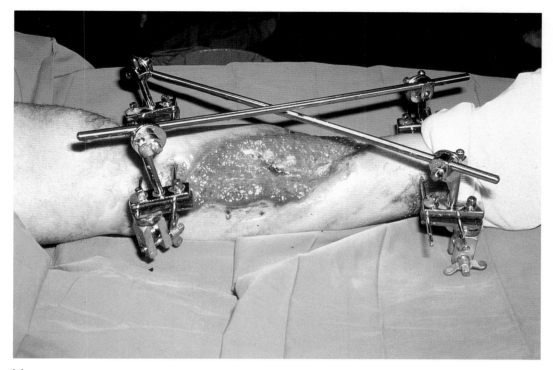

14
Nineteen-year-old man with active osteomyelitis in an unstable and exposed tibial
fracture. (Case of P.G. Arnold)

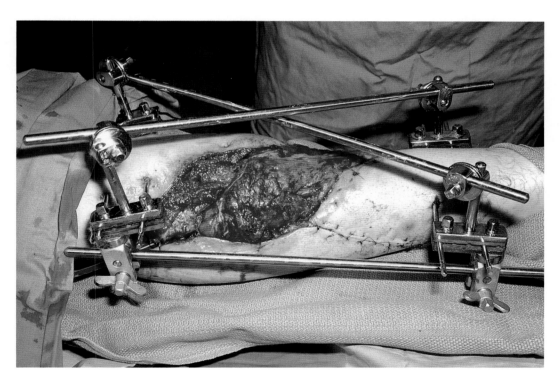

15
The soleus muscle was transposed at the
time of the initial debridement. The external fixation device was not removed.

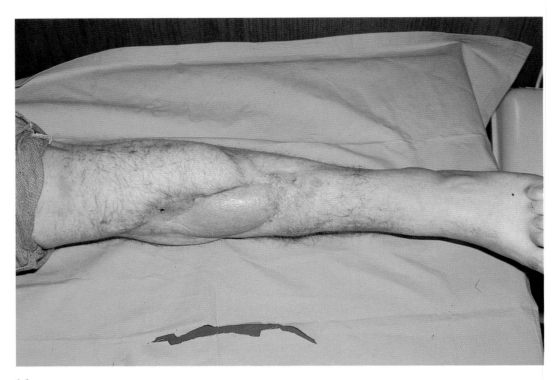

16

Stable wound and healed fracture at nine
months. The patient continues to do well
after seven years.

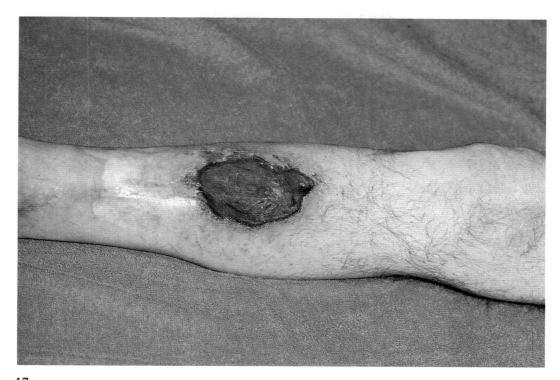

17

Fifty-seven-year-old man with a traumatic full-thickness loss of an old burn scar. The burn was sustained as a child and had been allowed to secondarily heal by epithelization. (Case of P.G. Arnold)

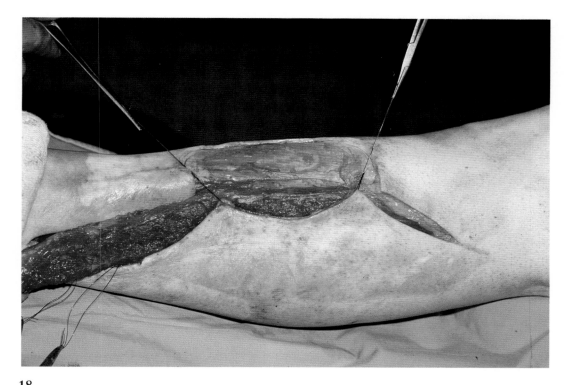

18

The debridement denuded the central one-third of the tibia. The soleus muscle was exposed by ''extending'' the medial margins of the wound.

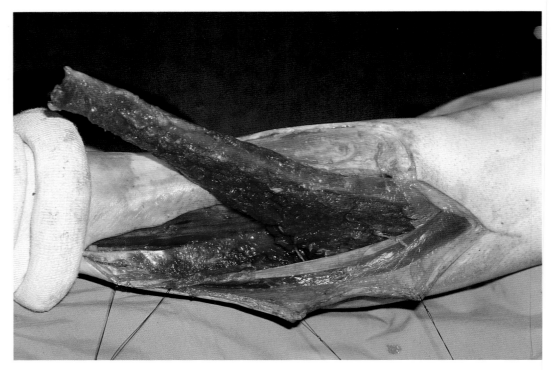

19

The distal soleus muscle was completely mobilized by sharply separating it from the Achilles tendon and the gastrocnemius muscle. Note the impressive length of the soleus muscle.

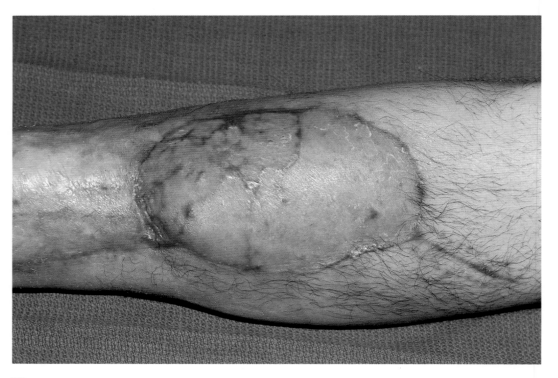

20

Three months following muscle transposition and skin grafting. The early graft appearance is irregular because the muscle was immediately grafted and the distal half of the graft was lost. A delayed skin graft would have been preferable. The wound has remained healed for five years.

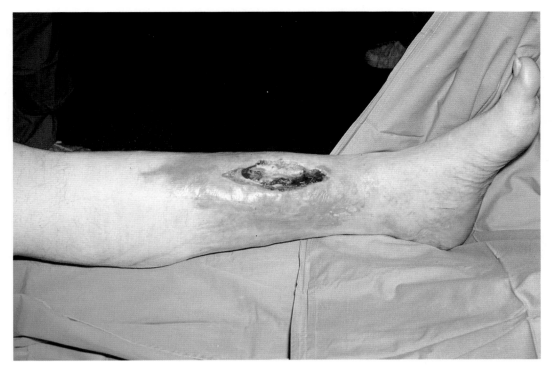

21

Osteomyelitis of the distal one-third of the tibia, which had continuously drained for five years. The surrounding venous stasis changes resulted from the complex injury of the tibia and fibula. (Case of P.G. Arnold)

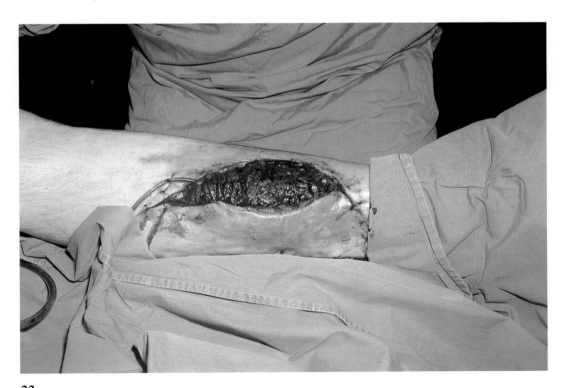

22

The proximal soleus muscle was explored and found to be a reasonable choice for this low tibial closure. A skin graft was placed forty-eight hours following the muscle transposition.

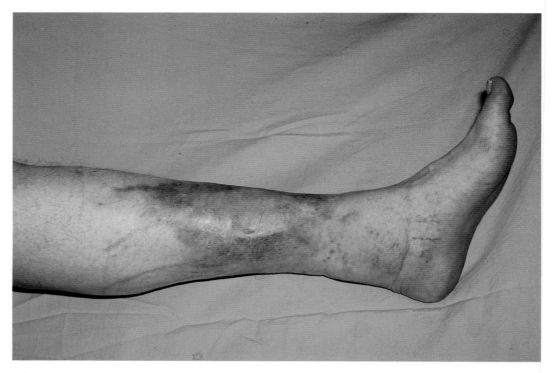

23

Eighteen months following the muscle flap closure. The venous hypertensive disease has not progressed, and the osteomyelitis has not recurred over a five year period.

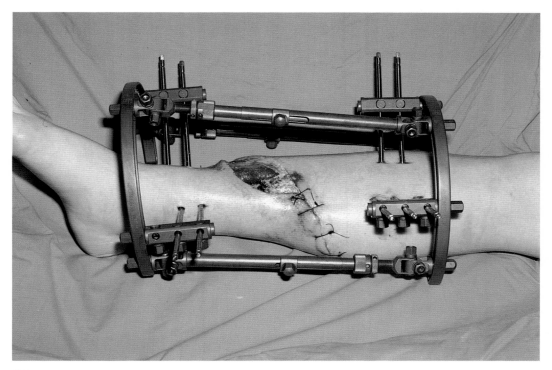

24

Nineteen-year-old female with an open tibial fracture forty-eight hours following
the initial debridement and placement of
an external fixation device. (Case of P.G.
Arnold)

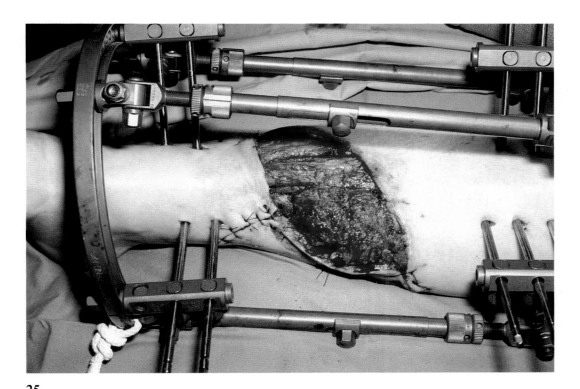

25

The proximal soleus muscle flap was explored and immediately transposed. Appearance of the muscle forty-eight hours
following transposition at the time of skin
grafting.

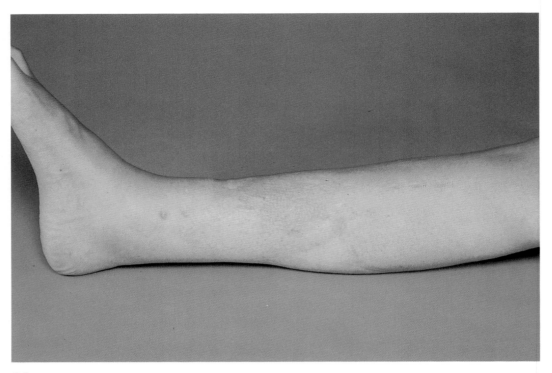

26

Healed muscle flap and tibial fracture at one year. The length of the soleus muscle was adequate to accommodate this low tibial defect.

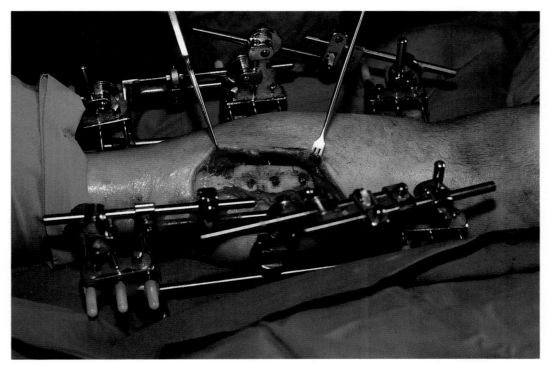

27

Thirty-one-year-old man eighteen months following an open fracture of the distal tibia. The fracture was first treated with an internal plate, but this was complicated by osteomyelitis and nonunion of the fracture. An external fixation device was placed at the time of our initial debridement. (Case of P.G. Arnold)

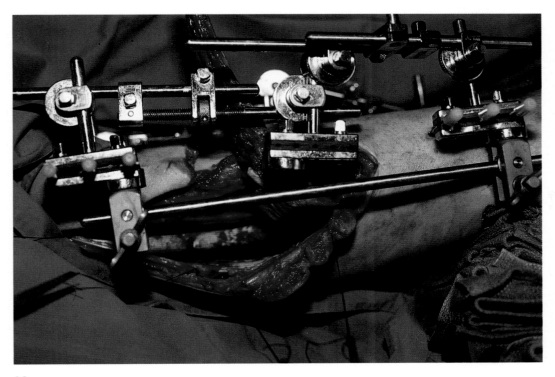

28

The soleus muscle flap is elevated with the fixation device in place. The necrotic tibia and the infected screw tracts were extensively debrided. A bone graft was not required.

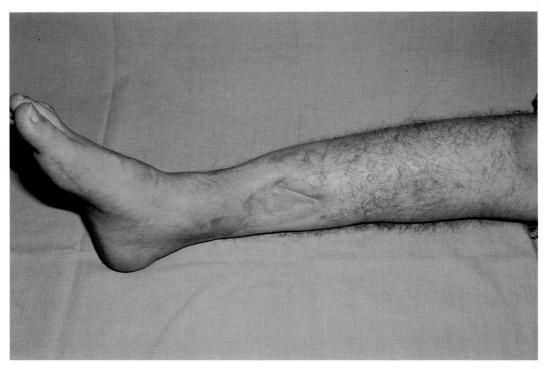

29

The tibia and the soleus muscle flap remain healed at two years. It is frequently worthwhile to explore the soleus muscle in these distal wounds, because it can offer a much simpler method of reconstruction than a ''free'' flap.

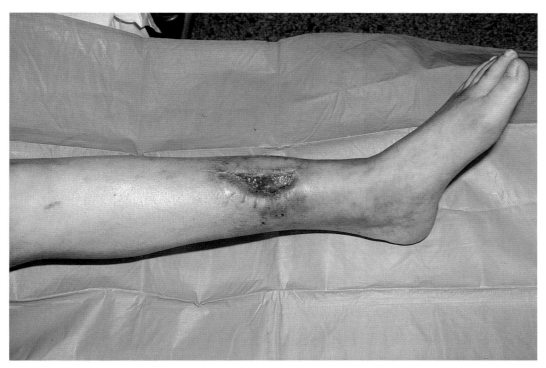

30

Thirty-two-year-old female with osteomyelitis of the distal one-third of the tibia
fourteen months after an open fracture.
(Case of P.G. Arnold)

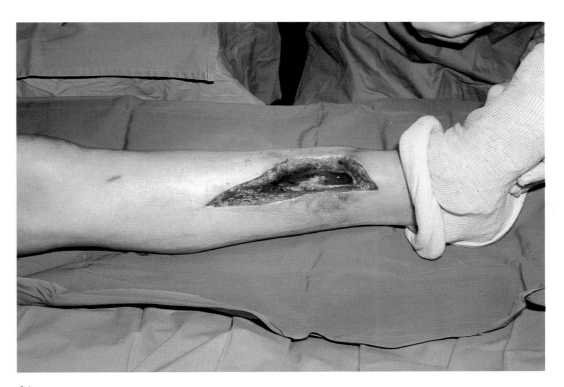

31

The initial debridement resulted in an extensive soft tissue defect and a deep
wound of the distal tibia.

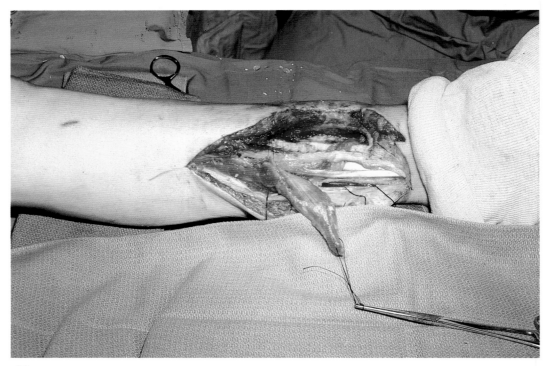

32

A proximal soleus muscle flap was elevated at the time of the initial
debridement.

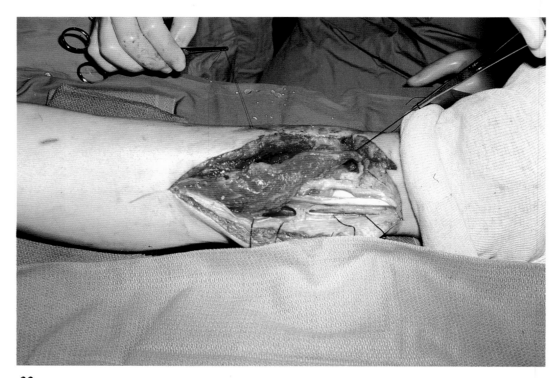

33

Transposed soleus muscle flap. Although
the soleus muscle was small, it was adequate to fill the tibial cavity.

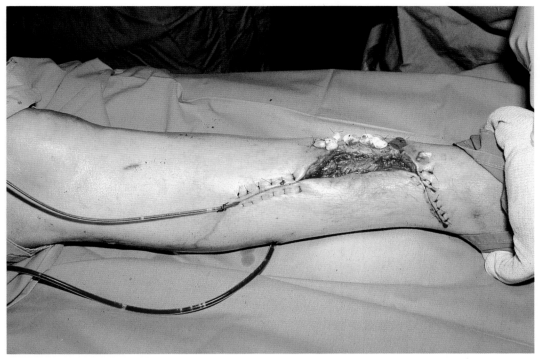

34
The patient was returned to the operating room for skin grafting after the viability of the muscle was assured.

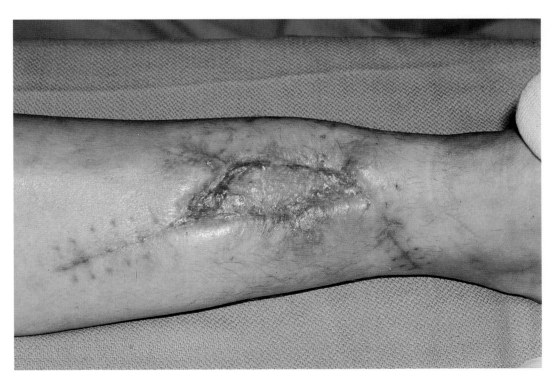

35
Healed soleus muscle flap at eleven months. The wound has remained stable for eight years.

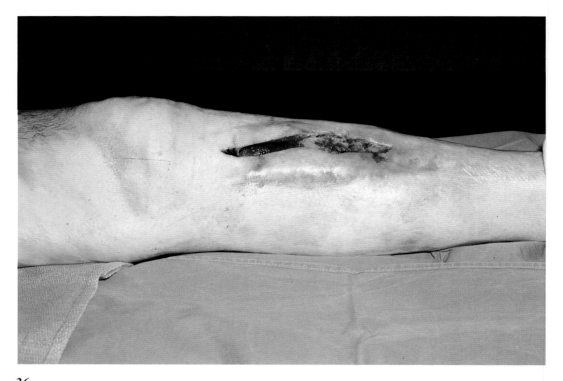

36

Severe osteomyelitis of the middle and upper tibia in a sixty-seven-year-old retired professional football player. The infection had been active for fifteen years. (Case of P.G. Arnold)

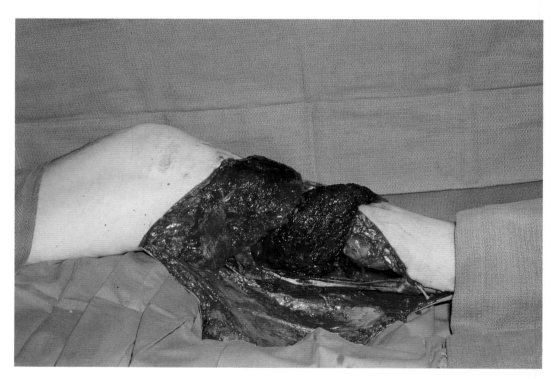

37

Because of the extensive nature of the soft tissue and bony defects, it was necessary to transpose both the soleus muscle and the medial head of the gastrocnemius muscle.

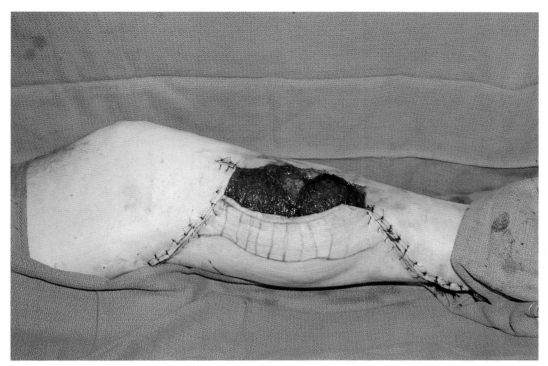

38

The patient was returned to the operating room for skin grafting forty-eight hours following the muscle flap procedure. The nonfluorescent medial calf skin (marked with cross hatches) was excised at this time.

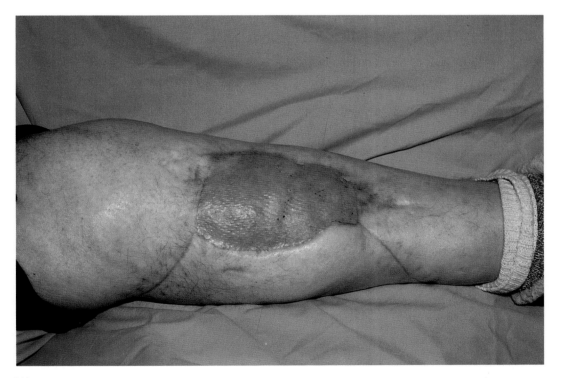

39

Healed wound eight months following the closure with soleus and gastrocnemius muscle flaps. As expected, there was no noticeable functional loss from the combined use of the soleus and gastrocnemius muscles. The osteomyelitis has not recurred over a seven year period.

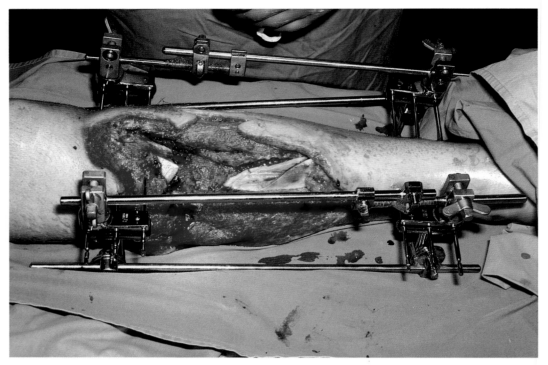

40

Twenty-seven-year-old man six weeks following an open fracture of the tibia with a large segment of missing bone. This case predated the ''free'' osteocutaneous flap era. (Case of P.G. Arnold)

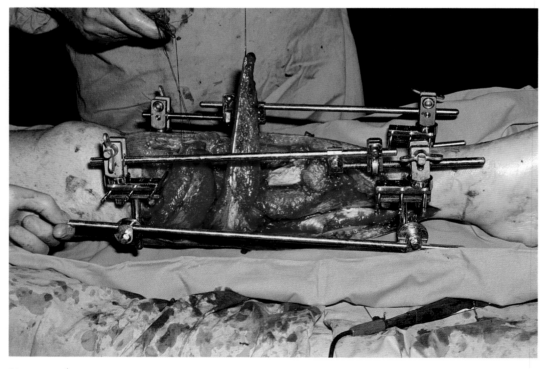

41

It was necessary to use the medial head of the gastrocnemius muscle as well as the soleus and tibialis anterior muscles to cover the massive tibial defect.

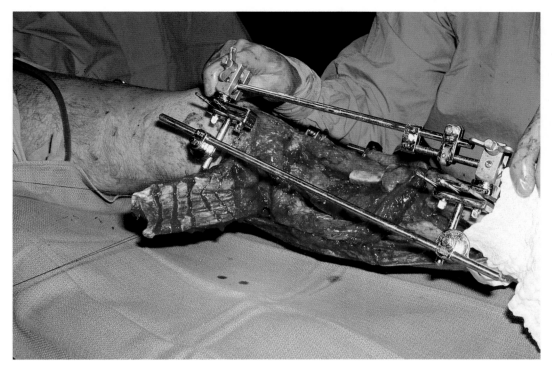

42

The deep fascia of the gastrocnemius muscle was "scored" to expand its coverage. It is just as easy to excise the muscular fascia. This also allows the "raw muscle" to be in direct contact with wound surface.

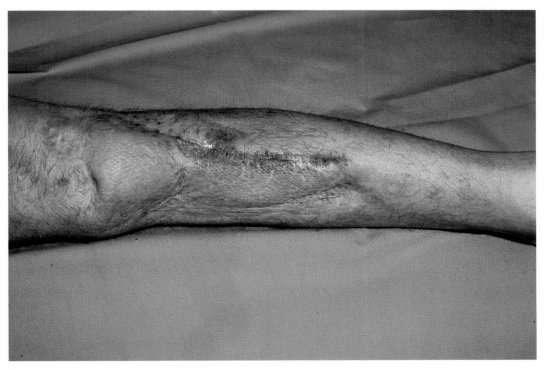

43

Appearance seven years following the surgery. The twenty centimeter tibial defect was reconstructed with a standard bone graft, which was introduced through a posterior approach after the muscle flap closure was secured.

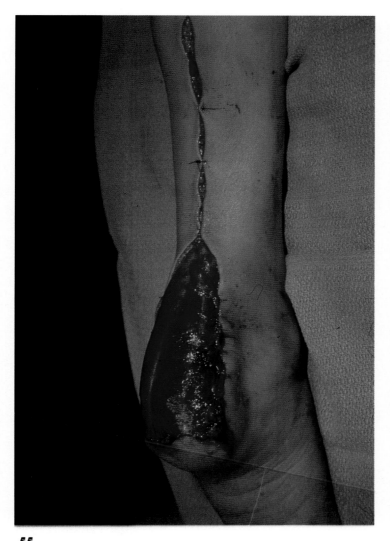

55

"Reversed" soleus muscle flap rotated inferiorly with its deep surface visible.

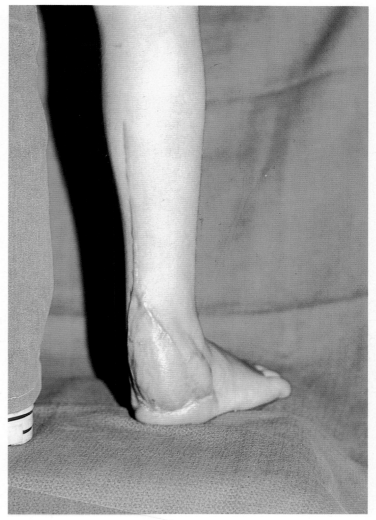

56

Skin-grafted muscle at five months. The
wound has been stable for six years. The
patient returned to full athletic activities,
including competitive soccer.

EXTENSOR DIGITORUM COMMUNIS

ANATOMICAL CONSIDERATIONS

Surface Markings

The extensor digitorum communis (EDC) muscle passes on a line from the head of the fibula to the midpoint of the anterior ankle. The EDC muscle is easily palpated in either the thin or the muscular individual.

Origin and Insertion

The EDC muscle originates from the lateral border of the upper two-thirds of the tibia and from the medial border of the fibula. The muscle becomes completely tendinous in its distal-third. After passing beneath the extensor retinaculum, the muscle inserts into the proximal phalanges of the second through the fifth toes. The function of the EDC muscle is duplicated by the extensor digitorum brevis muscle (short extensors) in all but the fifth toe. This long extensor toe function can also be replaced by a tenodesis of the extensor digitorum communis muscle to the extensor hallucis longus muscle.

Adjacent Muscle

Superiorly the EDC muscle lies between the tibialis anterior and the peroneus longus muscles. In the lower pretibial area the EDC muscle passes between the extensor hallucis longus and the peroneus brevis muscles. The superficial sensory branch of the peroneal nerve crosses over the EDC tendons just above the ankle.

Vascular Supply

The EDC muscle is supplied by multiple deep segmental perforating vessels from the anterior tibial artery. There are usually nine to fourteen distal perforators which can supply the distal two-thirds of the muscle as a distally based muscle flap. The number of deep perforators and the size of the "reversed" muscle flap are not anatomically precise because the effective size of the muscle flap is ultimately dependent upon the physiological nature of the intramuscular vascular arborization.

Motor Nerve

Peroneal nerve.

USES

The extensor digitorum communis muscle is used only as a distally based muscle flap to cover the lower one-third of the tibia. A proximally based extensor digitorum communis muscle flap is not even considered because there are better muscle flap options available. Although the "reversed" EDC muscle flap has a remarkable distal excursion, it will not reach the ankle joint nor the dorsum of the foot.

REGIONAL FLAP COMPARISON

A "free" microvascular transfer should always be considered when one is faced with a low pretibial defect. Although a "free" transfer necessitates a longer operative procedure, the time required for healing and the total length of the disability may be less than that of a "reversed" EDC muscle flap. Still, the properly chosen EDC muscle flap should routinely survive a distal transfer, and a "free" muscle transfer currently survives in only 85% to 95% of its pretibial applications. This difference in survivability is related primarily to the preexisting vascular damage within the "zone of injury." Intimal fibrosis of the recipient vessels may be even more extensive than suggested by the arteriogram, and the intimal damage may spread beyond the "zone of injury." An extensive "zone of injury" further diminishes the viability of a "free" flap if it forces one to use long interposition vein grafts between the recipient vessels and the "free" flap.

The proximally based (yes, proximally based) soleus muscle flap can frequently be used for small distal tibial defects. The proximal soleus muscle should always be explored before a "reversed" EDC flap is elevated. The distal excursion of the proximal soleus muscle flap can be surprising, and it may offer a simple solution to some difficult low pretibial problems.

Several other flaps will reach the distal tibia, but each has one or more significant disadvantages. The "island" dorsalis pedis skin flap is neither helpful in obliterating a cavity nor in eradicating infection. The already suspect "reversed" soleus muscle flap may be even more suspect because of preexisting harm to its deep perforating vessels in an extensive "zone of injury." Even when it is usable, the "reversed" soleus muscle flap offers an unsightly reconstruction and notable morbidity. Since the proximal portion of the tibialis anterior muscle originates from the tibia, a "reversed" tibialis anterior muscle flap can be used to "carry" the attached portion of the proximal tibia to a distal tibial bone defect. Other than this unusual transfer of the proximal tibia to the distal tibia, the unique functional importance of the tibialis anterior muscle precludes any other "reversed" flap applications.

DISADVANTAGES

Unlike the robust vitality of standard muscle flaps, any "reversed" muscle flap can be expected to have a markedly decreased blood flow. Fortunately, the distal vasculature of the EDC muscle is reasonably predictable and will generally sustain a "reversed" muscle flap. Muscle flap loss has not been a consistent problem, but the fragility of the "reversed" EDC muscle flap has to be respected. Acceptable toe extension can usually be reconstituted by a tenodesis, but some functional loss can be expected with the use of this muscle flap.

ADVANTAGES

The principal advantage of the "reversed" EDC muscle flap is that it can provide excellent muscle coverage for some of the most difficult problems in the lower third of the tibia without a prolonged microvascular procedure. The donor site is excellent, and the appearance of the skin-grafted muscle flap is quite acceptable.

COMPLICATIONS, PITFALLS, AND DONOR SITE

The EDC muscle does not have a well-delineated fascial covering so one must be very careful not to shred the muscle during its dissection. It is not clear exactly how many of the distal perforating vessels are necessary for the viability of this muscle flap, but one can safely take the proximal 30 to 40% of these vessels without harming the survival of the "reversed" muscle flap. If there is a question about the need to include certain deep perforators, microvascular clips can be placed on the suspect vessels, the muscle can be fluoresced, and then the muscle bleeding can be observed. If there is still a quandary, one can transpose the muscle and wait two to three days to excise any area of questionable viability. Skin grafting should preferably be completed in a delayed fashion.

The functional deficit from the use of the EDC muscle is not terribly significant if the extensor tendons are tenodesed. Only the fifth toe lacks an accessory short toe extensor. Since the primarily closed donor site is favorable, the known functional loss is a small price to pay for a healthy muscle flap transfer to these difficult pretibial defects of the lower leg. Presently the EDC muscle flap has a limited but very significant application. However, its usefulness may become less important as microvascular transfers become more effective.

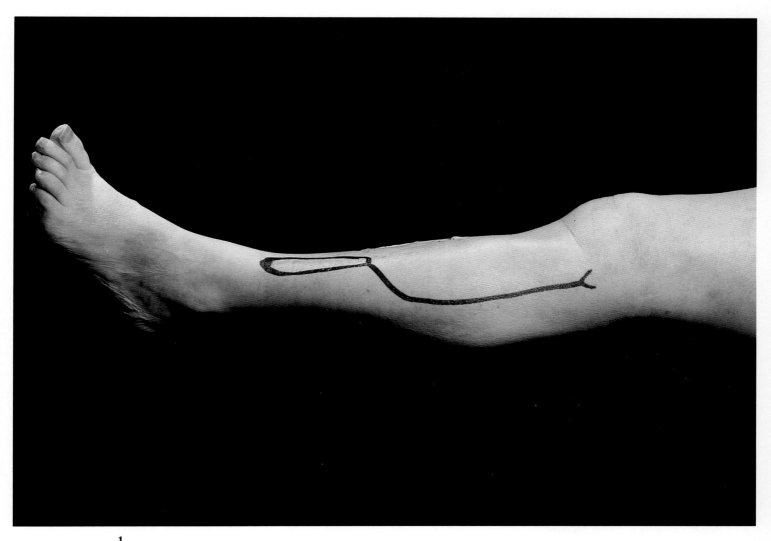

1

Outlined incision and a typical area of coverage for a distally based EDC muscle flap.

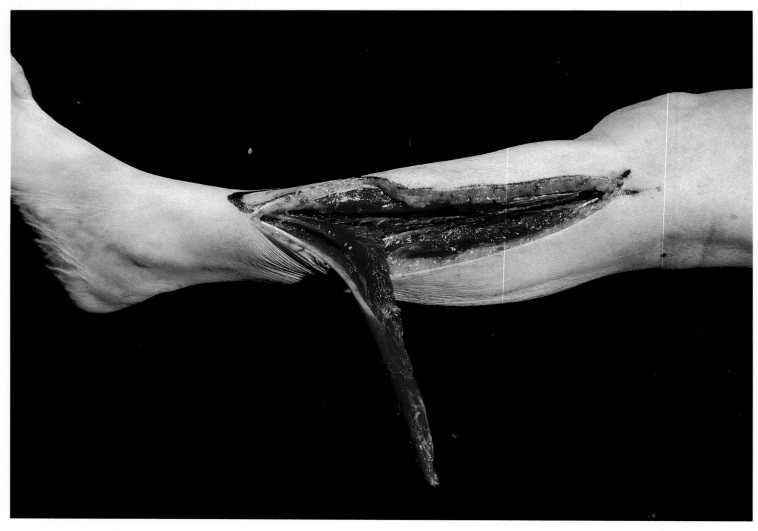

2

Multiple deep perforating vessels are seen entering the distal EDC muscle from the anterior tibial vessels.

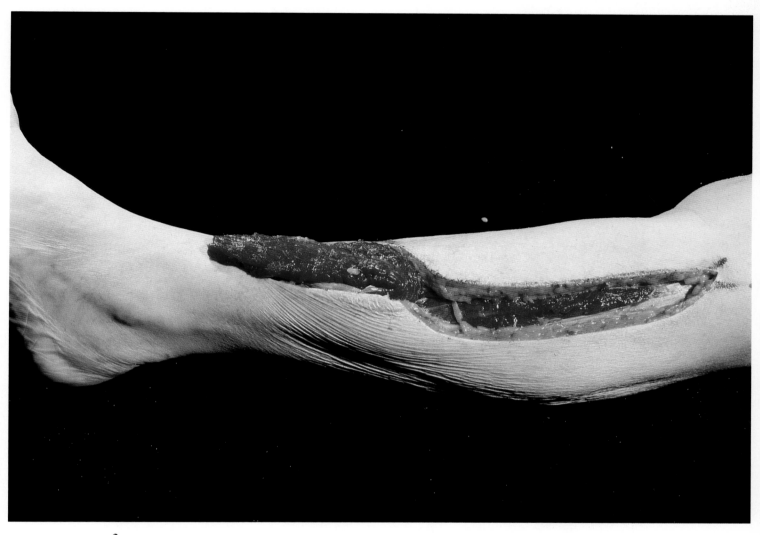

3

The EDC muscle is rotated distally to demonstrate the expected coverage for a lower pretibial defect. It does not reach the ankle joint nor the malleoli.

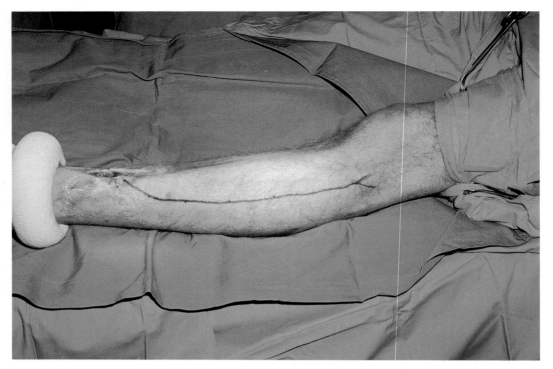

4

Twenty-seven-year-old male three years following an open fracture of the lower tibia. The osteomyelitic defect was small but the bone had been actively infected since the time of injury. The incision for the retrieval of the EDC muscle is outlined. (Case of P.G. Arnold)

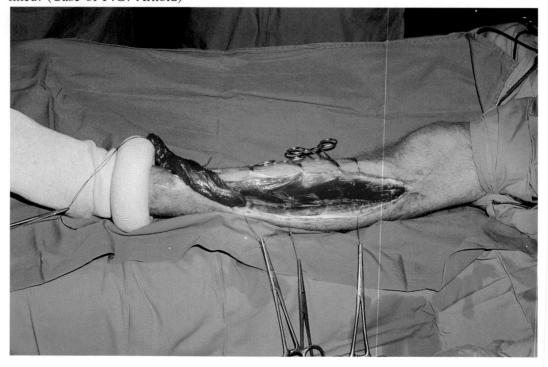

5

A "reversed" EDC muscle flap is transposed. The viable portion of the muscle flap extends well past the tibial defect.

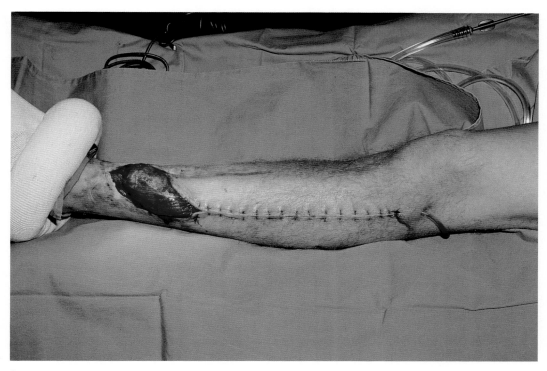

6

Appearance of the inset EDC muscle flap and the donor site closure. Grafting was delayed for forty-eight hours.

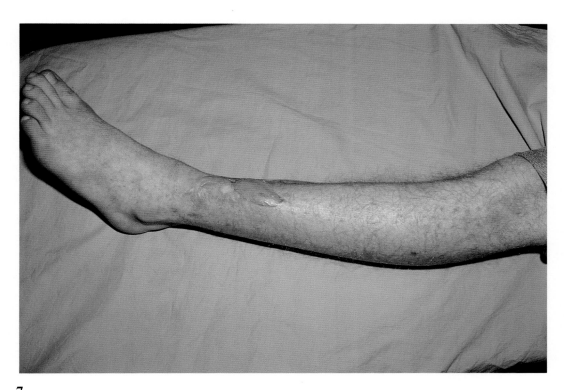

7

Appearance six years following the muscle flap closure. The wound has remained soundly healed and free of drainage.

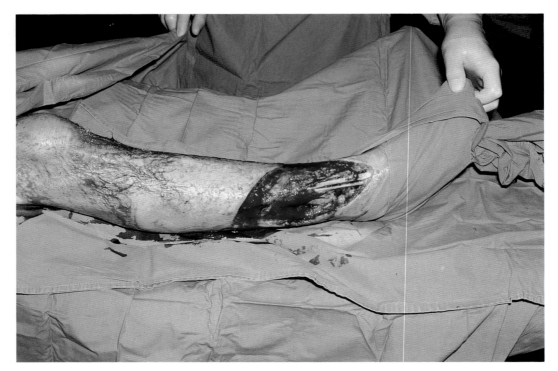

8

Twenty-three-year-old man with a grain auger injury, which exposed the anterior compartment. A distal fibular fracture is acutely infected. (Case of P.G. Arnold)

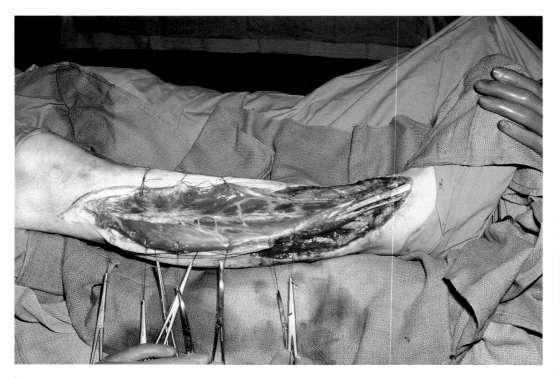

9

The extensor digitorum communis muscle is partially elevated. The multiple perforating vessels from the tibialis anterior vasculature are demonstrated between the retracted EDC muscle and the tibialis anterior muscle.

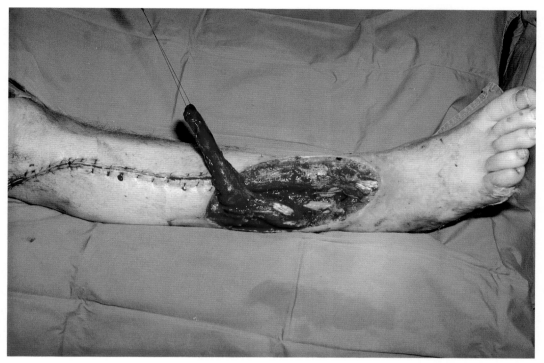

10

The extensor digitorum communis muscle is mobilized on the distal one-third of the perforating vessels.

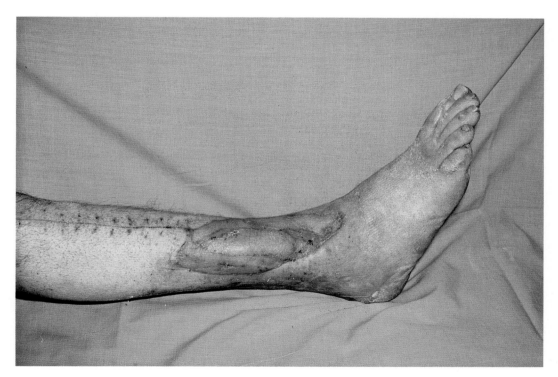

11

Healed wound approximately six weeks later. The fibular fracture healed, and the osteomyelitis has not recurred over a six year period.

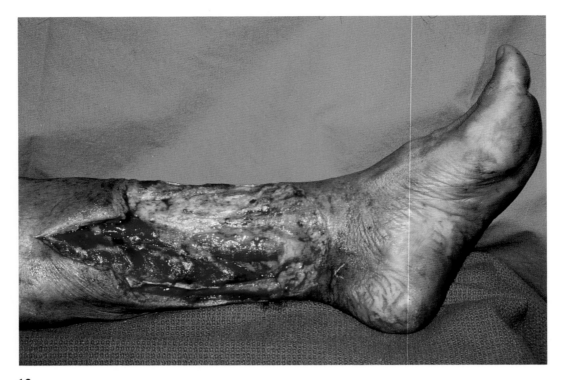

12

Skin loss of the anterior and medial calf following a Linton procedure for venous hypertensive disease. The patient had previously undergone more than twenty skin grafting procedures. She was strongly advised to have a very high below-knee amputation. (Case of J.B. McCraw)

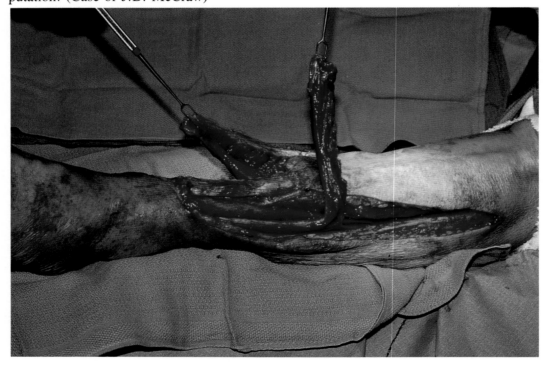

13

The wound was widely excised to remove all incompetent venous perforators. A proximally based soleus muscle flap is elevated medially, and a ''reversed'' EDC muscle flap is elevated laterally.

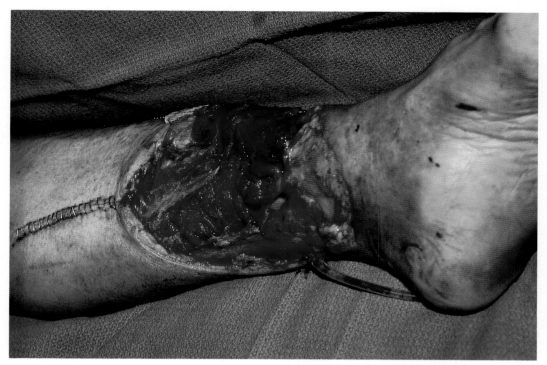

14

The soleus and EDC muscle flaps were approximated at the medial border of the tibia. Note that the "reversed" EDC muscle flap completely covers the distal tibia.

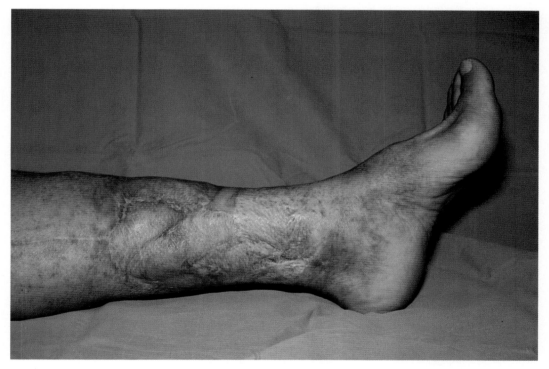

15

The split thickness skin grafts of the proximal soleus and distal EDC muscle flaps have remained healed for eight years.

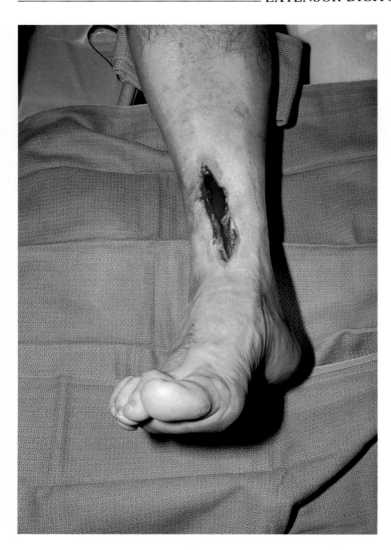

16

Extensive tibial osteomyelitic defect in a fifty-six-year-old man. The tibia is stable, but the infection has been progressive over a five year period. A sequestrectomy had been done forty-eight hours earlier. (Case of P.G. Arnold)

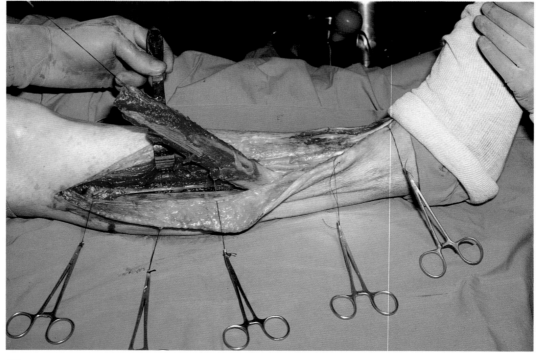

17

''Reversed'' EDC muscle flap elevated. Note the large size of the retracted muscle.

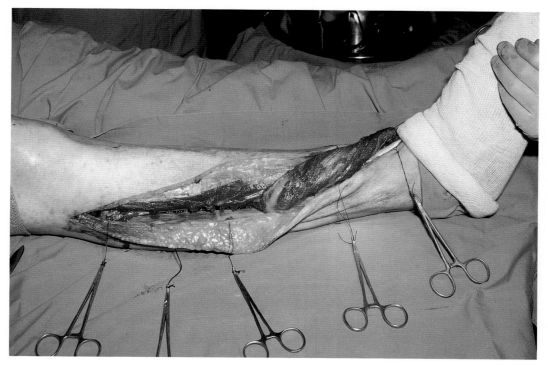

18

The tibial defect was completely obliterated by the EDC muscle flap. The EDC tendons were tenodesed.

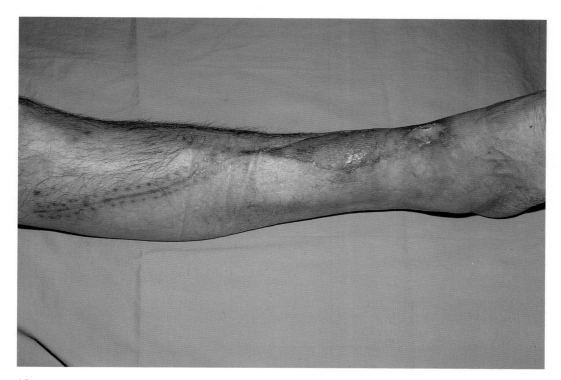

19

Healed muscle flap and STG at four months. The wound has remained healed for seven years. This wound certainly could be handled with a "free" flap today, but the EDC muscle flap still provides a useful alternative.

SMALL MUSCLES OF THE FOOT
ABDUCTOR HALLUCIS AND FLEXOR DIGITORUM BREVIS

ANATOMICAL CONSIDERATIONS

Surface Markings

The abductor hallucis muscle is located on the medial aspect of the foot and parallels the first metatarsal bone. It is easily palpated and consistent in its location. The flexor digitorum brevis (short flexor) muscle fans out from the midportion of the os calcis and parallels the long flexor tendons in its course to the toes.

Origin and Insertion

The abductor hallucis muscle originates from the medial aspect of the calcaneus and is adherent to the first metatarsal bone throughout its length. The muscle inserts into the medial condyle of the proximal phalanx of the great toe. The short flexors originate from the medial process of the calcaneus as well as from the plantar fascia. These small muscles individually insert into the middle phalanges of the second through fifth toes. Both the abductor hallucis and the short flexor muscles are completely expendable from a functional standpoint.

Adjacent Muscles

Although the abductor digiti quinti muscle may be large enough to use as a muscle flap, the adequacy of its volume must be confirmed by exploration. It can be used to cover a small lateral heel defect, if it is converted into a pure "island" flap, but it certainly does not reach the dorsum of the foot nor the lateral malleolus as has been diagrammatically suggested by others. An "island" extensor digitorum brevis muscle flap usually can be transposed from the dorsum of the foot to the lateral malleolus, but the length of the vascular leash is variable.

Vascular Pattern

As expected from their anatomical locations, the abductor hallucis muscle is supplied only by the medial plantar vessels, while the flexor digitorum brevis muscle is supplied by both the medial and lateral plantar vessels. The abductor hallucis muscle has a secondary vascular leash which penetrates the midportion of its muscular belly, but this can be sacrificed without fear of harm to its viability.

Motor Nerve

Medial plantar nerve.

Sensory Nerve

Medial plantar nerve.

USES

The abductor hallucis and the flexor digitorum brevis muscles are the two muscles which are consistently available for the transposition in the foot. These two muscles have limited arcs of rotation and can only be used to close small wounds, but they are quite helpful in certain situations. They have the added benefit of maintaining some pressure sensibility which is important in the ambulatory patient. They can also be used to augment the viability of local flaps of sole skin. For the most part the flexor digitorum brevis muscle flap is used for heel coverage and the abductor hallucis muscle flap is used for defects which lie between the medial malleolus and the heel. Neither muscle will consistently reach the Achilles area nor the flair of the medial malleolus.

REGIONAL FLAP COMPARISONS

These muscle flaps are best compared to the dorsalis pedis axial flap and the vascularized sole flap, which may or may not include the short flexor muscles. These cutaneous flaps offer the distinct advantage of providing surface sensibility but their donor sites usually require a skin graft. The dorsalis pedis flap provides the most predictable coverage for the medial and lateral malleoli which are beyond the reach of the small muscles of the foot. The dorsalis pedis flap is similarly useful for innervated heel coverage when the arterialized sole flap is unavailable. Unlike any other local foot flap, the "island" dorsalis pedis flap

597

can reach the Achilles tendon area. In children up to the age of ten, an ipsilateral buttock flap can be used because the knee joint in young children can be immobilized for two to three weeks and then rapidly remobilized. The donor site of this flap is good, but the gymnastics of the flap manipulations are not well tolerated by even young patients.

Although "free" microvascular transfers should always be considered as an option for these difficult foot defects, there are several unsolved problems. Flap viability is only 85% to 95% in good hands, usually because of the unsatisfactory nature of the recipient vessels. "Free" sensory innervated skin flaps have also been disappointing in the quality of their sensibility, which has generally not been good enough to protect the flap from late ambulatory loss. "Free" muscle transfers seem to be more durable than "free" skin transfers, even though they are less sensate. The conventional explanation for this is that the "shear" effect, which is normally prevented by the fibrous septa of heel skin, is more damaging to transferred subcutaneous fat than it is to transferred muscle. The "free" muscle transfer does become densely adherent to the os calcis, and perhaps this helps cushion any damaging "shear." There is little doubt that "free" transfers will become routine procedures in the future, but their anticipated advantages over local flaps have not yet been realized.

DISADVANTAGES

These transposed intrinsic muscles of the foot do not carry normal surface sensibility and they must be covered with a skin graft. Their dissection is tedious because they are intertwined with the sensory nerves of the sole of the foot. It should be recognized that they cover only small defects and certainly do not reach the dorsum of the foot nor the malleoli. These small muscles are frequently too atrophic to be usable at all in the denervated foot.

ADVANTAGES

The intrinsic muscles of the sole of the foot find their primary applications in the correction of heel ulcerations or in osteomyelitis of the os calcis. Even though their dissection is difficult, they provide a much simpler operation than most of the usual alternatives, such as the dorsalis pedis flap or a "free" microvascular transfer. Even though the local "island" cutaneous flaps provide better sensibility, these small muscle flaps maintain enough deep pressure sensibility to protect the walking surfaces of the foot.

COMPLICATIONS, PITFALLS, AND DONOR SITE

The safe dissection of these muscles depends on adequate exposure. In general a direct incision over the muscle belly is the most expeditious choice. Fortunately, the resulting scar is well tolerated in normal ambulation. The elevation of the abductor hallucis muscle is straightforward since it is primarily a dissection of the muscle away from the first metatarsal bone and the medial plantar nerve. The short flexors are more difficult to elevate because they need to be carefully separated from the intertwined digital nerves. The plantar fascia should always be elevated with the short flexors, to provide a fascial layer for suturing and to hold the small muscles together as a cohesive unit.

The donor site is inconsequential, unless a skin graft is required. The plantar skin flap donor site can frequently be primarily closed if enough of the os calcis is removed, but it is usually necessary to place a skin graft on the non-weight-bearing surface of the foot. The remaining weight-bearing skin will usually cornify and thicken enough to protect the ambulatory foot. The compound myocutaneous flap is preferred in the denervated foot since the small muscles of the foot may be atrophic to the point that they are difficult to identify.

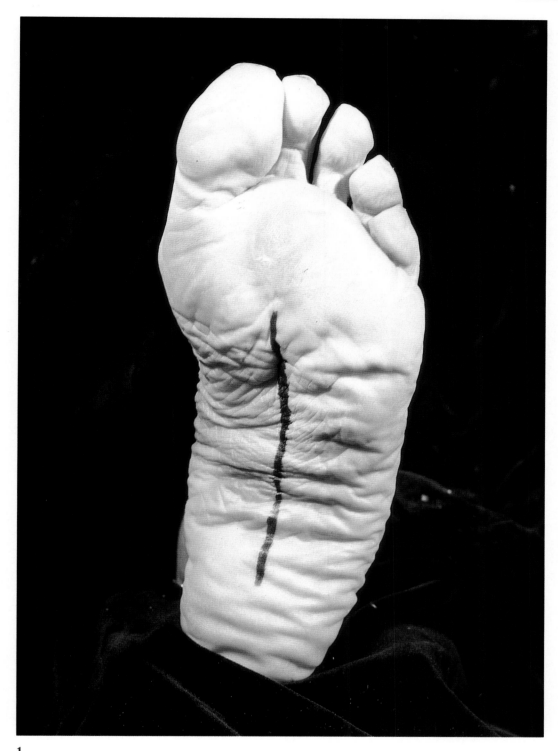

1

Midline plantar incision for retrieval of
the flexor digitorum brevis muscle in a
cadaver.

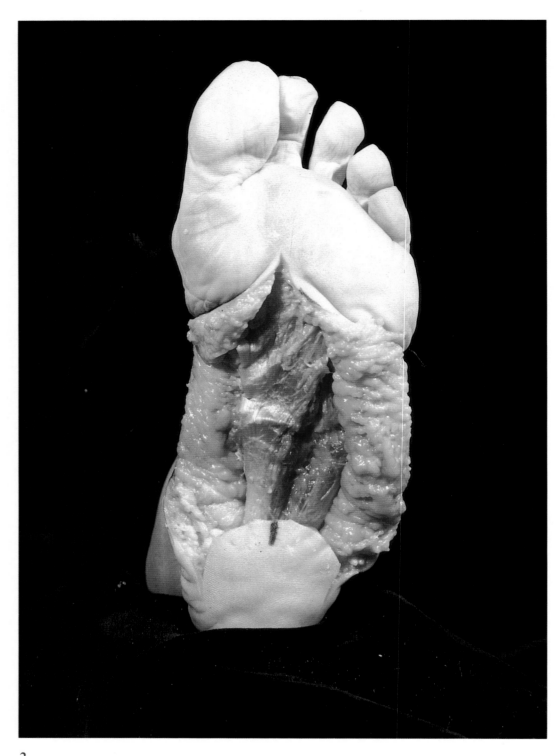

2

The plantar fascia is left attached to the
surface of the flexor digitorum brevis
muscle. Note how the muscle fans out
from its os calcis origin to the distal
insertion.

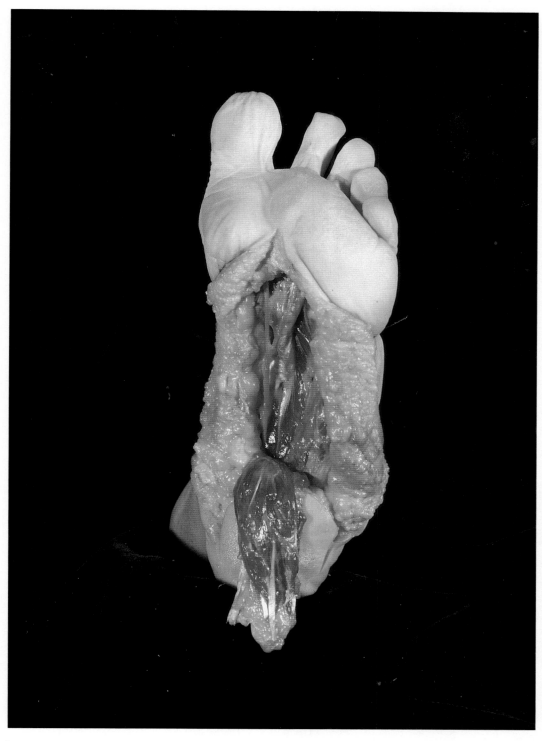

3

Short flexors transposed to the heel. The plantar nerves and vessels are protected in the course of the flap elevation.

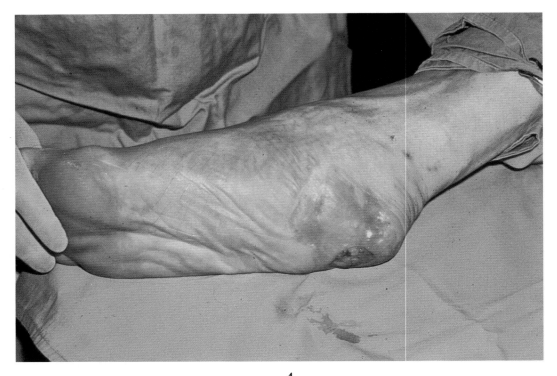

4

Chronic osteomyelitis of the os calis in a fifty-seven-year-old male. Multiple debridements failed to correct the osteomyelitis, and the skin-grafted heel was subject to constant ulceration. (Case of P.G. Arnold)

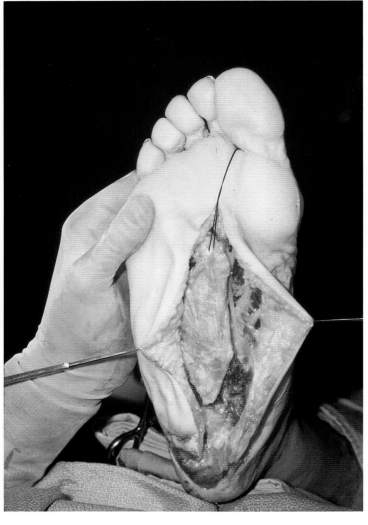

5

The short flexors are exposed through a midline plantar incision. The plantar fascia is left attached to the muscle.

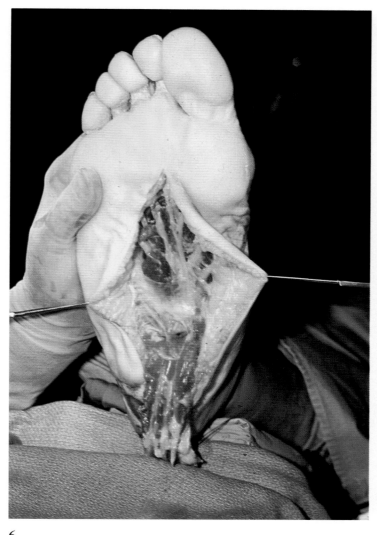

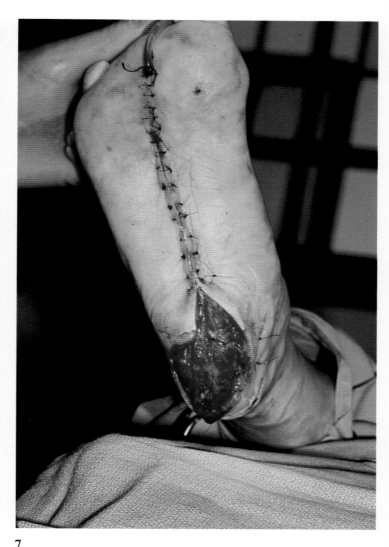

6

Short flexor muscle transposed to the heel. Note the medial and lateral plantar nerves and vessels above the lymbrical muscles and long flexor tendons.

7

Appearance of the flexor digitorum brevis muscle flap after forty-eight hours, at the time of skin grafting.

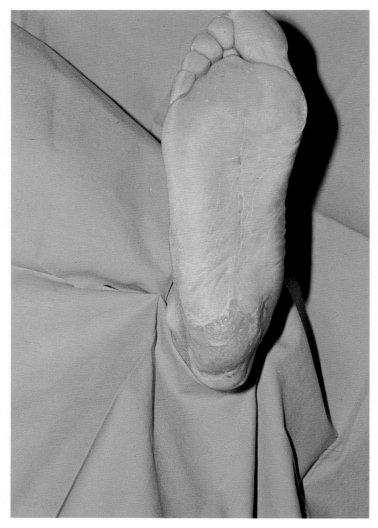

8

Eighteen months following the closure.
The osteomyelitis has not recurred, and
the patient has been able to work as a
machinist without further ulceration. Note
the midline donor site scar.

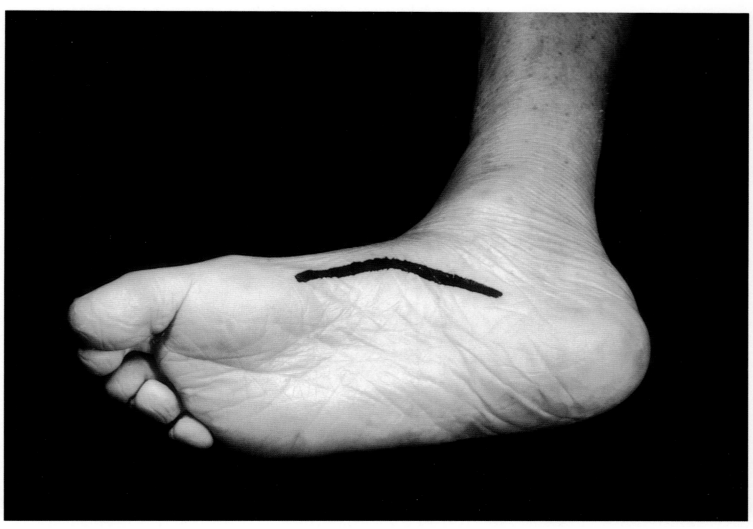

9

The usual incision for the retrieval of the abductor hallucis muscle is demonstrated in a cadaver.

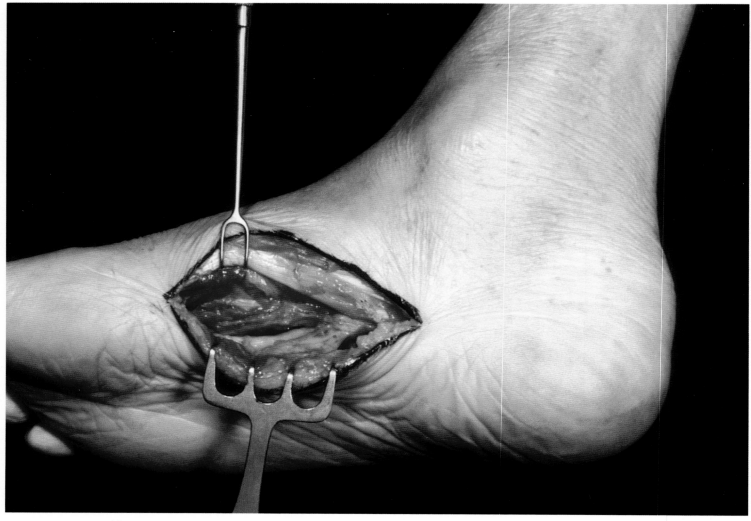

10

The abductor hallucis muscle is retracted superiorly. The short flexor muscle is exposed by retracting the plantar fascia inferiorly.

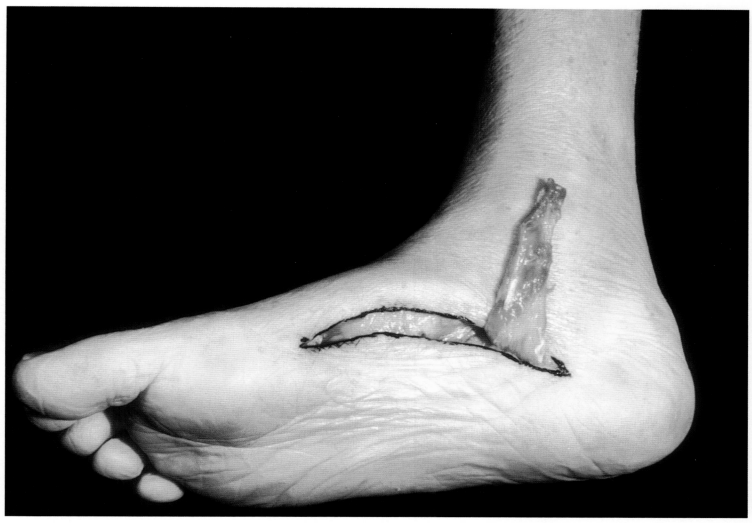

11

The small abductor hallucis muscle barely
reaches the medial malleolus.

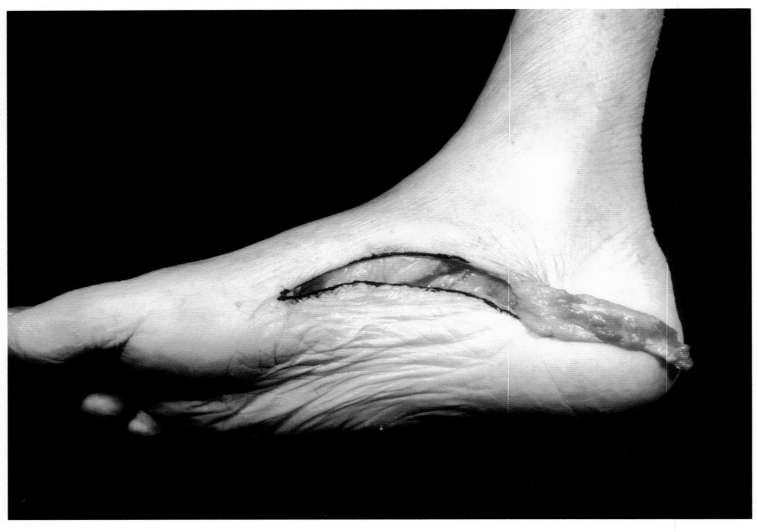

12

Posterior rotation of the abductor hallucis muscle. The size of this intrinsic muscle is variable and must be determined at exploration.

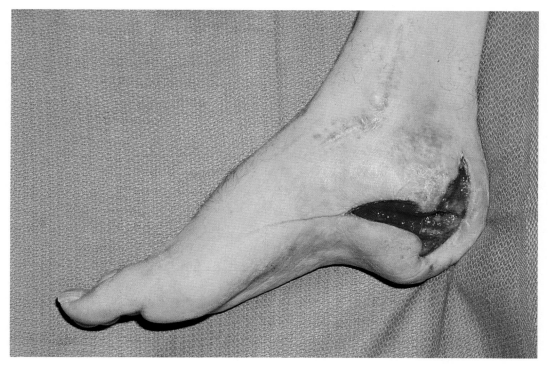

13

Osteomyelitis of the os calcis in a thirty-four-year-old airline pilot. The defect will be extended anteriorly to expose the abductor hallucis muscle. (Case of P.G. Arnold)

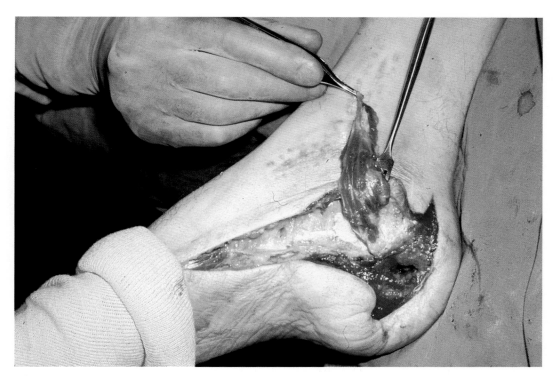

14

Elevated abductor hallucis muscle flap. The punched out sequestrectomy defect of the os calcis is seen centrally.

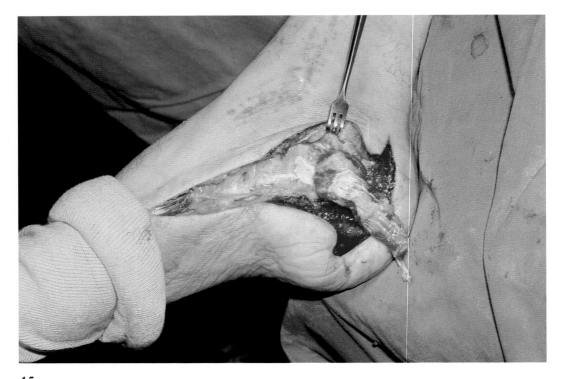

15

Muscle flap transposed into the bony
defect.

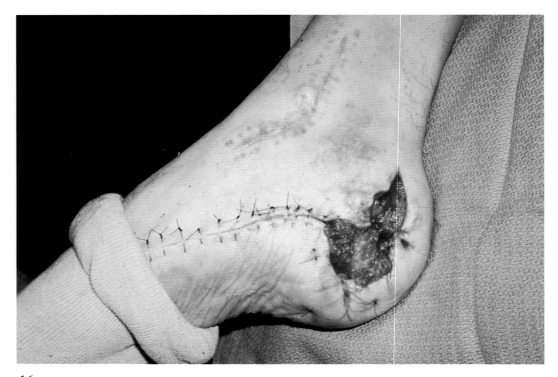

16

Appearance of the muscle flap at the time
of delayed skin grafting.

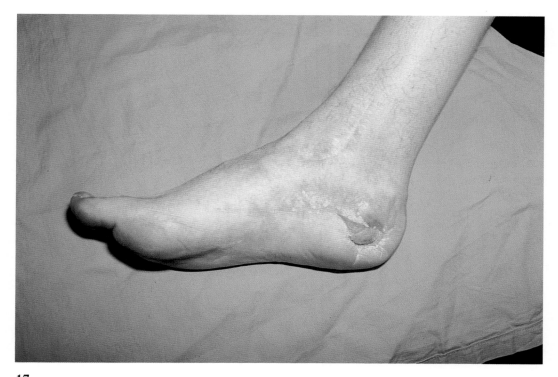

17

Five years following surgery. The patient wears a normal shoe, and the wound has remained healed for eight years.

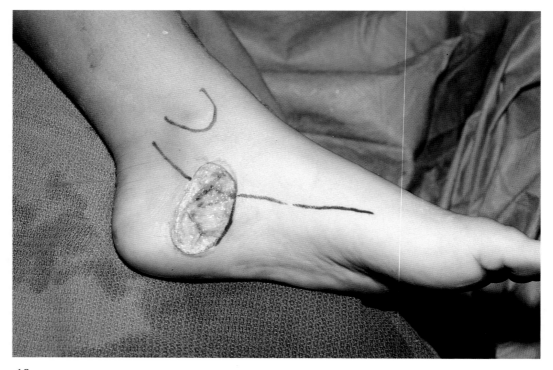

18

Resected hemangiopericytoma of the heel
in an eight-year-old girl. (Case of J.B.
McCraw)

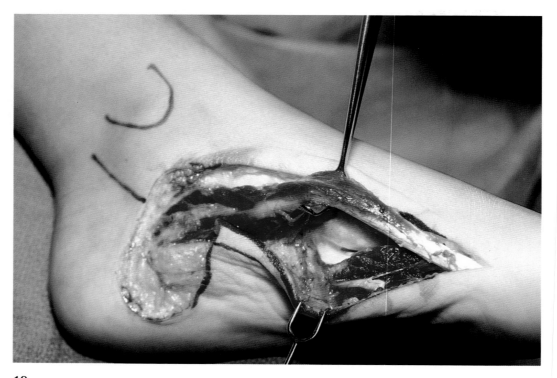

19

Retracted abductor hallucis muscle.

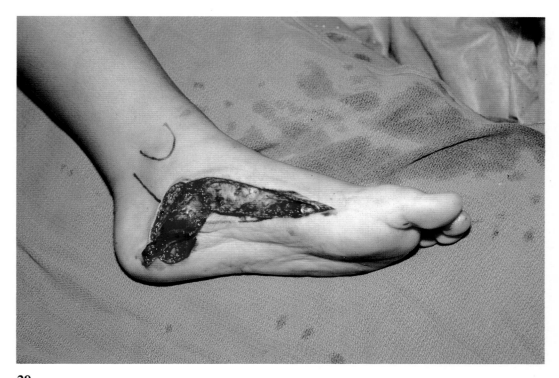

20
Abductor hallucis muscle transposed posteriorly.

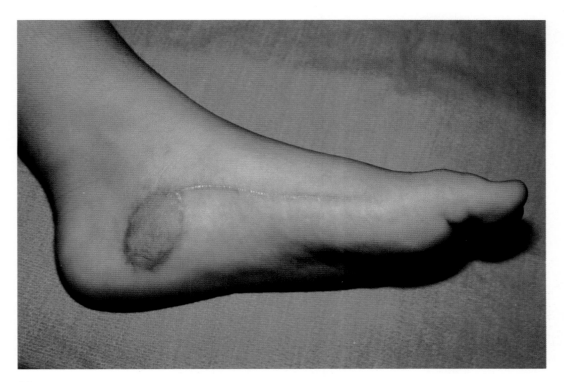

21
Skin-grafted muscle flap at four months. The full-thickness skin graft was harvested from the groin. Good pressure sensibility has been maintained in the muscle flap.

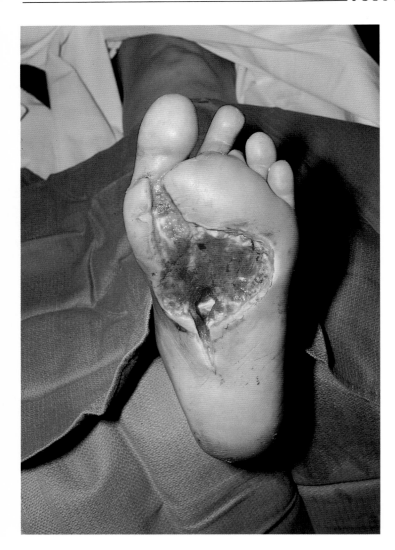

22

Fifty-year-old diabetic female with osteo-myelitis of the proximal first and second metatarsal bones following a deep plantar abscess. (Case of P.G. Arnold)

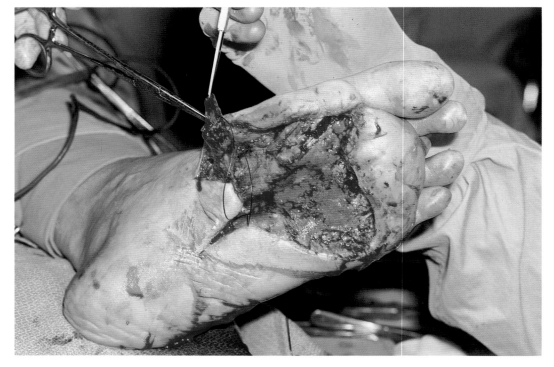

23

Elevated abductor hallucis muscle. The debrided distal sole wound will be skin grafted. The muscle flap will be used to obliterate the proximal metatarsal bone defects.

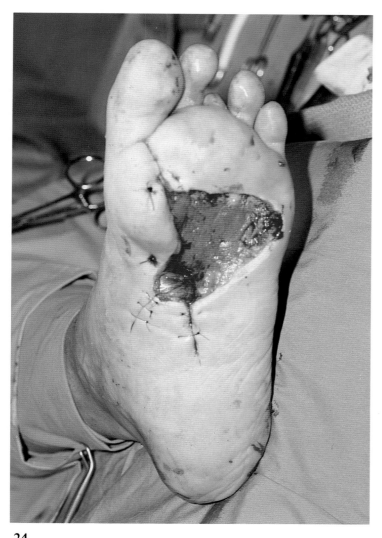

24
Abductor hallucis muscle transposed over the base of the second metatarsal bone. Skin grafting was delayed for forty-eight hours.

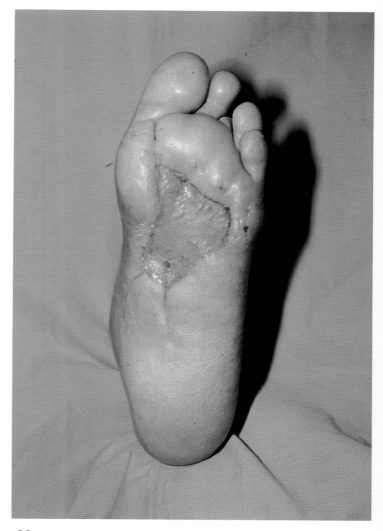

25
The osteomyelitis has not recurred, and the wound has remained healed for six years.

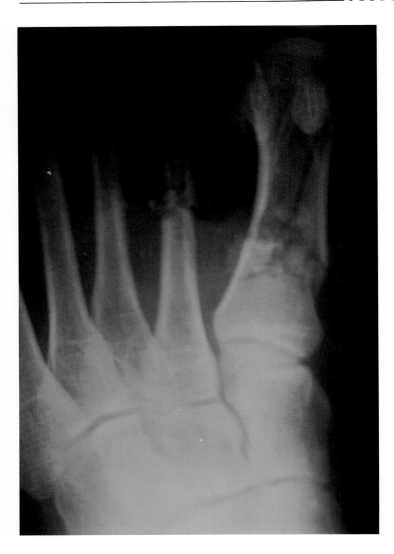

26
Open fractures of the first and second metatarsal bones from a riding lawn-mower injury. (Case of J.B. McCraw)

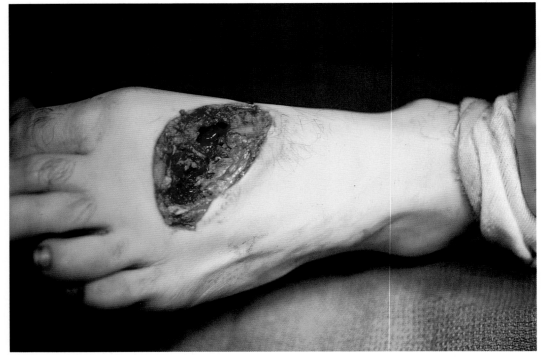

27
The anterior surfaces of the metatarsal bones were destroyed by the lawnmower blade. There was no loss of the dorsal foot skin.

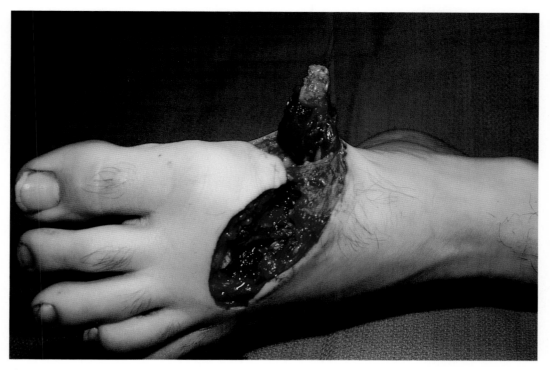

28

Abductor hallucis muscle elevated to cover the dorsal surface of the metatarsal bones. An immediate muscle flap was used to revascularize the contaminated fractures.

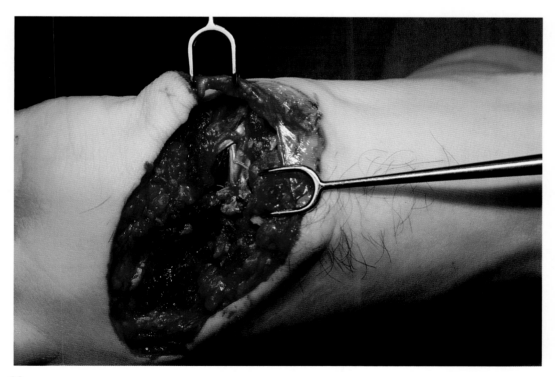

29

Transposed muscle flap. The fractures were stabilized with Kirschner wires.

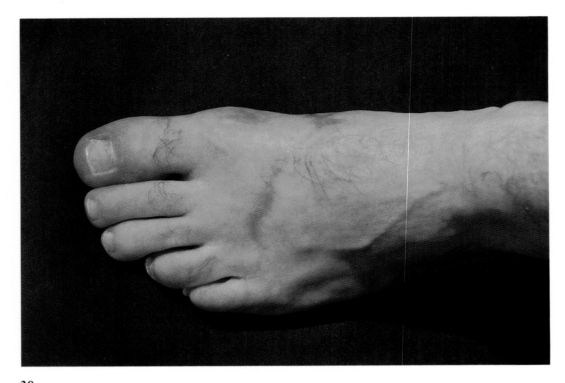

30

Healed wound at one year. The patient
returned to normal activities.

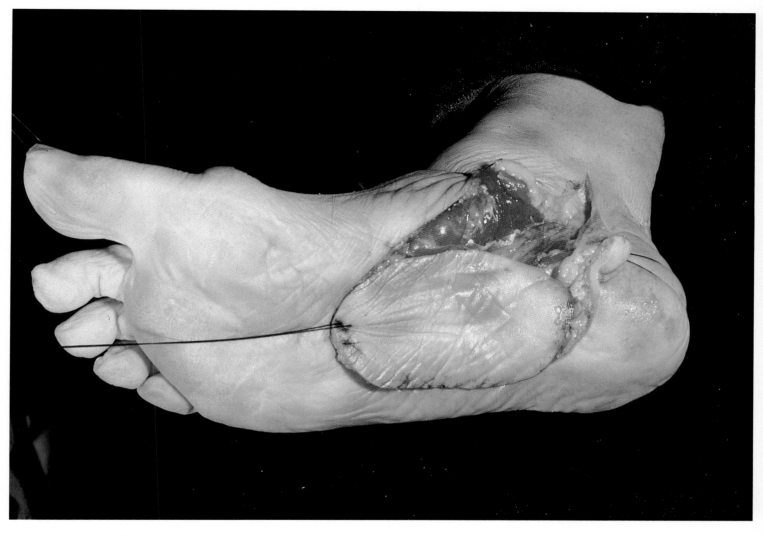

31

Cadaver dissection of the compound flexor digitorum brevis sole flap, which is based on the medial plantar artery and nerve. The posterior tibial nerve and vessels are first identified in the "tarsal tunnel" prior to elevation of the short flexor muscle and the sole skin.

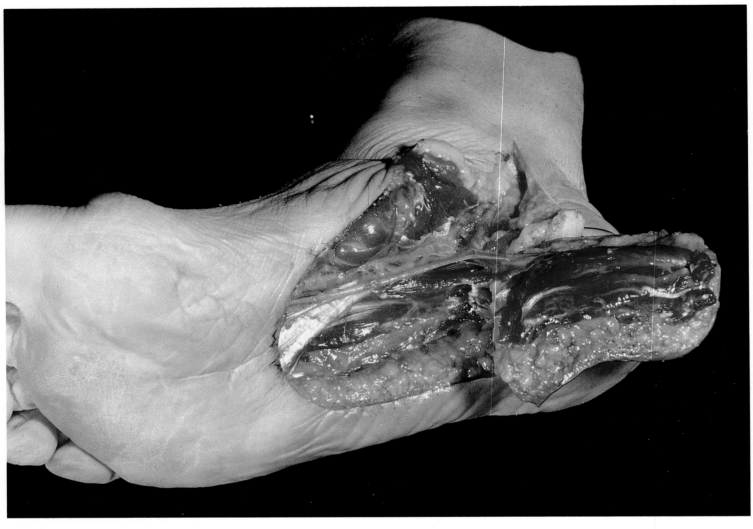

32

The compound flap is elevated with the
plantar fascia and the flexor digitorum
brevis muscles. Note the branch of the
medial plantar nerve which enters the flap
medially.

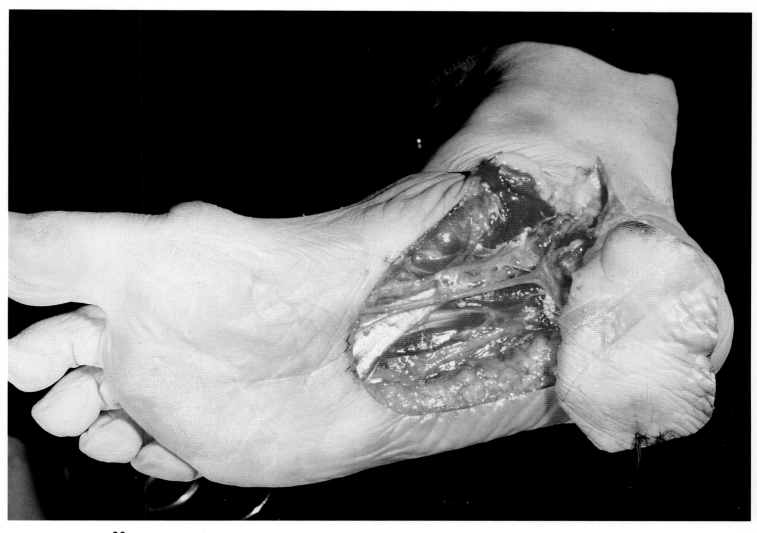

33

Transposition of the "island" flap to the
heel as a sensory innervated flap.

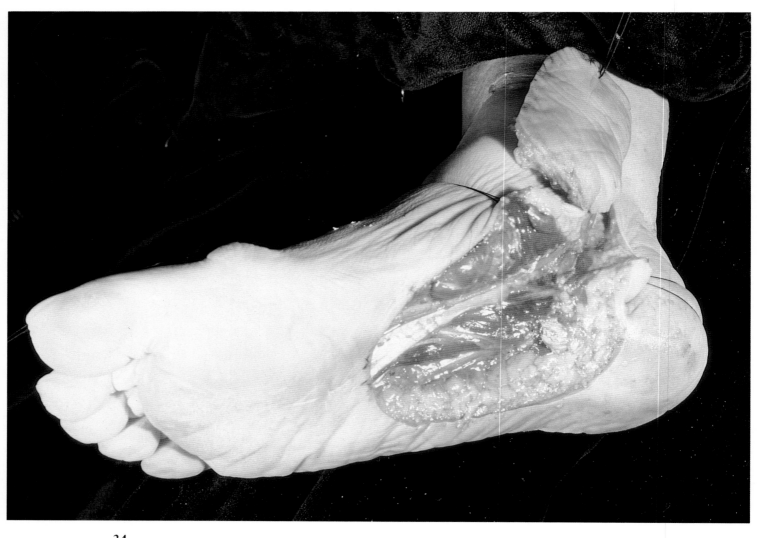

34

The ''island'' flap will reach the medial malleolus.

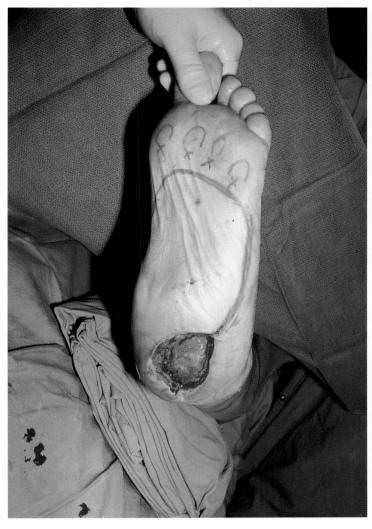

35

Fifty-nine-year-old paraplegic with a longstanding pressure sore of the heel. Outline of the medial plantar flap. (Case of P.G. Arnold)

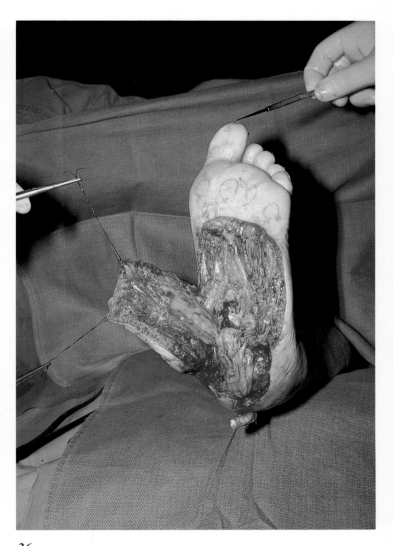

36

The short flexor muscles were first rotated into the os calcis defect. The innervated medial plantar fasciocutaneous flap was used for the overlying surface coverage of the heel.

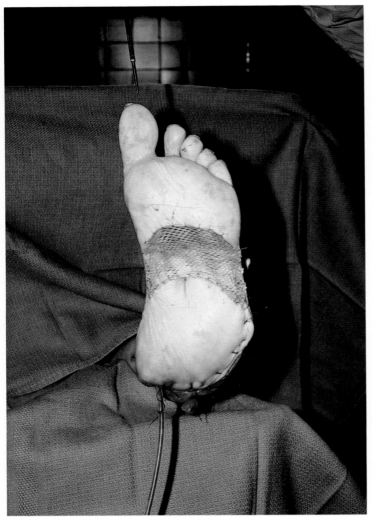

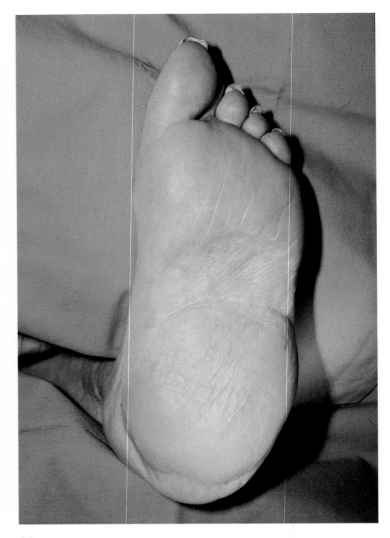

37

A meshed skin graft was used to cover
the donor site. In an ambulatory patient
more of the lateral weight-bearing surface
of the foot would have been left in the instep area, but this was not a consideration
in this paraplegic patient.

38

Four months following the closure. The
flap and the donor site skin graft have remained healed for six years.

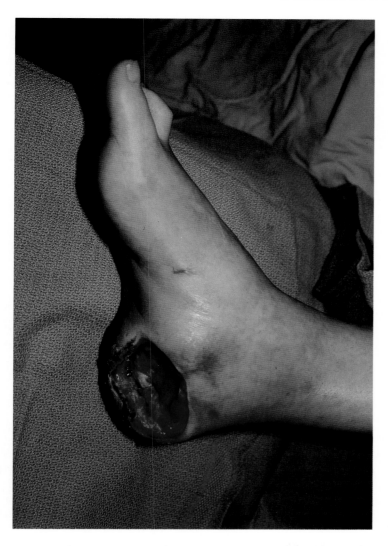

39

Osteomyelitis of the os calcis in a sixty-two-year-old diabetic patient with extremely poor sensation in the sole of the foot. The patient had been hospitalized elsewhere for over seven months for this heel problem, and multiple skin grafts had failed. (Case of J.B. McCraw)

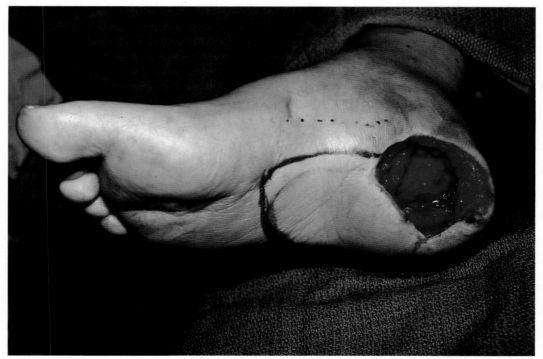

40

Appearance after one debridement of the heel ulcer. A laterally based flap was chosen because of the medial location of the heel defect.

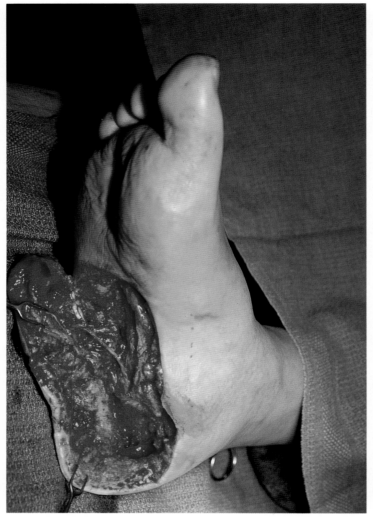

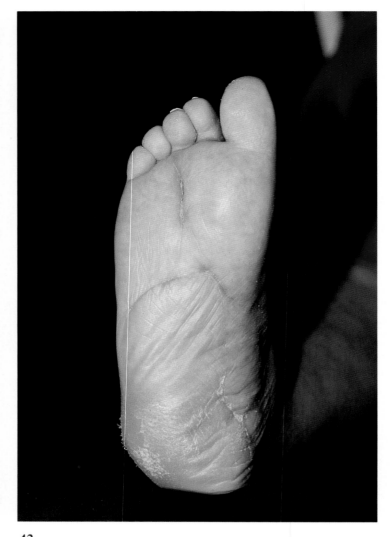

41

The sole flap included the lateral plantar vessels and nerve, which are visible near the lateral aspect of the flap. It was necessary to excise approximately one-half of the os calcis in order to eradicate the osteomyelitis.

42

Primary wound closure was possible because of the extensive removal of the os calcis.

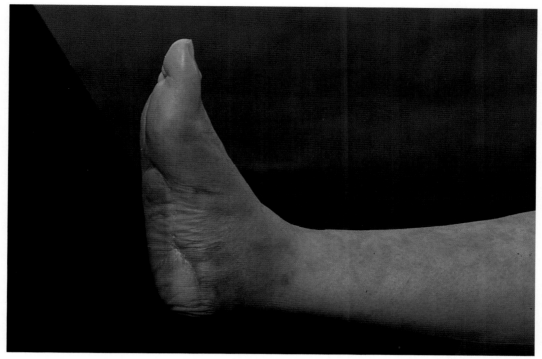

43

The lateral view demonstrates the reduced volume of the os calcis. The os calcis resection had no significant effect on ambulation with the use of special shoes. The osteomyelitis has not recurred during the six year follow-up period.

COMPLICATIONS

All of the early proponents of muscle flap surgery have emphasized the complications associated with these new procedures. Our honesty in these matters has not been derived from an inherent personal goodness, as much as it has come from the necessity to offer something which is reproducible in the hands of another surgeon. We have already shown the good results. It comes time for the bad news. As P.G. has said: "If a fellow does any single operation enough times, he can generate a full carousel of good results. It's the two carousels he left at home that we learn from." Many times a clearly understood complication is more instructive than a vast array of home runs. Obviously, the avoidance of problems is our best defense, and that is the purpose of this chapter.

There are several questions we should ask before we do any operation:

1) Should the surgery be done at all?
2) Will the flap survive?
3) Will the flap adequately cover the defect?
4) What happens if the flap fails?

SHOULD THE SURGERY BE DONE?

The question of *whether the surgery should be done at all* is the most difficult consideration. Is the deformity so large that it will not be corrected by the proposed flap? For instance, a 95% successful coverage of an open joint equates with a 100% failure. Sometimes, two major flaps should be used, rather than "pushing" one flap to its physiological limits and risking a major wound healing failure. *Can the patient cope with the prolonged reconstructive efforts?* All these procedures are difficult for both the patient and the surgeon, and all of the involved parties need to recognize this at the outset. A below-knee amputation may be an unattractive option, but months of suffering through multiple, unsuccessful reconstructive procedures may be a worse option in retrospect. It is frequently more difficult to make this fundamental decision about a reconstructive procedure than it is for an elective esthetic procedure. *Can the patient afford the loss of work* and the attendant expenses? These procedures are not free even if the surgeon accepts what the "third party" carriers allow. The patient may lose time from work or may be saddled with ancillary expenses which exceed the family's financial capabilities. When one member of the household is unable to perform his normal functions, additional non-medical expenses related to the running of the home will be incurred. Expenses for travel to the hospital, the doctor's office, or the therapy department may even be a problem. In the case of a long-term disability the worker stands to lose his or her senior position or, ultimately, his or her job. One must always ask whether the patient might be better off with a simpler procedure, which might correct the problem less elegantly, when the more complex procedure may be tied to a loss of economic independence.

Another consideration is *whether the procedure will fulfill the goals and expectations* of the patient. Patients must, obviously, be realistic in their expectations. There are occasions when no operation, even one devised by the most clever surgeon, can ever accomplish the patient's goals. It should also be recognized that any operation can be detrimental to the patient's existing condition. There are risks with all of these operations, and certain complications can precisely be viewed as catastrophic. The surgeon can offer rationalizations and even claim that he was "badgered into doing the operation." He can thereby blame the patient if there is a problem because it was the patient's decision. That never works for obvious reasons. From the standpoint of a legal "informed consent," the patient must be adequately informed about the goals, alternatives, risks, and benefits, so that he, as a "reasonable and prudent" person, can make an intelligent decision from the information given. Flip Wilson's comment, "The devil made me do it" doesn't hold up well in or out of court.

In every muscle flap operation one should always assess the anticipated *functional loss* and compare it to the expected benefits of the operation. This is usually not a major consideration, with the exception of certain flaps, but it should always be taken into account.

Finally, there is the *"unhappy patient."* The "unhappy patient" is not unhappy for the day, instead, this is the patient who has always been unhappy and will always be unhappy. This person never intends to have a happy result and should never be expected to have one. This negative attitude is a major source of discontent because these sad patients readily become angry. Clearly, the angry patient is the common denominator in the generation of lawsuits. Short of that eventuality, they make everyone in sight miserable and negate the benefits of these elegant procedures.

WILL THE FLAP SURVIVE?

The second major consideration is *whether or not the flap will survive.* If it won't reliably survive, then there is little reason to undertake the procedure. There are numerous causes of flap necrosis which are beyond the control of the surgeon, such as a *vascular compromise* of the lower extremity. It is obvious that one would not elect to sacrifice one of the two main vessels in the calf just to complete a muscle flap reconstruction. This is similar to the consideration of using a "free" flap in the one vessel leg. Usually, this is only a theoretical concern, but it can lead to a devastating problem. The possibility of a catastrophic complication must always be weighed against the chance that only the use of that procedure could save the extremity. In the case of the ischemic leg, a muscle flap is usually serviceable if it is non-tender and has a pink "muscular" appearance, even though the arteriorgram does not demonstrate any primary vessels to the flap. Uncomplicated *diabetes* is not a condition which has caused any noticeable changes in these "axial" flaps, with the exception of the distal cutaneous foot flaps. This is probably related to the fact that the very small, distal vessels are affected earlier in the course of the disease than are the major vessels. Advanced or long-standing diabetes is frequently associated with severe segmental arteriosclerosis of the major vessels, which can adversely affect the survival of a muscle flap or the survival of the entire extremity. *Denervation* makes some muscles unusable for soft tissue replacement because of atrophy. It does not seem to harm muscle flap viability. Denervation definitely diminishes the ability of certain long, thin muscles (e.g. the gracilis) to "carry" their overlying skin. Whether this is the direct result of denervation or is caused by the paralytic avascularity is a matter of conjecture. This effect is seldom seen in the flat muscles (e.g. the latissimus dorsi muscle) since their ability to form a compound myocutaneous flap is empirically undiminished. *Irradiation* does have a detrimental effect on the cutaneous segment of a myocutaneous flap, but it seldom results in flap necrosis. It is also unusual for irradiation to fatally harm the dominant vessels of the flap unless the irradiation dose has been truly massive. A more worrisome problem is the irradiated "random" skin at the site of inset. Loss of this skin is not at all uncommon, particularly when the progressive effects of the irradiation have had a long period of time to destroy the microcirculation of this skin. This may leave a viable myocutaneous flap stranded in a sea of surrounding dead "random" irradiated flaps. Necrosis of irradiated muscle flaps has not been observed even when there is "woody" fibrosis of the muscle. *Infection* can be a source of flap loss but it is most unusual and generally involves opportunistic bacterial invasion. It becomes effective, for the most part, in an already ischemic flap which is "fragile" enough to be lost with even the slightest additional insult. *Smoking* is a source of flap loss which is clearly recognized. One hates to incriminate a drug which is so commonly used, but nicotine ingestion is unequivocally harmful to flaps; and some patients are more sensitive to the peripheral vasoconstrictive and ischemic effects of nicotine than others. The harmful microcirculatory effect of nicotine may also persist for weeks after the cessation of smoking. There is no reliable preoperative cure for smoking, but there is an excellent postoperative cure. One simply maintains the patient on nasal oxygen and prohibits smoking. The "fire hazard" has proved to be a compelling motivator for these unfortunate addicts. When the cessation of smoking is critical to the survival of the flap, as in the case of the TRAM flap or a "free" flap, a preoperative urine nicotine level can be obtained to verify cessation. If the patient knows that the surgery will be cancelled because of the added risk of nicotine use, the urine nicotine test can act as a reasonable and civilized deterrent to continued smoking. *Cold* is a recognized cause of flap loss and should be avoided in both the operating room and the ward. There are certain flaps which are known to be cold-sensitive and they should be especially protected. The "core" body temperature can be maintained in the operating room by using warm ambient temperature, heated inspired air, heated intravenous fluids, a heating blanket, extremity wraps, and arctic body bags. Even the fluids to wash off the surface of the skin should be heated. The flap should also be protected with warm packs which are maintained at 37 degrees. We have passed the day when the "modern" operating room comes equipped with a heated Mayo basin which keeps the fluid temperature at 37 degrees. We have reinstated this antiquated practice, and until we did this, the too cold or too hot irrigation fluid temperature was determined by the nurse's gloved hand. This crude method of determining what is expected to be hot or cold to the patient's skin would never be tolerated by the awake patient. It has caused burns of the skin from steaming fluid and necrotic flaps from fluid which was too cold. The harmful effects of flap manipulation, in respect to *torsion* or *tension* which lead to vascular "spasm," are totally preventable. One must be very gentle in the amount of twist or stretch which is applied to both the vascular pedicle and the inset flap because this can make all the difference in the flap's survival. In addition, the *"crossing tension"* can be so excessive that it will result in the physical collapse of the subdermal plexus. When one fluoresces such a flap, it is easy to visualize the area of vascular compression, which appears as a blue streak across a nicely fluorescing "chartreuse" colored skin. This problem should be immediately corrected by "derotating" the flap and rearranging the closure.

WILL THE FLAP
COVER THE DEFECT?

A third question is *whether the flap will adequately cover the defect*. One must always have a secondary flap choice in mind as a ''back-up.'' This doesn't mean that when the primary flap fails, we start thinking about our alternative flap choice. Instead, it is the same mental processing which one should go through in the course of choosing a ''free'' flap. If a ''free'' flap is elected as the first line of defense, one should always have a ''back-up'' local flap available in the event of the loss of the ''free'' flap. If, as it turns out, the local ''back-up'' flap could do the job more efficaciously, then one should not use the ''free'' flap. Using a similar logic, if one loses a ''free'' flap and is not willing to use another ''free'' flap for exactly the same problem, a local flap should have been used in the first place. Secondary, ''back-up'' flaps must be deliberated with the same care as the primary flap choice.

WHAT HAPPENS IF IT FAILS?

Finally, *what happens if everything fails?* Do you do the same procedure again? Do you do a ''free'' flap? Do you quit? Of course this is an unanswerable question, but we think one should have some sort of parachute mechanism available. Luis Vasconez has said this best. Every year at the Flap Workshop he shows a case in which he used one TFL flap for an abdominal defect and half of it died. He then shows the opposite TFL flap transposed to the abdomen and half of it died. His conclusion to this is very simple: ''If Plan A is a complete and abject failure, do not make Plan B precisely the same as Plan A.'' If a local flap fails, it is certainly not unreasonable to consider a ''free'' flap. The reverse of this condition is equally valid. In fact, every time a local flap is considered a ''free'' flap should be considered as a reasonable possibility. The complication rates in the near future will be very similar, if they are not already. It should be emphasized that the *simplest solution is usually the best solution*. This may be a skin graft or a ''random'' flap, but it can also be a ''free'' flap. Neither should the operation be designed to fit a text book description. For that reason we have not listed the four ''best'' options for each area of the body in the order of our preference and prejudice. This is a final consideration which must be carefully thought out by the surgeon himself. The responsible surgeon must at least be conversant with the multiplicity of options to intelligently make this fundamental decision. Since any flap can fail, it is surgically naive to be familiar with only a single method of flap reconstruction. Instead, we should contemplate ''digging out'' before the die is cast.

SUMMATION

The basis for success with any muscle flap procedure is a precise knowledge of anatomy. One should be prepared for the anatomical variations in the blood supply of the proposed flap and the alternative flaps as well. Luis Vasconez was the first to suggest that the branches of the profunda femoris artery enter the anterior thigh muscles parallel to the inguinal ligament, approximately ten centimeters below this ligament. This is very helpful for planning purposes, but we have all found the vascular configuration to be either better or worse than we had expected.

It seems axiomatic that one should proceed with a definite plan, but the plan should be more flexible than rigid. The defect should be excised first, and then the flap should be designed to fit the problem. This premise must be tempered by the availability of an assuredly viable flap in the case of a life-threatening defect e.g. an open chest wall. One really needs to be able to think about a number of optional flaps at the same time, as though you have access to a built-in flap computer to weigh multiple simultaneous variables. For instance, the excision of an ischial ulcer or a pretibial osteomyelitis may yield a defect which is far different than what was expected. In this case one either has to have an alternative plan or be ready to pack the wound and go home. Although there is no compulsion to complete every reconstruction in a single setting, the lack of an alternative procedure should seldom be a reason for a delayed completion. The intraoperative design of the flap is something that should present a minimal problem, unless there are intervening circumstances such as heavy irradiation or previous scarring.

The elevation and manipulation of any flap should be technically gentle, even though some of the large sutures used for closure cast the surgeon as somewhat antediluvian. Obviously, shearing forces, torsion, and the separation of the skin from the muscle should be avoided. The transfer of the flap should be straightforward, but should be performed delicately. Because muscle is extremely sensitive to compression, constricting tunnels or a tight inset of the flap must be avoided.

The aftercare is fairly simple. The patient needs to be carefully followed in an environment conducive to the healing of the flap. This may mean special beds, positioning, and room temperature control. As important as aftercare is, it is usually of secondary importance because virtually all of our surgical misfortunes begin in the operating room. After seeing the same complications repeated over and over by subsequent generations of resident surgeons, Dr. Nathan Womack always tried to put an end to the repetition, when he said: ''Do we have to keep repeating this same clinical experiment? We all know that it will work.'' The mistakes have already been made by others. They should not need to be reinvented by each new generation of reconstructive surgeons.

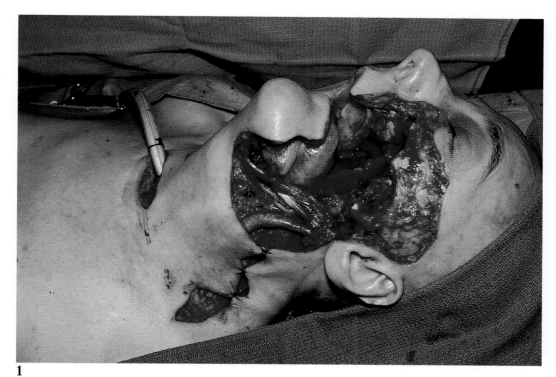

1

This seventy-four-year-old patient developed a well-differentiated squamous cell carcinoma of the buccal mucosa despite the absence of any history of alcohol or tobacco use. Positive frozen section margins were obtained throughout the procedure, and dictated the removal of half of the mandible and palate, the tonsillar area, the maxilla, and the cheek. Permanent pathological examination demonstrated microinvasion of vessels and involvement of six of twenty-six lymph nodes. An immunological deficiency and an unusually aggressive tumor should have been suspected in this elderly female who was a nonsmoker and a nondrinker. (Case of J.B. McCraw and G.L. Schecter)

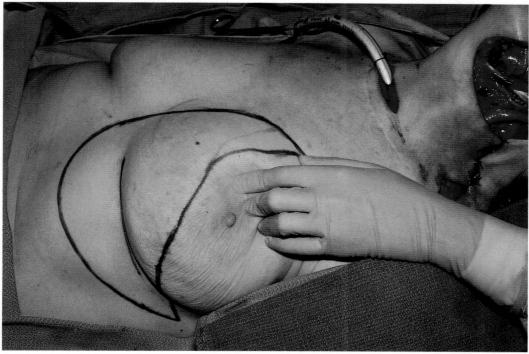

2

An extremely large pectoralis "paddle" was outlined. The flap carried virtually all of the breast tissue overlying the pectoralis major muscle. This was done to enhance the viability of the distal flap and to provide soft tissue "fill" for the cheek defect. During the extirpative procedure, the patient's core body temperature fell to 94 degrees, and it was not possible to raise the core temperature during the period of flap elevation.

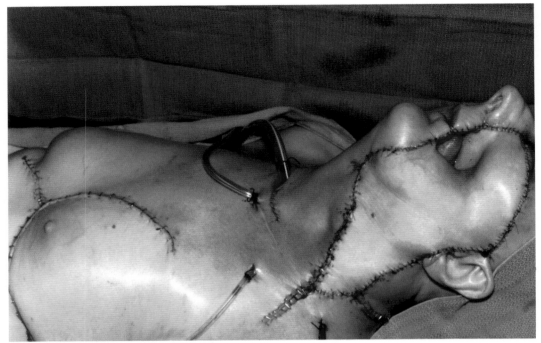

3

The donor site was primarily closed, and the flap was immediately inset. This particular flap design should be expected to be almost totally reliable, but the detrimental effects of the cold temperature resulted in very poor fluorescence. It was necessary to leave a large orocutaneous fistula so the palate, tonsil, and sulcus could be closed. It would have been preferable to have used a second flap to complete the reconstruction, but this was not possible for anesthetic reasons.

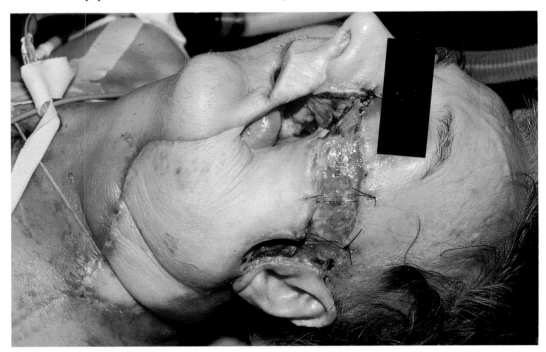

4

Only the distal one centimeter of the flap necrosed, but this completely disrupted the palatal and cheek closures. An opportunistic infection and gravity completed the disaster. The patient became desperately ill in the early postoperative course, and by the time it was possible to do a second flap, the aggressive tumor had recurred locally. She spent the rest of her days in the hospital in physical agony and emotional dejection, even to the exclusion of her family. This case raises a number of ''should'' questions about the advisability of this operation: 1) Should the procedure have been done in a single stage? 2) Should a marginally viable flap have been returned to the donor site? 3) Should the less cold-sensitive latissimus dorsi flap have been used instead of the pectoralis flap? and 4) What would the salvage procedure have been, if the patient had lived?

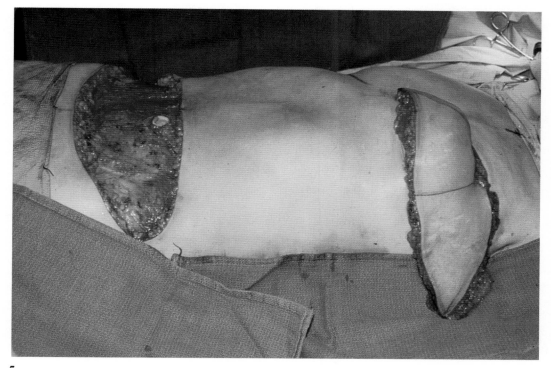

5

TRAM flap procedure in an ideal young candidate. The flap elevation was un-eventful. Intravenous florescein has been given and is visible in the flap. (Case of J.B. McCraw)

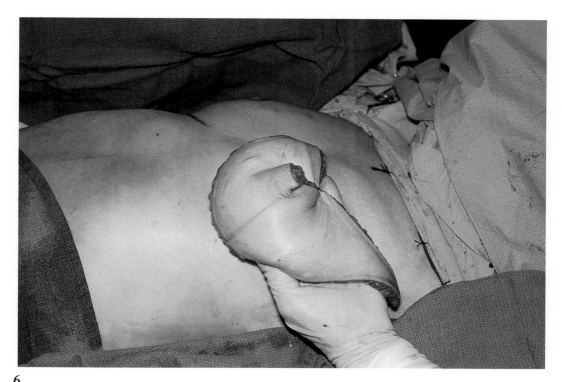

6

TRAM flap ready for insetting. The fluo-rescence of the entire flap is similar to the color of the surrounding skin.

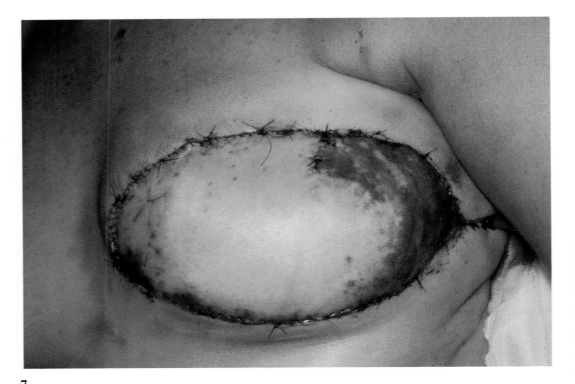

7

Appearance of the flap on the sixth post-operative day. The flap was pink and viable until the third postoperative day. The hospital room temperature dropped below 60 degrees, and the flap became totally blue over a six hour period. Warm packs corrected this cold-induced injury in the majority of the flap, but the lateral aspect of the flap was mortally wounded.

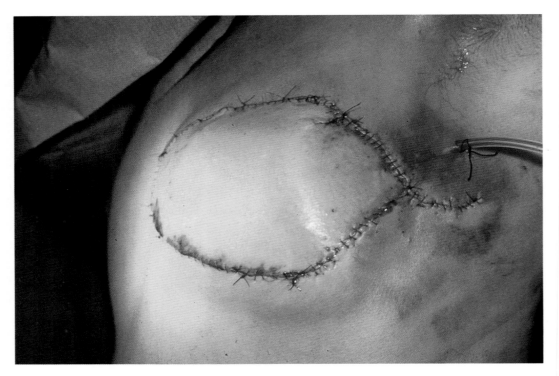

8

The lateral portion of the flap was excised and closed. This late loss of an initially healthy flap can only emphasize the fact that the TRAM flap is ''cold-sensitive.'' Protection of the flap from cold must be extended through the early postoperative period.

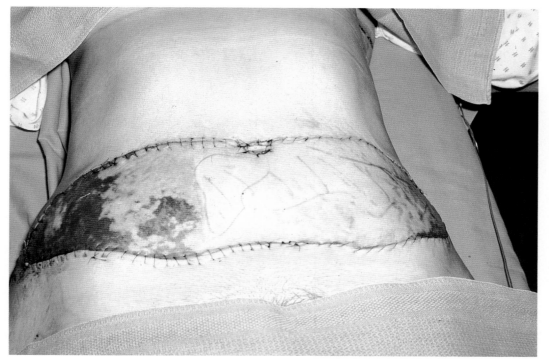

9

A left rectus abdominis myocutaneous flap was elevated and returned to the donor site because of very poor fluorescence. In this early case an attempt was made to remove very little anterior rectus fascia, and some obviously significant perforators were inadvertently excluded. Appearance of the flap at forty-eight hours. (Case of P.G. Arnold)

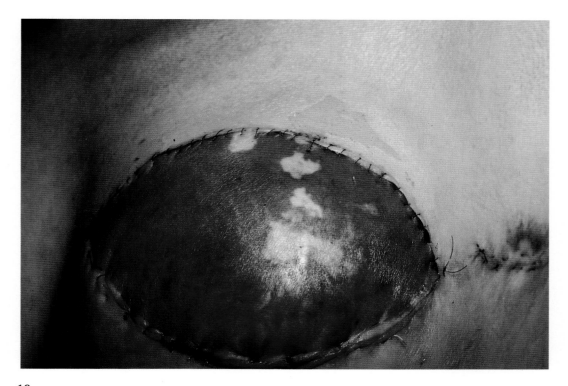

10

The flap was transferred at two days and was clearly nonviable at four days. The rectus abdominis flap was excised and replaced with a latissimus flap and an implant on the fourth day.

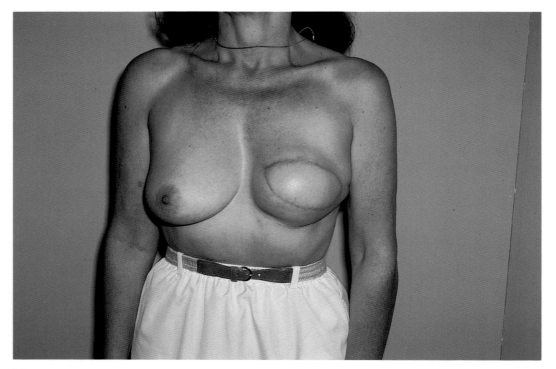

11

Appearance of nicely healed latissimus myocutaneous flap at six months. When a "salvage" flap is indicated, it should be done before the wound becomes stiff, unpliable, and infected.

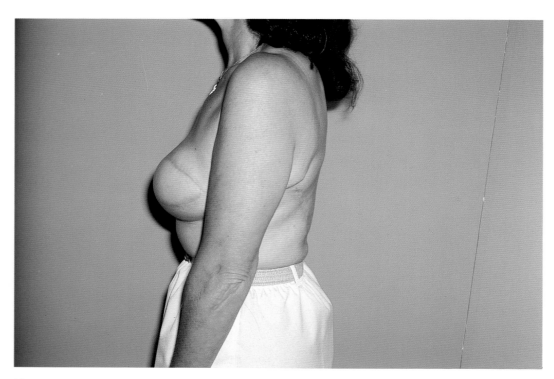

12

Lateral view at six months.

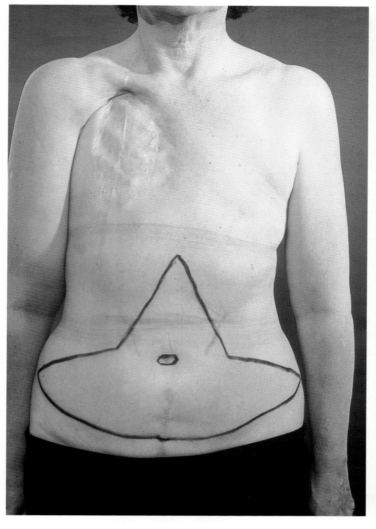

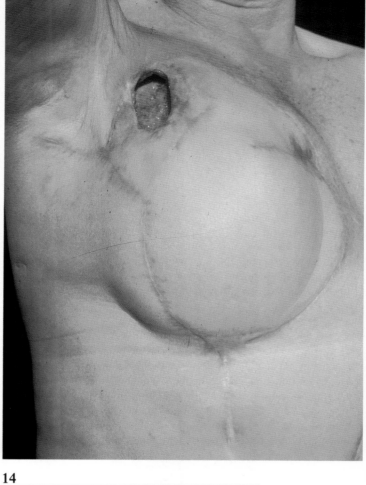

13

This patient offered every conceivable mastectomy deformity, including lymphedema. The breast and sternal areas had also been heavily irradiated. A combined vertical and horizontal TRAM flap was outlined because of the lower midline abdominal scar. This case predates the double muscle pedicle TRAM flap. (Case of J.B. McCraw)

14

The tip of the TRAM flap was lost. An attempt was made to retain a portion of the "opposite" abdominal skin in order to correct the axillary deformity. This flap ulceration started out as a one centimeter breakdown and evolved into a full-blown irradiation ulcer. Any flap introduced into a severely irradiated area must be totally self-sufficient since it will not receive any blood supply from the site of inset. It is also a futile exercise to hope that the "opposite" skin of a TRAM flap will survive beyond a midline scar.

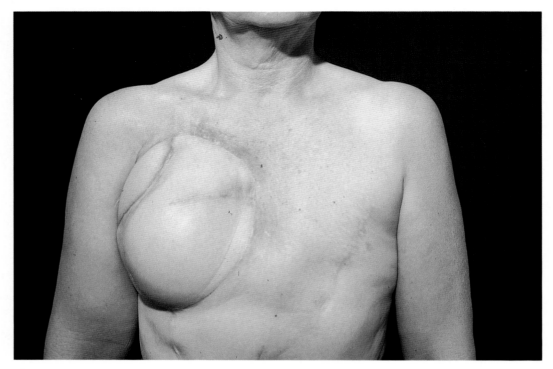

15

A small latissimus flap was brought into the axilla and the upper outer quadrant of the breast to repair the irradiation ulcer which we had created. In retrospect, it would have been advisable to have used both flaps in the initial operation because of the magnitude of the defect. Today, we would prefer a double muscle pedicle TRAM flap.

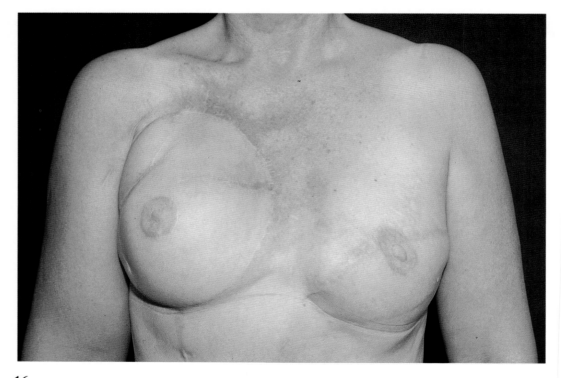

16

The rectus abdominis and latissimus dorsi flaps adequately reconstructed the massive right breast defect without an implant. Only the TRAM flap can be expected to correct such a complex deformity. The left breast was later reconstructed with a latissimus dorsi myocutaneous flap and an implant.

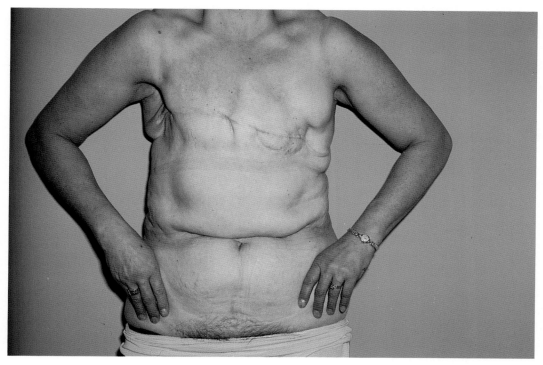

17

Fifty-eight-year-old female twelve years following a bilateral modified mastectomy. A lower midline scar extends from the umbilicus to the pubic area. Bilateral TRAM flaps were planned. (Case of P.G. Arnold)

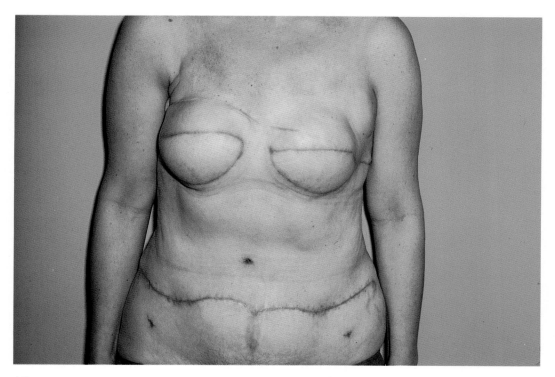

18

Appearance one year postoperatively. The level of flap inset at the "new" inframammary folds was chosen prior to the abdominal closure. The reconstructed breasts were positioned two to three centimeters lower than ideal. This could have been avoided by closing the abdominal donor site before a commitment had been made as to the level of the "new" inframammary fold. It is a difficult problem to correct after the fact.

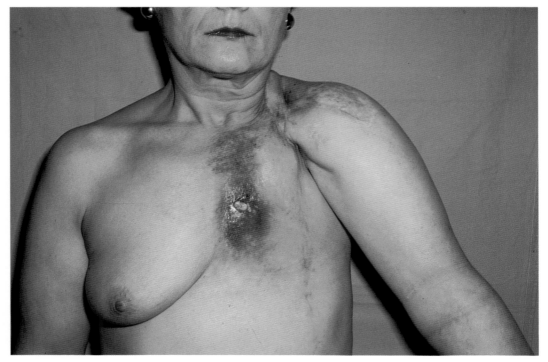

19

Fifty-seven-year-old female twenty-five years following a left radical mastectomy and irradiation therapy. Although the sternal ulceration had been present for only three weeks, the patient bled profusely from this ulcer on the day of admission. An emergency median sternotomy was re-quired for control of an eroded internal mammary vessel. Her consultant, P.G. Arnold, personally held pressure on this vessel in the vascular radiology suite, until operative control could be achieved. (Case of P.G. Arnold)

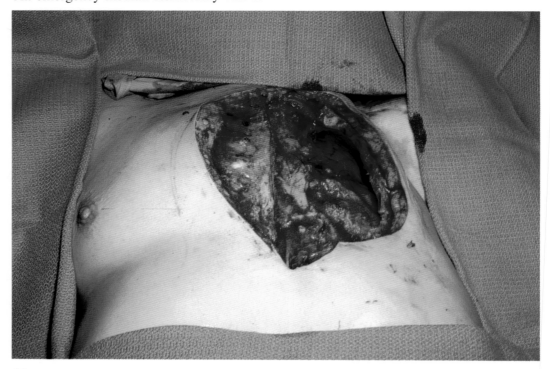

20

It was necessary to excise the left hemisternum and a major portion of the left anterior chest wall to remove the damaged tissue.

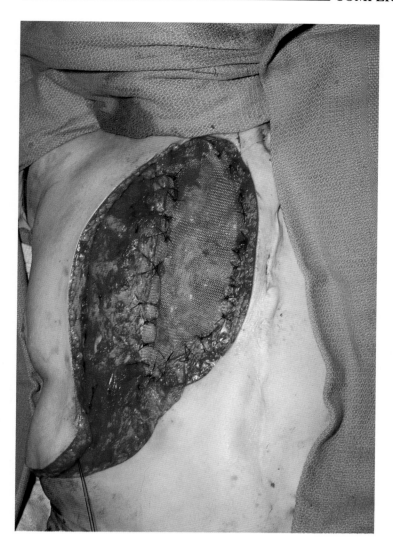

21

The thoracic skeleton was reconstructed with Prolene® mesh. The wound appeared to be "clean" following the debridement.

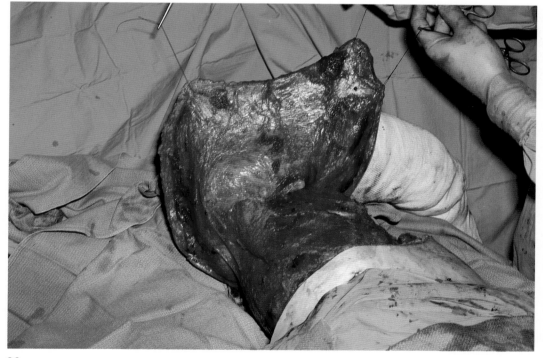

22

A massive myocutaneous flap was raised from the right chest wall. Both the pectoralis major and the latissimus dorsi muscles were included in the flap.

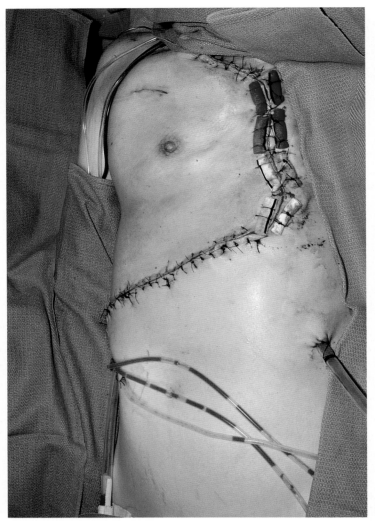

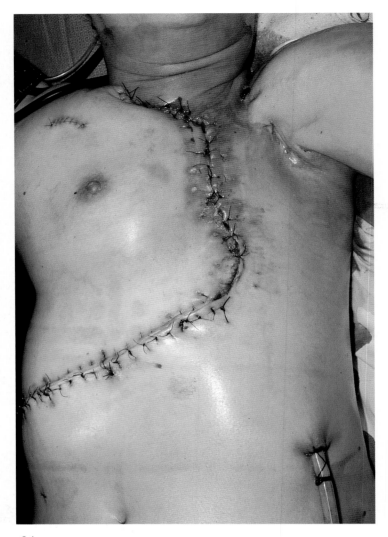

23

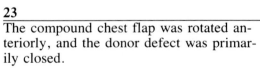

The compound chest flap was rotated anteriorly, and the donor defect was primarily closed.

24

Appearance five days postoperatively. The wound was frankly infected. The flap survived completely.

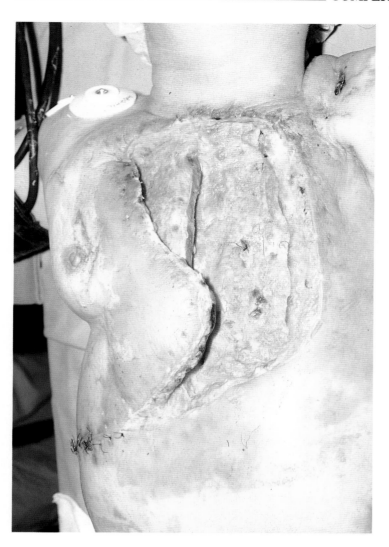

25

Even though the flap survived, the wound totally dehisced. The Prolene® mesh had to be removed. Serial debridements and saline dressings were used to prepare the wound for a secondary closure.

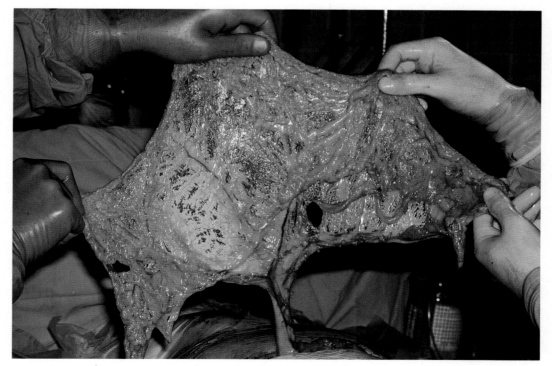

26

The omentum was elevated on the right gastroepiploic vessels to help "dig out" from this surgical maelstorm.

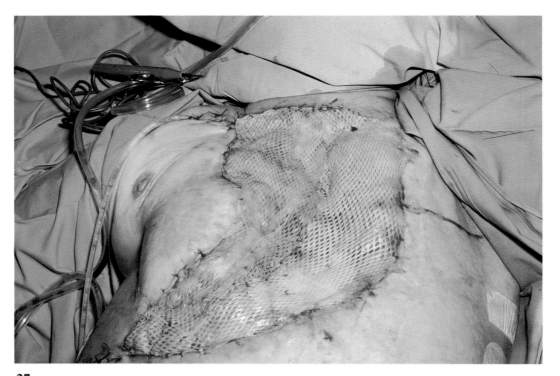

27

The omentum was passed through a subcutaneous tunnel and grafted in a delayed fashion.

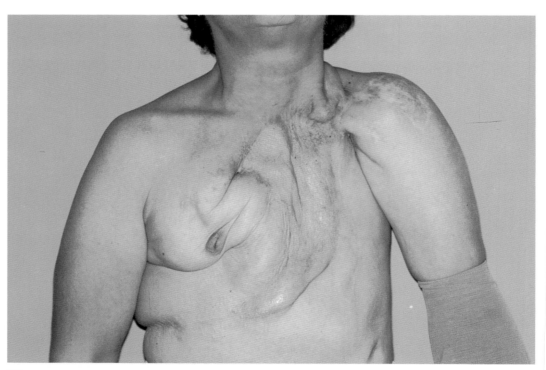

28

Appearance of the chest several months following a heroic but unattractive salvage. In retrospect, it was a mistake to place Prolene® mesh in an already infected wound. This problem would have been extremely difficult to solve if the omentum had not been available.

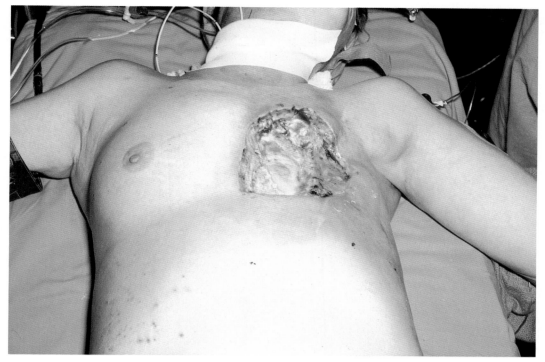

29

Forty-nine-year-old woman following a left radical mastectomy and chest wall irradiation. The ulcerated wound of the left anterior chest had been present for several months. The latissimus dorsi muscle was denervated and devascularized. This was the appearance at the time of the initial debridement. (Case of P.G. Arnold)

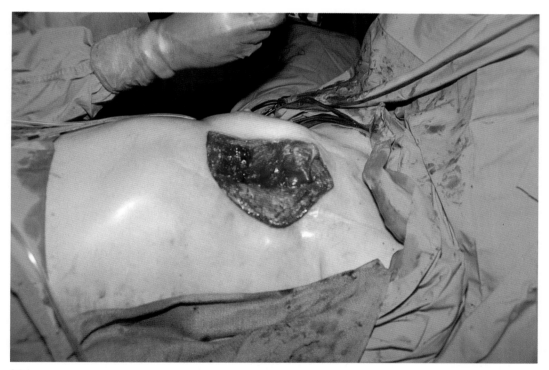

30

The right pectoralis major muscle was elevated on the internal mammary perforators and transposed into the left chest wall defect. This "turnover" pectoralis major flap was inadequate to close the wound.

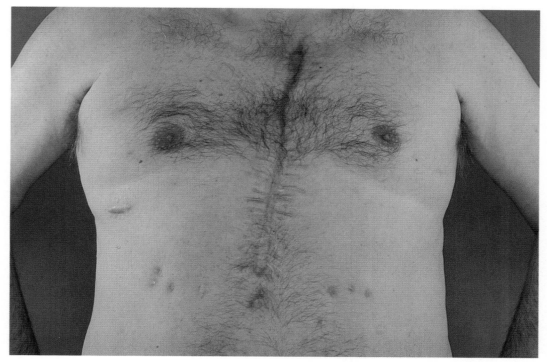

41

Appearance five months following the secondary closure with no further drainage. This represents the unfortunate case of an apparently adequate debridement and closure with muscle flaps and a delayed expression of a subclinical infection. Osteomyelitis of the sternum and the adjacent structures is similar to osteomyelitis of the long bones. It may be dormant for months or even years before it becomes clinically evident. It must be treated just as aggressively the second time around.

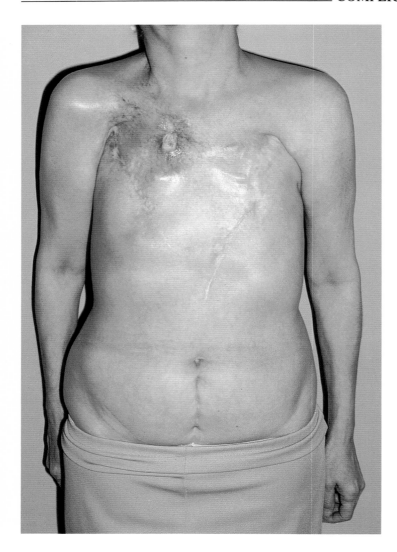

42

Fifty-four-year-old female who had undergone bilateral radical mastectomies with radiation therapy to the right chest. A painful ulceration had been present for several months. (Case of P.G. Arnold)

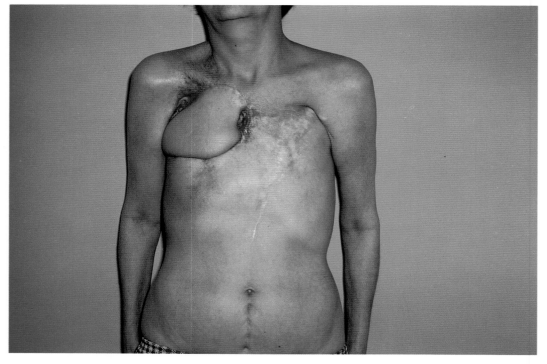

43

The irradiation ulcer was excised and closed with a latissimus dorsi flap. The patient was referred after three months of persistent drainage.

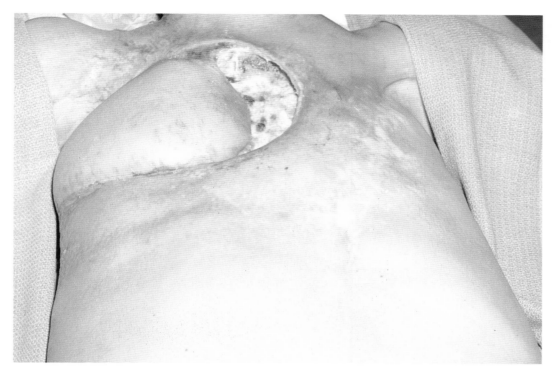

44

The stiffened latissimus flap was reelevated and advanced centrally in a V-Y maneuver in order to avoid a large secondary procedure. The advancement did not provide adequate muscular coverage of the sternum and disrupted because of the tense closure. This is a good example of a wasteful "small" procedure. This is usually done because someone says: "but doctor, I've already had a big operation."

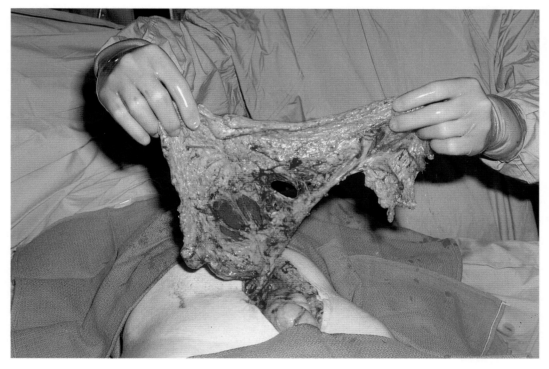

45

A celiotomy was performed, and the omentum was transposed into the remaining chest wall defect.

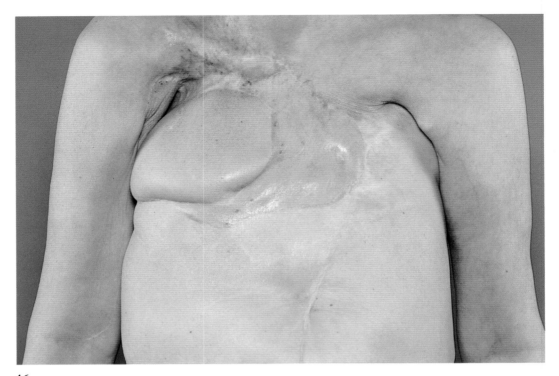

46

Appearance of the chest wall at ten months. The skin-grafted omental flap provided stable coverage.

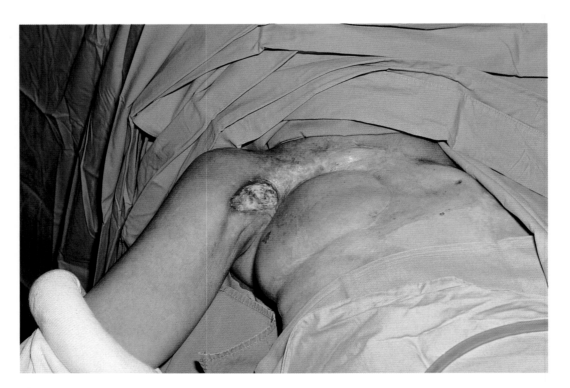

47

Two years later the patient had a new irradiation ulcer of the proximal humerus. The latissimus, pectoralis, serratus, and omental flaps were unavailable.

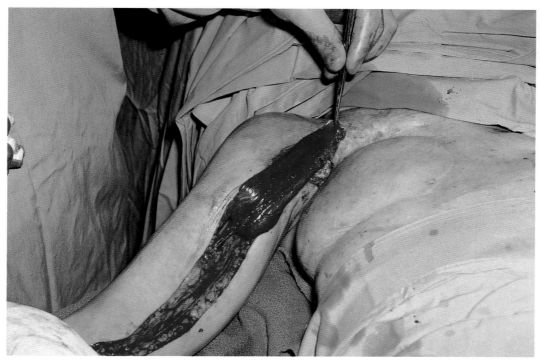

48

The long head of the biceps muscle is elevated on the proximal blood supply and transposed into the defect.

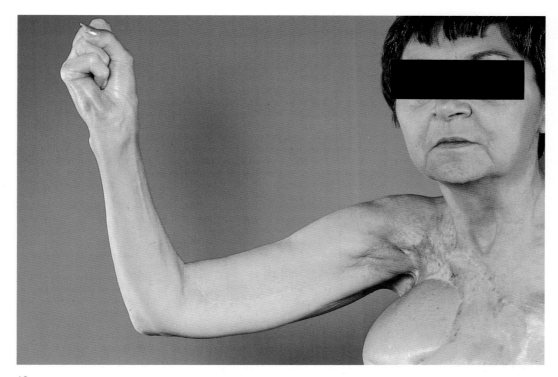

49

Two months following the biceps muscle flap reconstruction. The function of the arm was not harmed by the use of the biceps muscle flap.

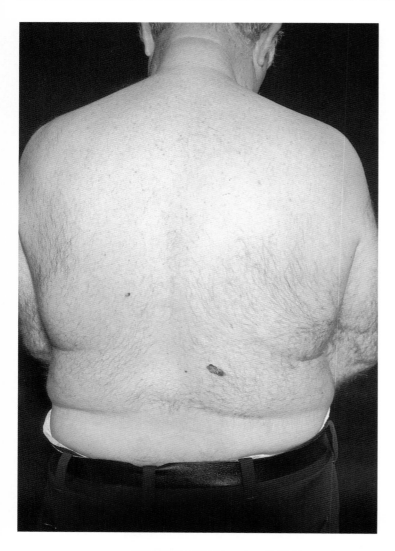

50

Forty-seven-year-old male with a level IV melanoma of the lower right back. Because the adipose layer was at least three inches in depth, it was felt that a skin graft would present a more difficult healing problem than a flap. (Case of J.B. McCraw)

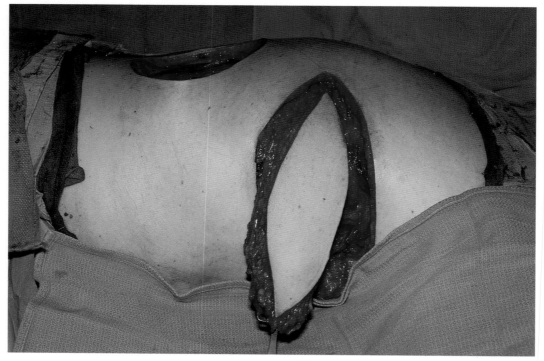

51

A ''reversed'' latissimus dorsi myocutaneous flap was elevated. No deep posterior perforating vessels were divided, and the flap fluorescence was excellent. All of the cutaneous segment was in direct contact with the underlying latissimus muscle. The proximal latissimus muscle itself was tunneled beneath the intervening skin bridge.

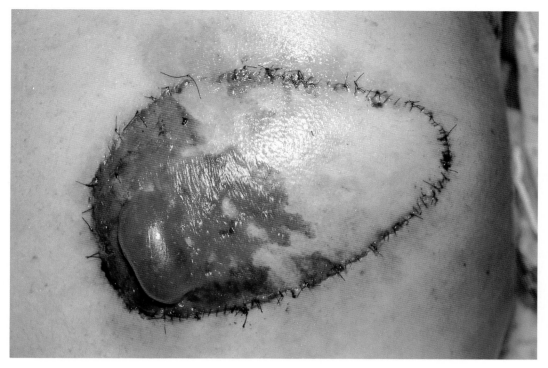

52

At five days the skin bridge constriction of the bulky muscle had caused the necrosis of the distal flap skin. Even the hardy latissimus muscle can be injured by external compression.

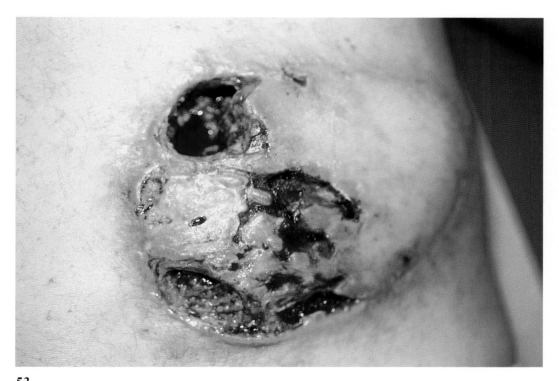

53

At three weeks this deep wound extended to the paraspinous muscles. This busy man had already returned to work and had chosen home care with the WaterPik® over further salvage surgery. Fortunately, he couldn't see his back.

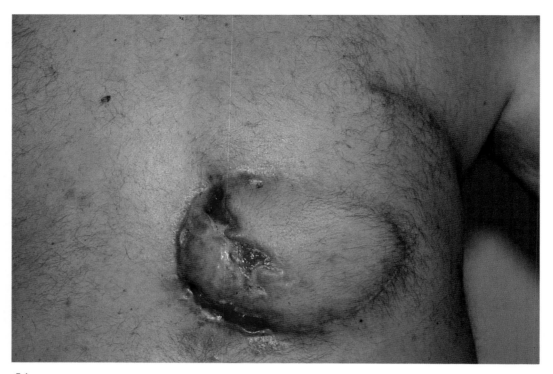

54

Over a period of two months the granulations reached the wound surface. Skin grafting was not required.

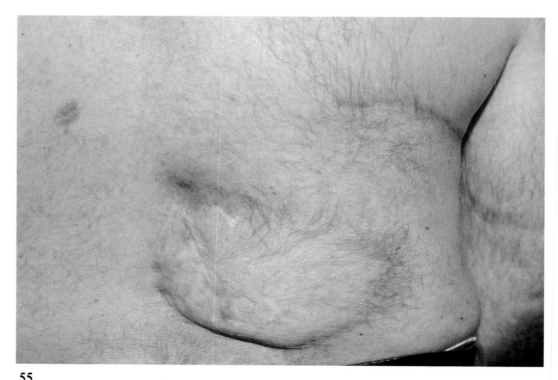

55

The wound eventually healed, but in this case a very simple technical error resulted in a greviously protracted postoperative course.

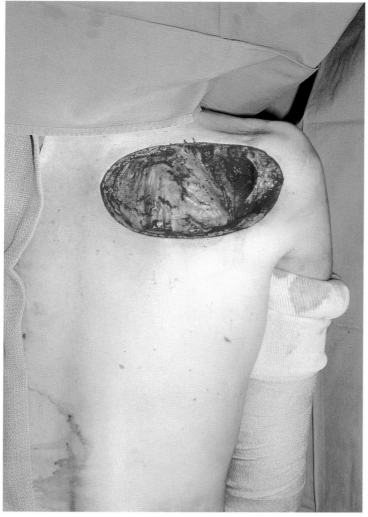

56

Fifty-seven-year-old woman with recurrent malignant fibrous histiocytoma following three previous resections and radiation therapy. The lower half of the scapula has been excised along with the paraspinous musculature. (Case of P.G. Arnold).

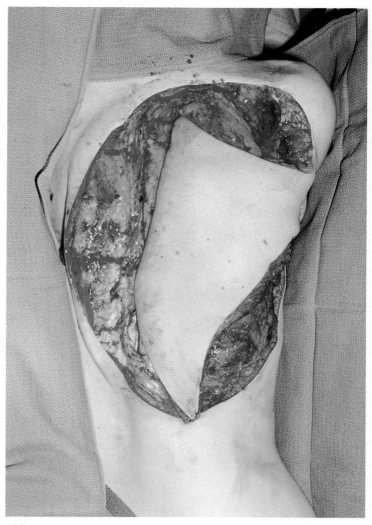

57

A latissimus dorsi musculocutaneous flap was elevated on the thoracodorsal vessels and advanced superiorly. The donor site was closed in a V-Y fashion.

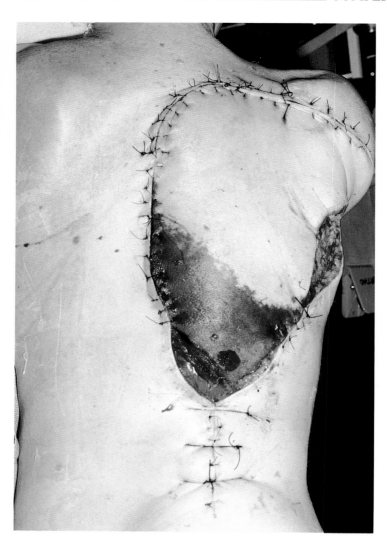

58
Appearance five days later. The lower half of the flap was lost.

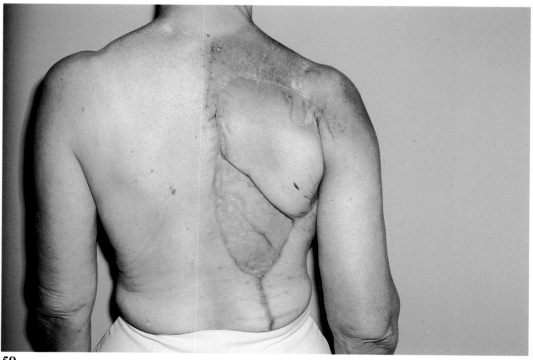

59
The necrotic flap was excised, and the remaining wound was closed with a skin graft. Although the reason for the flap loss is not known, it was undoubtedly related to the acute injury of one of the dominant flap vessels which had been heavily irradiated.

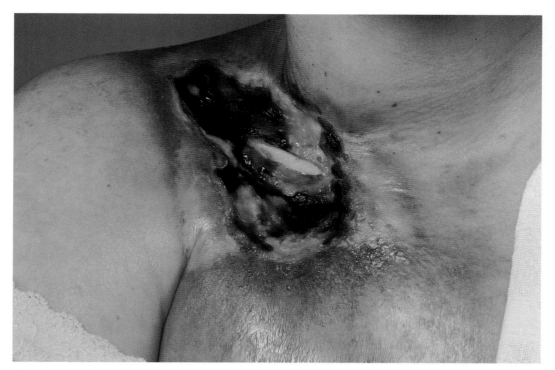

60

Forty-one-year-old female following a right modified radical mastectomy. Positive clavicular adenopathy had been treated with high-dose irradiation. Five months later the skin of the neck and upper chest necrosed and exposed the clavicle and the subclavian vessels. The right upper extremity was constantly painful and completely useless because of brachial plexopathy and lymphedema. (Case of P.G. Arnold)

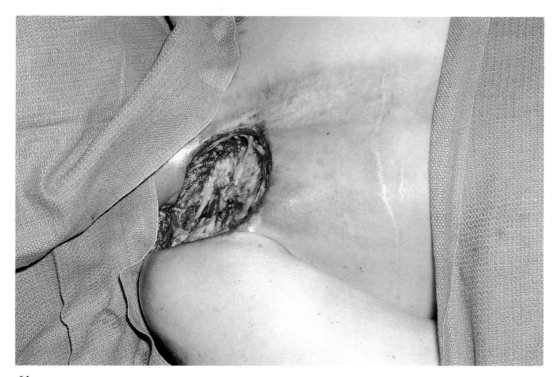

61

The wound was debrided, and the subclavian vessels were spared.

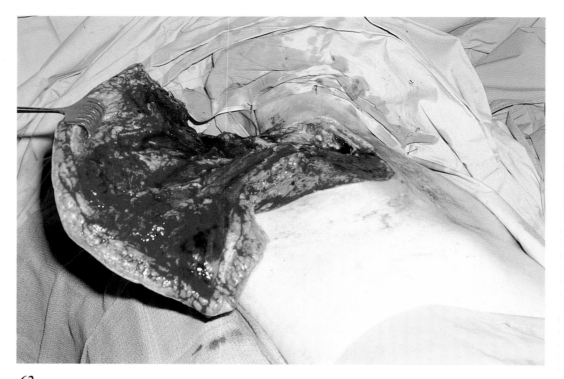

62

The humerus was removed, and the proximal upper extremity was treated as a large musculocutaneous flap. Forty-eight hours after the initial debridement the flap was inset.

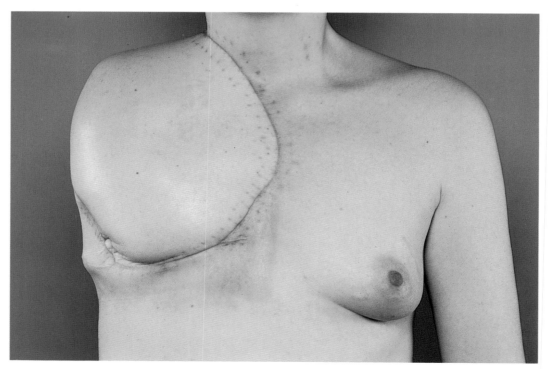

63

Appearance of the healed wound at four months. A reasonable contour of the shoulder was maintained, and the patient was relieved of her pain. The "total arm flap" seems drastic, but in this case, the arm was heavy, painful, insensate, and immobile.

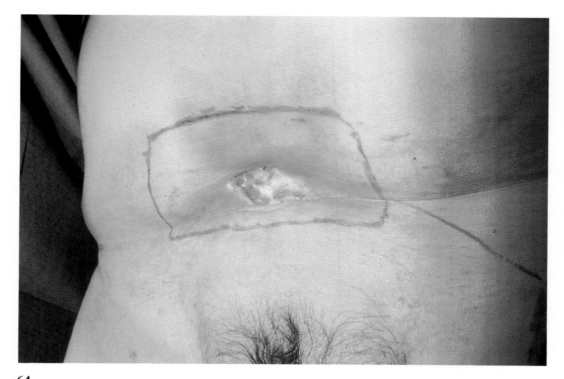

64

Eighty-year-old man with a painful irradiation ulcer of the suprapubic area following external beam therapy for a prostatic carcinoma. (Case of J.B. McCraw)

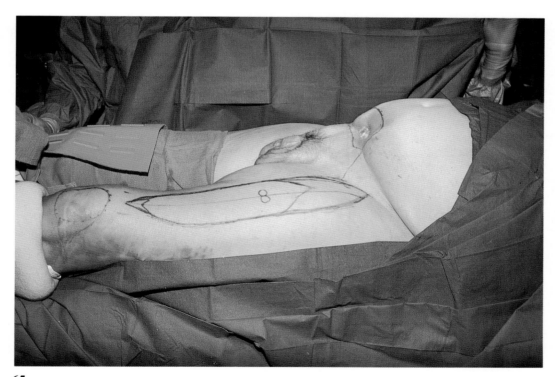

65

A left rectus femoris myocutaneous flap is outlined for coverage of the suprapubic ulcer.

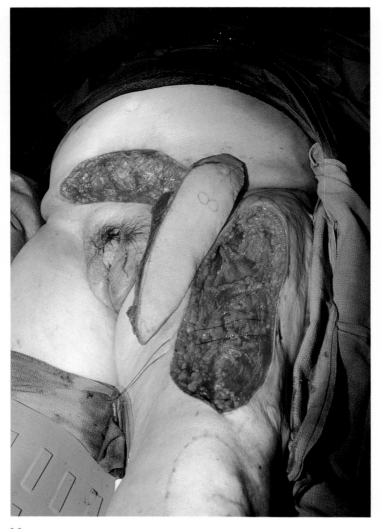

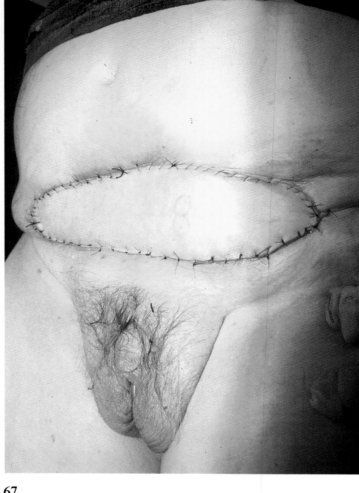

66

Two major mistakes were made in this case. The flap was raised as an ''island'' flap to avoid a bulge in the groin, which would have been a matter of little concern to this elderly man. The flap could have easily been inset into an incision passing between the donor site and the recipient site, leaving the proximal skin base of the flap intact. The dominant flap vessels were also placed under enough tension to result in vascular ''spasm.'' Rather than stretch the vessels of a single flap, it is preferable to use two flaps.

67

The second mistake was in the management of a ''sick'' flap. The cutaneous segment of the flap did not fluoresce well. At a minimum the flap should have been returned to the donor site. A better option would have been to discard the cutaneous segment and to skin graft the rectus femoris muscle immediately.

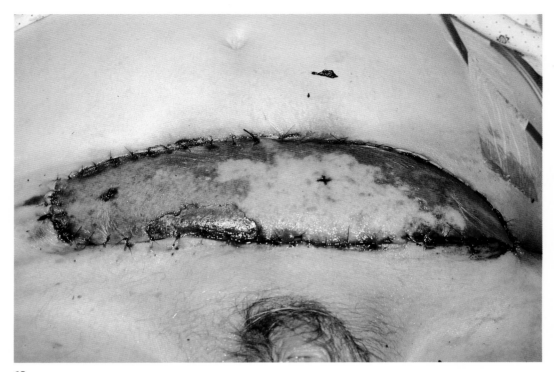

68

Four days following surgery, only the central portion of the myocutaneous flap was alive.

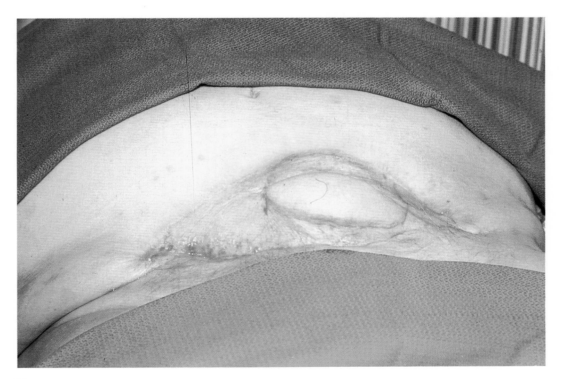

69

The necrotic margins of the flap skin were excised, and the exposed rectus femoris muscle was skin grafted. The flap loss could have been avoided by a better design and inset of the flap. Immediate acceptance of the flap failure and skin grafting of the rectus femoris muscle also could have yielded a primarily healed wound at the initial procedure.

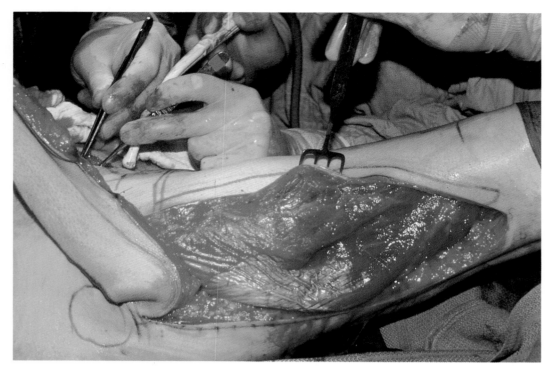

70

Elevated TFL fasciocutaneous flap and vastus lateralis muscle flap to cover an infected Dacron® vascular graft in the groin. (Case of J.B. McCraw and R.T. Gregory, Jr.)

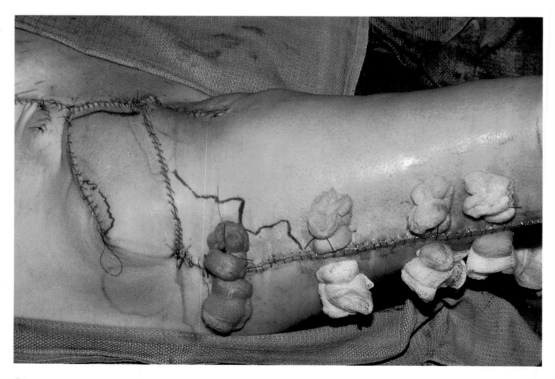

71

The vastus lateralis muscle was used to cover the area of the vascular "pseudosheath" excision which extended well above the inguinal ligament. The TFL flap was used for surface cover, rather than directly skin grafting the transposed vastus lateralis muscle flap. The fluorescein examination demonstrated three areas of probable non-viability of the skin flaps as outlined by the blue marking pen.

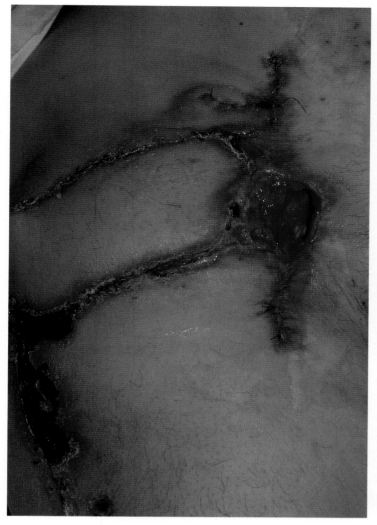

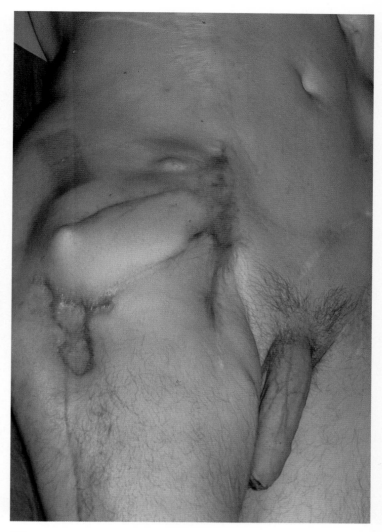

72

Anterior view of the groin at ten days. The pattern of skin loss predicted by the fluorescein test is precisely confirmed with time. Fluorescein is an excellent predictive test and should not be ignored. The basic mistake in this case was to use the TFL flap at all since a skin-grafted vastus lateralis muscle could have corrected this entire defect. The TFL flap was used to fulfill the old tenet of "replacing tissue with like tissue," but it resulted in a more extensive procedure and contributed to all of the wound healing problems.

73

Fortunately, the areas of flap necrosis were covered by the transposed vastus lateralis muscle and could be skin grafted. The vastus lateralis muscle flap did save the vascular graft so the Second Law of Vasconez (all of the flap survived except . . .) missed.

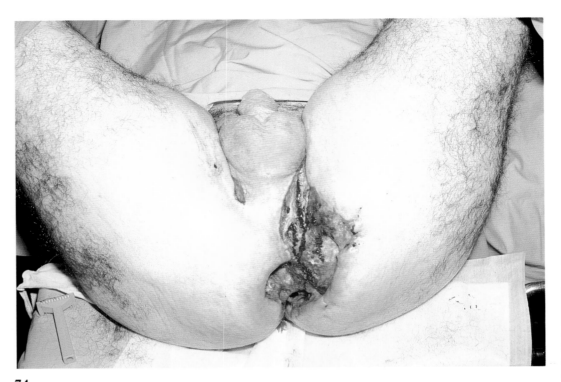

74

Infected abdominoperineal wound, ten days following a total colectomy for inflammatory bowel disease. (Case of P.G. Arnold)

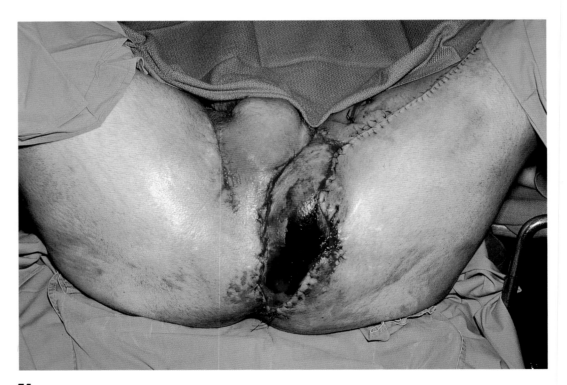

75

The perineal wound was closed with a left gracilis ''island'' myocutaneous flap. At five days it was apparent that the majority of the cutaneous segment was lost. Tension on the vascular pedicle resulted in vascular ''spasm'' and the subsequent necrosis of the flap. The entire gracilis muscle survived.

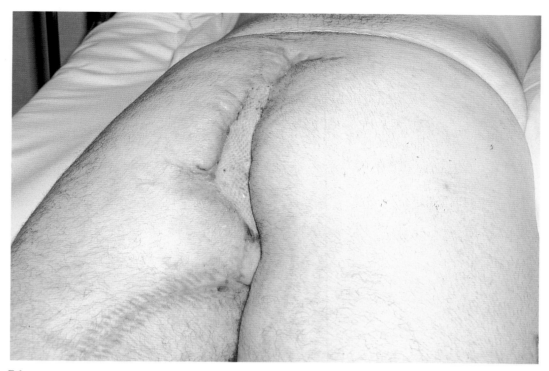

76

Posterior view of the skin-grafted gracilis muscle at two weeks. The skin graft provided a satisfactory closure.

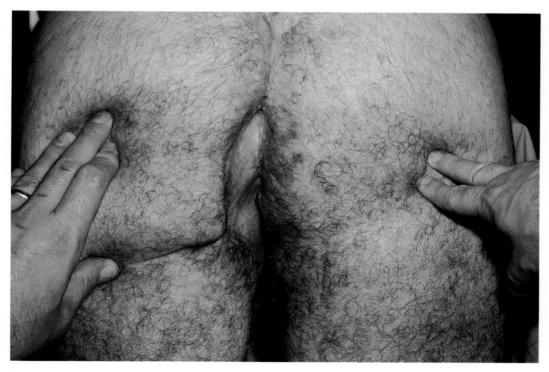

77

Appearance three years following surgery. The functional result is excellent. The grafted gracilis muscle is even less bulky than a gracilis myocutaneous flap.

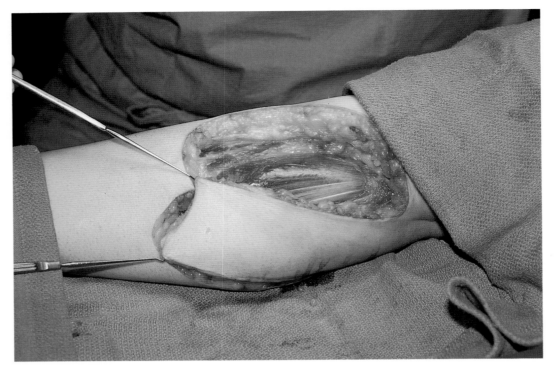

78

Twenty-four-year-old female following
the excision of a Level II melanoma from
the medial aspect of the upper calf. A
fasciocutaneous flap was raised from the
posterior calf in an effort to provide a
more durable closure for the pretibial
area. (Case of J.B. McCraw)

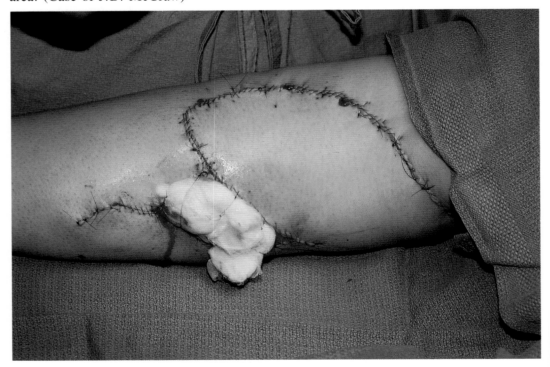

79

The transposed flap was closed under
moderate tension. The distal five centimeters of the flap did not fluoresce well
after transposition. A small skin graft was
placed on the posterior thigh donor site.

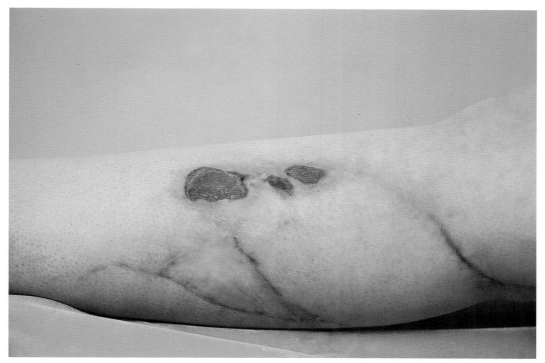

80

As predicted by the fluorescein examination, the distal portion of the flap was lost. At this juncture a healed primary skin graft on the area of excision would have looked better than the ulcers which required many months to heal.

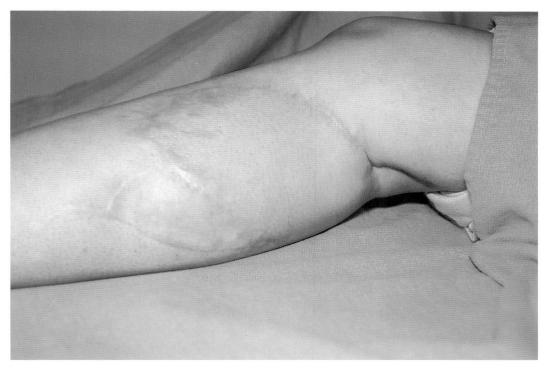

81

It is unclear what the technical error was in this case, but it is obvious that the elevation of the fasciocutaneous flap away from the gastrocnemius muscle and the tense flap closure were poorly tolerated.

Even the properly designed fasciocutaneous flap must be treated with care. We are also wary of the notion that fasciocutaneous flaps can be raised virtually "anywhere."

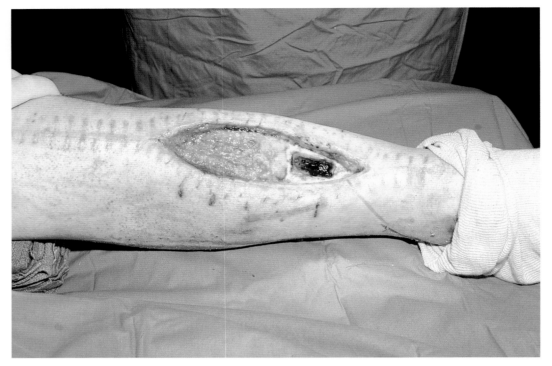

82

Twenty-seven-year-old male who presented with an acute osteomyelitis in an open tibial fracture. The tibial fracture was primarily covered with a proximal soleus muscle flap. Both the initial debridement and the size of the soleus muscle flap were inadequate to correct the problem. (Case of P.G. Arnold)

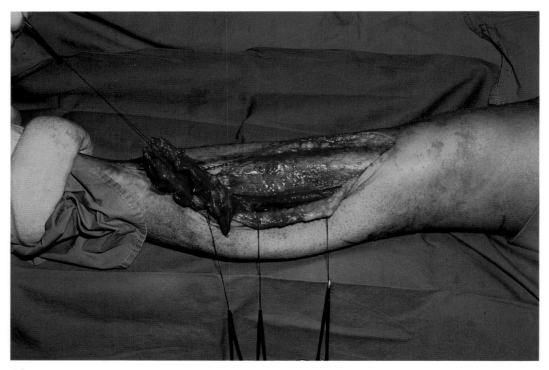

83

A further debridement was performed, and the EDC muscle was mobilized on its distal blood supply.

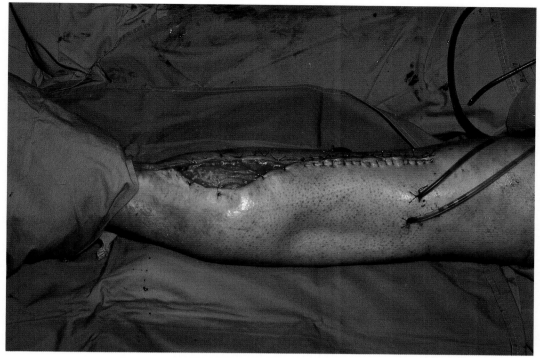

84

The EDC muscle flap was transposed into the distal tibial defect and skin grafted forty-eight hours later.

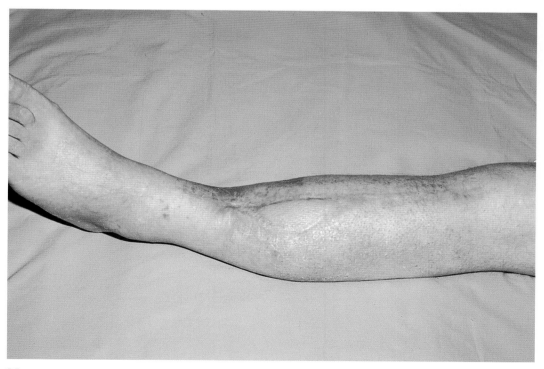

85

One year following the EDC muscle flap closure the distal tibial wound is stable. A return to the basic principles could have prevented the need for a second operation. One should feel completely comfortable with the initial debridement or it should be repeated prior to the definitive flap closure. Equally as important is the realistic assessment the ''zone of injury'' and the acceptance of the limitations of the soleus muscle in the distal third of the leg.

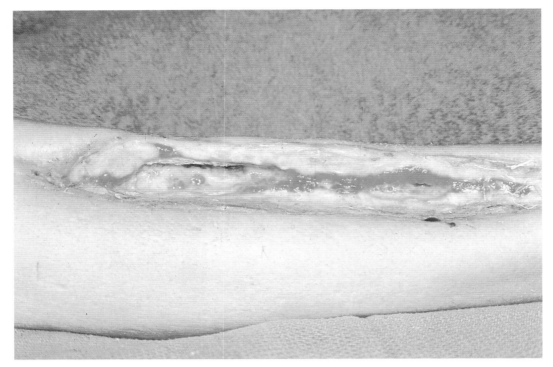

86

This fifty-nine-year-old patient had a long history of osteomyelitis which encompassed the middle portion of the tibia. The posterior two-thirds of the tibial cortex was desiccated, and the marrow had been lost. The peripheral pulses were palpable, but the patient was a diabetic and a smoker. This 1973 case predates our modern ''free'' flap capabilities. (Case of J.B. McCraw)

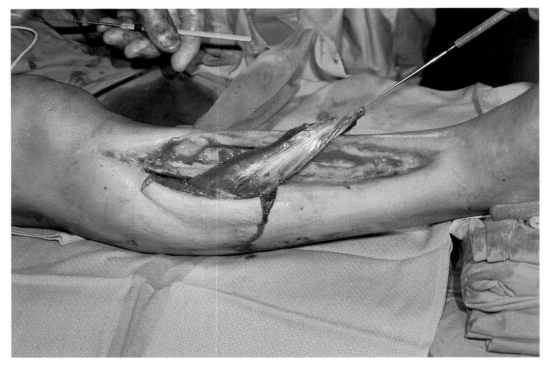

87

A proximal soleus muscle flap was passed through the interosseous membrane to gain better access to the lower tibial wound. This pitiful single muscle flap was obviously incapable of completely obliterating the huge pretibial dead space. This was a ''Shirley Temple'' solution to an ''atomic bomb'' problem.

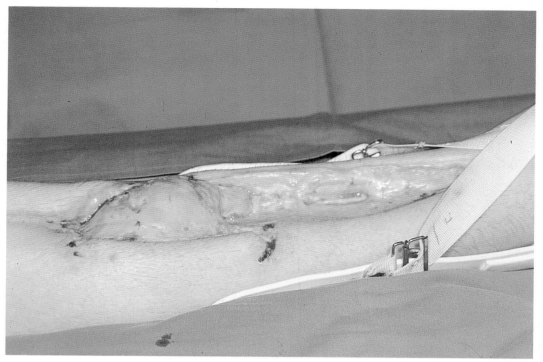

88

The soleus muscle was skin grafted and healed completely, but it had no effect on the osteomyelitis of the distal tibia. This type of "tubular" osteomyelitis is virtually incurable unless the dead bone is totally excised and completely covered with either a "free" muscle flap or multiple local muscle flaps. If this cannot be done an immediate amputation should be considered. Our lack of experience in 1973 was our sole excuse for this wasted operation. The disease has not changed.

BIBLIOGRAPHY

BASIC PRINCIPLES

Abbe, R. "A new plastic operation for the relief of deformity due to double hare lip." *Med. Rec.* 53: 477, 1898.

Abbe, R. "Case of plastic operation on the nose." *Med. Rec.* 87: 921, 1915.

Arnold, P.G. and Mixter, R.C. "Making the most of the gastrocnemius muscles." *Plast. and Reconstr. Surg.* 72(1): 38, 1983.

Arnold, P.G. and Pairolero, P.C. "Chest wall reconstruction: Experience with 100 consecutive patients." *Ann. Surg.* 199(6): 725, 1984.

Arnold, P.G. and Pairolero, P.C. "Use of pectoralis major muscle flaps to repair defects of the anterior chest wall." *Plast. Reconstr. Surg.* 63: 205, 1979.

Arnold, P.G., Pairolero, P.C. and Waldorf, J.C. "The serratus anterior muscle: intrathoracic and extrathoracic utilization." *Plast. and Reconstr. Surg.* 73(2): 240, 1984.

Bakamjian, V.Y. "A technique for primary reconstruction of the palate after radical maxillectomy for cancer." *Plast. Reconstr. Surg.* 31: 103, 1963.

Bakamjian, V.Y. "A two-stage method for pharyngoesophageal reconstruction with a primary pectoral skin flap." *Plast. Reconstr. Surg.* 36: 173, 1965.

Campbell, J. and Pennefather, C. "An investigation into the blood supply of muscle with special reference to war surgery." *Lancet*, 1: 294, 1919.

Cole, H.P. "Ununited fractures of the mandible: their incidence, causation, and treatment." *Br. J. Surg.* 6: 57, 1918-19.

Clark, W.E. and Blomfield, L.B. "The efficiency of intramuscular anastomoses with observations on the regeneration of devascularized muscle." *J. Anat.* 79: 15, 1945.

Cormack, G.C. and Lamberty, B.G.H. "A classification of fasciocutaneous flaps according to their patterns of vascularization." *Br. J. Plast. Surg.* 37: 80, 1984.

Cormack, G.C. and Lamberty, B.G.H. "Fasciocutaneous vessels in the upper arm: Application to the design of new fasciocutaneous flaps." *Plast. Reconstr. Surg.* 74: 244, 1984.

Cormack, G.C. and Lamberty, B.G.H. "The blood supply of the thigh skin." *Plast. Reconstr. Surg.* 75: 342, 1985.

Davis, J.S. "The story of plastic surgery." *Ann. Surg.* 113: 641, 1941.

Davis, J.S. *Plastic Surgery, Its Principles and Practice.* Philadelphia: P. Blakiston's Son and Co., 1919.

Davis, W.M., McCraw, J.B., and Carraway, J.H. "Use of a direct transverse thoracoabdominal flap to close difficult wounds of the thorax and upper extremity." *Plast. Reconstr. Surg.* 60(4): 526, 1977.

Dibbell, D.G. "Use of a long island flap to bring sensation to the sacral area in young paraplegics." *Plast Reconstr. Surg.* 54: 221, 1974.

Dibbell, D.G., McCraw, J.B. and Edstrom, L.E. "Providing useful and protective sensibility in patients with meningocele." *Plast. and Reconstr. Surg.* 64: 796. 1979.

Dowden, R.V., and McCraw, J.B. "The vastus lateralis muscle flap: technique and applications." *Annals of Plastic Surgery* 4: 396, 1980.

Erk, Y., Rhodes, F.A., and Spira, M. "Vascular augmentation of skin and musculocutaneous flaps." *Ann. Plast. Surg.* 10: 341, 1983.

Estlander, J.A. "Methode de autoplastic de la joul on d'une le've're." *Rev. Mens. de Med. Ed. Chir.* 1: 344, 1877.

Gallie, W.E. and LeMesurier, A.B. "The use of living sutures in operative surgery." *Can. Med. Assoc. J.* 11: 504, 1921.

Ger, R. and Levine, S.R. "The management of decubitus ulcers by muscle transposition." *Plast. Reconstr. Surg.* 58: 419, 1976.

Hester, T.R., McConnel, F.M.S., Nahai, F., Jurkiewicz, M.J., and Brown, R.G. "Reconstruction of the cervical esophagus, hypopharynx, and oral cavity using free jejunal transfer." *Amer. J. Surg.* 140: 487, 1980.

Hester, T.R., Nahai, F., Beegle, P.E., and Bostwick, J., III. "Blood supply of the abdomen revisited with emphasis on the superficial inferior epigastric artery." *Plast. Reconstr. Surg.* 74: 657, 1984.

Hudlicka, O. *Muscle blood flow (its relation to muscle metabolism and function).* Amsterdam: Swets en Zeitlinger, B.V., 1973.

Hueston, J.T. and McConchie, I.H. "A compound pectoral flap." *Aust. N.Z. J. Surg.* 38(1): 61, 1968.

Kanavel, A.B. "Plastic procedures for the obliteration of cavities with non-collapsible walls." *Surg. Gynecol. Obstet.* 32: 453, 1921.

Kaplan, I. "Neurovascular island flap in the treatment of trophic ulceration of the heel." *Br. J. Plast. Surg.* 22: 143, 1969.

Kitlowski, E.A. "The preservation of tendon function by the use of skin flaps." *Amer. J. Surg.* 51: 653, 1941.

Krizek, T.J., Tani, T., Desprez, J.D. and Kiehn, C.L. "Experimental transplantation of composite grafts by microsurgical vascular anastomoses." *Plast. Reconstr. Surg.* 36: 538, 1965.

Lamberty, B.G.H. and Cormack, G.C. "The anticubital fasciocutaneous flap." *Br. J. Plast. Surg.* 36: 428, 1983.

Lang, K. and Boyd, L.J. "The use of fluorescein to determine the adequacy of circulation." *Med. Clin. N. Am.* 26: 943, 1942.

BASIC PRINCIPLES

Littler, J.W. "Neurovascular pedicle method of digital transposition for reconstruction of the thumb." *Plast. Reconstr. Surg.* 12: 303, 1953.

Littler, J.W. "Neurovascular skin island transfer in reconstructive hand surgery." In *Transactions of the International Society of Plastic Surgeons.* Baltimore: Williams & Wilkins, 1960.

Littlewood, M. "Compound Flaps." In *Skin Flaps*, W.C. Grabb and M.R. Myers, Eds. Boston: Little, Brown and Co., 297-306, 1975.

Magee, W.P., McCraw, J.B., Horton, C.E., and McInnis, W.D. "Pectoralis 'paddle' myocutaneous flaps: the workhorse of head and neck reconstruction." *Amer. J. of Surg.* 140: 507, 1980.

Manchot, C. *Die Hautarteriern des Menschlichen Korpers.* Liepzig: F.C.W. Vogel, 1889.

Maruyama, Y., Ohnishi, K., and Takeuchi, S. "The lateral thigh fasciocutaneous flap in the repair of ischial and trochanteric defects." *Br. J. Plast. Surg.* 37: 103, 1984.

Mathes, S., Vasconez, L., and Jurkiewicz, M.J. "Extension and further applications of muscle flap transposition." *Plast. Reconstr. Surg.* 60: 6, 1977.

Mathes, S.J., Alpert, B., and Chang, N. "Use of the muscle flap in chronic osteomyelitis: experimental and clinical correlation." *Plast. Reconstr. Surg.* 69, 1982.

Mathes, S.J., McCraw, J.B., and Vanconez, L.O. "Muscle transposition flaps for coverage of lower extremity defects: anatomical considerations." *Surg. Clin. N. Amer.* 54: 1337, 1974.

Mathes, S.J. and Nahai, F. *Clinical Atlas of Muscle and Musculocutaneous Flaps.* St. Louis: C.V. Mosby Co. 1979.

Mathes, S.J. and Nahai, F. "Muscle flap transposition with function preservation: technical and clinical considerations." *Plast. Reconstr. Surg.* 66: 242, 1980.

Mathes, S.J. and Nahai, F. "Classification of the vascular anatomy of muscles: Experimental and clinical correlation." *Plast. Reconstr. Surg.* 67: 177, 1981.

Mathes, S.J. and Nahai, F. *Clinical Applications for Muscle and Musculocutaneous Flaps.* St. Louis: C.V. Mosby Co. 1982.

Mathes, S.J. and Nahai, F. *Clinical Applications for Muscle and Musculocutaneous Flaps.* St. Louis: The C.V. Mosby Co., 1982.

Mathes, S.J. and Nahai, F. *Clinical Atlas of Muscle and Musculocutaneous Flaps.* St. Louis: The C.V. Mosby Co., 1979.

McArthur, L.L. "Autoplastic suture in hernia and other diastases: preliminary report." *J. Amer. Med. Assoc.* 37: 1162, 1901.

McCraw, J.B., McDonald, W., McLeod, R., and Stephenson, H. Jr.: "A rapid test for intestinal perforation." *J.A.M.A.* 191: 934, 1965.

McCraw, J.B. "The recent history of myocutaneous flaps." *Clin. Plast. Surg.* 7: 3, 1980.

McCraw, J.B. "Intraoperative identification of the gracilis muscle for vaginal reconstruction." *Plast. Reconstr. Surg.* 65(3): 358, 1980.

McCraw, J.B. "You can call me Ray, you can call me Jay." (Letter): *Plast. and Reconstr. Surg.* 66: 857, 1980.

McCraw, J.B., and Dibbell, D.G. "Experimental definition of independent myocutaneous vascular territories." *Plast. Reconstr. Surg.* 60: 212, 1977.

McCraw, J.B., Dibbell, D.G., and Carraway, J.H. "Clinical definition of independent myocutaneous vascular territories." *Plast. Reconstr. Surg.* 60: 341, 1977.

McCraw, J.B., Fishman, J.H. and Sharzer, L.A. "The versatile gastrocnemius myocutaneous flap." *Plast. and Reconstr. Surg.* 62: 15, 1978.

McCraw, J.B. and Furlow, L.T., Jr. "The dorsalis pedis arterialized flap." *Plast. Reconstr. Surg.* 55: 177, 1975.

McCraw, J.B., Magee, W.P. and Kalwaic, H. "The use of the trapezius and sternomastoid myocutaneous flaps in head and neck reconstruction." *Plast. and Reconstr. Surg.* 63: 49, 1979.

McCraw, J.B., Massey, F.M., Shanklin, K.D. and Horton, C.E. Vaginal reconstruction with gracilis myocutaneous flaps." *Plast. Reconstr. Surg.* 58: 176, 1976.

McCraw, J.B., Myers, B., and Shanklin, K.D. "The value of fluorescein in predicting the viability of arterialized flaps." *Plast. Reconstr. Surg.* 60: 710, 1977.

McCraw, J.B., Penix, J.O. and Baker, J.W. "Repair of major defects of the chest wall and spine using the latissimus dorsi myocutaneous flap." *Plast. and Reconstr. Surg.* 62: 197, 1978.

McDowell, F. "Logs vs. harpsichords, blobby flaps vs. finished results (editorial)." *Plast. Reconstr. Surg.* 64: 249, 1979.

McGregor, I.A., and Jackson, I.T. "The Groin Flap." *Br. J. Plast. Surg.* 25: 3, 1972.

McGregor, I.A., and Morgan, G. "Axial and random pattern flaps." *Br. J. Plast. Surg.* 26: 202, 1973.

Moberg, E. "Evaluation and management of nerve injuries in the hand." *Surg. Clin. North Am.* 44: 1019, 1964.

Myers, M.B. "Prediction of skin sloughs at the time of operation with the use of fluorescein dye." *Surgery* 51: 158, 1962.

Nahai, F., Brown, R.G., and Vasconez, L.O. "Blood supply of the abdominal wall as related to planning abdominal incisions." *Am. Surg.* 42: 691, 1976.

Nahai, F., Silverton, J.S., Hill, H.L., and Vasconez, L.O. "The tensor fascia lata musculocutaneous flap." *Ann. Plast. Surg.* 1: 372, 1978.

Olivari, N. "The latissimus flap." *Br. J. Plast. Surg.* 29: 126, 1976.

Ortichocea, M. "The musculocutaneous flap method: an immediate and heroic substitute for the method of delay." *Br. J. Plast. Surg.* 25: 106, 1972.

BASIC PRINCIPLES

Ortichocea, M. "A new method of total reconstruction of the penis." *Br. J. Plast. Surg.* 25: 347, 1972.

Ortichocea, M. "History of the discovery of the musculo-cutaneous flap method as a universal and immediate substitute for the method of delay." *Br. J. Plast. Surg.* 36: 524, 1983.

Owens, N. "Compound neck pedicle designed for repair of massive facial defects." *Plast. Reconstr. Surg.* 15: 369, 1955.

Papp, C., McCraw, J.B., and Arnold, P.G. "Experimental reconstruction of the trachea with autogeneous materials." *J. of Throracic and Cardiovascular Surg.* 90(1): 13, 1985.

Papp, C., Parker, P., Boeheim, C. and McCraw, J.B. "Experimental use of intercostal muscle flaps for repair of induced cardiac defects." *J. of Thoracic and Cardiovascular Surg.* 90(2): 261, 1985.

Pers, M., and Medgyesi, S. "Pedicle muscle flaps and their application in the surgery of repair." *Br. J. Plast. Surg.* 26: 313, 1973.

Reid, C.D. and Taylor, G.I. "The vascular territory of the acromiothoracic axis." *Br. J. Plast. Surg.* 37: 194, 1984.

Ristic, J. and Morain, W.D. Translation of *The Cutaneous Arteries of the Human Body* by Carl Manchot. New York: Springer-Verlag, 1983.

Rowsell, A.R., Davies, D.M., Eisenberg, N., and Taylor, G.I. "The anatomy of the subscapular thorcacodorsal arterial system: Study of a hundred cadaver dissections." *Br. J. Plast. Surg.* 37: 574, 1984.

Salmon, M. *Arteres de la Peam* (Arteries of the skin). Masson, 1936.

Salmon, M. *Arteres des muscles de la tete et du cou* (Arteries of the muscles of the head and neck). Masson, 1936.

Salmon, M. and Dor, J. *Les arteres des muscles des membres et du tronc* (Arteries of muscles of the trunk and extremities). Masson, 1933.

Senior, H.D. "The development of the arteries of the human lower extremity." *Am. J. Anat.* 25: 55, 1919.

Shaw, D.T. and Payne R.L. "One stage tubed abdominal flaps." *Surg. Gynecol. Obstet.* 83: 205, 1946.

Smith, P.J. "The vascular basis of axial pattern flaps." *Br. J. Plast. Surg.* 26: 150, 1973.

Smith, P.J., Foley, B., McGregor, I.A., and Jackson, I.T. "The anatomical basis of the groin flap." *Plast. Reconstr. Surg.* 49: 41, 1972.

Snyder, G.B. and Edgerton, M.T. "The principle of the island neurovascular flap in the management of ulcerated anesthetic weight bearing areas of the lower extremity." *Plast. Reconstr. Surg.* 36: 518, 1965.

Stark, R.B. "Robert Abbe and his contributions to plastic surgery." *Plast. Reconstr. Surg.* 12: 14, 1953.

Stein, S. "Laebedannelse (Cheiloplastik) Udfort paa en my methode." *Hospitals Meddelser*, 1: 212, 1848.

Tamai, S., and co-workers. "Free muscle transplants in dogs with microsurgical neurovascular anastomoses." *Plast. Reconstr. Surg.* 46: 219, 1970.

Taylor, G.I. "A discussion of blood supply of the abdomen revisited with emphasis on the superficial inferior epigastric artery." *Plast. Reconstr. Surg.* 74: 667, 1984.

Tolhurst, D.E. "Surgical indications for fasciocutaneous flaps." *Ann. Plast. Surg.* 13: 495, 1984.

Tolhurst, D.E. "Discussion of fasciocutaneous vessels in the upper arm: Application to the design of new fasciocutaneous flaps." *Plast. Reconstr. Surg.* 74: 250, 1984.

Vasconez, L., Bostwick, J., III, and McCraw, J.B. "Coverage of exposed bone by muscle transposition and skin grafting." *Plast. Reconstr. Surg.* 53: 526, 1974.

Wangensteen, O.H. "Repair of recurrent and difficult hernias and other large defects of the abdominal wall employing the iliotibial tract of fascia lata as a pedicled flap." *Surg. Gynecol. Obstet.* 59: 766, 1934.

Wangensteen, O.H. "Repair of large abdominal defects by pedicled fascial flaps." *Surg. Gynecol. Obstet.* 82: 144, 1946.

Wee, J.T.K. "Reconstruction of the lower leg and foot with the reverse-pedicled anterior tibial flap: preliminary report of a new fasciocutaneous flap." *Br. J. Plast. Surg.* 39: 327, 1986.

Wei, W.I., Lan, K.H., and Wong, J. "The true pectoralis major myocutaneous island flap: An anatomic study." *Br. J. Plast. Surg.* 37: 578, 1984.

TEMPORALIS

Abul-Hassan, H.S., Ascher, G., and Acland, R.D. "Surgical anatomy and blood supply of the fascial layers of the temporal region." *Plast. Reconstr. Surg.* 77: 17, 1986.

Antonyshyn, O., Colclengh, R.C., Hurst, L.N., et al. "The temporalis myo-osseous flap: an experimental study." *Plast. Reconstr. Surg.* 77: 406, 1986.

Avelar, J.M. and Psillakis, J.M. "The use of fascial flaps in craniofacial deformities." *Ann. Plast. Surg.* 6: 464, 1981.

Bakamjian, V.Y. "A technique for primary reconstruction of the palate after radical maxillectomy for cancer." *Plast. Reconstr. Surg.* 31: 103, 1963.

Bakamjian, V.Y. and Souther, S.G. "Use of temporal muscle flap for reconstruction after orbito-maxillary resections for cancer." *Plast. Reconstr. Surg.* 56: 171, 1975.

Bosniak, S., Sachs, M., and Smith, B. "Temporalis muscle transfer: a vascular bed for autogenous dermis-fat orbital implantation." *Ophthalmology* 92(2): 292, 1985.

Bradley, P. and Brockbank, J. "The temporalis muscle flap in oral reconstruction." *J. Maxillofac. Surg.* 9(3): 139, 1981.

Brent, B., Upton, J., Acland, R., et al. "Experience with the temporoparietal fascial free flap." *Plast. Reconstr. Surg.* 76: 177, 1985.

Campbell, H.H. "Symposium on maxillo-facial surgery: surgery of lesions of the upper face." *Am. J. Surg.* 87: 676, 1954.

Campbell, H.H. "Reconstruction of the maxilla." *Plast. Reconstr. Surg.* 3: 66, 1984.

Conley, J. "Use of composite flaps containing bone for major repairs in the head and neck." *Plast. Reconstr. Surg.* 49: 522, 1972.

Cramer, L.M. "Surgical management of recurrent periorbital tumors." *Plast. Reconstr. Surg.* 29: 14, 1962.

Curioni, C., Toscano, P., Fioretti, C., and Salerno, G. "Reconstruction of the orbital floor with the muscle-bone flap (temporal muscle with coronoid process)." *J. Max. Fac. Surg.* 11: 263, 1983.

Cutting, C.B., McCarthy, J.B., and Berenstein, A. "Blood supply of the upper craniofacial skeleton: the search for composite calvarial bone flaps." *Plast. Reconstr. Surg.* 74: 603, 1981.

Deitch, R.D. and Callahan, A. "Temporal muscle transplant for tissue defects about the orbit." *Am. J. Ophth.* 58: 849, 1964.

Dupuis, A., Princ, G., and Gitton, E. "Palatal reconstruction using a sternocleidomastoid flap with an upper pedicle." *Ann. Chir. Plas. Esth.* 30: 251, 1985.

Edgerton, M.T., Tuerk, D.B., and Fisher, J.C. "Surgical treatment of Moebius syndrome by platysma and temporalis muscle transfer." *Plast. Reconstr. Surg.* 55(3): 305, 1975.

Gillies, H.D. In *Plastic Surgery on the Face*, Frowde, H. (Ed.) London: Oxford University Press, pp. 54-55, 1920.

Gillies, H.D. "Experiences with fascia lata grafts in the operative treatment of facial paralysis." *Pro. Soc. Med.* 27: 98, 1934.

Golovine, S.S. "Procede de cloture plastique de l'orbite apres l'estenteration." *Arch. Ophth.* 18: 679, 1898.

Gould, J.F. "Shortening of the temporalis tendon for hypermobility of the temporomandibular joint." *J. Oral Surg.* 36(10): 781, 1978.

Hallock, G.G. "Reconstruction of a lower eyelid defect using the temporalis muscle." *Ann. Plast. Surg.* 13(2): 157, 1984.

Harn, S.D. and Shackelford, L.S. "Further evaluation of the superficial and deep tendons of the human temporalis muscle." *Anat. Rec.* 202(4): 537, 1982.

Hauben, D.J. and van der Meulen, J.C. "Use of a temporal musculoperiosteal flap in the treatment of craniofacial abnormalities: experimental study." *Plast. Reconstr. Surg.* 74: 355, 1984.

Holmes, A.D. and Marshall, K.A. "Use of the temporalis muscle flap in blanking out orbits." *Plast. Reconstr. Surg.* 63(3): 336, 1979.

Horton, C.E., et al. "Tumors of the maxilla and orbit." In *Symposium on Cancer of the Head and Neck*. Gaisford, J.C. (Ed.) St. Louis: C.V. Mosby Co., p. 293, 1969.

Howowitz, J.H., Persing, J.A., Nichter, L.S., Morgan, R.F., and Edgerton, M.T. "Galeal-pericranial flaps in head and neck reconstruction: anatomy and application." *Am. J. Surg.* 148(4): 489, 1984.

Jones, R.W. "The repair of skull defects by a new pedicle bone-graft operation." *Brit. Med. Jrnl.* 780, 1933.

Konig, F. Quoted from Garre, Kuttner, and Lexer. *Handbuch der Praktischen Chirurgie*. Ed. 6 Stuttgart Enke, 1: 1106, 1926.

Longmore, R.B. and McRae, D.A. "Middle temporal veins — a potential hazard in the Gillies' operation." *Br. J. Oral Surg.* 19(2): 129, 1981.

McCarthy, J.G. and Zide, B.M. "The spectrum of calvarial bone grafting: introduction of the vascularized calvarial bone flap." *Plast. Reconstr. Surg.* 74: 10, 1984.

McGregor, I.A. and Reid, W.H. "The use of the temporal flaps in the primary repair of full thickness defects of the cheek." *Plast. Reconstr. Surg.* 38: 1, 1966.

McGregor, I.A. and Reid, W.H. "Simultaneous temporal and delto-pectoral flaps for full-thickness defects of the cheek." *Plast. Reconstr. Surg.* 45: 326, 1970.

Naquin, H.A. "Exenteration of the orbit." *Arch. Ophth.* 51: 850, 1954.

Naquin, H.A. "Orbital reconstruction utilizing temporalis muscle." *Am. J. Ophth.* 41: 519, 1956.

Rambo, J.H. "Musculoplasty: a new operation for suppurative middle ear deafness." *Transactions of the American Academy of Ophthalmology* 62: 166, 1958.

TEMPORALIS

Ranney, D.A. and Furness, M.A. "Results of temporalis transfer in lagophthalmos due to leprosy." *Plast. Reconstr. Surg.* 51(3): 301, 1973.

Reese, A.B. "Exenteration of the orbit: with transplantation of the temporalis muscle." *Am. J. Ophth.* 43: 386, 1958.

Reese, A.B. and Jones, I.S. "Exenteration of the orbit and repair of transplantation of the temporalis muscle." *Am. J. Ophth.* 51: 217, 1961.

Renner, G., Davis, W.E., and Templer, J. "Temporalis pericranial muscle flap for reconstruction of the lateral face and head." *Laryngoscope* 94(11 Part 1): 1418, 1984.

Savage, R.C. "Orbital exenteration and reconstruction for massive basal cell and squamous cell carcinoma of cutaneous origin." *Ann. Plast. Surg.* 10(6): 492, 1983.

Send, D.K. "Temporalis transplantation for paralytic lagophthalmos." *Br. J. Ophthalmol.* 54(10): 680, 1970.

Sevel, D. "Exenteration or the orbit using a frontal periosteal flap." *Head Neck Surg.* 4(2): 154, 1981.

Smith, R.A. "The free fascial scalp flap." *Plast. Reconstr. Surg.* 70: 204, 1982.

Van der Meulen, J.C.H., Hauben, D.J., Vaandrager, J.M., and Birgenhager-Frenkel, D.H. "The use of a temporal osteoperiosteal flap for the reconstruction of malar hypoplasia in Teacher Collins syndrome." *Plast. Reconstr. Surg.* 74: 687, 1984.

Verge, P., Raynaud, S., and Peri, G. "The use of the temporofrontal musculocutaneous flap in the reconstruction of the oropharynx after cancer." *Ann. Chir. Plas. Esth.* 30: 369, 1985.

Webster, J.P. "Refrigerated skin grafts." *Ann. Plast.* 120: 431, 1944.

Webster, J.P. "Temporalis muscle transplants for defects following orbital exenteration." *Tr. Internat. Soc. Plast. Surg.* 1: 291, 1955.

White, T.P., Faulkner, J.A., Markley, J.M., Jr., and Maxwell, L.C. "Translocation of the temporalis muscle for treatment of facial paralysis." *Muscle Nerve* 5(7): 500, 1982.

Wise, R.A. and Baker, H.W. "Orbital support." In *Surgery of Head and Neck*, Year Book Medical Publishers. 1st Ed., 1958. 2nd Ed., 1968.

STERNOCLEIDOMASTOID

Alvarez, G.E., Escamilla, J.T., and Carranza, A. "The split sternocleidomastoid myocutaneous flap." *Br. J. Plast. Surg.* 36(2): 183, 1983.

Ariyan, S. "One-stage reconstruction for defects of the mouth using a sternomastoid myocutaneous flap." *Plast. Reconstr. Surg.* 63: 618, 1979.

Ariyan, S. "One-stage repair of a cervical esophagostome with two myocutaneous flaps from the neck and shoulder." *Plast. Reconstr. Surg.* 63(3): 426, 1979.

Ariyan, S. "The sternocleidomastoid myocutaneous flap." *Laryngoscope* 90(4): 676, 1980.

Ariyan, S. "Functional radical neck dissection." *Plast. Reconstr. Surg.* 65(6): 768, 1980.

Bakamjian, V.Y. "A technique for primary reconstruction of the palate after radical maxillectomy for cancer." *Plast. Reconstr. Surg.* 31: 103, 1963.

Barnes, D.R., Ossoff, R.H., Pecaro, B., and Sisson, G.A. "Immediate reconstruction of mandibular defects with a composite sternocleidomastoid musculoclavicular graft." *Arch. Otolaryngol.* 107(11): 711, 1981.

Barnes, D.R., Ossoff, R.H., Pecaro, B., Sisson, G.A., Conley, J., and Gullane, P.J. "The sternocleidomastoid muscle flap." *Head Neck Surg.* 2(4): 308, 1980.

Caliot, P., Cabanie, P., Bousquet, V., and Midy, D. "A contribution to the study of the innervation of the sternocleidomastoid muscle." *Anat. Clin.* 6(1): 21, 1984.

Cole, H.P. "Ununited fractures of the mandible: their incidence, causation and treatment." *Br. J. Plast. Surg.* 6:57, 1918-19.

Conley, J. "Use of composite flaps containing bone for major repairs of the head and neck." *Plast. Reconstr. Surg.* 49: 522, 1972.

Conley, J. and Gullane, P.J. "The sternocleidomastoid muscle flap." *Head Neck Surg.* 2(4): 308, 1980.

Dupuis, A., Princ, G., and Gitton, E. "Palatal reconstruction using a sternocleidomastoid flap with an upper pedicle." *Ann. Chir. Plast. Esth.* 30: 251, 1985.

Eliachar, I. and Moscona, A.R. "Reconstruction of the laryngotracheal complex in children using the sternocleidomastoid myocutaneous flap." *Head Neck Surg.* 4(1): 16, 1981.

Gouet, O. "Interet du lambeau osteo-myo-cutane de clavicule dans les grands delabrements de la face: un cas clinique." *Ann. Chir. Plast. Esth.* 29(1): 35, 1984.

Gupta, A.K., Bhasin, D., and Shah, R. "Closure of post laryngectomy pharyngocutaneous fistula with sternocleidomastoid muscle flap." *Ann. Acad. Med.* Singapore 12(2 Suppl.): 407, 1983.

Hill, H.L. and Brown, R.G. "The sternocleidomastoid flap to restore facial contour in mandibular reconstruction." *Br. J. Plast. Surg.* 31(2): 143, 1978.

Jabaley, M.E., Heckler, F.R., Wallace, W.H., and Knott, L.H. "Sternocleidomastoid regional flaps: a new look at an old concept." *Br. J. Plast. Surg.* 32(2): 106, 1979.

Kanavel, A.B. "Plastic procedure for the obliteration of cavities with non-collapsible walls." *Surg. Gynecol. Obstet.* 32: 453, 1921.

Lagier, J.P., Lachard, A., Blanc, J.L., and Lachard, J. "Current trends in the treatment of mandibular osteoradionecrosis: use of a sternocleidomastoid osteomyocutaneous flap." *Reve. Stomatol. Chir. Maxillofac.* 86(1): 15, 1985.

Larson, D.L. and Goepfert, H. "Limitations of the sternocleidomastoid musculocutaneous flap in head and neck cancer reconstruction." *Plast. Reconstr. Surg.* 70(3): 328, 1982.

Littlewood, M. "Compound skin and sternomastoid flaps for repair in extensive carcinoma of the head and neck." *Br. J. Plast. Surg.* 20: 403, 1967.

Littlewood, M. "Compound flaps." In *Skin Flaps.* Grabb, W.C. and Myers, M.B. (Eds.) Boston: Little, Brown & Co., 1975, 297-306.

Marx, R.E. and McDonald, D.K. "The sternocleidomastoid muscle as a muscular or myocutaneous flap for oral and facial reconstruction." *J. Oral Maxillofac. Surg.* 43(3): 155, 1985.

Matulic, Z., Barlovic, M., Mikolji, V., and Virag, M. "Tongue reconstruction by means of the sternocleidomastoid muscle and a forehead flap." *Br. J. Plast. Surg.* 31(2): 147, 1978.

Mazzola, R.F., Oldini, C., and Sambataro, G. "Use of submandibular flaps to close pharyngostomes and other defects of lower anterior neck region." *Plast. Reconstr. Surg.* 64: 340, 1979.

McCraw, J.B., Dibbell, D.G., and Carraway, J.H. "Clinical definition of independent myocutaneous vascular territories." *Plast. Reconstr. Surg.* 60: 341, 1977.

McCraw, J.B., Magee, W.P., and Kalwaic, H. "Use of the trapezius and sternomastoid myocutaneous flaps in the head and neck reconstruction." *Plast. Reconstr. Surg.* 63: 49, 1979.

McKinley, L.M. and Hamilton, L.R. "Torticollis caused by absence of the right sternocleidomastoid muscle." *South Med. J.* 69(8): 1099, 1976.

Mikaelian, D.O. "Reconstruction of the tongue." *Laryngoscope* 94(1): 34, 1984.

O'Brien, B. "A muscle-skin pedicle for total reconstruction of the lower lip." *Plast. Reconstr. Surg.* 45: 395, 1970.

Owens, N. "A compound neck pedicle designed for repair of massive facial defects." *Plast. Reconstr. Surg.* 15: 369, 1955.

Rabson, J.A., Hurwitz, D.J., and Futrell, J.W. "The cutaneous blood supply of the neck: relevance to incision planning and surgical reconstruction." *Br. J. Plast. Surg.* 38(2): 208, 1985.

Sasaki, C.T. "The sternocleidomastoid myocutaneous flap." *Arch. Otolargyngol.* 106(2): 74, 1980.

STERNOCLEIDOMASTOID

Siemssen, S.O., Kirby, B., and O'Connor, T.P.F. "Immediate reconstruction of a resected segment of the lower jaw, using a compound flap of clavicle and sternomastoid muscle." *Plast. Reconstr. Surg.* 61: 724, 1978.

Snyder, C.C., et al. "Mandibulofacial restoration with live osteocutaneous flaps." *Plast. Reconstr. Surg.* 45: 14, 1970.

Toomey, J.M. and Jacobs, J.R. "The extended sternocleidomastoid flap for one stage repair of defects of the oral cavity." *Laryngoscope* 90: 886, 1980.

Tovi, F. and Gittot, A. "Sternocleidomastoid myoperiosteal flap for the repair of laryngeal and tracheal wall defects." *Head Neck Surg.* 5(5): 447, 1983.

Viti, M., Fujiwara, M., Basmanjian, J.M. and Iida, M. "The integrated roles of longus colli and sternocleidomastoid muscles: an electromyographic study." *Anat. Rec.* 177(4): 471, 1973.

Yamaguchi, K.T., Sanderson, R., and Turnbull, F. "Repair of the hemimandibulectomy defect with a sternocleidomastoid muscle rotation flap." *Trans Pac. Coast Otoophthalmol. Soc.* 58: 351, 1977.

PLATYSMA

Achard, E.M. *Les hermiatrophies faciales.* These pour le Doctorat en Medecine, Universite Paris VII, Paris, 1975, p. 49.

Cannon, C.R., Jones, M.E., Atkins, J.P., Jr., Keane, W.M., and Cantrell, R.W. "Reconstruction of the oral cavity using the platysma myocutaneous flap." *Arch. Otolaryngol.* 108(8): 491, 1982.

Coleman, J.J., III, Jurkiewicz, M.J., Nahai, F., and Mathes, S.J. "The platysma musculocutaneous flap: experience with 24 cases." *Plast. Reconstr. Surg.* 72(3): 315, 1983.

Coleman, J.J., Nahai, F., and Mathes, S.J. "Platysma musculocutaneous flap: clinical and anatomic considerations in head and neck reconstruction." *Am. J. Surg.* 144(4): 477, 1982.

de Castro, C.C. "The anatomy of the platysma muscle." *Plast. Reconstr. Surg.* 66(5): 680, 1980.

Delerm, A., Chevallier,H., and Albertini, F. "The platysma musculo-cutaneous flap in transmaxillary buccopharyngectomy." *Am. Chir. Plast. Esth.* 29: 38, 1984.

DesPrez, J.D. and Keihn, C.L. "Method of reconstruction following resection of anterior oral cavity and mandible for malignancy." *Plast. Reconstr. Surg.* 24: 238, 1959.

Edgerton, M.T. "Replacement of lining to oral cavity following surgery." *Cancer* 4: 110, 1951.

Farr, H.W., Jean-Gilles, B., and Die, A. "Cervical island skin flap repair of oral and pharyngeal defects in the composite operation for cancer." *Am. J. Surg.* 118: 759, 1969.

Freeland, A.P. and Rogers, J.H. "The vascular supply of the cervical skin with reference to incision planning." *Laryngoscope* 85: 714, 1975.

Futrell, J.W., Johns, M.E., Edgerton, M.T., Cantrell, R.W., and Fitz-Hugh, G.S. "Platysma myocutaneous flap for intraoral reconstruction." *Am. J. Surg.* 136(4): 504, 1978.

Gersuny, R. "Plastischer Ersatz der Wangenscheimhaut." *Zentralbl. Chir.* 14: 706, 1887.

Gluck, T. and Sorensen, H. "Die resektion und exstirpation des larynx, pharynx und oesophagus." In *Handbuch der Speziellen Chirugie des Ohres and der Oberen Luftwege.* Katz, L., Preysing, H. and Blumenfeld, F. (Eds.) Wurzburg: Verlag Curt Kabitsch, 1913, 68-69.

Hurwitz, D.J., Rabson, J.A., and Futrell, J.W. "The anatomic basis for the platysma skin flap." *Plast. Reconstr. Surg.* 72(3): 302, 1983.

Kanavel, A.B. "Plastic procedures for the obliteration of cavities with non-collapsible walls." *Surg. Gynecol. Obstet.* 32: 453, 1921.

Mazzola, R.F., Oldini, C., and Sambataro, G. "Use of submandibular flap to close pharyngostomas and other defects of lower anterior neck region." *Plast. Reconstr. Surg.* 64: 340, 1979.

Morestin, H. "Affections chirurgicales de la face." In *Nouveau Traite de Chirurgie Clinique et Operatoire.* Le Dentu, A. and Delbet, P. (Eds.) Paris: J.B. Bailliere et Fils, 1911, 217-222.

O'Brien, B. "A muscle-skin pedicle for total reconstruction of the lower lip." *Plast. Reconstr. Surg.* 45: 395, 1970.

Persky, M.S., Kaufman, D., and Cohen, N.L. "Platysma myocutaneous flap for intraoral defects." *Arch. Otolaryngol.* 109(7): 463, 1983.

Rabson, J.A., Hurwitz, D.J., and Futrell, J.W. "The cutaneous blood supply of the neck: relevance to incision planning and surgical reconstruction." *Br. J. Plast. Surg.* 38(2): 208, 1985.

Sanvanero-Rosselli, G. "Faringostomi e plastiche de chiusura." In *Trattato de Chirurgia Otorino-Laringologica.* Bologna: L. Cappelli, 1940, 1416-1423.

TRAPEZIUS

Ariyan, S. "One-stage repair of a cervical esophagostome with two myocutaneous flaps from the neck and shoulder." *Plast. Reconstr. Surg.* 63(3): 426, 1979.

Ariyan, S. "Discussion of the extended trapezius musculocutaneous flap for cranio-orbital fascial reconstruction." *Plast. Reconstr. Surg.* 75: 325, 1985.

Baek, S.M., Biller, H.F., Krespi, Y.P., and Lawson, W. "The lower trapezius island myocutaneous flap." *Ann. Plast. Surg.* 5(2): 108, 1980.

Bean, R.B. "A composite study of the subclavian artery in man." *Am. J. Anat.* 4: 303, 1905.

Bertotti, J.A. "Trapezius-musculocutaneous island flap in the repair of major head and neck cancer." *Plast. Reconstr. Surg.* 65(1): 16, 1980.

Chretien, P.B., Ketcham, A.S., Hoye, R.C., and Gertner, H.R. "Extended shoulder flap and its use in reconstruction of defects of the head and neck." *Am. J. Surg.* 118: 752, 1969.

Conley, J. "Use of composite flaps containing bone for major repairs in the head and neck." 49: 522, 1972.

Daseler, E.H. and Anson, B.J. "Surgical anatomy of the subclavian artery and its branches." *Surg. Gynecol. Obstet.* 108: 149, 1959.

Demergasso, F. "Colgajo cutaneo aislado a pediculo muscular: Neuva tecnica reconstructiva de cavidad oral en cancer de cabeza y cuello." *Actas de la Sociedad de Cirugia de Rusario.* 1976.

Demergasso, F. "Reconstruccion con colgajo osteo cutaneo trapecial en reseccion mandibulares segmentarias por cancer de cabeza y cuello." *Premio Annual Sociedad Argentina de Patologia de Cabeza y Cuello.* 1977.

Demergasso, F. and Piazza, M.V. "Colgajo cutaneo aislado a pediculo muscular en cirugia reconstructiva por cancer de cabeza y cuello: tecnica original." XLVII Congreso Argentino de Cirugia Forum de Investigaciones. *Rev. Argent. Cirug.* 32: 27, 1977.

Demergasso, F. and Piazza, M.V. "Trapezius myocutaneous flap in reconstructive surgery for head and neck cancer: an original technique." *Am. J. Surg.* 138(4): 533, 1979.

Dinner, M.I., Guyuron, B., and Labandter, H.P. "The lower trapezius myocutaneous flap for head and neck reconstruction." *Head Neck Surg.* 6(1): 613, 1983.

Guedon, C., Soussaline, M., and Gehanno, P. "The use of the trapezius musculocutaneous flap in reconstructive surgery of the head and neck." *Ann. Chir. Plast. Esth.* 29: 27, 1984.

Guillamondegui, O.M. and Larson, D.L. "The lateral trapezius musculocutaneous flap: its use in head and neck reconstruction." *Plast. Reconstr. Surg.* 67(2): 143, 1981.

Huelke, N.F. "A study of the transverse cervical and dorsal scapular arteries." *Anat. Rec.* 132: 233, 1958.

Kenyeres, M. "Experience with trapezius myocutaneous and osteomyocutaneous flaps." *Acta. Chir. Plast.* (Prague) 26(1): 39, 1984.

McCraw, J.B., Dibbell, D.G., and Carraway, J.H. "Clinical definition of independent myocutaneous vascular territories." *Plast. Reconstr. Surg.* 60: 341, 1977.

McCraw, J.B., Magee, W.P., and Kalwaic, H. "Use of the trapezius and sternomastoid myocutaneous flaps in head and neck reconstruction." *Plast. Reconstr. Surg.* 63(1): 49, 1979.

Mutter, T.C. "Cases of deformity from burns, relieved by operation." *Am. J. Med. Sci.* 4: 66, 1842.

Nichter, L.S., Morgan, R.F., Harman, D.M., Horowitz, J., and Edlich, R.F. "The trapezius musculocutaneous flap in head and neck reconstruction: potential pitfalls." *Head Neck Surg.* 7(2): 129, 1984.

Panje, W.R. "Myocutaneous trapezius flap." *Head Neck Surg.* 2(3): 206, 1980.

Panje, W.R. "A new method for total nasal reconstruction: the trapezius myocutaneous island 'paddle' flap." *Arch. Otolaryngol.* 108(3): 156, 1982.

Panje, W.R. "Mandible reconstruction with the trapezius osteomusculocutaneous flap." *Arch. Otolaryngol.* 111(4): 223, 1985.

Panje, W.R. and Cutting, C. "Trapezius osteomyocutaneous island flap for reconstruction of the anterior floor of the mouth and the mandible." *Head Neck Surg.* 3(1): 66, 1980.

Read, W.T. and Trotter, M. "The origins of transverse cervical and transverse scapular arteries in American whites and negroes." *Am. J. Phys. Anthropol.* 28: 239, 1941.

Rosen, H.M. "The extended trapezius musculocutaneous flap for cranio-orbital facial reconstruction." *Plast. Reconstr. Surg.* 75(3): 318, 1985.

Shapiro, M.J. "Use of trapezius myocutaneous flaps in the reconstruction of head and neck defects." *Arch. Otolaryngol.* 107(6): 333, 1981.

Tucker, H.M., Sobol, S.M., Levine, H., Wood, B., and Katz, R. "The transverse cervical trapezius myocutaneous island flap." *Arch. Otolaryngol.* 108(3): 194, 1982.

Zovickian, A. "Pharyngeal fistulas: repair and prevention using occiput based shoulder flaps." *Plast. Reconstr. Surg.* 19: 355, 1957.

PECTORALIS MUSCLE

Arnold, P.G. and Pairolero, P.C. "Chondrosarcoma of the manubrium: Resection and reconstruction with pectoralis major muscle." *Mayo Clin. Proc.* 53(1): 54, 1978.

Arnold, P.G. and Pairolero, P.C. "Use of pectoralis major muscle flaps to repair defects of anterior chest wall." *Plast. Reconstr. Surg.* 63: 205, 1979.

Arnold, P.G. and Pairolero, P.C. "Chest wall reconstruction: Experience with 100 consecutive patients." *Ann. Surg.* 199(6): 725, 1984.

Atkins, R.M., Bell, M.J., and Sharrard, W.J. "Pectoralis major transfer for paralysis of elbow flexion in children." *J. Bone Joint Surg.* (Br.) 67(4): 640, 1985.

Baek, S.M., Lawson, W., and Biller, H.F. "An analysis of 133 pectoralis major myocutaneous flaps." *Plast. Reconstr. Surg.* 69(3): 460, 1982.

Brown, R.G., Fleming, W.H., and Jurkiewicz, M.J. "An island flap of pectoralis major muscle." *Br. J. Plast. Surg.* 30: 161, 1977.

Burman, M. "The pectoralis major tendon as retinaculum of the long head of the biceps." *Bull. Hosp. Joint Dis.* 33(1): 80, 1972.

Calteux, N., Hamoir, M., de Coninck, A. "Mediastinal tracheostomy with a pectoralis major musculocutaneous island flap." *Am. Chir. Plast. Esth.* 30: 283, 1985.

Cantrell, R.W. "Myocutaneous flaps." *Otolaryngol Clin. North Am.* 16(2): 353, 1983.

Castilla, E.E., Paz, J.E., and Orioli, I.M. "Pectoralis major muscle defect and Poland complex." *Am. J. Med. Genet.* 4(3): 263, 1979.

Carroll, R.E. and Kleinman, W.B. "Pectoralis major transplantation to restore elbow flexion to the paralytic limb." *J. Hand Surg.* (Am.) 4(6): 501, 1979.

Coleman, J.J., III. "Complex thoracic wounds: muscle and musculocutaneous anatomy in closure." *South Med. J.* 78(2): 125, 1985.

Davis, R.K. and Price, J.C. "Bipedicled delay of the deltopectoral flap in raising the pectoral myocutaneous flap." *Laryngoscope* 94(4): 554, 1984.

Desphieux, J.L., Ducasse, A., and Lelattre, J.F. "The pectoralis major musculocutaneous flap: an anatomical study." *Ann. Chir. Plast. Esth.* 29: 23, 1984.

Dowden, R.V. and McCraw, J.B. "Muscle flap reconstruction of shoulder defects." *J. Hand Surg.* 5(4): 382, 1980.

Evans, P.H. and Das Gupta, A.R. "The use of the pectoralis major myocutaneous flap for one-stage reconstruction of the base of the tongue." *J. Laryngol. Otol.* 95(8): 809, 1981.

Frias, J.L. and Felman, A.H. "Absence of the pectoralis major, with ipsilateral aplasia of the radius, thumb, hemidiaphragm and lung: an extreme expression of Poland anomaly?" *Birth Defects* 10(5): 55, 1974.

Gardiner, L.J., Ariyan, S., and Pillsbury, H.C., III. "Myocutaneous flaps for challenging problems in head and neck reconstruction." *Arch. Otolaryngol* 109(6): 396, 1983.

Gudmundsson, B. "A case of rupture of the pectoralis major muscle." *Acta. Orthop. Scand.* 44(2): 213, 1973.

Harii, K., Ono, I., and Ebihara, S. "Closure of total cheek defects with two combined myocutaneous free flaps." *Arch. Otolaryngol.* 108(5): 303, 1982.

Harrison, D.H. "The pectoralis minor vascularized muscle graft for the treatment of unilateral facial palsy." *Plast. Reconstr. Surg.* 75(2): 206, 1985.

Hedge, H.R. and Shokeir, M.H. "Posterior shoulder girdle abnormalities with absence of pectoralis major muscle." *Am. J. Med. Genet.* 13(3): 285, 1982.

Hueston, J.T. and McConchie, I.H. "A compound pectoral flap." *Aust. N.Z. J. Surg.* 38(1): 61, 1968.

Johnsonbaugh, R.E., Catalano, J.D., and Meyer, B.P. "Congenital, unilateral absence of the breast and pectoralis major muscle." *South Med. J.* 64(4): 465, 1971.

Jonsson, B., Olofsson, B.M., and Steffner, L.C. "Function of the teres major latissimus dorsi and pectoralis major muscles: A preliminary study." *Acta. Morpho. Neerl. Scand.* 9(4): 275, 1972.

Jurkiewicz, M.J., and Arnold, P.G. "The omentum: an account of its use in reconstruction of the chest wall." *Ann. Surg.* 185: 548, 1977.

Jurkiewicz, M.J., Bostwick, J., III, and Hester, T.R. "Infected median sternotomy wound: successful treatment with muscle flap." *Am. Surg.* 191: 738, 1980.

Larson, D.L. and McMurtrey, M.J. "Musculocutaneous flap reconstruction of chest-wall defects: an experience with 50 patients." *Plast. Reconstr. Surg.* 73(5): 734, 1984.

Maier, H.C. and Luomanen, R.K.J. "Pectoral myoplasty for closure of residual empyema cavity and bronchial fistula." *Surgery* 25: 621, 1949.

Manktelow, R.T. "Discussion of the pectoralis minor vascularized muscle graft for the treatment of unilateral fascial palsy." *Plast. Reconstr. Surg.* 75: 214, 1985.

Manktelow, R.T., McKee, N.H., and Vettese, T. "An anatomical study of the pectoralis major muscle as related to functioning free muscle transplantation." *Plast. Reconstr. Surg.* 65(5): 610, 1980.

McCraw, J.B., Dibbell, D.G., and Carraway, J.H. "Clinical definition of independent myocutaneous vascular territories." *Plast. Reconstr. Surg.* 60: 341, 1977.

McEntire, J.E., Hess, W.E., and Coleman, S.S. "Rupture of the pectoralis major muscle: A report of eleven injuries and review of fifty-six." *J. Bone Joint Surg.* (Am.) 54(5): 1040, 1972.

Morain, W.D., Colen, L.B., and Hutchings, J.C. "The segmental pectoralis major muscle flap: a function-preserving procedure." *Plast. Reconstr. Surg.* 75(6): 825, 1985.

PECTORALIS MUSCLE

Morris, D.M., Reed, W., and Cunningham, M. "Primary head and neck reconstruction with a simultaneous ipsilateral pectoralis major myocutaneous flap and deltopectoral flap." *J. Surg. Oncol.* 25(1): 50, 1984.

Nahai, F., Morales, L., Jr., Bone, D.K., and Bostwick, J., III. "Pectoralis major muscle turnover flaps for closure of the infected sternotomy wound with preservation of form and function." *Plast. Reconstr. Surg.* 70(4): 471, 1982.

Pairolero, P.C. and Arnold, P.G. "Bronchopleural fistula: treatment by transportation of pectoralis major muscle." *J. Thorac. Cardiovasc. Surg.* 79(1): 142, 1980.

Pearl, S.N. and Dibbell, D.G. "Reconstruction after median sternotomy infection." *Surg. Gynecol. Obstet.* 159(1): 47, 1984.

Rees, R.S., Ivey, G.L., Shock, R.B., et al. "Pectoralis major myocutaneous flaps: long-term follow-up of hypopharyngeal reconstruction." *Plast. Reconstr. Surg.* 77: 586, 1986.

Reid, C.D. and Taylor, G.I. "The vascular territory of the acromiothoracic axis." *Br. J. Plast. Surg.* 37(2): 194, 1984.

Robertson, M.S. and Robinson, J.M. "Immediate pharyngoesophageal reconstruction. Use of a quilted skin-grafted pectoralis major muscle flap." *Arch. Otolaryngol.* 11(6): 386, 1984.

Sisson, G.A., Straehley, C.J., Jr., and Johnson, N.E. "Mediastinal dissection for recurrent cancer after laryngectomy." *Laryngoscope* 72: 1064, 1962.

Tobin, G.R. "Pectoralis major segmental anatomy and segmentally split pectoralis major flaps." *Plast. Reconstr. Surg.* 75: 814, 1985.

Tsai, T.M., Kalisman, M., Burns, J., and Kleinert, H.E. "Restoration of elbow flexion by pectoralis major and pectoralis minor transfer." *J. Hand Surg.* (Am.) 8(2): 186, 1983.

Urs, N.D. and Jani, D.M. "Surgical repair of rupture of the pectoralis major muscle: a case report." *J. Trauma* 16(9): 749, 1976.

Weber-Laumann, A. "Recurrent dislocation of the shoulder treated by transposition of the tendon to pectoralis minor: a follow-up of fifteen patients." *Acta. Orthop. Scand.* 41(2): 161, 1970.

Wilk, A., Balme, P., Keiling, R., et al. "The use of the pectoralis major flap in the cervicomaxillary surgery of irradiated patients." *Ann. Chir. Plast. Esth.* 30: 373, 1985.

Withers, E.H., Franklin, J.D., Madden, J.J., and Lynch, J.B. "Immediate reconstruction of the pharynx and cervical esophagus with the pectoralis major myocutaneous flap following laryngopharyngectomy." *Plast. Reconstr. Surg.* 68(6): 898, 1981.

PECTORALIS MYOCUTANEOUS FLAP

Acharya, G. and Johnson, M.L. "Use of pectoralis major myocutaneous flap in the Grillo procedure." *Ann. Plast. Surg.* 6(1): 11, 1981.

Ariyan, S. "The pectoralis major myocutaneous flap: a versatile flap for reconstruction in the head and neck." *Plast. Reconstr. Surg.* 63(1): 73, 1979.

Ariyan, S. "Further experiences with the pectoralis major myocutaneous flap for the immediate repair of defects from excisions of head and neck cancers." *Plast. Reconstr. Surg.* 64(5): 605, 1979.

Ariyan, S. "Pectoralis major, sternomastoid, and other musculocutaneous flaps for head and neck reconstruction." *Clin. Plast. Surg.* 7(1): 89, 1980.

Ariyan, S. "The donor site of the pectoralis myocutaneous flap (letter)." *Plast. Reconstr. Surg.* 66(1): 165, 1980.

Ariyan, S. "The pectoralis major for single-stage reconstruction of the difficult wounds of the orbit and pharyngoesophagus." *Plast. Reconstr. Surg.* 72(4): 468, 1983.

Ariyan, S. and Cuono, C.B. "Myocutaneous flaps for head and neck reconstruction." *Head Neck Surg.* 2(4): 321, 1980.

Ariyan, S. and Cuono, C.B. "Use of the pectoralis major myocutaneous flap for reconstruction of large cervical, facial or cranial defects." *Am. J. Surg.* 140(4): 503, 1980.

Baek, S.M., Biller, H.F., Krespi, Y.P., and Lawson, M. "The pectoralis major myocutaneous island flap for reconstruction of the head and neck." *Head Neck Surg.* 1: 293, 1979.

Baek, S.M., Lawson, W., and Biller, H.F. "An analysis of 133 pectoralis major myocutaneous flaps." *Plast. Reconstr. Surg.* 69(3): 460, 1982.

Baek, S.M., Lawson, W., and Biller, H.F. "Reconstruction of hypopharynx and cervical esophagus with pectoralis major island myocutaneous flap." *Ann. Plast. Surg.* 7(1): 18, 1981.

Bakamjian, V.Y. "A two-stage method for pharyngoesophageal reconstruction with a primary pectoral skin flap." *Plast. Reconstr. Surg.* 36: 173, 1984.

Bashie, A.H. "Transposition of the sterno-costal head of the pectoralis major in extensive burn contractures of the axilla." *Br. J. Plast. Surg.* 29(4): 377, 1976.

Bell, M.S. "Pectoralis major for mandibular reconstruction (letter)." *Plast. Reconstr. Surg.* 75(2): 281, 1985.

Bell, M.S. and Barron, P.T. "The rib-pectoralis major osteomyocutaneous flap." *Ann. Plast. Surg.* 6(5): 347, 1981.

Biller, H.F., Baek, S.M., Lawson, W., Krespi, Y.P., and Blaugrund, S.M. "Pectoralis major myocutaneous island flap in head and neck surgery: analysis of complication in 42 cases." *Arch. Otolaryngol.* 107(1): 23, 1981.

Biller, H.F., Krespi, Y.P., Lawson, W., and Baek, S.M. "A one-stage flap reconstruction following resection for stomal recurrence." *Otolaryngol Head Neck Surg.* 88(4): 357, 1980.

Brown, R.G., Fleming, W.H., and Jurkiewicz, M.J. "An island flap of the pectoralis major muscle." *Br. J. Plast. Surg.* 30(2): 161, 1977.

Calteux, N., Hamoir, M., and de Coninck, A. "Mediastinal tracheostomy with a pectoralis major musculocutaneous island flap." *Am. Chir. Plast. Esth.* 30: 283, 1985.

Coleman, J.J., III. "Complex thoracic wounds: muscle and musculocutaneous anatomy in closure." *South Med. J.* 78(2): 125, 1985.

Cuono, C.B. and Ariyan, S. "Immediate reconstruction of a composite mandibular defect with a regional osteomusculocutaneous flap." *Plast. Reconstr. Surg.* 65(4): 477, 1980.

Desphieux, J.L., Ducasse, A., and Delattre, J.F. "The pectoralis major musculocutaneous flap: an anatomical study." *Ann. Chir. Plast. Esth.* 29(1): 23, 1984.

Ducasse, A., Desphieux, J.L., Palot, J.R., Delattre, J.F., and Flament, J.B. "Anatomical basis for the use of the pectoralis major myocutaneous flap in reconstructive surgery." *Anat. Clin.* 5(4): 245, 1984.

Dvir, E. "The donor site of the pectoralis major myocutaneous flap (letter)." *Plast. Reconstr. Surg.* 66(1): 165, 1980.

Eliachar, I., Godlsher, M., Moscona, A.R., and Hurwitz, D.J. "Reconstruction of the larynx and cervical trachea with the pectoralis major myocutaneous island flap." *Head Neck Surg.* 6(4): 880, 1984.

Evans, P.H. and Das Gupta, A.R. "The use of the pectoralis major myocutaneous flap for one-stage reconstruction of the base of the tongue." *J. Laryngol. Otol.* 95(8): 809, 1981.

Freelander, E., Lee, K., and Vandervord, J.G. "Reconstruction of the axilla with a pectoralis major myocutaneous island flap." *Br. J. Plast. Surg.* 35(2): 144, 1982.

Freeman, J.L. "The pectoralis major myocutaneous flap." *J. Otolaryngol.* 10(5): 396, 1981.

Freeman, J.L., Gullane, P.J., and Rotstein, L.M. "The double paddle pectoralis major myocutaneous flap." *J. Otolaryngol.* 14(4): 237, 1985.

Freeman, J.L., Walker, E.P., Wilson, J.S.P., and Shaw, H.J. "The vascular anatomy of the pectoralis major myocutaneous flap." *Br. J. Plast. Surg.* 34(1): 3, 1981.

Frias, J.L. and Felman, A.H. "Absence of the pectoralis major, with ipsilateral aplasia of the radius, thumb, hemidiaphragm and lung: an extreme expression of Poland anomaly?" *Birth Defects* 10(5): 55, 1974.

Green, M.F., Gibson, J.R., Bryson, J.R., and Thomson, E. "A one-stage correction of mandibular defects using a split sternum pectoralis major osteomusculocutaneous transfer." *Br. J. Plast. Surg.* 34: 11, 1981.

Gregor, R.T. "The use of the pectoralis major myocutaneous island flap for reconstruction after major ablative head and neck surgery." *S. Afr. Med. J.* 61(21): 788, 1982.

PECTORALIS MYOCUTANEOUS FLAP

Harrison, D.H. "The pectoralis major vascularized muscle graft for the treatment of unilateral facial palsy." *Plast. Reconstr. Surg.* 75(2): 206, 1985.

Hedge, H.R. and Shokeir, M.H. "Posterior shoulder girdle abnormalities with absence of pectoralis major muscle." *Am. J. Med. Genet.* 13(3): 285, 1982.

Herrera, H.R. and Ginsburg, M.E. "The pectoralis major myocutaneous flap and omental transposition for closure of infected median sternotomy wounds." *Plast. Reconstr. Surg.* 70(4): 465, 1982.

Hodgkinson, D.J. "The pectoralis major myocutaneous flap for intraoral reconstruction: a word of warning." *Br. J. Plast. Surg.* 35: 80, 1982.

Hueston, J.J. and McConchie, D.H. "A compound pectoral flap." *Aust. N.Z. J. Surg.* 38: 61, 1968.

Hurwitz, D.J. "Complicated neck contracture treated with a pectoralis major myocutaneous flap." *Plast. Reconstr. Surg.* 63(6): 788, 1979.

Jones, N.F. and Sommerlad, B.C. "Reconstruction of the zygoma, temporo-mandibular joint, and mandible using a compound pectoralis major osteo-muscular flap." *Br. J. Plast. Surg.* 36(4): 491, 1983.

Joseph, C.A., Waner, M., Gregor, R.T., Davidge-Pitts, K.J., and Scott, N. "Pharyngo-esophageal reconstruction with the pectoralis major myocutaneous flap." *S. Afr. J. Surg.* 23(2): 67, 1985.

Kaplan, I.B. and Harwick, R.D. "Pectoralis major myocutaneous island flap revisited: a sentinel vessel simplifying dissection." *Head Neck Surg.* 5: 452, 1983.

Krishnan, M.M. and Canaganayagam, A. "The pectoralis major myocutaneous flap in the primary reconstruction of orofacial defects." *Med. J. Malaysia* 38(2): 126, 1983.

Kudo, K., Miyasawa, M., Fujioka, Y., and Sasaki, J. "Immediate repair of mandibular defects following surgery for carcinoma of the lower alveolus and gingiva using a pectoralis major osteomyocutaneous flap." *J. Maxillofac. Surg.* 13(3): 116, 1985.

Lam, K.H., Wei, W.I., and Sui, K.F. "The pectoralis major osteomyocutaneous flap for mandibular reconstruction." *Plast. Reconstr. Surg.* 73(6): 904, 1984.

Landra, A.P. "One-stage reconstruction of a massive gunshot wound of the lower face with a local compound osteomusculocutaneous flap." *Br. J. Plast. Surg.* 34: 395, 1981.

Little, J.W., III, McCollough, D.T., and Lyons, J.R. "The lateral pectoral composite flap in one-stage reconstruction of the irradiated mandible." *Plast. Reconstr. Surg.* 71(3): 326, 1981.

Luce, E.A. and Gottlieb, S.F. "The pectoralis major island flap for coverage in the upper extremity." *J. Hand Surg.* (Am.) 7(2): 156, 1982.

Magee, W.P., Jr., McCraw, J.B., Horton, C.E., and McInnis, W.D. "Pectoralis 'paddle' myocutaneous flaps: the workhorse of head and neck reconstruction." *Am. J. Surg.* 140: 507, 1980.

Maisel, R.H. and Liston, S.L. "Combined pectoralis major myocutaneous flap with medially based deltopectoral flap for closure of large pharyngocutaneous fistulas." *Ann. Otol. Rhinol. Laryngol.* 91(1 Pt. 1): 98, 1982.

Maisel, R.H., Liston, S.L., and Adams, G.L. "Complications of pectoralis myocutaneous flaps." *Laryngoscope* 93(7): 928, 1983.

Maruyama, Y., Fujino, T., Aoyagi, F., and Ozu, D. "One-stage reconstruction of oral cavity by use of pectoralis major myocutaneous island flap." *Keio, J. Med.* 27(2): 47, 1978.

Maruyama, Y., Nakajima, H., and Fujino, T. "A dynamic reconstruction of a facial defect with a pectoralis major myocutaneous flap." *Br. J. Plast. Surg.* 33: 145, 1980.

McCraw, J.B., Dibbell, D.G., and Carraway, J.H. "Clinical definition of independent myocutaneous vascular territories." *Plast. Reconstr. Surg.* 60: 341, 1977.

McGregor, I.A. "A 'defensive' approach to the island pectoralis flap myocutaneous flap." *Br. J. Plast. Surg.* 34(4): 435, 1981.

Mehrhof, A.I., Jr., Rosenstock, A., Neifeld, J.P., Merritt, W.H., Theogaraj, S.D., and Cohen, I.K. "The pectoralis major myocutaneous flap in head and neck reconstruction: analysis of complications." *Am. J. Surg.* 146(4): 478, 1983.

Mendelson, B.C. "The pectoralis major island flap: an important new flap for head and neck reconstruction." *Br. J. Plast. Surg.* 33(3): 318, 1980.

Morain, W.D., Colen, L.B., and Hutchings, J.C. "The segmental pectoralis major muscle flap: a function-preserving procedure." *Plast. Reconstr. Surg.* 75(6): 825, 1985.

Morain, W.D. and Geurkink, N.A. "Split pectoralis major myocutaneous flap." *Ann. Plast. Surg.* 5(5): 358, 1980.

Morgan, R.F., Sargent, L.A., and Hoopes, J.E. "Midfacial and total nasal reconstruction with bilateral pectoralis major myocutaneous flaps." *Plast. Reconstr. Surg.* 73(5): 824, 1984.

Murakami, Y., Saito, S., Ikari, T., Haraguchi, S., and Okada, K. "Esophageal reconstruction with a skin-grafted pectoralis major muscle flap." *Arch. Otolaryngol.* 108(1): 719, 1982.

Navarro-Vila, C., Zarate-Salazar, J., Molini-Dezotti, D., Martinez-Alegrio, J., Izaguirre-Espinozo, H., Suner-Machado, M., and Gil, J. "Reconstruction experience with myocutaneous and osteomyocutaneous skin flaps in oncological surgery of the head and neck." *J. Maxillofac. Surg.* 12(3): 107, 1984.

Neifeld, J.P., Merritt, W.A., Theogaraj, S.D., and Parker, G.A. "Tubed pectoralis major musculocutaneous flaps for cervical esophageal replacement." *Ann. Plast. Surg.* 11(1): 24, 1983.

Neifeld, J.P., Theogaraj, S.D., and Mehrhof, A.I. "Reconstruction after mediastinal tracheostomy." *Am. J. Surg.* 148(4): 505, 1984.

PECTORALIS MYOCUTANEOUS FLAP

Nicolai, J.P., Bruaset, I., and Manni, J.J. "Experiences with myocutaneous island flaps of the pectoralis major muscle for reconstruction of defects in the bucco-pharyngeal cavity." *Neth. J. Surg.* 35(1): 1, 1983.

Ossoff, R.H., Wurster, C.F., Berktold, R.E., Krespi, Y.P., and Sisson, G.A. "Complications after pectoralis major myocutaneous flap reconstruction of head and neck defects." *Arch. Otolaryngol.* 109(12): 812, 1983.

Pairolero, P.C. and Arnold, P.G. "Management of recalcitrant median sternotomy wounds." *J. Thorac. Cardiovasc. Surg.* 88(3): 357, 1984.

Price, J.C., Davis, R.K., and Koltai, P.J. "The pectoralis myocutaneous flap for salvage of necrotic wounds." *Laryngoscope* 95(2): 146, 1985.

Rees, R.S., Ivey, G.L., Shock, R.B., et al. "Pectoralis major myocutaneous flaps: long-term follow-up of hypopharyngeal reconstruction." *Plast. Reconstr. Surg.* 77: 586, 1986.

Reid, C.D. and Taylor, G.I. "The vascular territory of the acromiothoracic axis." *Br. J. Plast. Surg.* 37(2): 194, 1984.

Reid, C.D., Taylor, G.I., and Waterhouse, N. "The clavicular head of pectoralis major musculocutaneous free flap." *Br. J. Plast. Surg.* 39: 57, 1986.

Rosenberg, L. and Mahler, D. "Extended rotation-transportation of the pectoralis major myocutaneous flap in the repair of lesions over the shoulder." *Br. J. Plast. Surg.* 34(3): 322, 1981.

Rowsell, A.R., Davies, D.M., Eisenberg, N., and Taylor, G.I. "The anatomy of the subscapular-thoracodorsal arterial system: study of 100 cadaver dissections." *Br. J. Plast. Surg.* 37: 574, 1984.

Saraceno, C.A., Santini, H., Endicott, J.N., Martinez, C., and Shah, C. "The pectoralis major myocutaneous flap: an angiographic study." *Laryngoscope* 93(6): 756, 1983.

Saski, C.T., Ariyan, S., Spencer, D., and Buckwalter, J. "Pectoralis major myocutaneous reconstruction of the anterior skull base." *Laryngoscope* 95(2): 162, 1985.

Schuller, D.E. "Limitations of the pectoralis major myocutaneous flap in head and neck cancer reconstruction." *Arch. Otolaryngol.* 106(11): 709, 1980.

Schuller, D.E. "Pectoralis myocutaneous flap in head and neck cancer reconstruction." *Arch. Otolaryngol.* 109(3): 185, 1983.

Sharzer, L.A., Kalisman, M., Silver, C.E., and Strauch, B. "The parasternal paddle: a modification of the pectoralis major myocutaneous flap." *Plast. Reconstr. Surg.* 67(6): 753, 1981.

Sisson, G.A. and Goldman, M.E. "Pectoral myocutaneous island flap for reconstruction of stomal recurrence." *Arch. Otolaryngol.* 107(7): 446, 1981.

Smith, P.G. and Collins, S.L. "Repair of head and neck defects with thin and double-lined pectoralis flaps." *Arch. Otolaryngol.* 110: 468, 1984.

Soussaline, M., Guedon, C., Petoin, B., et al. "Assessment of the use of the pectoralis major musculocutaneous flaps in head and neck reconstruction." *Ann. Chir. Plast. Esth.* 29: 135, 1984.

Stiernberg, C.M. "Pectoralis myocutaneous flap modifications (letter)." *Arch. Otolaryngol.* 111(3): 208, 1985.

Strawberry, C.W., Jacobs, J.S., and McCraw, J.B. "Reconstruction for cervical irradiation ulcers with myocutaneous flaps." *Head Neck Surg.* 6(4): 836, 1984.

Theogaraj, S.D., Merritt, W.H., Acharya, G., and Cohen, I.K. "The pectoralis major musculocutaneous island flap in single-stage reconstruction of the pharyngoesophageal region." *Plast. Reconstr. Surg.* 65(3): 267, 1980.

Tiwari, R. and Snow, G.B. "Role of myocutaneous flaps in reconstruction of the head and neck." *J. Laryngol. Otol.* 97(5): 441, 1983.

Ueda, M., Torii, S., Nagayama, M., Kaneda, T., and Oka, T. "The pectoralis major myocutaneous flap for intraoral reconstruction: surgical complications and their treatment." *J. Maxillofac. Surg.* 13(1): 9, 1985.

Weaver, A.W., Vandenberg, H.J., Atkinson, D.P., and Wallace, J.R. "Modified bilobular ('gemini') pectoralis major myocutaneous flap." *Am. J. Surg.* 144(4): 482, 1982.

Wei, W.I., Lan, K.H., and Wong, J. "The true pectoralis major myocutaneous island flap: an anatomical study." *Br. J. Plast. Surg.* 37(4): 568, 1984.

Wilk, A., Balme, P., Keiling, R., et al. "The use of the pectoralis major flap in the cervico maxillary surgery of irradiated patients." *Ann. Chir. Plast. Esth.* 30: 373, 1985.

Wilson, J.S., Yiacoumettis, A.M., and O'Neill, J. "Some observations on 112 pectoralis major myocutaneous flaps." *Am. J. Surg.* 147(2): 273, 1984.

Withers, E.H., Franklin, J.D., Madden, J.J., and Lynch, J.B. "Pectoralis major musculocutaneous flap: a new flap in head and neck reconstruction." *Am. J. Surg.* 138(4): 537, 1979.

Withers, E.H., Franklin, J.D., Madden, J.J., and Lynch, J.B. "Immediate reconstruction of the pharynx and cervical esophagus with the pectoralis major myocutaneous flap following laryngopharyngectomy." *Plast. Reconstr. Surg.* 68(6): 898, 1981.

LATISSIMUS

Ali, S., Watson, J.S., and Bihari, J. "Use of the latissimus dorsi myocutaneous flap for total pharyngeal reconstruction." *J. Laryngol. Otol.* 96(9): 837, 1982.

Amoroso, P.J. and Angelats, J. "Latissimus dorsi myocutaneous flap in Poland syndrome." *Ann. Plast. Surg.* 6(4): 287, 1981.

Arianayagam, C. "Latissimus dorsi flap for the head and neck (letter)." *Plast. Reconstr. Surg.* 73(1): 156, 1984.

Arnold, P.G. and Pairolero, P.C. "Chest wall reconstruction: experience with 100 consecutive patients." *Ann. Surg.* 199(6): 725, 1984.

Asko-Seljavaara, S., Pitkanen, J., and Sundell, B. "Microvascular free flaps in early reconstruction of burns in the hand and forearm: case reports." *Scand. J. Plast. Surg.* 18(1): 139, 1984.

Asko-Seljavaara, S., Ryynanen, A., and Sundell, B. "Latissimus dorsi musculocutaneous flap used as a pedicle on free microvascular graft." *Ann. Chir. Gynaecol.* 71(1): 44, 1982.

Axer, A., Segal, D., and Elkon, A. "Partial transposition of the latissimus dorsi: a new operative technique to restore elbow and finger flexion." *J. Bone Joint Surg.* (Am.) 55(6): 1259, 1973.

Bailey, B.N. and Godfrey, A.M. "Latissimus dorsi muscle free flaps." *Br. J. Plast. Surg.* 35: 47, 1982.

Baker, S.R. "Closure of large orbital-maxillary defects with free latissimus dorsi myocutaneous flaps." *Head Neck Surg.* 6(4): 828, 1984.

Barrow, D.L., Nahai, F., and Fleischer, A.S. "Use of free latissimus dorsi musculocutaneous flaps in various neurosurgical disorders." *J. Neurosurg.* 58(2): 252, 1983.

Bartlett, S.P., May, J.W., Jr., and Yaremchuk, M.J. "The latissimus dorsi muscle: a fresh cadaver study of the primary neurovascular pedicle." *Plast. Reconstr. Surg.* 67(5): 631, 1981.

Barton, F.E., Jr., Spicer, T.E., and Byrd, H.S. "Head and neck reconstruction with the latissimus dorsi myocutaneous flap: anatomic observations and report of 60 cases." *Plast. Reconstr. Surg.* 71(2): 199, 1983.

Bianchi, A., Doig, C.M., and Cohen, S.J. "The reverse latissimus dorsi flap for congenital diaphragmatic hernia repair." *J. Pediatr. Surg.* 18(5): 560, 1983.

Biggs, T.M. and Cronin, E.D. "Technical aspects of the latissimus dorsi myocutaneous flap in breast reconstruction." *Ann. Plast. Surg.* 6(5): 381, 1981.

Blaiklock, C.R., Demetriou, E.L., and Rayner, C.R.W. "The use of a latissimus dorsi myocutaneous flap in the repair of spinal defects in spina bifida." *Br. J. Plast. Surg.* 34: 358, 1981.

Bostwick, J., III. "Reconstruction of the breast." *Acta. Chir. Belg.* 79(2): 125, 1980.

Bostwick, J., III. "Latissimus dorsi flap: current applications." *Ann. Plast. Surg.* 9(5): 377, 1982.

Bostwick, J., III, Nahai, F., Wallace, J.G., and Vasconez, L.O. "Sixty latissimus dorsi flaps." *Plast. Reconstr. Surg.* 63(1): 31, 1979.

Bostwick, J., III, and Scheflan, M. "The latissimus dorsi musculocutaneous flap: a one-stage breast reconstruction." *Clin. Plast. Surg.* 7(1): 71, 1980.

Bostwick, J., III, Scheflan, M., Nahai, F., and Jurkiewicz, M.J. "The 'reverse' latissimus dorsi muscle and musculotaneous flap: anatomical and clinical considerations." *Plast. Reconstr. Surg.* 65(4): 395, 1980.

Bostwick, J., III, Stevenson, T.R., Nahai, F., Hester, T.R., Coleman, J.J., and Jurkiewicz, M.J. "Radiation to the breast: complications amenable to surgical treatment." *Ann. Surg.* 200(4): 543, 1984.

Bostwick, J., III, Vasconez, L.O., and Jurkiewicz, M.J. "Breast reconstruction after a radical mastectomy." *Plast. Reconstr. Surg.* 61(5): 682, 1978.

Broadbent, T.R. and Woolf, R.M. "Breast reconstruction: a better skin pattern." *Aesthetic Plast. Surg.* 7(3): 145, 1983.

Brones, M.F., Wheeler, E.S., and Lesavoy, M.A. "Restoration of elbow flexion and arm contour with the latissimus dorsi myocutaneous flap." *Plast. Reconstr. Surg.* 69(2): 329, 1982.

Buncke, H.H. "Functional reconstruction of an extremity by free tissue transfer of the latissimus dorsi (letter)." *J. Bone Joint Surg.* (Am.) 66(5): 806, 1984.

Campbell, D.A. "Reconstruction of the anterior thoracic wall." *J. Thorac. Surg.* 19: 456, 1950.

Chaikhouni, A., Dyas, C.J., Jr., Robinson, J.H., and Kelleher, J.C. "Latissimus dorsi free myocutaneous flap." *J. Trauma* 21(5): 398, 1981.

Chicarilli, Z.N., Ariyan, S., Glenn, W.W., and Seashore, J.H. "Management of recalcitrant bronchopleural fistulas with muscle flap obliteration." *Plast. Reconstr. Surg.* 75(6): 882, 1985.

Christ, J.E. and Spira, M. "Application of the latissimus dorsi muscle to the heart." *Ann. Plast. Surg.* 8(2): 118, 1982.

Clovutivat, V. "Reconstruction of cheek and buccal mucosa with latissimus dorsi musculocutaneous flap." *Ann. Acad. Med.* Singapore 9(3): 342, 1980.

Cohen, B.E. "Shoulder defect correction with the island latissimus dorsi flap." *Plast. Reconstr. Surg.* 74(5): 650, 1984.

Cohen, B.E. and Cronin, E.D. "Breast reconstruction with the Latissimus dorsi musculocutaneous flap." *Clin. Plast. Surg.* 11(2): 287, 1984.

Cooper, G.G., Webster, M.H.C., and Bell, G. "The results of breast reconstruction following mastectomy." *Br. J. Plast. Surg.* 37: 369, 1984.

Dabb, R.W. and Conklin, W.T. "A sensory innervated latissimus dorsi musculocutaneous free flap: case report." *J. Microsurg.* 2(4): 289, 1981.

Davis, H.H., Tollman, J.P., and Brush, J.H. "Huge chondrosarcoma rib." *Surgery* 26: 699, 1949.

LATISSIMUS

Desprez, J.D., Kiehn, C.L., and Echstein, W. "Closure of large meningomyelocele defects by composite skin muscle flaps." *Plast. Reconstr. Surg.* 47: 234, 1971.

Dinner, M.I. "Value of angiography prior to use of the latissimus dorsi myocutaneous flap (letter)." *Plast. Reconstr. Surg.* 64(4): 553, 1979.

Doi, K., Ihara, K., Sakamoto, T., and Kawai, S. "Functional latissimus dorsi island pedicle musculocutaneous flap to restore finger function." *J. Hand Surg.* 10(5): 678, 1985.

Dowden, R.V., Horton, C.E., Rosato, F.E., and McCraw, J.B. "Reconstruction of the breast after mastectomy for cancer." *Surg. Gynecol. Obstet.* 149: 109, 1979.

Dowden, R.V. and McCraw, J.B. "Muscle flap reconstruction of shoulder defects." *J. Hand Surg.* 5(4): 382, 1980.

Fisher, J., Bostwick, J., III, and Powell, R. "Latissimus dorsi blood supply after thoracodorsal vessel division: the serratus collateral." *Plast. Reconstr. Surg.* 72(4): 502, 1983.

Fisher, J. and Wood, M.B. "The late necrosis of a latissimus dorsi free flap." *Plast. Reconstr. Surg.* 74(2): 274, 1984.

Fodor, P.B. and Khoury, F. "Latissimus dorsi muscle flap in reconstruction of congenitally absent breast and pectoralis muscle." *Ann. Plast. Surg.* 4(5): 422, 1980.

Gordon, L., Buncke, H.J., and Alpert, B.S. "Free latissimus dorsi muscle flap with split-thickness skin graft cover: a report of 16 cases." *Plast. Reconstr. Surg.* 70(2): 173, 1982.

Guly'as, G., Kartik, I., and Tak'acs, L. "Latissimus dorsi musculocutaneous island flap for the reconstruction of soft tissue defects of the upper arm." *Acta. Chir. Plast.* (Prague) 25(2): 72, 1983.

Hagan, K.F., Buncke, H.J., and Gonzalez, R. "Free latissimus dorsi muscle flap coverage of an electrical burn of the lower extremity." *Plast. Reconstr. Surg.* 69(1): 125, 1982.

Handel, N. and Post, G. "Latissimus dorsi musculocutaneous flap in postthoracotomy patient." *Ann. Plast. Surg.* 10(4): 314, 1983.

Haller, J.A., Jr., Colombani, P.M., Miller, D., and Manson, P. "Early reconstruction of Poland's syndrome using autologous rib grafts combined with a latissimus muscle flap." *J. Pediatr. Surg.* 19(4): 423, 1984.

Harashina, T., Takayama, S., Ikuta, Y., and Fujino, T. "Reconstruction of chest-wall radiation ulcer with free latissimus dorsi muscle flap and meshed skin graft." *Plast. Reconstr. Surg.* 71(6): 805, 1983.

Hochberg, J. and Fortes da Silva, F.B. "Latissimus dorsi myocutaneous flap to restore elbow flexion and axillary burn contracture: a report on two pediatric patients." *J. Pediatr. Orthop.* 2(5): 565, 1982.

Jamra, F.N.A., Akel, S.R., and Shamma, A.R. "Repair of major defect of the upper extremity with a latissimus dorsi myocutaneous flap: a case report." *Br. J. Plast. Surg.* 34: 121, 1981.

Jones, B.N., Manske, P.R., Schoenecker, P.L., and Dailey, L. "Latissimus dorsi transfer to restore elbow extension in obstetrical palsy." *J. Pediatr. Orthop.* 5(3): 287, 1985.

Johnson, B., Olofsson, B.M., and Steffner, L.C. "Function of the teres major, latissimus dorsi, and pectoralis major muscles: a preliminary study." *Acta. Morphol. Neerl. Scand.* 9(4): 275, 1972.

Jurkiewicz, M.J. and Arnold, P.G. "The omentum: an account of its use in reconstruction of the chest wall." *Ann. Surg.* 185(5): 548, 1977.

Kanavel, A.B. "Plastic procedures for the obliteration of cavities with non-collapsible walls." *Surg. Gynecol. Obstet.* 32: 453, 1921.

Katsaros, J., Gilbert, D., and Russell, R. "The use of a combined latissimus dorsi-groin flap as a direct flap for reconstruction of the upper extremity." *Br. J. Plast. Surg.* 36: 67, 1983.

Knowlton, E.W. "Release of axillary scar contracture with a latissimus dorsi flap." *Plast. Reconstr. Surg.* 74(1): 124, 1984.

Kobus, K., Stepniewski, J., and Charko, W. "History and remarks on clinical use of groin, dorsalis pedis, and musculocutaneous latissimus dorsi free flaps." *Acta. Chir. Plast.* (Prague) 24(2): 74, 1982.

Krishna, B.V. and Green, M.F. "Extended role of latissimus dorsi myocutaneous flap in reconstruction of the neck." *Br. J. Plast. Surg.* 33: 233, 1980.

Lai, M.F., Milroy, B.C., and Pennington, D.G. "Shoulder defect cover with functional restoration using the latissimus dorsi myocutaneous flap: a case report." *Br. J. Plast. Surg.* 35: 140, 1982.

Laitung, J.K. and Peck, F. "Shoulder function following the loss of the latissimus dorsi muscle." *Br. J. Plast. Surg.* 38(3): 375, 1985.

Landra, A.P. "The latissimus dorsi musculocutaneous flap used to resurface a defect on the upper arm and restore extension to the elbow." *Br. J. Plast. Surg.* 32(4): 275, 1979.

LaRossa, D., Mellissinos, E., Matthews, D., and Hamilton, R. "The use of microvascular free skin-muscle flaps in management of avulsion injuries of the lower leg." *J. Trauma* 20(7): 545, 1980.

Larson, D.L. and McMurtrey, M.J. "Musculocutaneous flap reconstruction of chest-wall defects: an experience with 50 patients." *Plast. Reconstr. Surg.* 73(5): 734, 1984.

Larson, D.L., McMurtrey, M.J., Howe, J.H., and Irish, C.E. "Major chest wall reconstruction after chest wall irradiation." *Cancer* 49(6): 1286, 1982.

Larsson, S., Pettersson, G., Eldh, J., and Eriksson, E. "Reconstruction of large anterior full-thickness defect in the chest wall after resection of chondrosarcoma." *Scand. J. Thorac. Cardiovasc. Surg.* 18(1): 63, 1984.

Lassen, M., Krag, C., and Nielsen, I.M. "The latissimus dorsi flap: an overview." *Scand. J. Plast. Reconstr. Surg.* 19(1): 41, 1985.

LATISSIMUS

Lehrman, A. and Owen, M.P. "Surgical repair of large meningomyeloceles." *Ann. Plast. Surg.* 12(6): 501, 1984.

Lejour, M., Alemanno, P., and DeMay, A. "Analysis of 56 breast reconstructions using the latissimus dorsi flap." *Ann. Chir. Plast. Esth.* 30: 7, 1985.

Levine, R.A. and DeFelice, C.A. "Possible explanation of successful latissimus dorsi flap without the thoracodorsal artery." *Plast. Reconstr. Surg.* 65(4): 532, 1980.

Lewinsky, B.S. "Latissimus dorsi myocutaneous flap (letter)." *Arch. Otolaryngol.* 110(5): 341, 1984.

Logan, A.M. and Black, M.J. "Injury to the brachial plexus resulting from shoulder positioning during latissimus dorsi flap pedicle dissection." *Br. J. Plast. Surg.* 38(3): 380, 1985.

Luce, E.A. and Walsh, J. "Wound closure of the myelomeningocoele defect." *Plast. Reconstr. Surg.* 75(3): 389, 1985.

MacKinnon, S.E., Weiland, A.J., and Godina, M. "Immediate forearm reconstruction with a functional latissimus dorsi island pedicle myocutaneous flap." *Plast. Reconstr. Surg.* 71(5): 706, 1983.

Magee, W.P., Jr., Gilbert, D.A. and McInnis, W.D. "Extended muscle and musculocutaneous flaps." *Clin. Plast. Surg.* 7(1): 57, 1980.

Marshall, D.R., Anstee, E.J., and Stapleton, M.J. "Immediate reconstruction of the breast following modified radical mastectomy for carcinoma." *Br. J. Plast. Surg.* 35: 438, 1982.

Marshall, D.R., Anstee, E.J., and Stapleton, M.J. "Soft tissue reconstruction of the breast using an extended composite latissimus dorsi myocutaneous flap." *Br. J. Plast. Surg.* 37(3): 361, 1984.

Maruyama, Y., Urita, Y., and Ohnishi, K. "Rib-latissimus dorsi osteomyocutaneous flap in reconstruction of a mandibular defect." *Br. J. Plast. Surg.* 38(2): 234, 1985.

Maves, M.D., Panje, W.R., and Shagets, F.W. "Extended latissimus dorsi myocutaneous flap reconstruction of major head and neck defects." *Otolaryngol. Head Neck Surg.* 92(5): 551, 1984.

Maxwell, G.P. "Iginio Tansini and the origin of the latissimus dorsi musculocutaneous flap." *Plast. Reconstr. Surg.* 65(5): 686, 1980.

Maxwell, G.P. "Latissimus dorsi breast reconstruction: an aesthetic assessment." *Clin. Plast. Surg.* 8(2): 373, 1981.

Maxwell, G.P., Horton, C.E., and McCraw, J.B. "Cancer trends: breast reconstruction after mastectomy." *Va. Med.* 108: 328, 1981.

Maxwell, G.P., Leonard, L.G., Manson, P.N., and Hoopes, J.E. "Craniofacial coverage using the latissimus dorsi myocutaneous island flap." *Ann. Plast. Surg.* 4(5): 410, 1980.

Maxwell, G.P., Manson, P.N., and Hoopes, J.E. "Experience with thirteen latissimus dorsi myocutaneous free flaps." *Plast. Reconstr. Surg.* 64(1): 1, 1979.

Maxwell, G.P., McGibbon, B.M., and Hoopes, J.E. "Vascular considerations in the use of a latissimus dorsi myocutaneous flap after a mastectomy with an axillary dissection." *Plast. Reconstr. Surg.* 64(6): 771, 1979.

Maxwell, G.P., Stueber, K., and Hoopes, J.E. "A free latissimus dorsi myocutaneous flap: case report." *Plast. Reconstr. Surg.* 62(3): 462, 1978.

May, J.W., Jr., Gallico, G.G., III, Jupiter, J., and Savage, R.C. "Free latissimus dorsi muscle flap with skin graft for treatment of traumatic chronic bony wounds." *Plast. Reconstr. Surg.* 73(4): 641, 1984.

McCraw, J.B., Bostwick, J. III, and Horton, C.E. "Methods of soft tissue coverage for the mastectomy defect." *Clin. Plast. Surg.* 6(1): 57, 1979.

McCraw, J.B., Dibbell, D.G., and Carraway, J.H. "Clinical definition of independent myocutaneous vascular territories." *Plast. Reconstr. Surg.*, 60: 341, 1977.

McCraw, J.B. and Horton, C.E. "Reconstruction of the breast." *Va. Med.* 109: 770, 1982.

McCraw, J.B., Maxwell, G.P., and Horton, C.E. "Reconstruction of the breast following mastectomy." *Acta Chir. Belg.* 2: 131, 1980.

McCraw, J.B., Penix, J.O., and Baker, J.W. "Repair of major defects of the chest wall and spine with the latissimus dorsi myocutaneous flap." *Plast. Reconstr. Surg.* 62(2): 197, 1978.

McGregor, J.C. "The 'reverse' latissimus dorsi musculocutaneous flap: case report." *J.R. Coll. Surg. Edinb.* 28(3): 154, 1983.

Medgyesi, S. "A successful operation for lymphaedema using a myocutaneous flap as a 'wick'." *Br. J. Plast. Surg.* 36: 64, 1983.

Mendelson, B.C. "The latissimus dorsi flap for breast reconstruction." *Aust. N.Z. J. Surg.* 50(2): 200, 1980.

Mendelson, B.C. "Latissimus dorsi breast reconstruction: refinement and results." *Br. J. Plast. Surg.* 70(3): 145, 1983.

Mendelson, B.C. and Masson, J.K. "Treatment of chronic radiation injury over the shoulder with a latissimus dorsi myocutaneous flap." *Plast. Reconstr. Surg.* 60(5): 681, 1977.

Millard, D.R., Jr. "Breast aesthetics when reconstructing with the latissimus dorsi musculocutaneous flap." *Plast. Reconstr. Surg.* 70(2): 161, 1982.

Moore, T.S., Dreyer, T.M., and Bevin, A.G. "Closure of large spina bifida cystica defects with bilateral bipedicled musculocutaneous flaps." *Plast. Reconstr. Surg.* 73(2): 288, 1984.

Morain, W.D. "Flaps of the latissimus dorsi muscle in difficult wounds of the trunk and arm." *Am. J. Surg.* 145(4): 520, 1983.

Morris, R.L., Given, K.S., and McCabe, J.S. "Repair of head and neck defects with the latissimus dorsi myocutaneous flap." *Am. Surg.* 47(4): 167, 1981.

LATISSIMUS

Muhlbauer, W. and Olbrisch, R. "The latissimus dorsi myocutaneous flap for breast reconstruction." *Chir. Plastica.* 4: 27, 1977.

Muldowney, J.B., Magi, E., Hein, K., and Birdsell, D. "The reverse latissimus dorsi myocutaneous flap with functional preservation: report of a case." *Ann. Plast. Surg.* 7(2): 150, 1981.

Nakajima, H. and Fujino, T. "Island fasciocutaneous flaps of dorsal trunk and their application to myocutaneous flaps." *Keio. J. Med.* 33(2): 59, 1984.

Narula, A.A. and Breach, N.C. "The use of the latissimus dorsi muscle flap for posterior scalp defects." *J. Laryngol. Otol.* 99(7): 693, 1985.

Nash, A.G. and Hurst, P.A. "Central breast carcinoma treated by simultaneous mastectomy and latissimus dorsi flap reconstruction." *Br. J. Surg.* 70(11): 654, 1983.

Nielsen, I.M., Lassen, M., Gregersen, B.N., and Krag, C. "Experience with the latissimus dorsi flap." *Scand. J. Rehabil. Med.* 17(2): 53, 1985.

O'Brien, B.M., Morrison, W.A., Lawler, D.L., MacLeod, A., and Newing, R.K. "The versatile latissimus dorsi myocutaneous flap in breast and other reconstruction." *Aust. N.Z. J. Surg.* 52(2): 174, 1982.

Ogawa, J., Inoue, H., Shohtsu, A., Tajima, T., Tanino, R., and Yamazaki, S. "Reconstruction of sternal defects with autologus bone grafts and myocutaneous flap of the latissimus dorsi muscle." *Tokai J. Exp. Clin. Med.* 7(1): 63, 1982.

Ohmori, K. and Takada, H. "Correction of Poland's pectoralis major muscle anomaly with latissimus dorsi musculocutaneous flaps." *Plast. Reconstr. Surg.* 65(4): 400, 1980.

Olivari, N. "The latissimus flap." *Br. J. Plast. Surg.* 29: 126, 1976.

Olivari, N. "Use of thirty latissimus dorsi flaps." *Plast. Reconstr. Surg.* 64(5): 654, 1979.

Pendergast, W.J., Jr., Bostwick, J., III, and Jurkiewicz, M.J. "The subcutaneous mastectomy cripple: surgical rehabilitation with the latissimus dorsi flap." *Plast. Reconstr. Surg.* 66(4): 554, 1980.

Pousset, C., Salmon, R.J., Soussaline, M., et al. "The use of a latissimus dorsi myocutaneous flap for the treatment of recurrent breast cancer." *Ann. Chir. Plast. Esth.* 31: 82, 1986.

Quillen, C.G. "Latissimus dorsi myocutaneous flaps in head and neck reconstruction." *Plast. Reconstr. Surg.* 63(5): 664, 1979.

Quillen, C.G., Shearin, J.C., Jr., and Georgiade, N.G. "Use of the latissimus dorsi myocutaneous island flap for reconstruction in the head and neck area: case report." *Plast. Reconstr. Surg.* 62(1): 113, 1978.

Ramming, K.P., Holmes, E.C., Zarem, H.A., Lesavoy, M.A., and Morton, D.L. "Surgical management and reconstruction of extensive chest wall malignancies." *Am. J. Surg.* 144(1): 146, 1982.

Reid, C.D. and Taylor, G.I. "The vascular territory of the acromiothoracic axis." *Br. J. Plast. Surg.* 37: 194, 1984.

Rosen, H.M. "Double island latissimus dorsi muscle-skin flap for through-and-through defects of the forefoot." *Plast. Reconstr. Surg.* 76(3): 461, 1985.

Rowsell, A.R., Davies, D.M., Eisenberg, N., and Taylor, G.I. "The anatomy of the subscapular-thoracodorsal arterial system: study of 100 cadaver dissections." *Br. J. Plast. Surg.* 37(4): 574, 1984.

Rubinstein, Z.J., Shafir, R., and Tsur, H. "The value of angiography prior to the use of the latissimus dorsi myocutaneous flap." *Plast. Reconstr. Surg.* 63(3): 374, 1979.

Sabatier, R.E. and Bakamjian, V.Y. "Transaxillary latissimus dorsi flap reconstruction in head and neck cancer: limitations and refinements in 56 cases." *Am. J. Surg.* 150(4): 427, 1985.

Scheflan, M., Mehrhof, A.I., Jr., and Ward, J.D. "Meningomyelocele closure with distally based latissimus dorsi flap." *Plast. Reconstr. Surg.* 73(6): 956, 1984.

Schmidt, D.R. and Robson, M.C. "One-stage composite reconstruction using the latissimus myoosteocutaneous free flap." *Am. J. Surg.* 144(4): 470, 1982.

Schneider, W.J., Hill, H.L., Jr., and Brown, R.G. "Latissimus dorsi myocutaneous flap for breast reconstruction." *Br. J. Plast. Surg.* 30(4): 277, 1977.

Schuller, D.E. "Latissimus dorsi myocutaneous flap for massive facial defects." *Arch. Otolaryngol.* 108(7): 414, 1982.

Shesol, B.F. and Clarke, J.S. "Intrathoracic application of the latissimus dorsi musculocutaneous flap." *Plast. Reconstr. Surg.* 66(6): 842, 1980.

Silverton, S., Nahai, F., and Jurkiewicz, M.J. "The latissimus dorsi myocutaneous flap to replace a defect on the upper arm." *Br. J. Plast. Surg.* 31(1): 29, 1978.

Smith, A.R., Sonneveld, G.J., and van Alphen, V.A. "The free latissimus dorsi flap in reconstructive microsurgery." *Neth. J. Surg.* 37(1): 7, 1985.

Stern, P.J., Neale, H.W., Gregory, R.O., and Kreilein, J.G. "Latissimus dorsi musculocutaneous flap for elbow flexion." *J. Hand Surg.* (Am.) 7(1): 25, 1982.

Stern, P.J., Neale, H.W., Gregory, R.O., and McDonough, J.J. "Functional reconstruction of an extremity by free tissue transfer of the latissimus dorsi." *J. Bone Joint Surg.* (Am.) 65(6): 729, 1983.

Stevenson, T.R., Duus, E.C., Greene, T.L., and Dingman, R.O. "Traumatic upper arm defect treated with latissimus dorsi muscle transposition." *J. Pediatr. Ortho.* 4(1): 111, 1984.

Stevenson, T.R., Rohrich, R.J., Pollock, R.A., Dingman, R.O., and Bostwick, J., III. "More experience with the 'reverse' latissimus dorsi musculocutaneous flap: precise location of blood supply." *Plast. Reconstr. Surg.* 74(2): 237, 1984.

LATISSIMUS

Takami, H., Takahashi, S., and Ando, M. "Latissimus dorsi transplantation to restore elbow flexion to the paralysed limb." *J. Hand Surg.* 9(1): 61, 1984.

Takami, H., Takahashi, S., and Ando, M. "Microvascular free musculocutaneous flaps for the treatment of avulsion injuries of the lower leg." *J. Trauma* 23(6): 473, 1983.

Takayanagi, S. and Tsukie, T. "Our experiences with the free latissimus dorsi myocutaneous flap." *Ann. Plast. Surg.* 5(6): 442, 1980.

Thomas, J.M. "Latissimus dorsi reconstruction of the breast (editorial)." *Br. Med. J.* (Clin. Res.) 287(6392): 569, 1983.

Tizian, C., Borst, H.G., and Berger, A. "Treatment of total sternal necrosis using the latissimus dorsi muscle flap." *Plast. Reconstr. Surg.* 76(5): 703, 1985.

Tobin, G.R., Mavroudis, C., Howe, W.R., and Gray, L.A., Jr. "Reconstruction of complex thoracic defects with myocutaneous and muscle flaps: applications of new flap refinements." *J. Thorac. Cardiovasc. Surg.* 85(2): 219, 1983.

Tobin, G.R., Moberg, A.W., DuBou, R.H., Weiner, L.J., and Bland, K.I. "The split latissimus dorsi myocutaneous flap." *Ann. Plast. Surg.* 7(4): 272, 1981.

Tobin, G.R., Schusterman, M., Peterson, G.H., Nichols, G., and Bland, K.I. "The intramuscular neurovascular anatomy of the latissimus dorsi muscle: the basis for splitting the flap." *Plast. Reconstr. Surg.* 67(5): 637, 1981.

Tomono, T., Hirose, T., Matsuo, K., and Matsui, T. "A denuded 'turn-over' deltopectoral flap combined with a latissimus dorsi myocutaneous flap in the repair of extensive radionecrosis of the chest wall." *Br. J. Plast. Surg.* 35: 63, 1982.

Vasconez, L.O., Johnson-Giebink, R., and Hall, E.J. "Breast reconstruction." *Clin. Plast. Surg.* 7(1): 79, 1980.

Vila, R. and Guinot, A. "Post-mastectomy breast reconstruction in an irradiated field using a contralateral latissimus dorsi free flap." *Br. J. Plast. Surg.* 35: 371, 1982.

Watson, J.S. "The use of the latissimus dorsi island flap for intra-oral reconstruction." *Br. J. Plast. Surg.* 35: 408, 1982.

Watson, J.S., Craig, R.D.P., and Orton, C.I. "The free latissimus dorsi myocutaneous flap." *Plast. Reconstr. Surg.* 64(3): 299, 1979.

Watson, J.S., and Lendrum, J. "One-stage pharyngeal reconstruction using a compound latissimus dorsi island flap." *Br. J. Plast. Surg.* 34: 87, 1981.

Wolf, L.E. and Biggs, T.M. "Aesthetic refinements in the use of the latissimus dorsi flap in breast reconstruction." *Plast. Reconstr. Surg.* 69(5): 788, 1982.

Yamamoto, K., Yokota, K., and Higaki, K. "Entire pharyngoesophageal reconstruction with latissimus dorsi myocutaneous island flap." *Head Neck Surg.* 7(6): 461, 1985.

Zancolli, E. and Mitre, H. "Latissimus dorsi transfer to restore elbow flexion: an appraisal of eight cases." *J. Bone Joint Surg.* (Am.) 55(6): 1265, 1973.

SERRATUS

Arnold, P.G. and Pairolero, P.C. "Chondrosarcoma of the manubrium: resection and reconstruction with pectoralis major muscle." *Mayo Clin. Proc.* 53(1): 54, 1978.

Arnold, P.G. and Pairolero, P.C. "Use of pectoralis major muscle flaps to repair defects of anterior chest wall." *Plast. Reconstr. Surg.* 63: 205, 1979.

Arnold, P.G. and Pairolero, P.C. "Chest wall reconstruction: experience with 100 consecutive patients." *Ann. Surg.* 199(6): 725, 1984.

Arnold, P.G., Pairolero, P.C., and Waldorf, J.C. "The serratus anterior muscle: intrathoracic and extrathoracic utilization." *Plast. Reconstr. Surg.* 73(2): 240, 1984.

Bartlett, S.P., May, J.W., Jr., and Yaremchuk, M.J. "The latissimus dorsi muscle: A fresh cadaver study of the primary neurovascular pedicle." *Plast. Reconstr. Surg.* 67: 631, 1981.

Duncan, M.A., Lotze, M.T., Gerber, L.H., and Rosenberg, S.A. "Incidence, recovery, and management of serratus anterior muscle palsy after axillary node dissection." *Phys. Ther.* 63(8): 1243, 1983.

Gregg, J.R., Labosky, D., Harty, M., Lotke, P., Ecker, M., DiStefano, V., and Das, M. "Serratus anterior paralysis in the young athlete." *J. Bone Joint Surg.* (Am.) 61: 825, 1979.

Gruber, R.P., Kahn, R.A., Lash, H., Maser, M.R., Apfelberg, D.B., and Laub, D.R. "Breast reconstruction following mastectomy: a comparison of submuscular and subcutaneous techniques." *Plast. Reconstr. Surg.* 67: 312, 1981.

Harii, K., Ono, I., and Ebihara, S. "Closure of total cheek defects with two combined myocutaneous free flaps." *Arch. Otolaryngol.* 108: 303, 1982.

Harii, K., Yamada, A., Ishihara, K., Miki, Y., and Itoh, M. "A free transfer of both latissimus dorsi and serratus anterior flaps with thoracodorsal vessel anastomoses." *Plast. Reconstr. Surg.* 70(5): 620, 1982.

Horwitz, M.T. and Tocantins, L.M. "Isolated paralysis of the serratus anterior (magnus) muscle." *J. Bone Joint Surg.* (Am.) 20: 720, 1938.

Jarrett, J.R., Cutler, R.G., and Teal, D.F. "Aesthetic refinements of prophylactic subcutaneous mastectomy with submuscular reconstruction." *Plast. Reconstr. Surg.* 69: 624, 1982.

Khoo, C.T.K. and Bailey, B.N. "The behaviour of free muscle and musculocutaneous flaps after early loss of axial blood supply." *Br. J. Plast. Surg.* 35: 43, 1982.

Pairolero, P.C. and Arnold, P.G. "Bronchopleural fistula: treatment by transportation of pectoralis major muscle." *J. Thorac. Cardiovasc. Surg.* 79(1): 142, 1980.

Pairolero, P.C. and Arnold, P.G. "Management of recalcitrant median sternotomy wounds." *J. Thorac. Cardiovasc. Surg.* 88(3): 357, 1984.

Pairolero, P.C., Arnold, P.G., and Piehler, J.M. "Intrathoracic transposition of extrathoracic skeletal muscle." *J. Thorac. Cardiovasc. Surg.* 86(6): 809, 1983.

Rasch, P.J. and Burke, R.K. *Kinesiology and Applied Anatomy: The Science of Human Movement*, 6th Ed. Philadelphia: Lea & Febiger, 1978.

Takayanagi, S. and Tsukie, T. "Free serratus anterior muscle and myocutaneous flaps." *Ann. Plast. Surg.* 8(4): 277, 1982.

Woods, J.E., Irons, G.B., Jr., and Arnold, P.G. "The case for submuscular implantation of prostheses in reconstructive breast surgery." *Ann. Plast. Surg.* 5: 115, 1980.

INTRATHORACIC

Abrashanoff. "Plastische Methode der Schiessung von Fistelgangen, welche von inneren Organen kommen." *Zentralbl. Chir.* 38: 186, 1911.

Arnold, P.G. "Reconstruction of the Chest Wall." *Clinical Applications for Muscle and Musculocutaneous Flaps.* S.J. Mathes & F. Nahai, Eds. St. Louis: C.V. Mosby Company, 1982, pp. 236-268.

Arnold, P.G., and Pairolero, P.C. "Chondrosarcoma of the manubrium: Resection and reconstruction with pectoralis major muscle." *Mayo Clin. Proc.* 53(1): 54, 1978.

Arnold, P.G., and Pairolero, P.C. "Use of pectoralis major muscle flaps to repair defects of anterior chest wall." *Plast. Reconstr. Surg.* 63: 205, 1979.

Arnold, P.G., and Pairolero, P.C. "Chest wall reconstruction: Experience with 100 consecutive patients." *Ann. Surg.* 199(6): 725, 1984.

Arnold, P.G., Paierolero, P.C., and Waldorf, J.C. "The serratus anterior muscle: Intrathoracic and extrathoracic utilization." *Plast. Reconstr. Surg.* 73(2): 240, 1984.

Barker, W.L., Faber, L.P., Ostermiller, W.E., and Langston, H.T. "Management of persistent bronchopleural fistulas." *J. Thorac. Cardiovasc. Surg.* 62: 393, 1971.

Chang, N., and Mathes, S.J. "Comparison of the effect of bacterial inoculation in musculocutaneous and random-pattern flaps." *Plast. Reconstr. Surg.* 70: 1, 1982.

Clagett, O.T., and Geraci, J.E. "A Procedure for the management of postpneumonectomy empyema." *J. Thorac. Cardiovasc. Surg.* 45: 141, 1963.

Dellon, A.L., Wells, J.H., and Cowley, R.A. "A surgical procedure to prevent tracheo-innominate artery erosion." *J. Trauma* 18: 550, 1978.

Demos, N.J., and Timmes, J.J. "Myoplasty for closure of tracheobroncial fistula." *Ann. Thorac. Surg.* 15: 88, 1973.

Eggers, C. "The treatment of bronchial fistulae." *Ann. Surg.* 72: 345, 1920.

Hankins, J.R., Miller, J.E., Attar, S., Satterfield, J.R., and McLaughlin, J.S. "Bronchopleural fistula: Thirteen year experience with 77 cases." *J. Thorac. Cardiovasc. Surg.* 76: 755, 1978.

Hankins, J.R., Miller, J.E., and McLaughlin, J.S. "The use of chest wall muscle flaps to close bronchopleural fistulas: Experience with 21 patients." *Ann. Thorac. Surg.* 25: 491, 1978.

Harashina, T., Takayama, S., Ikuta, Y., and Fujino, T. "Reconstruction of chest-wall radiation ulcer with free latissimus dorsi muscle flap and meshed skin graft." *Plast. Reconstr. Surg.* 71(6): 805, 1983.

Jurkiewicz, M.J. "Infected median sternotomy wound: successful treatment of muscle flap." *Am. Surg.* 191: 738, 1980.

Jurkiewicz, M.J. and Arnold, P.G. "The omentum: an account of its use in reconstruction of the chest wall." *Ann. Surg.* 185: 548, 1977.

Kanavel, A.B. "Plastic procedures for the obliteration of cavities with noncollapsible walls." *Surg. Gynecol. Obstet.* 32: 453, 1921.

Kirsh, M.M., Rotman, H., Behrendt, D.M., Orringer, M.B., and Sloan, H. "Complications of pulmonary resection." *Ann. Thorac. Surg.* 20: 215, 1975.

Larson, D.L., and McMurtrey, M.J. "Musculocutaneous flap reconstruction of chest-wall defects: an experience with 50 patients." *Plast. Reconstr. Surg.* 73(5): 734, 1984.

Maier, H.C., and Luomanen, R.K.J. "Pectoral myoplasty for closure of residual empyema cavity and bronchial fistula." *Surgery* 25: 621, 1949.

Meadows, J.A., III, Staats, B.A., Pairolero, P.C., Rodarte, J.R., and Arnold, P.G. "Effect of resection of the sternum and manubrium in conjection with muscle transposition on pulmonary function." *Mayo Clin. Proc.* 60(9): 604, 1985.

Miyamoto, Y., Hattori, T., and Nosoh, Y. "One-stage antethoracic reconstruction of the thoracic oesophagus using myocutaneous flaps." *Br. J. Plast. Surg.* 37(4): 577, 1984.

Nahai, F., Morales, L., Jr., Bone, D.K., and Bostwick, J., III. "Pectoralis major muscle turnover flaps for closure of the infected sternotomy wound with preservation of form and function." *Plast. Reconstr. Surg.* 70(4): 471, 1982.

Pairolero, P.C., and Arnold, P.G. "Bronchopleural Fistula: Treatment by transposition of pectoralis major muscle." *J. Thorac. Cardiovasc. Surg.* 79(1): 142, 1980.

Pairolero, P.C., and Arnold, P.G. "Management of recalcitrant median sternotomy wounds." *J. Thorac. Cardiovasc. Surg.* 88(3): 357, 1984.

Pairolero, P.C., Arnold, P.G., and Piehler, J.M. "Intrathoracic transposition of extrathoracic skeletal muscle." *J. Thorac. Cardiovasc. Surg.* 86(6): 809, 1983.

Pairolero, P.C., and Payne, W.S. "Postoperative care and complications in the thoracic surgical patient." *J. Thorac. Cardiovasc. Surg. Ed. 4.* W.W.L. Glenn & A.E. Baue, Eds. Norwalk, CN: Appleton-Century Crofts, 1983, pp. 335-351.

Papp, C., Klima, G., and McCraw, J.B. "Reconstruction of aorta and atrium by intercostal muscle flap." *Chir. Plastica.* 8: 165, 1986.

Papp, C., McCraw, J.B., and Arnold, P.G. "Experimental reconstruction of the trachea with autogenous materials." *J. Thorac. Cardiovasc. Surg.* 90(1): 13, 1985.

Papp, C., Parker, P., Boeheim, C., and McCraw, J.B. "Experimental use of intercostal muscle flaps for repair of induced cardiac defects." *J. Thorac. Cardiovasc. Surg.* 90(2): 261, 1985.

INTRATHORACIC

Pool, E.H., and Garlock, J.H. "A treatment of persistent bronchial fistula: An experimental and clinical study." *Ann. Surg.* 90: 213, 1929.

Schaff, H.V., Arnold, P.G., and Reeder, G.S. "Late mediastinal infection and pseudoaneurysm following left ventricular aneurysmectomy: Repair utilizing a pectoralis major muscle flap." *J. Thorac. Cardiovasc. Surg.* 84: 912, 1982.

Shesol, B.F., and Clarke, J.S. "Intrathoracic application of the latissimus dorsi musculocutaneous flap." *Plast. Reconstr. Surg.* 66: 842, 1980.

Stafford, E.G., and Clagett, O.T. "Postpneumonectomy empyema: Neomycin instillation and definitive closure." *J. Thorac. Cardiovasc. Surg.* 63: 771, 1972.

Takayanagi, S., and Tsukie, T. "Free serratus anterior muscle and myocutaneous flaps." *Ann. Plast. Surg.* 8: 277, 1982.

Virkkula, L. "Treatment of the bronchopleural fistual (editorial)." *Ann. Thorac. Surg.* 25: 489, 1978.

Virkkula, L., and Eorola, S. "Use of pectoralis skin pedicle flap for closure of large bronchial fistula connected with postphenumonectomy empyema." *Scan. J. Thorac. Cardiovasc. Surg.* 9: 144, 1975.

Wangensteen, O.H. "The pedicled muscle flap in the closure of persistent bronchopleural fistula: With description of preservation and employment of the intercostal muscle bundles by a process of ribboning (for the avoidance of adominal hernia) in the obliteration of large chronic empyema cavities." *J. Thorac. Surg.* 5: 27, 1935.

VERTICAL RECTUS

Arnold, M. "The surgical anatomy of sternal blood supply." *J. Thorac. Cardiovasc. Surg.* 64: 596, 1972.

Baroudi, R., Pinotti, J.A., and Keppke, E.M. "A transverse thoraco-abdominal skin flap for closure after radical mastectomy." *Plast. Reconstr. Surg.* 61: 547, 1978.

Bostwick, J., Stevenson, T.R., Nahai, F., Hester, T.R., Coleman, J.J., and Jurkiewicz, M.J. "Radiation to the breast: complications amenable to surgical treatment." *Ann. Surg.* 200(4): 543, 1984.

Boyd, J., Taylor, G., and Corlett, R. "The vascular territories of the superior epigastric and deep inferior epigastric systems." *Plast. Reconstr. Surg.* 73(1): 1, 1984.

Brown, R.G., Vasconez, L.O., and Jurkiewicz, M.J. "Transverse abdominal flaps and the deep epigastric arcade." *Plast. Reconstr. Surg.* 55: 417, 1975.

Bunkis, J., Walton, R.L., and Mathes, S.J. "The rectus abdominis free flap for lower extremity reconstruction." *Ann. Plast. Surg.* 11(5): 373, 1983.

Bunkis, J., Walton, R.L., Mathes, S.J., Krizek, T.J., and Vasconez, L.O. "Experience with the transverse lower rectus abdominis operation for breast reconstruction." *Plast. Reconstr. Surg.* 72(6): 819, 1983.

Davis, W.M., McCraw, J.B., and Carraway, J.H. "Use of a direct, transverse, thoracoabdominal flap to close difficult wounds of the thorax and upper extremity." *Plast. Reconstr. Surg.* 60: 526, 1977.

De Troyer, A. "Mechanical role of the abdominal muscles in relation to posture." *Respir. Physiol.* 53(53): 341, 1983.

Dinner, M.I. and Dowden, R.V. "The L-shaped combined vertical and transverse abdominal island flap for breast reconstruction." *Plast. Reconstr. Surg.* 72(6): 894, 1983.

Dinner, M.I., Labandter, H.P., and Dowden, R.V. "The role of the rectus abdominis myocutaneous flap in breast reconstruction." *Plast. Reconstr. Surg.* 69(2): 209, 1982.

Drever, J.M. "The epigastric island flap." *Plast. Reconstr. Surg.* 59: 343, 1977.

Drever, J.M. "Total breast reconstruction." *Ann. Plast. Surg.* 7: 54, 1981.

Drever, J.M. "The lower abdominal transverse rectus abdominis myocutaneous flap for breast reconstruction." *Ann. Plast. Surg.* 10(3): 179, 1983.

Drever, J.M. and Hodson-Walker, N. "Closure of the donor defect for breast reconstruction with rectus abdominis myocutaneous flaps." *Plast. Reconstr. Surg.* 76(4): 558, 1985.

Ford, T.D. "Rectus abdominis myocutaneous flap used to close a median sternotomy chest defect: a case report." *S. Afr. Med. J.* 68(2): 115, 1985.

Galvao, M.S. "Transplant of an inferiorly based rectus abdominis myocutaneous flap to the calf (letter)." *Plast. Reconstr. Surg.* 75(3): 437, 1985.

Giampapa, V., Keller, A., Shaw, W.W., and Colen, S.R. "Pelvic floor reconstruction using the rectus abdominis muscle flap." *Ann. Plast. Surg.* 13(1): 56, 1984.

Heckler, F.R. "Gracilis myocutaneous and muscle flaps." *Clin. Plast. Surg.* 7: 27, 1980.

Hughes, G.S., Jr., Treadwell, E.L., and Miller, J. "Syndrome of the rectus abdominis muscle mimicking the acute abdomen." *Ann. Emerg. Med.* 14(7): 694, 1985.

Hurwitz, D.J. "Closure of a large defect of the pelvic cavity by an extended compound myocutaneous flap based on the inferior gluteal artery." *Br. J. Plast. Surg.* 33: 256, 1980.

Hurwitz, D.J., Schwartz, W.M., and Mathes, S.J. "A reliable sensate flap for the closure of buttock and perineal wounds." *Plast. Reconstr. Surg.* 68: 40, 1981.

Irons, G.B. "Rectus abdominis muscle flaps for closure of osteomyelitis hip defects." *Ann. Plast. Surg.* 11(6): 469, 1983.

Ishii, C.H., Jr., Bostwick, J., III, Raine, T.J., Coleman, J.J., III, and Hester, T.R. "Double-pedicle transverse rectus abdominis myocutaneous flap for unilateral breast and chest-wall reconstruction." *Plast. Reconstr. Surg.* 76(6): 901, 1985.

Jurkiewicz, M.J. and Arnold, P.G. "The omentum: an account of its use in reconstruction of the chest wall." *Ann. Surg.* 185: 548, 1977.

Kanavel, A.B. "Plastic procedures for the obliteration of cavities with noncollapsible walls." *Surg. Gynecol. Obstet.* 32: 453, 1921.

Kaufman, T., Hurwitz, D.J., Boehnke, M., and Futrell, J.W. "The microcirculatory pattern of the transverse-abdominal flap: a cross-sectional xerographic and CAT scanning study." *Ann. Plast. Surg.* 14(4): 340, 1985.

K'om'ar, J. and Varga, B. "Syndrome of the rectus abdominis muscle: a peripheral neurological condition causing abdominal diagnostic problems." *J. Neurol.* 210(2): 121, 1975.

Logan, S.E. and Mathes, S.J. "The use of rectus abdominis myocutaneous flap to reconstruct a groin defect." *Br. J. Plast. Surg.* 37(3): 351, 1984.

Mathes, S.J. and Bostwick, J., III. "A rectus abdominis myocutaneous flap to reconstruct abdominal wall defects." *Br. J. Plast. Surg.* 30(4): 282, 1977.

McCraw, J.B. and Dibbell, D.G. "Experimental definition of independent myocutaneous vascular territories." *Plast. Reconstr. Surg.* 60: 212, 1977.

McCraw, J.B., Dibbell, D.G., and Carraway, J.H. "Clinical definition of independent myocutaneous vascular territories." *Plast. Reconstr. Surg.*, 60: 341, 1977.

McCraw, J.B., Massey, F.M., Shanklin, K.D., and Horton, C.E. "Vaginal reconstruction with gracilis myocutaneous flaps." *Plast. Reconstr. Surg.* 58(2): 176, 1976.

McGregor, I.A. and Jackson, I.T. "The groin flap." *Br. J. Plast. Surg.* 35: 3, 1972.

VERTICAL RECTUS

Milloy, F.J., Anson, B.J., and McAfee, D.K. "The rectus abdominis muscle and the epigastric arteries." *Surg. Gynecol. Obstet.* 122: 293, 1960.

Miyamoto, Y., Hattori, T., and Nosoh, Y. "One-stage antethoracic reconstruction of the thoracic esophagus using myocutaneous flaps." *Br. J. Plast. Surg.* 37(4): 577, 1984.

Neal, H.W., Kreilein, J.G., Schreiber, J.T., and Gregory, R.O. "Complete sternectomy for chronic osteomyelitis with reconstruction using a rectus abdominis myocutaneous island flap." *Ann. Plast. Surg.* 6(4): 305, 1981.

Parkash, S. and Bhandari, M. "Rectus abdominis myocutaneous island flap for bridging defect after cystectomy for bladder extrophy." *Urology* 20(5): 536, 1982.

Parkash, S. and Palepu, J. "Rectus abdominis myocutaneous island flap: clinical experience with ipsilateral and contralateral flaps." *Br. J. Surg.* 70(2): 68, 1983.

Pennington, D.G. and Pelly, A.D. "The rectus abdominis myocutaneous free flap." *Br. J. Plast. Surg.* 33(2): 277, 1980.

Psillakis, J.M., Woisky, R., and Saracut, G. "Rectus abdominis deepithealized musculocutaneous island flap as a silicone substitute in breast reconstruction." *Ann. Plast. Surg.* 10(6): 492, 1983.

Robbins, T.H. "Rectus abdominis myocutaneous flap for breast reconstruction." *Aust. N.Z. J. Surg.* 49(5): 527, 1979.

Robbins, T.H. "Post-mastectomy breast reconstruction using a rectus abdominis musculocutaneous island flap." *Br. J. Plast. Surg.* 34: 286, 1981.

Robbins, T.H. "Breast reconstruction using a rectus abdominis musculocutaneous flap: 5 year follow-up." *Aust. N.Z. J. Surg.* 55(1): 65, 1985.

Scheflan, M. "Rectus abdominis myocutaneous flaps (letter)." *Plast. Reconstr. Surg.* 72(5): 737, 1983.

Shaw, D.T., and Payne, R.L. "One-stage tubed abdominal flaps." *Surg. Gynecol. Obstet.* 83: 205, 1946.

Shaw, W.W. "Breast reconstruction by superior gluteal microvascular free flaps without silicone implants." *Plast. Reconstr. Surg.* 72(4): 490, 1983.

Shukla, H.S. and Hughes, L.E. "The rectus abdominis flap for perineal wounds." *Ann. R. Coll. Surg. Engl.* 66(5): 337, 1984.

Tai, Y. and Hasegawa, H.A. "A transverse abdominal flap for reconstruction after radical operations for recurrent breast cancer." *Plast. Reconstr. Surg.* 53: 52, 1974.

Taylor, G.I., Corlett, R.J., and Boyd, J.B. "The extended deep inferior epigastric flap: a clinical technique." *Plast. Reconstr. Surg.* 72(6): 751, 1983.

Taylor, G.I., Corlett, R.J., and Boyd, J.B. "The versatile deep inferior epigastric (inferior rectus abdominis) flap." *Br. J. Plast. Surg.* 37(3): 330, 1984.

Temple, W.J., Mnaymneh, W., and Ketcham, A.S. "The total thigh and rectus abdominis myocutaneous flap for closure of extensive hemipelvectomy defects." *Cancer* 50(11): 2524, 1982.

Webster, D.J. and Hughes, L.E. "The rectus abdominis myocutaneous island flap in breast cancer." *Br. J. Plast. Surg.* 70(2): 71, 1983.

HORIZONTAL RECTUS

Arnold, M. "The surgical anatomy of sternal blood supply." *J. Thorac. Cardiovasc. Surg.* 64: 596, 1972.

Baroudi, R., Pinotti, J.A., Keppke, E.M. "A transverse thoraco-abdominal skin flap for closure after radical mastectomy." *Plast. Reconstr. Surg.* 61: 547, 1978.

Boyd, J.B., Taylor, G.I., and Corlett, R. "The vascular territories of the superior epigastric and the deep inferior epigastric systems." *Plast. Reconstr. Surg.* 73(1): 1, 1984.

Bricout, N. and Banzet, P. "The use of the lower rectus abdominis musculocutaneous flap in breast reconstruction." *Ann. Chir. Plast. Esth.* 30: 111, 1985.

Bunkis, J., Walton, R.L., and Mathes, S.J. "The rectus abdominis free flap for lower extremity reconstruction." *Ann. Plast. Surg.* 11(5): 373, 1983.

Bunkis, J., Walton, R.L., Mathes, S.J., Krizek, T.J., and Vasconez, L.O. "Experience with the transverse lower rectus abdominis operation for breast reconstruction." *Plast. Reconstr. Surg.* 72(6): 819, 1983.

Caix, M., Outrequin, G., Descottes, B., Kalfon, M., and Pouget, V. "The muscles of the abdominal wall: a new functional approach with anatomoclinical deductions." *Anat. Clin.* 6(2): 101, 1984.

Davis, W.M., McCraw, J.B., and Carraway, J.H. "Use of a direct transverse thoracoabdominal flap to close difficult wounds of the thorax and upper extremity." *Plast. Reconstr. Surg.* 60(4): 526, 1977.

De la Plaza, R., Arroyo, J.M., and Vasconez, L.O. "Upper transverse rectus abdominis flap: the flag flap." *Ann. Plast. Surg.* 12(5): 410, 1984.

Dinner, M.I. and Dowden, R.V. "Rectus abdominis flaps (letter)." *Plast. Reconstr. Surg.* 72(2): 268, 1983.

Dinner, M.I. and Dowden, R.V. "The value of the anterior rectus sheath in the transverse abdominal island flap." *Plast. Reconstr. Surg.* 72(5): 724, 1983.

Dinner, M.I. and Dowden, R.V. "The L-shaped combined vertical and transverse abdominal island flap for breast reconstruction." *Plast. Reconstr. Surg.* 72(6): 894, 1983.

Dinner, M.I., Dowden, R.V., and Scheflan, M. "Refinements in the use of the transverse abdominal island flap for postmastectomy reconstruction." *Ann. Plast. Surg.* 11(5): 362, 1983.

Dinner, M.I. and Hartrampf, C.R., Jr. "Re: Drever: lower abdominal transverse rectus abdominis myocutaneous flap for breast reconstruction (letter)." *Ann. Plast. Surg.* 11(5): 453, 1983.

Dinner, M.I., Labandter, H.P., and Dowden, R.V. "The role of the rectus abdominis myocutaneous flap in breast reconstruction." *Plast. Reconstr. Surg.* 69(2): 209, 1982.

Drever, J.M. "The epigastric island flap." *Plast. Reconstr. Surg.* 59: 343, 1977.

Drever, J.M. "Total breast reconstruction." *Ann. Plast. Surg.* 7: 54, 1981.

Drever, J.M. "The lower abdominal transverse rectus abdominis myocutaneous flap for breast reconstruction." *Ann. Plast. Surg.* 10(3): 179, 1983.

Drever, J.M. "Letter to the editor. Re: Dinner et al: refinements in use of transverse abdominal island flap." *Ann. Plast. Surg.* 11(5): 453, 1985.

Drever, J.M. and Hodson-Walker, N. "Immediate breast reconstruction after mastectomy using a rectus abdominis myodermal flap without an implant." *Can. J. Surg.* 25(4): 429, 1982.

Drever, J.M. and Hodson-Walker, N. "Closure of the donor defect for breast reconstruction with rectus abdominis myocutaneous flaps." *Plast. Reconstr. Surg.* 76(4): 558, 1985.

Elliot, L.F. and Hartrampf, C.R., Jr. "Tailoring of the new breast using the transverse abdominal island flap." *Plast. Reconstr. Surg.* 72(6): 887, 1983.

Gandolfo, E.A. "Breast reconstruction with a lower abdominal myocutaneous flap." *Br. J. Plast. Surg.* 25: 452, 1982.

Georgiade, G.S., Voci, V.E., Riefkohl, R., and Scheflan, M. "Potential problems with the transverse rectus abdominis myocutaneous flap in breast reconstruction and how to avoid them." *Br. J. Plast. Surg.* 37: 121, 1984.

Giampapa, V., Keller, A., Shaw, W.W., and Colen, S.R. "Pelvic floor reconstruction using the rectus abdominis muscle flap." *Ann. Plast. Surg.* 13(1): 56, 1984.

Hartrampf, C.R., Jr. *Transverse Abdominal Island Flap Technique for Breast Reconstruction after Mastectomy.* Baltimore: University Park Press, 1984.

Hartrampf, C.R., Jr. "Abdominal wall competence in transverse abdominal island flap operations." *Ann. Plast. Surg.* 12(2): 139, 1984.

Hartrampf, C.R., Jr., Scheflan, M., and Black, P.W. "Breast reconstruction with a transverse abdominal island flap." *Plast. Reconstr. Surg.* 69(2): 216, 1982.

Hester, T.R., Jr., Nahai, F., Beegle, P.E., and Bostwick, J., III. "Blood supply of the abdomen revisited, with emphasis on the superficial inferior epigastric artery." *Plast. Reconstr. Surg.* 74(5): 657, 1984.

Hueston, J.T. "The evolution of breast reconstruction after mastectomy for cancer." *Aust. N.Z. J. Surg.* 49(5): 527, 1979.

Lejour, M. and De May, A. "Experience with 33 epigastric rectus flaps in breast reconstruction." *Handchir. Mikrochir. Plast. Chir.* 15(4): 257, 1983.

Logan, S.E. and Mathes, S.J. "The use of a rectus abdominis myocutaneous flap to reconstruct a groin defect." *Br. J. Plast. Surg.* 37: 351, 1984.

Kaufman, T., Hurwitz, D.J., Boehnke, M., and Futrell, J.W. "The microcirculatory pattern of the transverse-abdominal flap: a cross-sectional xerographic and CAT scanning study." *Ann. Plast. Surg.* 14(4): 340, 1985.

HORIZONTAL RECTUS

McCraw, J.B. and Dibbell, D.G. "Experimental definition of independent myocutaneous vascular territories." *Plast. Reconstr. Surg.* 60: 212, 1977.

McCraw, J.B., Dibbell, D.G., and Carraway, J.H. "Clinical definition of independent myocutaneous vascular territories." *Plast. Reconstr. Surg.* 60: 341, 1977.

Milloy, F.J., Anson, B.J., and McAfee, D.K. "The rectus abdominis muscle and the epigastric arteries." *Surg. Gynecol. Obstet.* 122: 293, 1960.

Parkash, S. and Palepu, J. "Rectus abdominis myocutaneous flap: clinical experience with ipsilateral and contralateral flaps." *Br. J. Plast. Surg.* 70(2): 68, 1983.

Parkash, S. and Ramakrishnan, K. "A myocutaneous island flap in the treatment of a chronic radionecrotic ulcer of the abdominal wall." *Br. J. Plast. Surg.* 33: 138, 1980.

Pennington, D.G., Lai, M.F., and Pelly, A.D. "The rectus abdominis myocutaneous free flap." *Br. J. Plast. Surg.* 33: 277, 1980.

Psillakis, J.M., Woisky, R., and Saracut, G. "Rectus abdominis deepithelialized musculocutaneous island flap as a silicone substitute in breast reconstruction." *Ann. Plast. Surg.* 10(6): 492, 1983.

Robbins, T.H. "Rectus abdominis myocutaneous flap for breast reconstruction." *Aust. N.Z. J. Surg.* 49(5): 527, 1979.

Robbins, T.H. "Breast reconstruction using a rectus abdominis musculocutaneous flap: 5 yr. follow-up." *Aust. N.Z. J. Surg.* 34(2): 286, 1981.

Robbins, T.H. "Post-mastectomy breast reconstruction using a rectus abdominis musculocutaneous island flap." *Br. J. Plast. Surg.* 34(2): 286, 1981.

Scheflan, M. "Rectus abdominis myocutaneous flaps (letter)." *Plast. Reconstr. Surg.* 72(5): 737, 1983.

Scheflan, M. and Dinner, M.I. "The transverse abdominal island flap. Part I. Indications, contraindications, results, and complications." *Ann. Plast. Surg.* 10(1): 24, 1983.

Scheflan, M. and Dinner, M.I. "The transverse abdominal island flap. Part II. Surgical technique." *Ann. Plast. Surg.* 10(2): 120, 1983.

Shaw, W.W. "Breast reconstruction by superior gluteal microvascular free flaps without silicone implants." *Plast. Reconstr. Surg.* 72(4): 490, 1983.

Slavin, S.A. "The rectus abdominis myocutaneous flap: observation and refinements (letter)." *Plast. Reconstr. Surg.* 71(2): 280, 1983.

Smith, P.J., Foley, B., McGregor, I.A., and Jackson, I.T. "The anatomical basis of the groin flap." *Plast. Reconstr. Surg.* 49: 41, 1972.

Tai, Y. and Hasegawa, H. "A transverse abdominal flap for reconstruction after radical operations for recurrent breast cancer." *Plast. Reconstr. Surg.* 53(1): 52, 1974.

Taylor, G.I., Corlett, R.J., and Boyd, J.B. "The extended deep inferior epigastric flap: a clinical technique." *Plast. Reconstr. Surg.* 72(6): 751, 1983.

Taylor, G.I., Corlett, R.J., and Boyd, J.B. "The versatile deep inferior epigastric (inferior rectus abdominis) flap." *Br. J. Plast. Surg.* 37: 330, 1984.

Vasconez, L.O., Grotting, J.C., Calderon, W., and Mathes, S.J. "Reconstruction of the breast: where do we fall short? An evolution of ideas." *Am. J. Surg.* 148(1): 103, 1984.

Vasconez, L.O., Psillakis, J., and Johnson-Giebeik, R. "Breast reconstruction with contralateral rectus abdominis myocutaneous flap." *Plast. Reconstr. Surg.* 71(5): 668, 1983.

Webster, D.J. and Hughes, L.E. "The rectus abdominis myocutaneous island flap in breast cancer." *Br. J. Plast. Surg.* 70(2): 71, 1983.

EXTERNAL OBLIQUE

Fisher, J. "External oblique fasciocutaneous flap for elbow coverage." *Plast. Reconstr. Surg.* 75(1): 51, 1985.

Hershey, F.B. and Butcher, H.R. "Repair of defects after partial resection of the abdominal wall." *Amer. J. Surg.* 107: 586, 1964.

Hodgkinson, D.J. and Arnold, P.G. "Chest-wall reconstruction using the external oblique muscle." *Br. J. Plast. Surg.* 33: 216, 1980.

Holle, J. and Pierini, A. "Breast reconstruction with an external oblique abdominis muscle turnover flap and a bipedicled abdominal skin flap." *Plast. Reconstr. Surg.* 73(3): 469, 1984.

Lesnick, G.J. and Davids, A.M. "Repair of surgical abdominal wall defect with a pedicled musculofascial flap." *Ann. Surg.* 137: 569, 1953.

Marshall, D.R., Anstee, E.J., and Stapleton, M.J. "Soft tissue reconstruction of the breast using an external oblique myocutaneous abdominal flap." *Br. J. Plast. Surg.* 35: 443, 1982.

Mialhe, C. and Brice, M. "A new compound osteo-myocutaneous free flap: the posterior iliac artery flap." *Br. J. Plast. Surg.* 38(1): 30, 1985.

Parkash, S. and Ramakrishnan, K. "A myocutaneous island flap in the treatment of a chronic radionecrotic ulcer of the abdominal wall." *Br. J. Plast. Surg.* 33: 138, 1980.

Wangensteen, O.H. "Repair of recurrent and difficult hernias and other large defects of the abdominal wall employing the iliotibial tract of fascia lata as a pedicle flap." *Surg. Gynecol. Obstet.* 59: 766, 1934.

Wangensteen, O.H. "Repair of large abdominal defects by pedicled fascial flaps." *Surg. Gynecol. Obstet.* 82: 144, 1946.

GLUTEUS MAXIMUS

Baek, S.M., Williams, G.D., McElhinney, A.J., and Simon, B.E. "The gluteus maximum myocutaneous flap in the management of pressure sores." *Ann. Plast. Surg.* 5(6): 471, 1980.

Baker, D.C., Barton, F.E., and Converse, J.M. "A combined biceps and semitendinosus muscle flap in repair of ischial sores." *Br. J. Plast. Surg.* 31: 26, 1978.

Becker, H. "The distally-based gluteus maximus muscle flap." *Plast. Reconstr. Surg.* 63(5): 653, 1979.

Block, I.R. "Levator ani as substitute puborectalis sling." *Surg. Gynecol. Obstet.* 141: 611, 1975.

Brandesky, G. and Holschneider, A.M. "Operations for the improvement of faecal incontinence." *Prog. Pediatr. Surg.* 9: 105, 1976.

Bruining, H.A., Box, K.E., Colthoff, E.G., and Tolhurst, D.E. "Creation of an anal sphincter mechanism by bilateral proximally based gluteal muscle transposition." *Plast. Reconstr. Surg.* 67(1): 70, 1981.

Chantraine, A., Lloyd, K. and Swinyard, C. "The sphincter ani externus in spina bifida and myelomeningocoele." *J. Urol.* 95: 250, 1966.

Chittenden, A.S. "Reconstruction of anal sphincter by muscle slips from glutei." *Ann. Surg.* 92: 152, 1930.

Daniel, R.K., Terzis, J.K., and Cunningham, D.M. "Sensory skin flaps for coverage of pressure sores in paraplegic patients." *Plast. Reconstr. Surg.* 58: 317, 1976.

Daniel, R.K., Kerrigan, C.L., and Gard, D.A. "The great potential of the intercostal flap for torso reconstruction." *Plast. Reconstr. Surg.* 61: 653, 1978.

Davis, W.M., McCraw, J.B., and Carraway, J.H. "Use of a direct transverse thoracoabdominal flap to close difficult wounds of the thorax and upper extremity." *Plast. Reconstr. Surg.* 60(4): 526, 1977.

Dibbell, D.G. "Use of a large island flap to bring sensation to the sacral area in young paraplegics." *Plast. Reconstr. Surg.* 54: 221, 1974.

Dibbell, D.G., McCraw, J.B., and Edstrom, L.E. "Providing useful and protective sensibility in patients with meningocele." *Plast. Reconstr. Surg.* 64: 796, 1979.

Erk, Y., Spira, M., Parsa, F.D., and Stal, S. "A modified gluteus maximus musculocutaneous free flap based on the inferior gluteal vessels." *Ann. Plast. Surg.* 11(4): 344, 1983.

Fisher, J., Arnold, P.G., Waldorf, J., and Woods, J.E. "The gluteus maximus musculocutaneous V-Y advancement flap for large sacral defects." *Ann. Plast. Surg.* 11(6): 517, 1983.

Ger, R. "The surgical management of decubitus ulcers by muscle transposition." *Surgery* 69: 106, 1971.

Ger, R. and Levine, S.A. "The management of decubitus ulcers by muscle transposition: an 8 year review." *Plast. Reconstr. Surg.* 58: 419, 1976.

Hang, Y.S. "Contracture of the hip secondary to fibrosis of the gluteus maximus muscle." *J. Bone Joint Surg.* (Am). 61(1): 52, 1979.

Hentz, V.R. "Construction of a rectal sphincter using the origin of the gluteus maximum muscle." *Plast. Reconstr. Surg.* 70(1): 82, 1982.

Hill, H.L., Brown, R.G., and Jurkiewicz, M.J. "The transverse lumbosacral back flap." *Plast. Reconstr. Surg.* 63: 177, 1978.

Hurwitz, D.J. "Closure of a large defect of the pelvic cavity by an extended compound flap based on the inferior gluteal artery." *Br. J. Plast. Surg.* 33: 256, 1980.

Hurwitz, D.J., Swartz, W.M., and Mathes, S.J. "The gluteal thigh flap: A reliable, sensate flap for the closure of buttock and perineal wounds." *Plast. Reconstr. Surg.* 68: 521, 1981.

Jacob, E.T., Shapira, Z., Bar-Natan, N., and Berant, M. "Total anorectal reconstruction following congenital anorectal anomaly: report of a case." *Dis. Colon Rectum*, 19(2): 172, 1976.

Janecki, C.J. "The gluteus maximus femoral insertion: a guide in surgery about the hip." *Clin. Orthop.* 123: 16, 1977.

Joseph, J. and Williams, P.L. "Electromyography of certain hip muscles." *J. Anat.* 91: 286, 1957.

Labandter, H.P. "The gracilis muscle flap and musculocutaneous flap in the repair of perineal and ischial defects." *Br. J. Plast. Surg.* 33: 95, 1980.

Little, J.W., III, and Lyons, J.R. "The gluteus medius-tensor fasciae latae flap." *Plast. Reconstr. Surg.* 71(3): 366, 1983.

Maruyama, Y., Nakajima, H., Wada, M., Imai, T., and Fujino, T. "A gluteus maximus myocutaneous island flap for the repair of a sacral decubitus ulcer." *Br. J. Plast. Surg.* 33: 150, 1980.

Maruyama, Y. and Tajima, S. "Gluteus maximus muscle island flaps for repair of sacral radiation ulcers." *Keio. J. Med.* 27(2): 53, 1978.

Mathes, S.J., Vasconez, L.O., and Jurkiewicz, M.J. "Extensions and further applications of muscle flap transposition." *Plast. Reconstr. Surg.* 60: 6, 1977.

McCraw, J.B., Dibbell, D.G. and Carraway, J.H. "Clinical definition of independent myocutaneous vascular territories." *Plast. Reconstr. Surg.* 60: 341, 1977.

Minami, R.T., Mills, R., and Pardoe, R. "Gluteus maximus myocutaneous flaps for repair of pressure sores." *Plast. Reconstr. Surg.* 60(2): 242, 1977.

Mustarde, J.C. "Reconstruction of the spinal canal in severe spina bifida." *Plast. Reconstr. Surg.* 42: 109, 1968.

Nahai, F. "The tensor fascia lata flap." *Clin. Plast. Surg.* 7: 51, 1980.

Nahai, F., Hill, L., and Hester, T.R. "Experiences with the tensor fascia lata flap." *Plast. Reconstr. Surg.* 63: 788, 1979.

Napier, J. "The antiquity of human walking." *Sci. Am.* 216: 56, 1967.

Orgel, M.G. and Kucan, J.D. "A double-split gluteus maximus muscle flap for reconstruction of the rectal sphincter." *Plast. Reconstr. Surg.* 75(1): 62, 1985.

GLUTEUS MAXIMUS

Parkash, S. and Banerjee, S. "The total gluteus maximus rotation and other gluteus maximus musculocutaneous flaps in the treatment of pressure ulcers." *Br. J. Plast. Surg.* 39: 66, 1986.

Parry, S.W. and Mathes, S.J. "Bilateral gluteus maximus myocutaneous advancement flaps: sacral coverage for ambulatory patients." *Ann. Plast. Surg.* 8(6): 443, 1982.

Perez-Gurri, J.A., Temple, W.J., and Ketcham, A.S. "Gluteus maximus myocutaneous flap for the treatment of recalcitrant pilonidal disease." *Dis. Colon Rectum*, 27(4): 262, 1984.

Prochiantz, A. and Gross, P. "Gluteal myoplasty for sphincter replacement: principles, results and prospects." *J. Pediatr. Surg.* 17(1): 25, 1982.

Ramirez, O.M., Hurwitz, D.J., and Futrell, J.W. "The expansive gluteus maximus flap." *Plast. Reconstr. Surg.* 74(6): 757, 1984.

Ramirez, O.M., Orlando, J.C., and Hurwitz, D.J. "The sliding gluteus maximus myocutaneous flap: its relevance in ambulatory patients." *Plast. Reconstr. Surg.* 74(1): 68, 1984.

Rees, R.S., Reilley, A.F., Nanney, L.B., and Lynch, J.B. "Sacral pressure sores: treatment with island gluteus maximus musculocutaneous flaps." *South Med. J.* 78(10): 1147, 1985.

Salibian, A.H., Anzel, S.H., and Rogers, F.R. "The gluteus medius-tensor fasciae latae myocutaneous flap for infected gridlestone procedures: Report of two cases." *J. Bone Joint Surg.* 66(9): 1466, 1984.

Scheflan, M., Nahai, F., and Bostwick, J., III. "Gluteus maximus island musculocutaneous flap for closure of sacral and ischial ulcers." *Plast. Reconstr. Surg.* 68(4): 533, 1981.

Senior, H.D. "The development of the arteries of the human lower extremity." *Am. J. Anat.* 25: 55, 1919.

Shaw, A. and Futrell, J.W. "Cure of chronic perineal sinus with gluteus maximus flap." *Surg. Gynecol. Obstet.* 147(3): 417, 1978.

Shaw, W.W. "Breast reconstruction by superior gluteal microvascular free flaps without silicone implants." *Plast. Reconstr. Surg.* 72(4): 490, 1983.

Simonsen, O.S., Stolf, N.A., Aun, F., Raia, A., and Habrgama, A. "Rectal sphincter reconstruction in perineal colostomies after abdominoperineal resection for cancer." *Br. J. Surg.* 63(5): 389, 1976.

Skef, Z., Radhakrishnan, J., and Reyes, H.M. "Anorectal continence following sphincter reconstruction utilizing the gluteus maximus muscle: a case report." *J. Pediatr. Surg.* 19(6): 779, 1983.

Stallings, J.O., Delgrado, J.P., and Converse, J.M. "Turnover island flap of gluteus maximus muscle for the repair of sacral decubitus ulcer." *Plast. Reconstr. Surg.* 54(1): 52, 1974.

Stern, J.T., Jr. "Anatomical and functional specializations of the human gluteus maximus." *Am. J. Phys. Anthropol.* 36(3): 315, 1972.

Twisk, R. van and Borghouds, J.M.H.M. "The gluteus maximus musculocutaneous flap as bilateral V-Y sliding flap or as pendulum flap for closure of sacral and ischial pressure sores." *Acta. Chir. Plast.* 8: 215, 1986.

Uszynski, H., Jethon, J., and Towpik, E. "Muscle and myocutaneous flaps in the treatment of pressure sores in paraplegics." *Acta. Chir. Plast.* 27(3): 185, 1985.

Vasconez, L.O., Schneider, W.J., and Jurkiewicz, M.J. "Pressure sores." *Curr. Probl. Surg.* 14: 1, 1977.

Wheatley, M.D. and Jahnke, W.D. "Electromyographic study of the superficial thigh and hip muscles in normal individuals." *Arch. Phys. Med.* 32: 508, 1951.

Wingate, G.B. and Friedland, J.A. "Repair of ischial pressure ulcers with gracilis musculocutaneous island flaps." *Plast. Reconstr. Surg.* 62: 245, 1978.

BICEPS FEMORIS

Baker, D.C., Barton, F.E., Jr., and Converse, J.M. "A combined biceps and semitendinosus muscle flap in the repair of ischial sores." *Br. J. Plast. Surg.* 31: 26, 1978.

Becker, H. "The distally based gluteus maximus muscle flap." *Plast. Reconstr. Surg.* 63: 653, 1979.

Blocksma, R., Kostrubala, J.G., and Greely, P.W. "The surgical repair of decubitus ulcer in paraplegics." *Plast. Reconstr. Surg.* 4: 123, 1949.

Conway, H. and Griffin, B.H. "Plastic surgery for closure of decubitius patients with paraplegia." *Am. J. Surg.* 91: 946, 1956.

Duchenne, G.B.A. *Physiology of Motion.* E.B. Kaplan (Ed.) Philadelphia: Lippincott, 1949.

Hurwitz, D.J. "Closure of a large defect of the pelvic cavity by an extended compound myocutaneous flap based on the inferior gluteal artery." *Br. J. Plast. Surg.* 33: 256, 1980.

Hurwitz, D.J., Schwartz, W.M.. and Mathes, S.J. "A reliable sensate flap for the closure of buttock and perineal wounds." *Plast. Reconstr. Surg.* 68: 40, 1981.

James, J.H. and Moir, I.H. "The biceps femoris musculocutaneous flap in the repair of pressure sores around the hip." *Plast. Reconstr. Surg.* 66(5): 736, 1980.

Kaplan, E.B. "Factors responsible for the stability of the knee." *Bull. Hosp. Joint Dis.* 18: 51, 1957.

Kennedy, J.C. and Fowler, P.J. "Medial and anterior instability of the knee." *J. Bone Joint Surg.* 53(A): 1257, 1971.

Marshall, J.K., Girgis, F., and Zelko, R.R. "The biceps femoris tendon and its functional significance." *J. Bone Joint Surg.* (Am.). 54(7): 1444, 1972.

McCraw, J.B. and Dibbell, D.G. "Experimental definition of independent myocutaneous vascular territories." *Plast. Reconstr. Surg.* 60(2): 212, 1977.

McCraw, J.B., Dibbell, D.G., and Carraway, J.H. "Clinical definition of independent myocutaneous vascular territories." *Plast. Reconstr. Surg.* 60: 341, 1977.

Sneath, R.S. "The insertion of the biceps femoris." *J. Anat.* 89: 550, 1955.

Sugarbaker, P.H. and Lampert, M.H. "Excision of quadriceps muscle group." *Surgery* 93(3): 462, 1983.

Tobin, G.R., Sanders, B.P., Man, D., and Weiner, L.J. "The biceps femoris myocutaneous advancement flap: a useful modification for ischial pressure ulcer reconstruction." *Ann. Plast. Surg.* 6(5): 396, 1981.

GRACILIS

Achauer, B.M., Braly, P., Berman, M.L., and DiSaia, P.J. "Immediate vaginal reconstruction following resection for malignancy using the gluteal thigh flap." *Gynecol. Oncol.* 19(1): 79, 1984.

Apfelberg, D. and Finseth, F. "Double-muscle gracilis and sartorius myocutaneous flap." *Br. J. Plast. Surg.* 34: 41, 1981.

Atri, S.P. "The treatment of complete rectal prolapses by graciloplasty." *Br. J. Plast. Surg.* 67(6): 431, 1980.

Baek, S.M., Greenstein, A., McElhinney, A.J., and Aufses, A.H., Jr. "The gracilis myocutaneous flap for persistent perineal sinus after proctocolectomy." *Surg. Gynecol. Obstet.* 153(5): 713, 1981.

Bartholdson, L. and Hulten, L. "Repair of persistent perineal sinuses by means of a pedicle flap of musculus gracilis: Case report." *Scand. J. Plast. Reconstr. Surg.* 9(1): 74, 1975.

Becker, D.W., Jr., Massey, F.M., and McCraw, J.B. "Musculocutaneous flaps in reconstructive pelvic surgery." *Obstet. Gynecol.* 54(2): 178, 1979.

Bell, J.G., Weiser, E.B., Metz, P., and Hoskins, W.J. "Gracilis muscle repair of perineal hernia following pelvic exenteration." *Obstet. Gynecol.* 56(3): 377, 1980.

Ben-Hur, N., Gilai, A., Golan, J., Sagher, U., and Issac, M. "Reconstruction of the anal sphincter by gracilis muscle transfer: the value of electromyography in the preoperative assessment and postoperative management of the patient." *Br. J. Plast. Surg.* 33(2): 256, 1980.

Berek, J.S., Hacker, N.F., and Lagasse, L.D. "Vaginal reconstruction performed simultaneously with pelvic exenteration." *Obstet. Gynecol.* 63(3): 318, 1984.

Block, I.R. "Levator ani as substitute puborectalis sling." *Surg. Gynecol. Obstet.* 141: 611, 1975.

Bricker, E.M., Kraybill, W.G., and Lopez, M.J. "Combined reconstruction of the rectum and vagina following irradiation and surgical treatment for clear cell carcinoma." *Surg. Gynecol. Obstet.* 159(2): 166, 1984.

Chantraine, A., Lloyd, K., and Swinyard, C. "The sphincter ani externus in spina bifida and myelomeningocoele." *J. Urol.* 95: 250, 1966.

Cohen, B.E., and Ryan, J.A., Jr. "Gracilis muscle flap for closure of the persistent perineal sinus." *Surg. Gynecol. Obstet.* 148(1): 33, 1979.

Corman, M.L. "Gracilis muscle transposition for anal incontinence: late results." *Br. J. Plast. Surg.* 72 Supp: S21, 1985.

Dibbell, D.G. "Dynamic correction of intractable vaginal prolapse." *Ann. Plast. Surg.* 2: 254, 1979.

Furnas, D.W. and McCraw, J.B. "Resurfacing the genital area." *Clin. Plast. Surg.* 7(2): 235, 1980.

Harii, K., Ohmori, K., and Sekiguchi, J. "The free musculocutaneous flap." *Plast. Reconstr. Surg.* 57(3): 294, 1976.

Harii, K., Ohmori, K., and Torii, S. "Free gracilis muscle transplantation, with microneurovascular anastomoses for the treatment of facial paralysis: A preliminary report." *Plast. Reconstr. Surg.* 57(2): 133, 1976.

Hatch, K.D. "Construction of a neovagina after exenteration using the vulvobulbocavernosus myocutaneous graft." *Obstet. Gynecol.* 63(1): 110, 1984.

Heath, P.M., Woods, J.E., Podratz, K.C., Arnold, P.G., and Irons, G.B., Jr. "Gracilis myocutaneous vaginal reconstruction." *Mayo Clin. Proc.* 59(1): 21, 1984.

Heckler, F.R. "Gracilis myocutaneous and muscle flaps." *Clin. Plast. Surg.* 71(1): 27, 1980.

Heckler, F.R., Dibbell, D.G., and McCraw, J.B. "Successful use of muscle flaps or myocutaneous flaps in patients with sickle cell disease." *Plast. Reconstr. Surg.* 59: 902, 1977.

Hester, T.R., Hill, H.L., and Jurkiewicz, M.J. "One-stage reconstruction of the penis." *Br. J. Plast. Surg.* 31: 279, 1978.

Horton, C.E., McCraw, J.B., Devine, C.J., Jr., and Devine, P.C. "Secondary reconstruction of the genital area." *Urol. Clin. North Am.* 4(1): 133, 1977.

Hoskins, W.J., Park, R.C., Long, R., Artman, L.E., and McMahon, E.B. "Repair of urinary tract fistulas with bulbocavernosus myocutaneous flaps." *Obstet. Gynecol.* 63(4): 588, 1984.

Hurwitz, D.J. "Closure of a large defect of the pelvic cavity by an extended compound myocutaneous flap based on the inferior gluteal artery." *Br. J. Plast. Surg.* 33: 256, 1980.

Hurwitz, D.J., Schwartz, W.M., and Mathes, S.J. "A reliable sensate flap for the closure of buttock and perineal wounds." *Plast. Reconstr. Surg.* 68: 40, 1981.

Kalisman, M. and Sharzer, L.A. "Anal sphincter reconstruction and perineal resurfacing with a gracilis myocutaneous flap." *Dis. Colon Rectum* 24(7): 529, 1981.

Kaplan, I. and Alfandary, H. "The surgical treatment of rectal incontinence by gracilis muscle transplant." *Am. J. Protocol* 22(2): 102, 1971.

Krzeski, T. and Borkowski, A. "Bladder flap for reconstruction of congenital absence of the vagina." *Eur. Urol.* 9(2): 125, 1983.

Labandter, H.P. "The gracilis muscle flap and musculocutaneous flap in the repair of perineal and ischial defects." *Br. J. Plast. Surg.* 33(1): 95, 1980.

Landeen, J.M. and Habal, M.B. "The rejuvenation of the anal sphincteroplasty." *Surg. Gynecol. Obstet.* 149(1): 78, 1979.

Larson, D.L. and Bracken, R.B. "Use of gracilis musculocutaneous flap in urologic cancer surgery." *Urology* 19(2): 148, 1982.

Leguit, P., Jr., van Baal, J.G., and Brummelkamp, W.H. "Gracilis muscle transposition in the treatment of fecal incontinence: Long-term follow-up and evaluation of anal pressure recordings." *Dis. Colon Rectum* 29(1): 1, 1985.

GRACILIS

Lesavoy, M.A. "Vaginal reconstruction." *Urol. Clin. North Am.* 12(2): 369, 1985.

Lesavoy, M.A. "Vaginal reconstruction." *Clin. Obstet. Gynecol.* 12(2): 515, 1985.

Lewis, M.I. "Gracilis muscle transplant for the correction of anal incontinence: report of a case." *Dis. Colon Rectum* 15(4): 292, 1972.

Magrina, J.F. and Masterson, B.J. "Vaginal reconstruction in gynecological oncology: a review of techniques." *Obstet. Gynecol. Surg.* 36(1): 1, 1981.

Magrina, J.F. and Masterson, B.J. "Vaginal reconstruction: procedures following radical pelvic surgery." *J. Kans. Med. Soc.* 82(2): 61, 1981.

Manktelow, R. and McKee, N.H. "Free muscle transplantation to provide active finger flexion." *J. Hand Surg.* 3: 416, 1978.

Markland, C. and Hastings, D. "Vaginal reconstruction using cecal and sigmoid bowel segments in transsexual patients." *J. Urol.* 111(2): 217, 1974.

Maruyama, Y., Ohnishi, K., and Hashimura, C. "Functional reconstruction of anal constriction using a gracilis musculocutaneous flap." *Acta. Chir. Plast.* (Prague), 225(2): 76, 1983.

Mathes, S.J. and Albert, B.S. "Advances in muscle and musculocutaneous flaps." *Clin. Plast. Surg.* 7(1): 15, 1980.

McComas, B.C., Reddick, L.P., and Donaldson, R.C. "Gracilis myocutaneous flap reconstruction after radical vulvectomy and posterior exenteration." *J. Tenn. Med. Assoc.* 77(1): 17, 1984.

McCraw, J.B. "Flaps for perineal reconstruction." *Weekly Urology Update* 1978.

McCraw, J.B. "Intraoperative identification of the gracilis muscle for vaginal reconstruction (Letter)." *Plast. Reconstr. Surg.* 65(3): 358, 1980.

McCraw, J.B., Dibbell, D.G., and Carraway, J.H. "Clinical definition of independent myocutaneous vascular territories." *Plast. Reconstr. Surg.* 60: 341, 1977.

McCraw, J.B., Massey, F.M., Shanklin, K.D., and Horton, C.E. "Vaginal reconstruction with gracilis myocutaneous flaps." *Plast. Reconstr. Surg.* 58(2): 176, 1976.

McGregor, J.C. "The gracilis musculocutaneous flap as a method of closure of ischial pressure sores: preliminary report." *Paraplegia* 20(4): 217, 1982.

Morrow, C.P., Lacey, C.G., and Lucas, W.E. "Reconstructive surgery in gynecology cancer employing the gracilis myocutaneous pedicle graft." *Gynecol. Oncol.* 7(2): 176, 1979.

Nahai, F. "Muscle and musculocutaneous flaps in gynecologic surgery." *Clin. Obstet. Gynecol.* 24(4): 1277, 1981.

Nakajima, T., Naide, Y., and Kami, T. "Repair of a prostatomembranous urethral stricture with a gracilis myocutaneous flap." *Br. J. Plast. Surg.* 37(4): 539, 1984.

Ng, H.T., Kan, Y.Y., Chao, K.C., and Yuan, C.C. "Vaginal reconstruction with a sigmoid loop in pelvic exenteration." *Asia Oceania. J. Obstet. Gynaecol.* 10(3): 341, 1984.

Nieves, P.M., Valles, G., Arang'uren, G., and Maldonado, D. "Gracilis muscle transplant for correction of traumatic anal incontinence: report of a case." *Dis. Colon Rectum* 18(4): 349, 1975.

Obrink, A. and Bunne, G. "Gracilis interposition in fistulas following radiotherapy for cervical cancer: A retrospective study." *Urol. Int.* 33(5): 370, 1978.

Orticochea, M. "A new method of total reconstruction of the penis." *Br. J. Plast. Surg.* 25: 347, 1972.

Orticochea, M. "The musculocutaneous flap method: an immediate and heroic substitute for the method of delay." *Br. J. Plast. Surg.* 15: 106, 1972.

Parkask, S. "The use of myocutaneous flaps in block dissections of the groin in cases with gross skin involvement." *Br. J. Plast. Surg.* 35(4): 413, 1982.

Persky, L., Resnick, M., and Despres, J. "Penile reconstruction with gracilis pedicle grafts." *J. Urol.* 129(3): 603, 1983.

Pickrell, K.L., Broadbent, T.R., and Masters, F.S. "Construction of rectal sphincter and restoration of anal continence by transplanting gracilis muscle." *Ann. Surg.* 135: 853, 1952.

Pickrell, K.L., Georgiade, N., Maguire, C., and Crawford, H. "Gracilis muscle transplant for rectal incontinence." *Surgery* 40: 349, 1956.

Pickrell, K.L., Masters, F.W., Georgiade, N., and Horton, C.E. "Rectal sphincter reconstruction, using gracilis muscle transplant." *Plast. Reconstr. Surg.* 13: 46, 1954.

Raffensperger, J. "The gracilis sling for fecal incontinence." *J. Pediatr. Surg.* 14(6): 794, 1979.

Ramos, R.R., Andrews, J.M., and Ferreira, L.M. "A gracilis myocutaneous flap for reconstruction of the scrotum." *Br. J. Plast. Surg.* 37(2): 171, 1984.

Raven, R.W. "Rectal prolapse and incontinence treated by reconstruction of the anorectal sphincters." *Proc. R. Soc. Med.* 63 P Suppl: 94, 1970.

Ryan, J.A., Jr. "Gracilis muscle flap for the persistent perineal sinus of inflammatory bowel disease." *Am. J. Surg.* 148(1): 64: 1984.

Ryan, J.A., Jr., Beebe, H.G., and Gibbons, R.P. "Gracilis muscle flap for closure of rectourethral fistula." *J. Urol.* 122(1): 124, 1979.

Schellhas, H.F. and Fidler, J.P. "Vaginal reconstruction after total pelvic exenteration using a modification of the William's procedure." *Gynecol. Oncol.* 3(1): 21, 1976.

Shubailat, G.F., Ajluni, N.J., and Shahateet, M.A. "Repair of a lower leg defect with an ipsilateral gracilis myocutaneous flap." *Plast. Reconstr. Surg.* 64(4): 560, 1979.

GRACILIS

Song, I.C., Cramer, M.S., and Bromberg, B.E. "Primary vaginal reconstruction after pelvic exenteration." *Plast. Reconstr. Surg.* 51(5): 509, 1973.

Song, R., Wang, X., and Zhou, G. "Reconstruction of the vagina with sensory function." *Clin. Plast. Surg.* 9(1): 105, 1982.

Sorosky, J.I., Bass, D.M., Curry, S.L., and Hewett, W.J. "Gracilis myocutaneous flap as a life-saving procedure in control of necrosis following radiotherapy and radical surgery for pelvic malignancy." *Gynecol. Oncol.* 13(3): 405, 1982.

Venugopalan, S. "Repair of midline abdominal incisional hernia by gracilis muscle transfer." *Br. J. Plast. Surg.* 33(1): 43, 1980.

Wee, J.T. and Wong, C.S. "Functional and sphincter reconstruction with the gracilis muscle after abdominoperineal resection (letter)." *Lancet* 2(8361): 1245, 1983.

Westfall, C.T. and Keller, H.B. "Scrotal reconstruction utilizing bilateral gracilis myocutaneous flaps." *Plast. Reconstr. Surg.* 68(6): 945, 1981.

Wheeless, C.R., McGibbon, B., Dorsey, J.H., et al. "Gracilis myocutaneous flap in reconstruction of the vulva and female perineum." *Obstet. Gynecol.* 54: 97, 1979.

Wingate, G.B. and Friedland, J.A. "Repair of ischial pressure ulcers with gracilis myocutaneous island flaps." *Plast. Reconstr. Surg.* 62(2): 245, 1978.

Woods, J.E. and Beard, R.W., Jr. "Reconstruction of non-healing perineal wounds with gracilis muscle flaps." *Ann. Plast. Surg.* 11(6): 513, 1983.

TENSOR FASCIA LATA

Airhart, R.A., deKernion, J.B., and Guillermo, E.O. "Tensor fascia lata myocutaneous flap for coverage of skin defects after radical groin dissection for metastatic penile carcinoma." *J. Urol.* 128(3): 599, 1982.

Caffee, H.H. "Reconstruction of the abdominal wall by variations of the tensor fasciae latae flap." *Plast. Reconstr. Surg.* 71(3): 348, 1983.

Caffee, H.H. and Asokan, R. "Tensor fascia lata myocutaneous free flaps." *Plast. Reconstr. Surg.* 68(2): 195, 1981.

Chafe, W., Fowler, W.C., Walton, L.A., and Currie, J.L. "Radical vulvectomy with use of tensor fascia lata myocutaneous flap." *Am. J. Obstet. Gynecol.* 145(2): 207, 1983.

Chiu, H.W. "Tensor fasciae latae free flap for full-thickness abdominal wall reconstruction utilizing the greater omentum as a vascular supply (letter)." *Plast. Reconstr. Surg.* 75(4): 607, 1985.

Dibbell, D.G. "Use of a large island flap to bring sensation to the sacral area in young paraplegics." *Plast. Reconstr. Surg.* 54: 221, 1974.

Dibbell, D.G., McCraw, J.B., and Edstrom, L.E. "Providing useful and protective sensibility in patients with meningocele." *Plast. Reconstr. Surg.* 64: 796, 1979.

Echinard, C., Latrl, F., Roffe, J.L., et al. "The use of a fascia lata myocutaneous flap to repair lesions of the abdominal wall after radiation therapy." *Ann. Chir. Plast. Esth.* 32: 42, 1985.

Hershey, F.B. and Butcher, H.R., Jr. "Repair of defects after partial resection of the abdominal wall." *Am. J. Surg.* 107: 586, 1964.

Hill, H.L., Hester, R., and Nahai, F. "Covering large groin defects with the tensor fascia lata musculocutaneous flap." *Br. J. Plast. Surg.* 32(1): 12, 1979.

Hill, L.H., Nahai, F., and Vasconez, L.O. "The tensor fascia lata myocutaneous free flap." *Plast. Reconstr. Surg.* 61(4): 517, 1978.

Kastaros, J. "Use of the island tensor fasciae latae flap to cover a chest wall defect." *Plast. Reconstr. Surg.* 6: 1007, 1982.

Lesnick, G.J. and Davids, A.M. "Repair of surgical abdominal wall defect with a pedicled musculofascial flap." *Ann. Surg.* 137: 569, 1953.

Lynch, S.M. "The bilobed tensor fascia lata myocutaneous flap." *Plast. Reconstr. Surg.* 67(6): 796, 1981.

Mairesse, J.L., Mestdagh, H., Bailleul, J.P., and Depreux, R. "Contribution to the study of vascularization of the fascia lata tensor muscle." *Acta. Anat.* (Basel) 110(3): 270, 1981.

Maruyama, Y. and Nakajima, H. "One-stage reconstruction of a massive buttock and sacroperineal defect with multiple myocutaneous flaps." *Br. J. Plast. Surg.* 36: 116, 1983.

Maruyama, Y., Ohnishi, K. and Takeuchi, S. "The lateral thigh fascio-cutaneous flap in the repair of ischial and trochanteric defects." *Br. J. Plast. Surg.* 37(1): 103, 1984.

Mathes, S.J. and Buchanan, R.T. "Tensor fascia lata: neurosensory musculocutaneous free flap." *Br. J. Plast. Surg.* 32: 184, 1979.

McCraw, J.B. "Flaps for perineal reconstruction." *Weekly Urology Update.* 1978.

McCraw, J.B., Dibbell, D.G., and Carraway, J.H. "Clinical definition of independent myocutaneous vascular territories." *Plast. Reconstr. Surg.* 60: 341, 1977.

McGregor, J.C. and Buchan, A.C. "Our clinical experience with the tensor fasciae latae myocutaneous flap." *Br. J. Plast. Surg.* 33(2): 270, 1980.

Nahai, F. "The tensor fascia lata flap." *Clin. Plast. Surg.* 7(1): 51, 1980.

Nahai, F., Hill, L., and Hester, T.R. "Experiences with the tensor fascia lata flap." *Plast. Reconstr. Surg.* 63(6): 788, 1979.

Nahai, F., Silverton, J.S., Hill, H.L., and Vasconez, L.O. "The tensor fascia lata musculocutaneous flap." *Ann. Plast. Surg.* 1(4): 372, 1978.

Nappi, J.F., Ruberg, R.L., and Berggren, R.B. "Innervated cross-leg tensor fascia lata fasciocutaneous flap for foot reconstruction." *Ann. Plast. Surg.* 10(5): 411, 1983.

O'Hare, P.M., and Leonard, A.G. "Reconstruction of major abdominal wall defects using the tensor fasciae latae myocutaneous flap." *Br. J. Plast. Surg.* 35: 361, 1982.

O'Hare, P.M., Leonard, A.G., and Brennen, M.D. "Experience with the tensor fasciae latae free flap." *Br. J. Plast. Surg.* 36(1): 98, 1983.

Peled, I.J., Kaplan, H.Y., Herson, M., and Wexler, M.R. "Tensor fascia lata musculocutaneous flap for abdominal wall reconstruction." *Ann. Plast. Surg.* 11(2): 141, 1983.

Riebelova, V. "The tensor fasciae latae musculocutaneous flap in operations for trochanteric decubitus ulcers." *Acta. Chir. Plast.* (Prague) 27(1): 17, 1985.

Salibian, A.H., Anzel, S.H., and Rogers, F.R. "The gluteus medius-tensor fasciae latae myocutaneous flap for infected girdlestone procedures: report of two cases." *J. Bone Joint Surg.* 66(9): 1466, 1984.

Scholtz, J.F. and Coetzee, P.F. "Reconstruction of the abdominal wall using a tensor fasciae latae musculocutaneous island flap: A case report." *S. Afr. Med. J.* 64(22): 873, 1983.

Shubailat, G.F., Ajluni, N.J., and Kirresh, B.S. "Reconstruction of heel with ipsilateral tensor fascia lata myocutaneous flap." *Ann. Plast. Surg.* 4: 323, 1979.

TENSOR FASCIA LATA

Stair, J.M. and Petty, P.M. "Clinical uses of the tensor fasciae latae myocutaneous flap." *J. Arkansas Med. Soc.* 81(9): 475, 1985.

Wangensteen, O.H. "Repair of recurrent and difficult hernias and other large defects of the abdominal wall employing the iliotibial tract of fascia lata as a pedicled flap." *Surg. Gynecol. Obstet.* 59: 766, 1934.

Watson, A.C.H. and McGregor, J.C. "The simultaneous use of a groin flap and a tensor fasciae latae myocutaneous flap to provide tissue cover for a completely degloved hand." *Br. J. Plast. Surg.* 34: 349, 1981.

Watson, J.S. "Reconstruction of the anterior abdominal wall above the umbilicus using a tensor fasciae latae myocutaneous island flap." *Br. J. Plast. Surg.* 36: 334, 1983.

Withers, E.H., Franklin, J.D., Madden, J.J., et al. "Further experience with the tensor fascia lata musculocutaneous flap." *Ann. Plast. Surg.* 4: 31, 1980.

RECTUS FEMORIS

Arnold, P.G. and Witzke, D.J. "Management of failed total hip arthroplasty with muscle flaps." *Ann. Plast. Surg.* 11(6): 474, 1983.

Bell, M.S. and Earnshaw, P.H. "Rectus femoris myocutaneous flaps for trochanteric ulcers." *Can. J. Surg.* 24(5): 496, 1981.

Bhagwat, B.M., Pearl, R.M., and Laub, D.R. "Uses of the rectus femoris myocutaneous flap." *Plast. Reconstr. Surg.* 62: 698, 1978.

Bostwick, J., III, Hill, H.L., and Nahai, F. "Repairs in the lower abdomen, groin, or perineum with myocutaneous or omental flaps." *Plast. Reconstr. Surg.* 63: 186, 1979.

Brandell, B.R. "Functional roles of the calf and vastus muscles in locomotion." *Am. J. Phys. Med.* 56(2): 59, 1977.

Ikuta, Y., Kubo, T., and Tsuge, K. "Free muscle transplantation by microsurgical technique to treat severe Volkmann's contracture." *Plast. Reconstr. Surg.* 58(4): 407, 1976.

Knight, K.L., Martin, J.A., and Londeree, B.R. "EMG comparison of quadriceps femoris activity during knee extension and straight leg raises." *Am. J. Phys. Med.* 58(2): 57, 1979.

Lotze, M.T. and Sugarbaker, P.H. "Femoral artery based myocutaneous flap for hemipelvectomy closure: amputation after failed limb-sparing surgery and radiotherapy." *Am. J. Surg.* 150(5): 625, 1985.

Manktelow, R.T. and McKee, N.H. "Free muscle transplantation to provide active finger flexion." *J. Hand Surg.* (Am.) 3(5): 416, 1978.

McCraw, J.B., Dibbell, D.G., and Carraway, J.H. "Clinical definition of independent myocutaneous vascular territories." *Plast. Reconstr. Surg.* 60: 341, 1977.

McGregor, I.A. and Jackson, I.T. "The groin flap." *Br. J. Plast. Surg.* 25: 3, 1972.

Renstrom, P., Grimby, G., and Larsson, E. "Thigh muscle strength in below-knee amputees." *Scand. J. Rehabil. Med.* (Suppl.) 9: 163, 1983.

Schenck, R.R. "Rectus femoris muscle and composite skin transplantation by microneurovascular anastomoses for avulsion of forearm muscles: a case report." *J. Hand Surg.* (Am.) 3(1): 60, 1978.

Sugarbaker, P.H. and Chretien, P.A. "Hemipelvectomy for buttock tumors utilizing an anterior myocutaneous flap of quadriceps femoris muscle." *Ann. Surg.* 197(1): 106, 1983.

Titone, C., Lipsius, M., and Krakauer, J.S. " 'Spontaneous' hematoma of the rectus abdominis muscle: critical review of 50 cases with emphasis on early diagnosis and treatment." *Surgery* 72(4): 568, 1972.

VASTUS LATERALIS

Arnold, P.G. and Witzke, D.J. "Management of failed total hip arthroplasty with muscle flaps." *Ann. Plast. Surg.* 11(6): 474, 1983.

Bovet, J.L., Nassif, T.M., Guimberteau, J.C., and Baudet, J. "The vastus lateralis musculocutaneous flap in the repair of trochanteric pressure sores: technique and indications." *Plast. Reconstr. Surg.* 69(5): 830, 1982.

Dowden, R.V. and McCraw, J.B. "The vastus lateralis muscle flap: technique and applications." *Ann. Plast. Surg.* 4(5): 396, 1980.

Ecker, M.L., Lotke, P.A., and Glazer, R.M. "Late reconstruction of the patellar tendon." *J. Bone Joint Surg.* (Am.), 61(6A): 884, 1979.

Eltorai, I. "The girdlestone procedure in spinal cord injured patients: a ten year experience." *J. Am. Paraplegia Soc.* 6(4): 85, 1983.

Francis, R.S. and Scott, D.E. "Hypertrophy of the vastus medialis in knee extension." *Phys. Ther.* 54(10): 1066, 1974.

Hauben, D.J., Smith, A.R., Sonneveld, G.J., and Van der Meulen, J.C. "The use of vastus lateralis musculocutaneous flap for the repair of trochanteric pressure sores." *Ann. Plast. Surg.* 10(5): 359, 1983.

Jamra, F.N.A., Afeiche, N., and Sumrani, N.B. "The use of a vastus lateralis muscle flap to repair a gluteal defect." *Br. J. Plast. Surg.* 36: 319, 1983.

Larson, D.L. and Liang, M.D. "The quadriceps musculocutaneous flap: a reliable, sensate flap for the hemipelvectomy defect." *Plast. Reconstr. Surg.* 72(3): 347, 1983.

Minami, R.T., Hentz, V.R., and Vistnes, L.M. "Use of vastus lateralis muscle flap for repair of trochanteric pressure sores." *Plast. Reconstr. Surg.* 60(3): 364, 1977.

Murray, M.P., Jacobs, P.A., Mollinger, L.A., and Gore, D.R. "Functional performance after excision of the vastus lateralis and vastus intermedius: a case report." *J. Bone Joint Surg.* (Am.), 65(6): 856, 1983.

Oni, O.O. and Ahmad, S.H. "The vastus lateralis derived flap for repair of neglected rupture of the quadriceps femoris tendon." *Surg. Gynecol. Obstet.* 161(4): 385, 1985.

Tobin, G.R. "Vastus medialis myocutaneous and myocutaneous tendinous composite flaps." *Plast. Reconstr. Surg.* 75: 677, 1985.

VASTUS MEDIALIS

Arnold, P.G., and Pruner-Carrillo, F. "Vastus medialis muscle flap for functional closure of the exposed knee joint." *Plast. Reconstr. Surg.* 68: 69, 1981.

Francis, R.S. and Scott, D.E. "Hypertrophy of the vastus medialis in knee extension." *Phys. Ther.* 54(10): 1066, 1974.

Hunter, S.C., Marascalco, R., and Hughston, J.C. "Disruption of the vastus medialis obliqus with medial knee ligament injuries." *Am. J. Sports Med.* 11(6): 427, 1983.

Kanavel, A.B. "Plastic procedures for the obliteration of cavities with non-collapsible walls." *Surg. Gynecol. Obstet.* 32: 453, 1921.

Santavirta, S. "Integrated electromyography of the vastus medialis muscle after meniscectomy." *Am. J. Sports Med.* 7(1): 40, 1979.

Speakman, H.G. and Weisberg, J. "The vastus medialis controversy." *Physiotherapy* 63(8): 249, 1977.

Tobin, G.R. "Vastus medialis myocutaneous and myocutaneous tendinous composite flaps." *Plast. Reconstr. Surg.* 75: 677, 1985.

GASTROCNEMIUS

Aiache, A.E. "A gastrocnemius muscle flap to fill an osteomyelitic hole in the femur." *Br. J. Plast. Surg.* 31(3): 214, 1978.

Arnold, P.G. and Mixter, R.C. "Making the most of the gastrocnemius muscles." *Plast. Reconstr. Surg.* 72(1): 38, 1983.

Asko-Seljavaara, S. and Haajanen, J. "The exposed knee joint: five case reports." *J. Trauma* 22(12): 1021, 1982.

Barclay, T.L., Cardoso, E., Sharpe, D.T., and Crockett, D.J. "Repair of lower leg injuries with fascio-cutaneous flaps." *Br. J. Plast. Surg.* 35: 127, 1982.

Barfod, B. and Pers, M. "Gastrocnemius-plasty for primary closure of compound injuries of the knee." *J. Bone Joint Surg.* 52: 124, 1970.

Barfred, T. and Reumert, T. "Myoplasty for covering exposed bone or joint on the lower leg." *Acta. Orthop. Scand.* 44: 532, 1973.

Bashir, A.H. "A gastrocnemius tenocutaneous island flap." *Br. J. Plast. Surg.* 35: 436, 1982.

Bashir, A.H. "Inferiorly based gastrocnemius muscle flap in the treatment of war wounds of the middle and lower third of the leg." *Br. J. Plast. Surg.* 36(3): 307, 1983.

Byrd, H.S., Spicer, T.E., and Cierny, G., III. "Management of open tibial fractures." *Plast. Reconstr. Surg.* 76(5): 719, 1985.

Byrd, H.S., Cierny, G., and Tebbetts, J.B. "The management of open tibial fractures with associated soft-tissue loss: external pin fixation with early flap coverage." *Plast. Reconstr. Surg.* 68: 73, 1981.

Cormack, G.C. and Lamberty, B.G.H. "The anatomical vascular basis of the axillary fascio-cutaneous pedicled flap." *Br. J. Plast. Surg.* 37: 425, 1983.

Cormack, G.C. and Lamberty, B.G.H. "A classification for fascio-cutaneous flaps according to their patterns of vascularization." *Br. J. Plast. Surg.* 37: 80, 1984.

Cormack, G.C. and Lamberty, B.G.H. "The anatomical vascular basis of the axillary fascio-cutaneous pedicled flap." *Br. J. Plast. Surg.* 37: 425, 1983.

Dibbell, D.G. and Edstrom, L.E. "The gastrocnemius myocutaneous flap." *Clin. Plast. Surg.* 7(1): 45, 1980.

Durig, M., Schuppisser, J.P., Gauer, E.F., and Muller, W. "Spontaneous rupture of the gastrocnemius muscle." *Injury* 9(2): 143, 1977.

Elsahy, N.I. "Cover of the exposed knee joint by the lateral head of the gastrocnemius." *Br. J. Plast. Surg.* 31(2): 136, 1978.

Ersek, R.A., Abell, J.M., Jr., and Calhoon, J.H. "The island pedicle rotation advancement gastrocnemius musculocutaneous flap for complete coverage of the popliteal fossa." *Ann. Plast. Surg.* 12(6): 533, 1984.

Feldman, J.J., Cohen, B.E., and May, J.W., Jr. "The medial gastrocnemius myocutaneous flap." *Plast. Reconstr. Surg.* 61(4): 531, 1978.

Furnas, D.W. and Anzel, S.H. "Two consecutive repairs of the lower limb with a single gastrocnemius musculocutaneous cross-leg flap." *Plast. Reconstr. Surg.* 66(1): 137, 1980.

Ger, R. "The management of pretibial skin loss." *Surgery* 63: 757, 1968.

Ger, R. "The technique of muscle transposition and the operative treatment of traumatic and ulcerative lesions." *J. Trauma* 2: 502, 1971.

Ger, R. "Surgical management of ulcerative lesions of the leg." *Curr. Prob. Surg.* (3): 1, 1972.

Ger, R. "Muscle transposition for treatment and prevention of chronic post-traumatic osteomyelitis of the tibia." *J. Bone Joint Surg.* 59A: 784, 1977.

Gryskiewicz, J.M., Edstrom, I.E., and Dibbell, D.G. "The gastrocnemius myocutaneous flap in lower-extremity injuries." *J. Trauma* 24(6): 539, 1984.

Halar, E.M., Stolov, W.C., Venkatesh, B., Brozovich, F.V., and Harley, J. "Gastrocnemius muscle belly and tendon length in stroke patients and able-bodied persons." *Arch. Phys. Med. Rehabil.* 59(10): 476, 1978.

Hallock, G. "Cutaneous coverage for the difficult lower extremity wound." *Cont. Orthop.* 10(2): 17, 1985.

Keller, A., Allen, R., and Shaw, W. "The medial gastrocnemius muscle flap: a local free flap." *Plast. Reconstr. Surg.* 73(6): 974, 1984.

Kojima, T., Kohno, T., and Ito, T. "Muscle flap with simultaneous mesh skin graft for skin defects of the lower leg." *J. Trauma* 19: 724, 1979.

Landra, A.P. "Salvage of a seriously injured lower limb with a musculocutaneous cross-leg flap." *Br. J. Plast. Surg.* 35: 40, 1982.

Lentz, M.W., Noyes, F.R., and Neale, H.W. "Muscle flap transposition for traumatic soft tissue defects of the lower extremity." *Clin. Orthop.* 143: 200, 1979.

Linton, P.C. "The combined medial and lateral gastrocnemius musculocutaneous V-Y island advancement flap." *Plast. Reconstr. Surg.* 70(4): 490, 1982.

Malawer, M.M. and Price, W.M. "Gastrocnemius transposition flap in conjunction with limb-sparing surgery for primary bone sarcomas around the knee." *Plast. Reconstr. Surg.* 73(5): 741, 1984.

Mathes, S.J., Alpert, B.S., and Chang, N. "Use of the muscle flap in chronic osteomyelitis: experimental and clinical correlation." *Plast. Reconstr. Surg.* 69(5): 815, 1982.

Mathes, S.J. and Nahai, F. "Muscle flap transposition with function preservation: technical and clinical considerations." *Plast. Reconstr. Surg.* 66: 242, 1980.

Mathes, S.J., Nahai, F., and Vasconez, L.O. "Myocutaneous free flap transfer, anatomical and experimental considerations." *Plast. Reconstr. Surg.* 62: 162, 1978.

Mathes, S.J., Vasconez, L.O., and Jurkiewicz, M.J. "Extension and further applications of muscle flap transposition." *Plast. Reconstr. Surg.* 60: 6, 1977.

GASTROCNEMIUS

Mathes, S.J., Vasconez, L.O., and McCraw, J.B. "Muscle transposition flaps for coverage of lower extremity defects: anatomical considerations." *Surg. Clin. North Am.* 54: 1337, 1974.

McCraw, J.B., Dibbell, D.G., and Carraway, J.H. "Clinical definition of independent myocutaneous vascular territories." *Plast. Reconstr. Surg.* 60: 341, 1977.

McCraw, J.B., Fishman, J.H., and Sharzer, L.A. "The versatile gastrocnemius myocutaneous flap." *Plast. Reconstr. Surg.* 62(1): 15, 1978.

McHugh, M. and Prendiville, J.B. "Muscle flap in the repair of skin defects and the exposed tibia." *Br. J. Plast. Surg.* 28: 205, 1975.

Miller, W.A. "Rupture of the musculotendinous juncture of the medial heal of the gastrocnemius muscle." *Am. J. Sports Med.* 5(5): 191, 1977.

Morris, A.M. "A gastrocnemius musculocutaneous flap." *Br. J. Plast. Surg.* 31(3): 216, 1978.

Morris, A.M. and Buchanan, A.C. "The place of the cross-leg flap in reconstructive surgery of the lower leg and foot: a review of 165 cases." *Br. J. Plast. Surg.* 31: 138, 1978.

Moscona, A.R., Keret, D., and Reis, N.D. "The gastrocnemius muscle flap in the correction of severe flexion contracture of the knee." *Arch. Orthop. Trauma Surg.* 100(2): 139, 1982.

Nahai, F. and Mathes, S.J. "Musculocutaneous flap or muscle flap and skin graft?" *Ann. Plast. Surg.* 12(2): 199, 1984.

Neale, H.W., Stern, P.J., Kreilein, J.G., Gregory, R.O., and Webster, K.L. "Complications of muscle-flap transposition for traumatic defects of the leg." *Plast. Reconstr. Surg.* 72(4): 512, 1983.

Orticochea, M. "Immediate (undelayed) musculocutaneous island cross-leg flaps." *Br. J. Plast. Surg.* 31: 205, 1978.

Pers, M. and Medgyesi, S. "Pedicle muscle flaps and their applications in the surgery of repair." *Br. J. Plast. Surg.* 26: 313, 1973.

Petty, C. and Hogue, R., Jr. "Closure of an exposed knee joint by use of a sartorius muscle flap: case report." *Plast. Reconstr. Surg.* 62: 458, 1978.

Ponten, B. "The fasciocutaneous flap: its use in the soft tissue defects of the lower leg." *Br. J. Plast. Surg.* 34: 215, 1981.

Robbins, T.H. "Use of fascio-muscle flaps to repair defects in the lower leg." *Plast. Reconstr. Surg.* 57: 460, 1976.

Rosenfeld, S.R. and Anzel, S.H. "Use of the Hoffmann apparatus in myocutaneous pedicle flap." *J. Trauma* 21(12): 1045, 1981.

Salibian, A.H. and Anzel, S.H. "Salvage of an infected total knee prothesis with medial and lateral gastrocnemius muscle flaps: a case report." *J. Bone Joint Surg.* (Am.), 65(5): 681, 1983.

Salibian, A.H. and Menick, F.J. "Bipedicle gastrocnemius musculocutaneous flap for defects of the distal one-third of the leg." *Plast. Reconstr. Surg.* 70(1): 17, 1982.

Sanders, R. and O'Neill, T. "The gastrocnemius myocutaneous flap used as a cover for exposed knee prosthesis." *J. Bone Joint Surg.* (Br.) 63-B(3): 383, 1981.

Schoenhaus, H.D. and Jay, R.M. "A modified gastrocnemius lengthening." *J. Am. Podiatry Assoc.* 68(1): 31, 1978.

Sharrard, W.J. and Bernstein, S. "Equinus deformity in cerebral palsy: a comparison between elongation of the tendocalcaneus and gastrocnemius recession." *J. Bone Joint Surg.* (Br.) 54(2): 272, 1972.

Stark, R.B. "Blood supply of cross-leg pedicle flaps." *Plast. Reconstr. Surg.* 3: 694, 1948.

Stark, R.B. "The cross-leg flap procedure." *Plast. Reconstr. Surg.* 9: 173, 1952.

Sundell, B. and Asko-Seljavaara, S. "Transposition of muscle flaps for covering exposed bone in the leg." *Ann. Chir. Gynaecol.* 68(1): 1, 1979.

Thatte, R.L. and Laud, N. "The use of the fascia of the lower leg as a roll-over flap: its possible clinical applications in reconstructive surgery." *Br. J. Plast. Surg.* 37: 88, 1984.

Tolhurst, D.E. "Surgical indications for fasciocutaneous flaps." *Ann. Plast. Surg.* 13(6): 495, 1984.

Tolhurst, D.E., Haeseker, B., and Zeeman, R.J. "The development of the fasciocutaneous flap and its clinical applications." *Plast. Reconstr. Surg.* 71): 597, 1983.

Vasconez, L.O., Bostwick, J., III, and McCraw, J.B. "Coverage of exposed bone by muscle transplantation and skin grafting." *Plast. Reconstr. Surg.* 53: 526, 1974.

Yoshimura, M., Imura, S., Shimamura, K., Yamauchi, S., and Nomura, S. "Peroneal flap for reconstruction in the extremity: preliminary report." *Plast. Reconstr. Surg.* 74(3): 402, 1984.

SOLEUS

Byrd, H.S., Spicer, T.E., and Cierney, G., III. "Management of open tibial fractures." *Plast. Reconstr. Surg.* 76(5): 719, 1985.

Chen, Y. "Microsurgical anatomy of the lateral skin flap of the lag." *Ann. Plast. Surg.* 15(4): 313, 1985.

Fitzgerald, R.H., Jr., Ruttle, P.E., Arnold, P.G., Kelly, P.G., and Irons, G.B. "Local muscle flaps in the treatment of chronic osteomyelitis." *J. Bone Joint Surg.* (Am.) 67(2): 175, 1985.

Fugl-Meyer, A.R., Sostrom, M., and Wahlby, L. "Human plantar flexion strength and structure." *Acta. Physiol. Scand.* 107(1): 47, 1979.

Ger, R. "The operative treatment of the advanced stasis ulcer." *Am. J. Surg.* 111: 659, 1966.

Ger, R. "Operative treatment of the advanced stasis ulcer using muscle transposition." *Am. J. Surg.* 120: 376, 1970.

Ger, R. "The management of open fracture of the tibia with skin loss." *J. Trauma* 10(2): 112, 1970.

Ger, R. "The technique of muscle transposition in the operative treatment of traumatic and ulcerative lesions of the leg." *J. Trauma* 2(6): 502, 1971.

Ger, R. "Surgical management of ulcerative lesions of the leg." *Curr. Prob. Surg.* (3): 1, 1972.

Ger, R. and Sedlin, E. "The accessory soleus muscle." *Clin. Orthop.* 116: 200, 1976.

Magee, W.P., Jr., Gilbert, D.A., and McInnis, W.D. "Extended muscle and muscolocutaneous flaps." *Clin. Plast. Surg.* 7(1): 57, 1980.

Markhede, G. and Nistor, L. "Strength of plantar flexion and function after resection of various parts of the triceps surae muscle." *Acta. Orthop. Scand.* 50(6 Pt. 1): 693, 1979.

Mathes, S., Vasconez, L.O., and Jurkiewicz, M.J. "Extension and further applications of muscle flap transposition." *Plast. Reconstr. Surg.* 60: 6, 1977.

Mathes, S., Vasconez, L.O., and McCraw, J.B. "Muscle transposition flaps for coverage of lower extremity defects: anatomical considerations." *Surg. Clin. North Am.* 54: 1337, 1974.

McCraw, J.B., Dibbell, D.G., and Carraway, J.H. "Clinical definition of independent myocutaneous vascular territories." *Plast. Reconstr. Surg.* 60: 341, 1977.

McCraw, J.B., Fishman, J.H., and Scharzer, L.A. "The versatile gastrocnemius myocutaneous flap." *Plast. Reconstr. Surg.* 62: 15, 1978.

McHugh, M. and Prendiville, J.B. "Muscle flaps in the repair of skin defects and the exposed tibia." *Br. J. Plast. Surg.* 28: 205, 1975.

Murray, M.P., Guten, G.N., Sepic, S.B., Gardner, G.M., and Baldwin, J.M. "Function of the triceps surae during gait: Compensatory mechanisms for unilateral loss." *J. Bone Joint Surg.* (Am.) 60(4): 473, 1978.

Pers, M. and Medgyesi, S. "Pedicle muscle flaps and their applications in the surgery of repair." *Br. J. Plast. Surg.* 26: 313, 1973.

Ponten, B. "The fasciocutaneous flap: its use in soft tissue defects of the lower leg." *Br. J. Plast. Surg.* 34: 215, 1981.

Sjostom, M., Fugl-Meyer, A.R., and Wahlby, L. "Achilles tendon injury: Plantar flexion strength and structure of the soleus muscle after surgical repair." *Act. Chir. Scand.* 144(4): 219, 1978.

Stein, S.R. and Luekens, C.A., Jr. "Closed treatment of Achilles tendon ruptures." *Orthop. Clin. North Am.* 7(1): 241, 1976.

Tobin, G.R. "Myocutaneous and muscle flap reconstruction of problem wounds." *Surg. Clin. North Am.* 64(4): 667, 1984.

Tobin, G.R. "Hemisoleus and reversed hemisoleus flaps." *Plast. Reconstr. Surg.* 76(1): 87, 1985.

Townsend, P.L.G. "An inferiorly based soleus muscle flap." *Br. J. Plast. Surg.* 31(3): 210, 1978.

Thiemeyer, J.S., Jr. "The role of muscle flaps in the treatment of chronic osteomyelitis." *The Military Surgeon.* 107(5): 374, 1950.

Vasconez, L.O., Bostwick, J., III, and McCraw, J.B. "Coverage of exposed bone by muscle transplantation and skin grafting." *Plast. Reconstr. Surg.* 53: 526, 1974.

Weber-Laumann, A. "Recurrent dislocation of the shoulder treated by transposition of the tendon to pectoralis minor: A follow-up of fifteen patients." *Acta. Orthop. Scand.* 41(2): 161, 1970.

Wright, J.K. and Watkins, R.P. "Use of the soleus muscle flap to cover part of the distal tibia." *Plast. Reconstr. Surg.* 68(6): 957, 1981.

EXTENSOR DIGITORUM COMMUNIS

Daniel, R.K. and Williams, H.B. "The free transfer of skin flaps by microvascular anastomoses: An experimental study and a reappraisal." *Plast. Reconstr. Surg.* 52(1): 1973.

Hill, H.L., Nahai, F., and Vasconez, L.O. "The tensor fascia lata myocutaneous free flap." *Plast. Reconstr. Surg.* 61(4): 517, 1978.

Mathes, S.J. and Buchanan, R.T. "Tensor fascia lata: neurosensory musculocutaneous free flaps." *Br. J. Plast. Surg.* 32: 184, 1979.

Mathes, S.J., Vasconez, L.O., and Jurkiewicz, M.J. "Extension and further applications of muscle flap transposition." *Plast. Reconstr. Surg.* 60: 6, 1977.

Maxwell, G.P., Manson, P.N., and Hoopes, J.E. "Experience with 13 latissimus dorsi myocutaneous free flaps." *Plast. Reconstr. Surg.* 64: 1, 1979.

McCraw, J.B., Fishman, J.H., and Scharzer, L.A. "The versatile gastrocnemius myocutaneous flap." *Plast. Reconstr. Surg.* 62: 15, 1978.

O'Brien, B.M., et al. "Successful transfer of a large island flap from the groin to the foot by microvascular anastomosis." *Plast. Reconstr. Surg.* 52: 271, 1973.

Pers, M. and Medgyesi, S. "Pedicle muscle flaps and their applications in surgery of repair." *Br. J. Plast. Surg.* 26: 313, 1973.

Ponten, B. "The fasciocutaneous flap: its use in soft tissue defects of the lower leg." *Br. J. Plast. Surg.* 34: 215, 1981.

Vasconez, L.O., Bostwick, J., III, and McCraw, J.B. "Coverage of exposed bone by muscle transplantation and skin grafting." *Plast. Reconstr. Surg.* 53: 526, 1974.

FOOT FLAPS

Bennett, J.E. and Kahn, R.A. "Surgical management of soft tissue defects of the ankle-heel region." *J. of Trauma* 12(8): 696, 1971.

Bostwick, J., III. "Reconstruction of the heel pad by muscle transposition and split skin graft." *Surg. Gynecol. Obstet.* 143(6): 973, 1976.

Buncke, H.J., Jr. and Colen, L.B. "An island flap from the first web space of the foot to cover plantar ulcers." *Br. J. Plast. Surg.* 33: 242, 1980.

Colen, L.B. and Buncke, H.J., Jr. "Neurovascular island flaps from the plantar vessels and nerves for foot reconstruction." *Ann. Plast. Surg.* (4): 327, 1984.

Daniel, R.K. and Taylor, G.I. "Distant transfer of an island flap by microvascular anastomosis: a clinical technique." *Plast. Reconstr. Surg.* 52: 111, 1973.

Drabyn, G.A. and Avedian L. "Ipsilateral buttock flap for coverage of a foot and ankle defect in a young child." *Plast. Reconstr. Surg.* 63: 422, 1979.

Duncan, M.J., Zuker, R.M., and Manktelow, R.T. "Resurfacing weight bearing areas of the heel: The role of the dorsalis pedis innervated free tissue transfer." *J. Reconstr. Micro.* 1(3): 201, 1984.

Ger, R. "Surgical management of ulcerative lesions of the leg." *Curr. Prob. Surg.* (3): 1, 1972.

Ger, R. "The management of chronic ulcers of the dorsum of the foot by muscle transposition with free skin grafting." *Br. J. Plast. Surg.* 29: 199, 1976.

Ger, R. "The surgical management of ulcers of the heel." *Surg. Gynecol. Obstet.* 140: 909, 1975.

Grabb, W.C. and Argenta, L.C. "The lateral calcaneal artery skin flap (the lateral calcaneal artery, lesser saphenous vein, and sural nerve skin flap)." *Plast. Reconstr. Surg.* 68(5): 723, 1981.

Gulyas, G., Mate, F., and Kartik, I. "A neurovascular island flap from the first web space of the foot to repair a defect over the heel: case report." *Br. J. Plast. Surg.* 37: 398, 1984.

Harii, K. and Ohmori, K. "Free groin flaps in children." *Plast. Reconstr. Surg.* 55: 588, 1975.

Harrison, D.H. and Morgan, B.D.G. "The instep island flap to resurface plantar defects." *Br. J. Plast. Surg.* 34: 315, 1981.

Hartrampf, C.R., Jr., Scheflan, M., and Bostwick, J., III. "The flexor digitorum brevis muscle island pedicle flap: a new dimension in heel reconstruction." *Plast. Reconstr. Surg.* 66(2): 264, 1980.

Holmes, J. and Rayner, C.R.W. "Lateral calcaneal artery island flaps." *Br. J. Plast. Surg.* 37: 402, 1984.

Huber, J.F. "The arterial network supplying the dorsum of the foot." *Anat. Rec.* 80: 373, 1941.

Ikuta, Y., Murakami, T., Yoshioka, K., and Tsuge, K. "Reconstruction of the heel pad by flexor digitorum brevis musculocutaneous flap transfer." *Plast. Reconstr. Surg.* 74(1): 86, 1984.

Kaplan, I. "Neurovascular island flap in the treatment of trophic ulceration of the heel." *Br. J. Plast. Surg.* 22: 143, 1969.

Leitner, D.W., Gordon, L., and Buncke, H.J. "The extensor digitorum brevis as a muscle island flap." *Plast. Reconstr. Surg.* 76(5): 77, 1985.

Lichtblau, S. "Section of the abductor hallucis tendon for correction of metatarsus varus deformity." *Clin. Orthop.* (110): 227, 1975.

Littler, J.W. "Neurovascular skin island transfer in reconstructive hand surgery." In *Transactions of the International Society of Plastic Surgeons.* Baltimore: Williams & Wilkins, 1960.

MacLeod, A.M. and Robinson, D.W. "Reconstruction of defects involving the mandible and floor of mouth by free osteocutaneous flaps derived from the foot." *Br. J. Plast. Surg.* 35: 239, 1982.

Maisels, D.O. "Repairs of the heel." *Br. J. Plast. Surg.* 117, 1961.

May, J.W., Lakash, F.N., and Gallico, G.G. "Latissimus dorsi free muscle flap in lower extremity reconstruction." *Plast. Reconstr. Surg.* 68: 603, 1981.

McCraw, J.B. "On the transfer of a free dorsalis pedis sensory flap to the hand." (Letter) *Plast. Reconstr. Surg.* 59: 738, 1977.

McCraw, J.B. and Furlow, L.T., Jr. "The dorsalis pedis arterialized flap." *Plast. Reconstr. Surg.* 55(2): 177, 1975.

Mitchell, G.P. "Abductor hallucis release in congenital metatarsus varus." *Int. Orthop.* 3(4): 229, 1980.

Moberg, E. "Evaluation and management of nerve injuries in the hand." *Surg. Clin. North Am.* 44: 1019, 1964.

Morain, W.D. "Island toe flaps in neurotrophic ulcers of the foot and ankle." *Ann. Plast. Surg.* 13(1): 1, 1984.

Morrison, W.A., Crabb, D., O'Brien, B., and Jenkins, A. "The instep of the foot as a fasciocutaneous island and as a free flap for heel defects." *Plast. Reconstr. Surg.* 72(1): 56, 1983.

O'Brien, B.M., et al. "Successful transfer of a large island flap from the groin to the foot by microvascular anastomosis." *Plast. Reconstr. Surg.* 52: 271, 1973.

Panconi, B., Vidal, L., Bovet, J.L., et al. "The use of the medial plantar flap to cover heel defects." *Ann. Chir. Plast. Esth.* 30: 78, 1985.

Reiffel, R.S. and McCarthy, J.G. "Coverage of heel and sole defects: a new subfascial arterialized flap." *Plast. Reconstr. Surg.* 66(2): 250, 1980.

Scheflan, M., Nahai, F., and Hartrampf, C.R., Jr. "Surgical management of heel ulcers — a comprehensive approach." *Ann. Plast. Surg.* 7: 385, 1981.

Shah, A. and Pandit, S. "Reconstruction of the heel with chronic ulceration with flexor digitorum brevis myocutaneous flap." *Lepr. Rev.* 56(1): 41, 1985.

FOOT FLAPS

Shanahan, R.E. and Gingrass, R.P. "Medial plantar sensory flap for coverage of heel defects." *Plast. Reconstr. Surg.* 64(3): 295, 1979.

Shubailat, G.F., Ajluni, N.J., and Kirresh, B.S. "Reconstruction of heel with ipsilateral tensor fascia lata myocutaneous flap." *Ann. Plast. Surg.* 4: 323, 1979.

Shubailat, G.F., Ajluni, N.J., Shahateet, M.A. "Repair of a lower leg defect with an ipsilateral gracilis myocutaneous flap." *Plast. Reconstr. Surg.* 64: 560, 1979.

Skef, Z., Ecker, H.A., Jr., and Graham, W.P., III. "Heel coverage by a plantar myocutaneous island pedicle flap." *J. Trauma* 23(6): 466, 1983.

Snyder, G.B. and Edgerton, M.T. "The principle of the island neurovascular flap in the management of ulcerated anesthetic weightbearing areas of the lower extremity." *Plast. Reconstr. Surg.* 36: 518, 1965.

Sommerlad, B.C. and McGrouther, D.A. "Resurfacing the sole: long-term follow-up and comparison of techniques." *Br. J. Plast. Surg.* 31: 107, 1978.

Stark, R.B. "Blood supply of cross-leg pedicle flaps." *Plast. Reconstr. Surg.* 3: 694, 1948.

Stark, R.B. "The cross-leg flap procedure." *Plast. Reconstr. Surg.* 9: 173, 1952.

Taylor, G.A. and Hopson, W.L.G. "The cross-foot flap." *Plast. Reconstr. Surg.* 55(6): 677, 1975.

Thatte, R.L. "One-stage random-pattern de-epithelialised 'turn over' flaps in the leg." *Br. J. Plast. Surg.* 35: 287, 1982.

Thatte, R.L., Dhami, L.D., and Patil, U.A. "De-epithelialised turn-over flaps for 'salvage' operations." *Br. J. Plast. Surg.* 36: 178, 1983.

Vann, H.M. "A note on the formation of the plantar arterial arch of the human foot." *Anat. Rec.* 85: 269, 1943.

Vasconez, L.O., Bostwick, J., III, and McCraw, J.B. "Coverage of exposed bone by muscle transposition and skin grafting." *Plast. Reconstr. Surg.* 53(5): 526, 1974.

Watson, J.S., Brough, M.D., and Orton, C. "Simultaneous coverage of both heels with one free flap." *Plast. Reconstr. Surg.* 269, 1979.

Woltering, E.A., and co-workers. "Split-thickness skin grafting of the plantar surface of the foot after wide excision of neoplasms of the skin." *Surg. Gynecol. Obstet.* 149: 229, 1979.

INDEX

Vastus Lateralis Muscle
adjacent muscles to
463, 465, 467-468
arc of rotation
463-464, 469-472
fascia of
464
function of
463
insertion of
463
nerve supply of
463, 466
origin of
463
surface markings of
463
vascular supply of
463, 466, 468
width of
470

Vastus Medialis Flap
advantages of
483
arc of rotation
483, 485
combined with vastus lateralis
489-490
comparison with
gastrocnemius
483
vastus lateralis
483
complications of
483
disadvantages of
483
donor site of
483
inclusion of fascia with
483, 485
nerve supply of
483
use in knee reconstruction
483, 486-488
use with vastus lateralis
483
uses of
483
V-Y advancement of
483

Vastus Medialis Muscle
adjacent muscles to
483-484
function of
483
insertion of
483-484
origin of
483
surface markings of
483
vascular supply of
483

Vertical Rectus Abdominis
abdominal morbidity with
267
abdominal reconstruction with
266, 294
adjacent muscles of
265
advantages of
267
arc of rotation of
269-270, 274-275

breast reconstruction with
265-267, 282-285
cadaver dissection of
269-275
chest wall reconstruction with
265-267, 269-270, 276-281,
286-291
cold sensitivity of
267
combined with thoracoepigastric flap
266
comparison with
distally based latissimus flap
266
pectoralis flap
266
T.R.A.M. flap
265-267
complications of
267, 278
coverage for exposed vessels
294
delay of
278
disadvantages of
237, 266-267
donor site of
266-267, 277, 285, 287, 291,
293, 295
function of
265, 267
functional loss of
267
hernia with the use of
267
insertion of
265
nerve supply of
265
origin of
265
perineal reconstruction with
266-267, 292-293
repair of facial defect of
266
surface markings of
265, 268
use of muscle flap
288, 290, 292
use in irradiated patient
267
use when common femoral vessels are
injured
267, 294
uses of
60, 237, 265
vaginal reconstruction with
266
vascular supply of
265, 272

Vertical Rectus Inferiorly Based
arc of rotation of
266, 267, 274-275
cadaver dissection of
271-275
uses of
265-266
vascular supply of
265

Vertical Rectus Superiorly Based
arc of rotation of
265, 267, 269-270
cadaver dissection of
269-270
uses of
265-267

vascular supply of
265
Vertical Trapezius Flap
advantages of
61
arc of rotation of
60, 71-74
cadaver dissection of
67-74
comparison to adjacent muscles
59
complications of
60-61
disadvantages of
60-61
donor site
complications of
60-61
disruption of
61
nerve supply of
59
surface markings of
59
use following radical neck dissection
61
use in
occipital coverage
87-90
orbital reconstruction
91-93
scalp reconstruction
87-90
uses of
59-61
vascular supply of
59, 70

Wangensteen
procedure described by
440
use of flaps of
423

Wound Care
3-4

Wound Preparation
3-4

Zone of Injury
assessment of
5, 677
vascular damage in
583

Zygomatic Arch
coverage of
32, 34

ACKNOWLEDGEMENTS

Permission was granted by *Annals of Plastic Surgery* for the use of the following photographs:

> Page 473-474, figures 9-12 from Arnold, P.G. and Witzke, D.J. "Management of failed total hip arthroplasty with muscle flaps." *Ann. Plast. Surg.* 11: 474-478.

> Page 669, figure 13 from Dowden, R.V. and McCraw, J.B. "The vastus lateralis muscle flap: technique and applications." *Ann. Plast. Surg.* 4: 396-404.

Permission was granted by *Annals of Surgery* for the use of the following photographs:

> Pages 106-108, figures 9 and 14 and pages 290-291, figures 33-36 from Arnold, P.G. and Pairolero, P.C. "Chest wall reconstruction: experience with 100 consecutive patients." *Ann. Surg.* 199: 725-732.

Permission was granted by *Journal of Bone and Joint Surgery* for the use of the following photographs:

> Pages 522-524, figures 37-42; pages 557-558, figures 14-16; and pages 609-611, figures 13-17 from Fitzgerald, R.H., Jr., et al. "Local muscle flaps in the treatment of chronic osteomyelitis." *J. Bone Joint Surg.* 67A: 175-185.

Permission was granted by *Journal of Hand Surgery* for the use of the following photographs:

> Pages 115-118, figures 26-33 and pages 215-217, figures 99-104 from Dowden, R.V. and McCraw, J.B. "Muscle flap reconstruction of shoulder defects." *J. Hand Surg.* 5: 382.

Permission was granted by *Journal of Thoracic and Cardiovascular Surgery* for the use of the following photographs:

> Pages 256-257, figures 33-36 from Schaff, H.V., Arnold, P.G., and Reeder, G.S. "Late mediastinal infection and pseudoaneurysm following left ventricular aneurysmectomy: repair utilizing a pectoralis major muscle flap." *J. Thorac. Cardiovasc. Surg.* 84: 912-916.

> Page 251, figures 23-24 from Pairolero, P.C., et al. "Intrathoracic transposition of extrathoracic skeletal muscle." *J. Thorac. Cardiovasc. Surg.* 86: 809-817.

> Page 107, figure 12 from Pairolero, P.C. and Arnold, P.G. "Management of recalcitrant median sternotomy wounds." *J. Thorac. Cardiovasc. Surg.* 88: 357-364.

Permission was granted by *Plastic and Reconstructive Surgery* for the use of the following photographs:

> Pages 404-405, figures 176-183 from McCraw, J.B., et al. "Vaginal reconstruction with gracilis myocutaneous flaps." *Plast. Reconstr. Surg.* 58: 176-183.

> Pages 170-174, figures 11-19 from McCraw, J.B., Penix, J.O., and Baker, J.W. "Repair of major defects of the chest wall and spine with the latissimus dorsi myocutaneous flap." *Plast. Reconstr. Surg.* 62: 197-206.

> Pages 535-536, figures 63-66 from McCraw, J.B., Fishman, J.H., and Sharzer, L.E. " The versatile gastrocnemius flap." *Plast. Reconstr. Surg.* 62: 15-23.

> Pages 47-48, figures 14-17 and pages 75-80, figures 14-25 from McCraw, J.B., Magee, W.P., and Kalwaic, H. "Uses of the trapezius and sternomastoid myocutaneous flaps in head and neck reconstruction." *Plast. Reconstr. Surg.* 63: 49-57.

> Pages 594-595, figures 17-19 from Arnold, P.G. and Hodgkinson, D.J. "Extensor digitorum turn-down muscle flap." *Plast. Reconstr. Surg.* 66: 599-604.

> Pages 112-114, figures 20-25 from Arnold, P.G. and Irons, G.B. "The greater omentum: extensions in transposition and free transfer." *Plast. Reconstr. Surg.* 67: 169-176.

> Page 242, figures 5-6 from Arnold, P.G., Pairolero, P.C., and Waldorf, J.C. "The serratus anterior muscle: Intrathoracic and extrathoracic utilization." *Plast. Reconstr. Surg.* 173: 240-246.

> Pages 514-521, figures 21-36; pages 533-534, figures 59-62; and pages 572-573, figures 31-36 from Arnold, P.G. and Mixter, R.C. "Making the most of the gastrocnemius muscles." *Plast. Reconstr. Surg.* 72: 38-48.

> Pages 91-93, figures 43-47 from Rosen, H.M. "The extended trapezius musculocutaneous flap for cranio-orbital facial reconstruction." *Plast. Reconstr. Surg.* 75: 318-327.